Gastrointestinal Emergencies

Autumn Graham • David J. Carlberg

Editors

Gastrointestinal Emergencies

Evidence-Based Answers to Key Clinical Questions

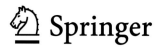

Editors
Autumn Graham
Department of Emergency Medicine
MedStar Georgetown University Hospital
Washington, DC
USA

David J. Carlberg
Department of Emergency Medicine
MedStar Georgetown University Hospital
Washington, DC
USA

ISBN 978-3-319-98342-4   ISBN 978-3-319-98343-1   (eBook)
https://doi.org/10.1007/978-3-319-98343-1

Library of Congress Control Number: 2018967969

This Springer imprint is published by the registered company Springer Nature Switzerland AG
The registered company address is: Gewerbestrasse 11, 6330 Cham, Switzerland

Preface

Abdominal pain is the most common complaint in emergency medicine. In developing this textbook, we wanted to provide evidence-based answers to specific clinical questions encountered during the evaluation and management of patients with abdominal pain. While each part, read in total, provides a comprehensive review of the topic (e.g., gallbladder disease), each chapter can be read individually as a real-time clinical reference (e.g., is a negative CT good enough to rule out acute cholecystitis?).

In the era of team-based care, understanding a consultant's approach to a clinical problem can make conversations easier and facilitate patient care. Therefore, each part includes a Consultant Corner chapter, which answers some of the same questions from the standpoint of the consultant.

We included an "Additional Reading" section at the end of each chapter, allowing our authors to highlight landmark interesting articles from the medical literature as well as free open access medical education (FOAM) resources, such as podcasts and blogs.

While editing the book, we played the role of both learner and educator. Each part taught us interesting, useful, and sometimes funny facts that broadened our knowledge of gastrointestinal emergencies. Below we list one or two things we learned from editing each part of the book.

Part	Things we learned
General Approach to Acute Abdominal Pain	Abdominal pain cases with a recognized diagnostic error were more likely to have (1) inadequately addressed abnormalities on laboratory studies, (2) a shorter initial length of stay, (3) a differential diagnosis that did not include the final diagnosis, or (4) discrepancies/omissions of history documented by nursing and emergency medicine provider.
Gastrointestinal Bleeding	Of those patients with ascites, 60% will have varices. Antibiotic administration, specifically ceftriaxone 1 gm IV, decreases morbidity and mortality in patients with variceal bleeding.
Abdominal Aortic Aneurysm and Aortic Dissection	Permissive hypotension for ruptured abdominal aortic aneurysm involves restricting fluid administration with a goal systolic blood pressure (SBP) of 50–100 mm Hg. The optimal target SBP is unclear.
Mesenteric Ischemia	Lactate represents evidence of late disease and corresponds with irreversible bowel necrosis. D-dimer may play a role in early diagnosis, but it is still unclear what role it plays. Young, female patients with chronic, intermittent abdominal and an extensive negative work-up may have chronic mesenteric ischemia from vasculitis or rheumatologic disease.
Abdominal Pain and Vomiting	Topical abdominal application of capsaicin is a noninvasive, low-risk treatment for cannabis hyperemesis syndrome. The only proven long-term treatment is cessation of cannabis use.
Pancreatitis	The probability of a common bile duct (CBD) stone increases from 28% to 50% when the diameter cutoff of the CBD is changed from 6 mm to 10 mm; gallstone pancreatitis warrants cholecystectomy during their index presentation.
Bowel Obstruction	Bedside ultrasound performed by emergency physicians can rule in and rule out small bowel obstruction with a specificity of 90–96% and a sensitivity of 93–97%.

Part	Things we learned
Gallbladder Disease	Among those who did not undergo cholecystectomy for acute cholecystitis during their index admission, 19% had a gallstone-related emergency department visit or hospital admission within 3 months.
Liver Disease	Patients with acute liver failure should be considered for early transfer to a liver transplant center, ideally prior to elevation in intracranial pressure or the development of severe coagulopathy.
Appendicitis	Appendicitis in pregnancy may lack the classic pain presentation due to downregulation of pain receptors and increased distance from the inflamed appendix to the parietal peritoneum.
Diverticulitis	No antibiotics for uncomplicated diverticulitis is recommended by many European practice guidelines and a growing body of literature supports this "watchful waiting" management.
Inflammatory Bowel Disease	Budesonide is the steroid of choice for treating inflammatory bowel disease flares because its extensive first-pass metabolism decreases systemic exposure. Budesonide is optimal for mild flares and patients at high risk for complications from prednisone. Prednisone should be used in moderate flares and for those who have failed budesonide.
Diarrhea	Vancomycin 125 mg four times a day is the new first-line treatment for *Clostridium difficile* infections.
Abdominal Pain in the Pregnant Patient	Up to 1% of women need an operation during pregnancy for a non-obstetric abdominal emergency.
Abdominal Pain in the Immunocompromised Patient	In transplant patients, time from transplant guides the choice of empiric antimicrobial therapy; in the first 6 months when patients are on high doses of immunosuppression, antimicrobial treatments are directed toward opportunistic infections such as CMV and hospital acquired infections; after 6 months when the immunosuppressive regimens are lessened, community acquired infections predominate.
Abdominal Pain in the Bariatric Patient	Bowel obstruction with history of RYGB is an internal hernia until proven otherwise; vague neurologic symptoms in any bariatric patient, particularly following malabsorptive procedures, should prompt consideration for B1/Thiamine deficiency (Wernicke's encephalopathy).
Abdominal Pain in the Post-Procedure Patient	An uncommon complication of colonoscopy is intracolonic explosion due to electrocautery-induced ignition of methane.
Chronic Abdominal Pain	Anterior cutaneous nerve entrapment syndrome (ACNES) is a commonly undiagnosed cause of chronic abdominal pain and injection of local anesthetic can be both diagnostic and therapeutic.

Washington, DC, USA   Autumn Graham
                                                                                               David J. Carlberg

Contents

Contributors

Lindsea Abbott, MD MedStar Washington Hospital Center, Department of Emergency Medicine, Washington, DC, USA

Ainsley Adams, MD Department of Emergency Medicine, George Washington University School of Medicine & Health Sciences, Washington, DC, USA

Essa M. Aleassa, MD Bariatric and Metabolic Institute, Cleveland Clinic Foundation, Cleveland, OH, USA

Department of Surgery, College of Medicine and Health Sciences, United Arab Emirates University, Al-Ain, United Arab Emirates

M. Aamir Ali, MD, AGAF Division of Gastroenterology, George Washington University, Washington, DC, USA

Matthias Barden, MD Department of Emergency Medicine, Eisenhower Medical Center, Rancho Mirage, CA, USA

John C. Beauchamp, MD Department of Emergency Medicine, McGovern Medical School at The University of Texas Health Science Center at Houston (UTHealth), Houston, TX, USA

Brent A. Becker, MD Wellspan York Hospital, Department of Emergency Medicine, York, PA, USA

Eric Benoit, MD Division of Trauma & Surgical Critical Care, Alpert Medical School of Brown University, Providence, RI, USA

Joelle Borhart, MD, FACEP, FAAEM Department of Emergency Medicine, MedStar Washington Hospital Center & MedStar Georgetown University Hospital, Washington, DC, USA

Matthew P. Borloz, MD Virginia Tech Carilion School of Medicine, Department of Emergency Medicine, Roanoke, VA, USA

Stacy Brethauer, MD Bariatric and Metabolic Institute, Cleveland Clinic Foundation, Cleveland, OH, USA

Robert M. Brickley, MD UPMC Department of Emergency Medicine, Pittsburgh, PA, USA

Elaine Bromberek, MD MedStar Washington Hospital Center, MedStar Georgetown University Hospital, Washington, DC, USA

John David Buek, MD MedStar Washington Hospital Center, Department of Obstetrics and Gynecology, Washington, DC, USA

Jaclyn Caffrey, MD Department of Emergency Medicine, Alpert Medical School of Brown University, Providence, RI, USA

David Carlberg, MD Department of Emergency Medicine, MedStar Georgetown University Hospital & Washington Hospital Center, Washington, DC, USA

Kimberly A. Chambers, MD Department of Emergency Medicine, McGovern Medical School at The University of Texas Health Science Center at Houston (UTHealth), Houston, TX, USA

Karin Chase, MD University of Rochester Medical Center, Rochester, NY, USA

KinWah Chew, MD WellSpan York Hospital Department of Emergency Medicine, York, PA, USA

Cullen Clark, MD Emergency Medicine/Pediatrics Resident, Louisiana State University Health Sciences Center – New Orleans, New Orleans, LA, USA

Michelle Clinton, MD Virginia Tech – Carilion Clinic, Department of Emergency Medicine, Roanoke, VA, USA

Mark Collin, MD Section of Emergency Ultrasound, York Hospital Emergency Ultrasound Fellowship, York Hospital Emergency Medicine Residency, York Hospital Department of Emergency Medicine, York, PA, USA

Catherine Cummings, MD, FACEP Department of Emergency Medicine, Alpert Medical School of Brown University, Providence, RI, USA

Krishna Dass, MD MedStar Washington Hospital Center, Department of Infectious Disease, Washington, DC, USA

I. David Shocket, MD MedStar Washington Hospital Center, Washington, DC, USA

W. Nathan Davis, MD Department of Emergency Medicine, University of Pittsburgh Medical Center, Pittsburgh, PA, USA

John Davitt, MD MedStar Washington Hospital Center, Department of Obstetrics and Gynecology, Washington, DC, USA

Lindsey DeGeorge, MD Department of Emergency Medicine, MedStar Washington Hospital Center, Washington, DC, USA

Edward A. Descallar, MD Department of Emergency Medicine, MedStar Washington Hospital Center, MedStar Georgetown University Hospital, Washington, DC, USA

Maria Dynin, MD Department of Emergency Medicine, MedStar Washington Hospital Center & MedStar Georgetown University Hospital, Washington, DC, USA

Adam C. Ehrlich, MD, MPH Section of Gastroenterology, Department of Medicine, Lewis Katz School of Medicine at Temple University, Philadelphia, PA, USA

Daniel Eum, MD Keck School of Medicine of the University of Southern California, Los Angeles County/University of Southern California (LAC+USC) Department of Emergency Medicine, Los Angeles, CA, USA

Lindley E. Folkerson, MD Department of Emergency Medicine, McGovern Medical School at The University of Texas Health Science Center at Houston (UTHealth), Houston, TX, USA

Timothy J. Fortuna, DO Virginia Tech Carilion School of Medicine, Department of Emergency Medicine, Roanoke, VA, USA

Alexa R. Gale, MD, MS FACEP, FAAEM Georgetown University School of Medicine, MedStar Washington Hospital Center, Department of Emergency Medicine, Washington, DC, USA

Cameron Gettel, MD Department of Emergency Medicine, Alpert Medical School of Brown University, Providence, RI, USA

Daniel B. Gingold, MD, MPH University of Maryland School of Medicine, Department of Emergency Medicine, Baltimore, MD, USA

Jonathan Giordano, DO, MS Department of Emergency Medicine, McGovern Medical School at The University of Texas Health Science Center at Houston (UTHealth), Houston, TX, USA

Kelle Goranson, MD Department of Emergency Medicine, McGovern Medical School at The University of Texas Health Science Center at Houston (UTHealth), Houston, TX, USA

Autumn Graham, MD Department of Emergency Medicine, MedStar Washington Hospital Center, MedStar Georgetown University Hospital, Washington, DC, USA

Ashley Gray, MD Department of Emergency Medicine, Alpert Medical School of Brown University, Providence, RI, USA

Richard T. Griffey, MD, MPH Washington University School of Medicine, St. Louis, MO, USA

Mohamed Hagahmed, MD Department of Emergency Medicine, University of Pittsburgh Medical Center, Pittsburgh, PA, USA

Jonathan L. Hansen, MD, MBA, FACEP MedStar Franklin Square Medical Center, Baltimore, MD, USA

Georgetown University School of Medicine, Washington, DC, USA

Michelle A. Hieger, DO Section of Toxicology, Department of Emergency Medicine, Wellspan Health, York Hospital, York, PA, USA

Matthew Hinton, PharmD, BCPS Department of Pharmacy, Temple University Hospital, Philadelphia, PA, USA

Andrea J. Hladik, MD Department of Emergency Medicine, Eisenhower Medical Center, Rancho Mirage, CA, USA

Christina S. Houser, MD MedStar Washington Hospital Center, MedStar Georgetown University Hospital, Washington, DC, USA

Joseph Izzo, MD Department of Emergency Medicine, MedStar Georgetown University Hospital, Washington, DC, USA

Patrick G. Jackson, MD MedStar Georgetown University Hospital, Washington, DC, USA

MedStar Washington Hospital Center, Washington, DC, USA

Timothy Jang, MD Harbor-UCLA Medical Center, David Geffen School of Medicine at UCLA, Torrance, CA, USA

Adam Janicki, MD Department of Emergency Medicine, University of Pittsburgh Medical Center, Pittsburgh, PA, USA

Angela F. Jarman, MD Department of Emergency Medicine, Alpert School of Medicine of Brown University, Providence, RI, USA

Kelli L. Jarrell, MD University of Cincinnati College of Medicine, Department of Emergency Medicine, Cincinnati, OH, USA

Laura S. Johnson, MD Georgetown University School of Medicine, Washington, DC, USA

Herman Kalsi, MD Department of Emergency Medicine, MedStar Georgetown University Hospital, Washington, DC, USA

Theodore Katz, MD Department of Emergency Medicine, MedStar Georgetown University Hospital, Washington, DC, USA

Efrat Rosenzweig Kean, MD Temple University Hospital, Philadelphia, PA, USA

Thompson Kehrl, MD, FACEP, RDMS Section of Emergency Ultrasound, York Hospital Emergency Ultrasound Fellowship, York Hospital Emergency Medicine Residency, York Hospital Department of Emergency Medicine, York, PA, USA

Shawna Kettyle, MD MedStar Washington Hospital Center, Washington, DC, USA

Basil Z. Khalaf, MD Department of Emergency Medicine, McGovern Medical School at The University of Texas Health Science Center at Houston (UTHealth), Houston, TX, USA

Eric S. Kiechle, MD MPH MedStar Washington Hospital Center, Department of Emergency Medicine, Washington, DC, USA

Evan Kingsley, MD Department of Emergency Medicine, Temple University Hospital, Philadelphia, PA, USA

Ahnika Kline, MD PhD National Institute of Health, Bethesda, MD, USA

Adeola A. Kosoko, MD Department of Emergency Medicine, McGovern Medical School at The University of Texas Health Science Center at Houston (UTHealth), Houston, TX, USA

Alex Koyfman, MD The University of Texas Southwestern Medical Center, Department of Emergency Medicine, Dallas, TX, USA

Anita Kumar, MD George Washington University School of Medicine & Health Sciences, Department of Medicine, Division of Gastroenterology, Washington, DC, USA

Diana Ladkany, MD Department of Emergency Medicine, MedStar Washington Hospital Center & MedStar Georgetown University Hospital, Washington, DC, USA

Kerri Layman, MD Department of Emergency Medicine, MedStar Washington Hospital Center & MedStar Georgetown University Hospital, Washington, DC, USA

Maxine Le Saux, BS Department of Emergency Medicine, George Washington University School of Medicine & Health Sciences, Washington, DC, USA

Mary Carroll Lee, MD Virginia Tech Carilion Emergency Medicine Residency, Roanoke, VA, USA

Stephen D. Lee, MD Department of Emergency Medicine, University of Maryland School of Medicine, Baltimore, MD, USA

Zone-En Lee, MD, FACG Division of Gastroenterology, MedStar Georgetown University Hospital, Washington, DC, USA
MedStar Georgetown University Hospital, Washington, DC, USA

Erin Leiman, MD Division of Emergency Medicine, Department of Surgery, Duke University Medical Center, Durham, NC, USA

Kevin Vincent Leonard, MD UPMC Department of Emergency Medicine, Pittsburgh, PA, USA

Mark Levine, MD Washington University School of Medicine, St. Louis, MO, USA

Kerrie Lind, MD, MSc MedStar Southern Maryland Hospital Center, Department of Emergency Medicine, Clinton, MD, USA

Yiju Teresa Liu, MD Harbor-UCLA Medical Center, David Geffen School of Medicine at UCLA, Torrance, CA, USA

Robert Loflin, MD University of Rochester Medical Center, Rochester, NY, USA

Brit Long, MD Brooke Army Medical Center, Department of Emergency Medicine, Fort Sam Houston, San Antonio, TX, USA

Emily Lovallo, MD UPMC Department of Emergency Medicine, Pittsburgh, PA, USA

Samuel D. Luber, MD, MPH, FACEP Department of Emergency Medicine, McGovern Medical School at The University of Texas Health Science Center at Houston (UTHealth), Houston, TX, USA

Charles Maddow, MD, FACEP McGovern Medical School at the University of Texas Health Science Center at Houston, Department of Emergency Medicine, Houston, TX, USA

Nidhi Malhotra, MD MedStar Washington Hospital Center, Washington, DC, USA

Sara Manning, MD Department of Emergency Medicine, University of Maryland School of Medicine, Baltimore, MD, USA

Joseph P. Martinez, MD University of Maryland School of Medicine, Baltimore, MD, USA

Mariana Martinez, MD Department of Emergency Medicine, Los Angeles County + USC Medical Center, Los Angeles, CA, USA

Caroline Massarelli, BS Georgetown University School of Medicine, Washington, DC, USA

Courtney H. McKee, MD University of Cincinnati College of Medicine, Department of Emergency Medicine, Cincinnati, OH, USA

Andrew C. Meltzer, MD MS Department of Emergency Medicine, George Washington University School of Medicine & Health Sciences, Washington, DC, USA

Katharine Meyer, MD Department of Emergency Medicine, MedStar Georgetown University Hospital & Washington Hospital Center, Washington, DC, USA

Tracy M. Moore, MD, MS Department of Emergency Medicine, University of Pittsburgh Medical Center, Pittsburgh, PA, USA

Chad Mosby, MD Virginia Tech Carilion School of Medicine, Department of Emergency Medicine, Roanoke, VA, USA

James Murrett, MD, MBE Temple University Hospital, Philadelphia, PA, USA

Bennett A. Myers, MD Department of Emergency Medicine, University of Maryland School of Medicine, Baltimore, MD, USA

Sandeep Nadella, MBBS, MD Division of Gastroenterology, MedStar Georgetown University Hospital, Washington, DC, USA

Sreeja Natesan, MD Duke University Medical Center, Durham, NC, USA

Alejandro Negrete, MPH Case-Western Reserve University, Cleveland, OH, USA

Michael O'Keefe, MD Division of Emergency Medicine, Duke University Medical Center, Durham, NC, USA

Kathleen Ogle, MD Department of Emergency Medicine, George Washington University School of Medicine & Health Sciences, Washington, DC, USA

Susan Owens, MD University of Cincinnati College of Medicine, Department of Emergency Medicine, Cincinnati, OH, USA

Jessica Palmer, MD Department of Emergency Medicine, MedStar Washington Hospital Center & MedStar Georgetown University Hospital, Washington, DC, USA

Rajesh Panchwagh, DO WellSpan Gastroenterology, WellSpan Population Health Services, WellSpan York Hospital, York, PA, USA

Scott H. Pasichow, MD, MPH Department of Emergency Medicine, Alpert School of Medicine of Brown University, Providence, RI, USA

Seema Patil, MD Division of Gastroenterology and Hepatology, University of Maryland School of Medicine, Baltimore, MD, USA

Gita Pensa, MD Department of Emergency Medicine, Alpert Medical School of Brown University, Providence, RI, USA

Jack Perkins, MD Virginia Tech Carilion School of Medicine, Roanoke, VA, USA

Alanna Peterson, MD UPMC Department of Emergency Medicine, Pittsburgh, PA, USA

John B. Pierson, MD Virginia Tech – Carilion Clinic, Department of Emergency Medicine, Roanoke, VA, USA

Elizabeth Pontius, MD, RDMS Georgetown University School of Medicine, Washington, DC, USA

Department of Emergency Medicine, MedStar Georgetown University Hospital and MedStar Washington Hospital Center, Washington, DC, USA

Kenneth Potter, MD Department of Anesthesiology and Perioperative Medicine, Penn State Hershey Medical Center, Hershey, PA, USA

Jane Preotle, MD Department of Emergency Medicine, Alpert Medical School of Brown University, Providence, RI, USA

Heather A. Prunty, MD, FACEP UPMC Department of Emergency Medicine, Pittsburgh, PA, USA

Sandra Quezada, MD, MS Division of Gastroenterology and Hepatology, University of Maryland School of Medicine, Baltimore, MD, USA

Ghady Rahhal, MD Washington University School of Medicine, St. Louis, MO, USA

Jennifer Repanshek, MD Temple University Hospital, Philadelphia, PA, USA

Zachary Repanshek, MD Lewis Katz School of Medicine, Temple University Hospital, Philadelphia, PA, USA

Jessica Riley, MD, FACEP WellSpan York Hospital, Department of Emergency Medicine, York, PA, USA

Robert Riviello, MD, MPH Harvard University School of Medicine, Brigham and Women's Hospital, Boston, MA, USA

Clare Roepke, MD Lewis Katz School of Medicine at Temple University Hospital, Philadelphia, PA, USA

Sarah Ronan-Bentle, MD, MS University of Cincinnati College of Medicine, Department of Emergency Medicine, Cincinnati, OH, USA

Emily Rose, MD Department of Emergency Medicine, Los Angeles County + USC Medical Center, Los Angeles, CA, USA

Keck School of Medicine of the University of Southern California, Department of Emergency Medicine, Los Angeles County + USC Medical Center, Los Angeles, CA, USA

Brandon Ruderman, MD Duke University Medical Center, Durham, NC, USA

Amber Ruest, MD Department of Emergency Medicine, Wellspan York Hospital, York, PA, USA

Patrick Sandiford, MD, MPH Emergency Medicine Residency, University of Rochester Medical Center, Rochester, NY, USA

Anthony Scarcella, MD, JD Department of Emergency Medicine, Eisenhower Medical Center, Rancho Mirage, CA, USA

Jordan B. Schooler, MD, PhD Department of Anesthesiology and Perioperative Medicine, Penn State Hershey Medical Center, Hershey, PA, USA

Department of Emergency Medicine, Penn State Hershey Medical Center, Hershey, PA, USA

Kraftin E. Schreyer, MD Department of Emergency Medicine, Temple University Hospital, Philadelphia, PA, USA

Sara Scott, MD, FACEP Department of Surgery and Perioperative Care, University of Texas at Austin Dell Medical School, Austin, TX, USA

Bradley J. Serack, MD Department of Emergency Medicine, McGovern Medical School at The University of Texas Health Science Center at Houston (UTHealth), Houston, TX, USA

Krystle Shafer, MD Department of Emergency Medicine, Critical Care Intensivist, OHICU and MSICU, Wellspan York Hospital, York, PA, USA

Stephen Shaheen, MD Duke University Medical Center, Durham, NC, USA

Zachary Shaub, DO Virginia Tech Carilion School of Medicine, Department of Emergency Medicine, Roanoke, VA, USA

Manpreet Singh, MD Department of Emergency Medicine, David Geffen School of Medicine at UCLA, Harbor-UCLA Medical Center, Torrance, CA, USA

Bryan Sloane, MD Department of Emergency Medicine, Harbor-UCLA Medical Center, Torrance, CA, USA

Janet Smereck, MD Department of Emergency Medicine, MedStar Georgetown University Hospital, Washington, DC, USA

Jessica L. Smith, MD, FACEP Department of Emergency Medicine, Alpert Medical School of Brown University, Providence, RI, USA

Veronica Solorio, MD, MPH Department of Emergency Medicine, Harbor-UCLA Medical Center, Torrance, CA, USA

Philippa N. Soskin, MD, MPP MedStar Georgetown University Hospital and Washington Hospital Center, Washington, DC, USA

F. James Squadrito, MD Lewis Katz School of Medicine at Temple University Hospital, Philadelphia, PA, USA

Stephanie Streit United States Air Force, Washington, DC, USA

Nellis Air Force Base, Las Vegas, NV, USA

University of Nevada Las Vegas, Las Vegas, NV, USA

Bob Stuntz, MD, RD, MS, FAAEM, FACEP Department of Emergency Medicine, WellSpan York Hospital, York, PA, USA

Mark E. Sutherland, MD University of Maryland Medical Center, Departments of Emergency Medicine, Internal Medicine, and Critical Care, Baltimore, MD, USA

Katrin Takenaka, MD, MEd McGovern Medical School (part of UT Health/The University of Texas Health Science Center at Houston), Houston, TX, USA

Shawn Tejiram, MD MedStar Georgetown University Hospital – Washington Hospital Center Residency Program in General Surgery, Department of Surgery, MedStar Washington Hospital Center, Washington, DC, USA

Meredith C. Thompson, MD Department of Emergency Medicine, University of Virginia Health System, Charlottesville, VA, USA

Travis A. Thompson, MD MedStar Washington Hospital Center, Department of Emergency Medicine, Washington, DC, USA

Traci Thoureen, MD, MHS-CL, MMCi, FACEP Division of Emergency Medicine, Duke University Medical Center, Durham, NC, USA

Shahab Toursavadakohi, MD Department of Surgery, Division of Vascular Surgery, University of Maryland School of Medicine, Baltimore, MD, USA

Aortic Center, University of Maryland Medical Center, Baltimore, MD, USA

Nick Tsipis, MD MPH MedStar Washington Hospital Center, Department of Emergency Medicine, Washington, DC, USA

Andrew Victory, MD UPMC Department of Emergency Medicine, Pittsburgh, PA, USA

Julie T. Vieth, MBChB Canton-Potsdam Hospital, Potsdam, NY, USA

Angelina Vishnyakova, MD McGovern Medical School at the University of Texas Health Science Center at Houston, Department of Emergency Medicine, Houston, TX, USA

Kathryn Voss, MD MedStar Georgetown University and Washington Hospital Center, Washington, DC, USA

Jonathan Wagner, MD Keck School of Medicine of the University of Southern California, Los Angeles County/University of Southern California (LAC+USC) Department of Emergency Medicine, Los Angeles, CA, USA

Anne Walker, MD University of Maryland Medical Center, Baltimore, MD, USA

Deena D. Wasserman, MD, FAWM Department of Emergency Medicine, Temple University Hospital, Philadelphia, PA, USA

Jonathan Watson, MD Department of Emergency Medicine, MedStar Georgetown University Hospital and Washington Hospital Center, Washington, DC, USA

Patrick D. Webb, MD Centers for Gastroenterology, Fort Collins, CO, USA

Lindsay A. Weiner, MD University of Maryland School of Medicine, Department of Emergency Medicine, Baltimore, MD, USA

Jennifer Wellington, DO Division of Gastroenterology and Hepatology, University of Maryland School of Medicine, Baltimore, MD, USA

Jessie Werner, MD Department of Emergency Medicine, Alpert Medical School of Brown University, Providence, RI, USA

Lauren M. Westafer, DO, MPH Department of Emergency Medicine, Baystate Medical Center/UMMS, Springfield, MA, USA

Lauren Westover, MD Department of Emergency Medicine, University of Pittsburgh Medical Center, Pittsburgh, PA, USA

Lauren Wiesner, MD Georgetown University School of Medicine, Department of Emergency Medicine, Washington, DC, USA

MedStar Washington Hospital Center, Washington, DC, USA

Matthew Wilson, MD, FACEP Georgetown University School of Medicine, MedStar Washington Hospital Center, Department of Emergency Medicine, Washington, DC, USA

Richard Wroblewski, MD Temple University Hospital, Philadelphia, PA, USA

Andrea Wu, MD, MMM Department of Emergency Medicine, David Geffen School of Medicine at UCLA, Harbor-UCLA Medical Center, Torrance, CA, USA

Zhaoxin Yang MedStar Georgetown University Hospital, Department of Emergency Medicine, Washington, DC, USA

Thomas Yeich, MD, FACEP Department of Emergency Medicine, Wellspan York Hospital, York, PA, USA

Hani Zamil, MD, CMQ McGovern Medical School, UT Health, Houston, TX, USA

Anna Zelivianskaia, MD MedStar Washington Hospital Center, Department of Obstetrics and Gynecology, Washington, DC, USA

Part I

General Approach to Acute Abdominal Pain

What Are the "Rules of the Road" When Approaching Patients with Acute Abdominal Pain? What Are Common Diagnostic Errors and Who Are High-Risk Patients?

Kelle Goranson and Samuel D. Luber

Pearls and Pitfalls
- Approach acute abdominal pain by obtaining a history that elicits the patient's symptoms (location, quality, and progression of symptoms) and perform a thorough physical exam.
- The vertical level of visceral (dull, midline) pain suggests the organs involved while parietal (sharp, localized) pain identifies the location or quadrant involved.
- Cases with a recognized diagnostic error were more likely to have (1) inadequately addressed abnormalities on laboratory studies, (2) a shorter initial length of stay, or (3) a differential diagnosis that did not include the final diagnosis.
- Elderly, female, and immunocompromised patients with acute abdominal pain may present atypically.

Acute abdominal pain is a complicated chief complaint that can be approached with an organized thought process and a thorough history and physical exam. An evaluation of the patient's complaint begins with a history that allows the clinician to characterize the patient's symptoms in terms of location, quality, and progression of symptoms [1]. Subsequently, the findings of the physical exam can further characterize the patient's overall presentation to develop a differential diagnosis (Fig. 1.1) that will guide the provider in creating an appropriate diagnostic evaluation and treatment plan. Throughout the patient assessment, the clinician should be mindful of potential diagnostic errors and give special consideration to high-risk populations that may present atypically or harbor acute surgical pathology.

What Are the "Rules of the Road" When Approaching Patients with Acute Abdominal Pain?

A focused history is the first step to determine the location and quality of acute abdominal pain. An understanding of the innervation of the abdomen prioritizes the clinician's management and lends diagnostic insight into the etiology of the patient's symptoms.

When abdominal organs are disturbed by pathologic processes leading to organ wall stretch from distension, ischemia, or inflammation, the patient develops *visceral pain*, often described as dull or gnawing [1, 2]. The abdominal organs are bilaterally innervated which leads to pain perceived in the midline [1, 2]. The vertical level of visceral pain helps localize the source [1, 2]. Visceral pain originating from the stomach, proximal duodenum, liver, pancreas, and biliary structures is generally appreciated in the epigastrium [1, 2]. Pain arising from the distal small intestine and proximal colon is manifested in a periumbilical distribution [1, 2]. Finally, visceral pain produced by the distal colon, rectum, and intraperitoneal genitourinary organs is felt in the suprapubic region [1, 2].

As a disease process evolves, inflammation of the nearby peritoneum may result in focal *parietal pain*, described as sharp and localized. Parietal pain may guide the clinician to a specific location of pathology [1, 2]. Often the progression of symptoms can yield insight into the underlying disease process. For example, appendicitis may initially manifest as midline pain in a periumbilical distribution reflecting visceral pain due to intestinal wall stretching. With time, the overlying abdominal peritoneum may become inflamed, and the patient can develop parietal pain perceived specifi-

K. Goranson · S. D. Luber (✉)
Department of Emergency Medicine, McGovern Medical School at The University of Texas Health Science Center at Houston (UTHealth), Houston, TX, USA
e-mail: Samuel.D.Luber@uth.tmc.edu

© Springer Nature Switzerland AG 2019
A. Graham, D. J. Carlberg (eds.), *Gastrointestinal Emergencies*, https://doi.org/10.1007/978-3-319-98343-1_1

Fig. 1.1 Abdominal pain differential diagnosis by abdominal quadrant

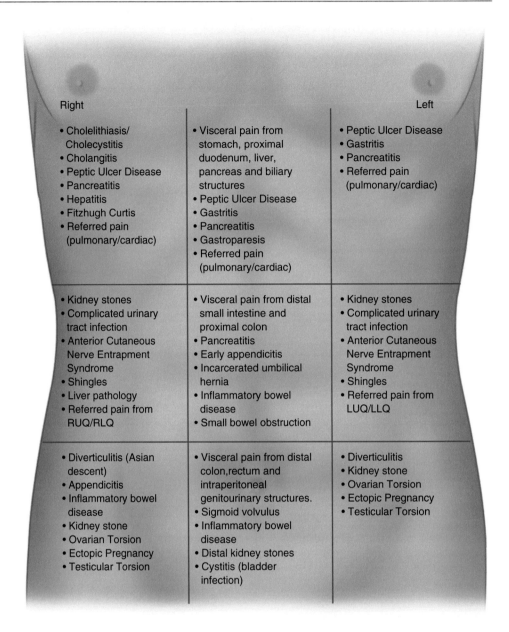

Right

- Cholelithiasis/ Cholecystitis
- Cholangitis
- Peptic Ulcer Disease
- Pancreatitis
- Hepatitis
- Fitzhugh Curtis
- Referred pain (pulmonary/cardiac)

- Visceral pain from stomach, proximal duodenum, liver, pancreas and biliary structures
- Peptic Ulcer Disease
- Gastritis
- Pancreatitis
- Gastroparesis
- Referred pain (pulmonary/cardiac)

Left

- Peptic Ulcer Disease
- Gastritis
- Pancreatitis
- Referred pain (pulmonary/cardiac)

- Kidney stones
- Complicated urinary tract infection
- Anterior Cutaneous Nerve Entrapment Syndrome
- Shingles
- Liver pathology
- Referred pain from RUQ/RLQ

- Visceral pain from distal small intestine and proximal colon
- Pancreatitis
- Early appendicitis
- Incarcerated umbilical hernia
- Inflammatory bowel disease
- Small bowel obstruction

- Kidney stones
- Complicated urinary tract infection
- Anterior Cutaneous Nerve Entrapment Syndrome
- Shingles
- Referred pain from LUQ/LLQ

- Diverticulitis (Asian descent)
- Appendicitis
- Inflammatory bowel disease
- Kidney stone
- Ovarian Torsion
- Ectopic Pregnancy
- Testicular Torsion

- Visceral pain from distal colon,rectum and intraperitoneal genitourinary structures.
- Sigmoid volvulus
- Inflammatory bowel disease
- Distal kidney stones
- Cystitis (bladder infection)

- Diverticulitis
- Kidney stone
- Ovarian Torsion
- Ectopic Pregnancy
- Testicular Torsion

cally in the right lower quadrant [1]. Pain perceived as distant from the abdomen can be the result of intra-abdominal pathology and is known as referred pain. For instance, pain stemming from the pancreas can present as back pain, and biliary or diaphragmatic irritation can be perceived as shoulder pain [1, 3, 4].

During the physical exam, palpation may localize the region of maximal tenderness, allowing the clinician to narrow the differential diagnosis [2]. Abdominal muscle contraction (guarding) can be reduced by having the patient bend their knees during the exam [2]. Severe guarding (rigidity) and pain with movement or sudden release of applied pressure (rebound) often is the result of parietal pain from an underlying pathologic process [2]. Tenderness localized to a

specific quadrant of the abdomen can aid the clinician in determining the anatomic origin of the patient's symptoms. For example, pain specific to the right upper quadrant often results from a biliary or hepatic etiology [2].

What Are The Common Diagnostic Errors and High-Risk Patients?

Common Diagnostic Errors

A comprehensive history and physical exam are powerful tools. Their importance was demonstrated by Medford-Davis et al. in a study that explored the cause of diagnostic error during the evaluation of abdominal pain in the emergency department. Thirty-five diagnostic errors were singled out in 100 high-risk cases. The authors identified diagnostic errors after reviewing charts of emergency department patients who (1) were evaluated for abdominal pain and subsequently discharged and (2) returned within 10 days and were hospitalized. The authors described process breakdowns during the initial emergency department visit that may have contributed to the errors. Many of the identified breakdowns were due to history taking and to a lesser extent, the physical exam. Breakdowns in history taking occurred when clinical information contradicted nursing documentation or was obtained without the aid of a language interpreter. One breakdown during the physical exam occurred in a patient with abdominal pain where the documented exam did not find lower abdominal tenderness. The patient was discharged and returned later with ruptured appendicitis. Cases with a recognized diagnostic error were more likely to have (1) inadequately addressed abnormalities on laboratory studies, (2) a shorter initial length of stay, and (3) a differential diagnosis that did not include the final diagnosis. Regarding inadequately addressed laboratory abnormalities, the authors suggested breakdowns frequently occurred when the provider failed to obtain abdominal imaging studies to further evaluate abnormal liver function tests. In an effort to reduce common diagnostic errors, the clinician should place emphasis on taking adequate time to obtain a thorough history and physical exam, explain laboratory abnormalities, and generate a robust differential diagnosis [5].

High-Risk Populations

Elderly Patients

Elderly patients presenting with acute abdominal pain warrant special consideration due to their propensity to present atypically as well as their increased mortality rate [4, 6–8]. In one report, only 21% of patients over the age of 70 with gastrointestinal perforation presented with epigastric rigidity on exam [7]. As another example of atypical presentation, only about half of elderly patients with cholecystitis will have a positive Murphy's sign or right upper quadrant pain [4, 8]. Importantly, gallbladder and biliary pathology are common in the elderly. One study of autopsy reports revealed gallstones in over 50% of patients over the age of 70 [9, 10]. Acute cholecystitis is a leading cause of surgical emergency in the elderly, and in one series, 40% of operative procedures in patients over the age of 65 with acute abdominal complaints were attributable to gallbladder and biliary disease [6, 11]. Advanced age is also associated with potentially catastrophic abdominal disease processes includ-

ing abdominal aortic aneurysm and acute mesenteric ischemia, with the latter carrying a mortality rate of approximately 70% [12–14]. Given the potential for atypical presentation, acute surgical pathology, and the magnitude of morbidity and mortality, the clinician should approach elderly patients complaining of abdominal pain with a high degree of suspicion for severe underlying illness.

Female Patients

Among female patients presenting with acute abdominal pain, the clinician should keep in mind several considerations. In females of reproductive age, complications of pregnancy must be considered, and an ectopic pregnancy must be included on the clinician's differential. The Centers for Disease Control reported that up to 13% of pregnancy-related deaths were associated with ectopic pregnancy complications [15]. Additionally, the clinician must consider genitourinary processes such as pelvic inflammatory disease and ovarian torsion if the clinical picture suggests these diagnoses [16].

Immunocompromised Patients

When evaluating the immunocompromised patient presenting with abdominal pain, the clinician must give special consideration to potential infectious and neoplastic processes. Among patients infected with HIV, a low CD4 count can predispose patients to opportunistic infections such as *Cytomegalovirus* (CMV) and *Cryptosporidium* [17–19]. *Cytomegalovirus* is a pathogen that can cause abdominal pain, fever, and diarrhea; however gastrointestinal hemorrhage and intestinal perforation have been documented [20–24]. *Cryptosporidium* can cause similar symptoms such as abdominal pain, fever, and diarrhea and has been associated specifically with acalculous cholecystitis in immunocompromised patients [25–27]. Finally, neoplastic processes such as lymphoma are known complications of HIV infection [27, 28]. Gastrointestinal involvement has been documented in up to 44% of HIV-infected patients with lymphoma and can present with acute abdominal pain, perforation, and obstruction [27–30].

Summary

Ultimately, acute abdominal pain can be caused by an extensive list of possible etiologies, but a thorough history and physical exam with attention to high-risk populations can assist the clinician narrow the differential, avoid potential diagnostic errors, and initiate an appropriate diagnostic and therapeutic plan.

References

1. McNamara D, Dean AJ. Approach to acute abdominal pain. Emerg Med Clin North Am. 2011;29(2):159–73.
2. Mary CO. Acute abdominal pain. In: Tintinalli JE, Stapczynski JS, Ma OJ, Yealy DM, Meckler GD, Cline DM, editors. Tintinalli's emergency medicine: a comprehensive study guide [internet]. 8th ed. New York: McGraw-Hill Education; 2016. Available from: http://accessmedicine.mhmedical.com/Book.aspx?bookid=1658.
3. Kendall JL, Moreira, ME. Evaluation of the adult with abdominal pain in the emergency department [Internet]. 2016 [Updated 2016 Sep 29; cited 2017 Sep 11]. Available from: https://www.uptodate.com/contents/evaluation-of-the-adult-with-abdominal-pain-in-the-emergency-department.
4. Lyon C, Clark DC. Diagnosis of acute abdominal pain in older patients. Am Fam Physician. 2006;74(9):1537–44.
5. Medford-Davis L, Park E, Shlamovitz G, Suliburk J, Meyer AN, Singh H. Diagnostic errors related to acute abdominal pain in the emergency department. Emerg Med J. 2016;33(4):253–9.
6. Kizer KW, Vassar MJ. Emergency department diagnosis of abdominal disorders in the elderly. Am J Emerg Med. 1998;16(4):357–62.
7. Fenyo G. Acute abdominal disease in the elderly: experience from two series in Stockholm. Am J Surg. 1982;143(6):751–4.
8. Rothrock SG, Greenfield R, Falk JL. Acute abdominal emergencies in the elderly: clinical evaluation and management. Part II – diagnosis and management of common conditions. Emerg Med Reports. 1992;13:185–92.
9. Crump C. The incidence of gallstones and gallbladder disease. Surg Gynecol Obstet. 1931;53:447–55.
10. Huber DF, Martin EW Jr, Cooperman M. Cholecystectomy in elderly patients. Am J Surg. 1983;146(6):719–22.
11. Gurleyik G, Gurleyik E, Unalmiser S. Abdominal surgical emergency in the elderly. Turk J Gastroenterol. 2002;13(1):47–52.
12. Lederle FA, Johnson GR, Wilson SE, Chute EP, Littooy FN, Bandyk D, et al. Prevalence and associations of abdominal aortic aneurysm detected through screening. Ann Intern Med. 1997;126(6):441–9.
13. Greenwald DA, Brandt LJ, Reinus JF. Ischemic bowel disease in the elderly. Gastroenterol Clin N Am. 2001;30(2):445–73.
14. Brandt LJ, Boley SJ. AGA technical review on intestinal ischemia. Gastroenterology. 2000;118(5):954–68.
15. Goldner TE, Lawson HW, Xia Z, Atrash HK. Surveillance for ectopic pregnancy – United States, 1970–1989 [Internet]. 1993 Dec 17 [Cited 2017 Sep 11]. Available from: https://www.cdc.gov/mmwr/preview/mmwrhtml/00031632.htm.
16. Kamin RA, Nowicki TA, Courtney DS, Powers RD. Pearls and pitfalls in the emergency department evaluation of abdominal pain. Emerg Med Clin North Am. 2003;21(1):61–72.
17. Guidelines for prevention and treatment of opportunistic infections in HIV-infected adults and adolescents. 2013 [Updated 2013 Jun 17; cited 2018 Jan 25]. Available from: https://aidsinfo.nih.gov/contentfiles/lvguidelines/adult_oi.pdf.
18. Arribas JR, Storch GA, Clifford DB, Tselis AC. Cytomegalovirus encephalitis. Ann Intern Med. 1996;125(7):577–87.
19. Flanigan T, Whalen C, Turner J, Soave R, Toerner J, Havlir D, Kotler D. Cryptosporidium infection and CD4 counts. Ann Intern Med. 1992;116(10):840–2.
20. Whitley RJ, Jacobson MA, Friedberg DN, Holland GN, Jabs DA, Dieterich DT, et al. Guidelines for the treatment of cytomegalovirus diseases in patients with AIDS in the era of potent antiretroviral therapy: recommendations of an international panel. International AIDS Society – USA. Arch Intern Med. 1998;158(9):957–69.
21. Dieterich DT, Rahmin M. Cytomegalovirus colitis in AIDS: presentation in 44 patients and a review of the literature. J Acquir Immune Defic Syndr. 1991;4(Suppl 1):S29–35.
22. Wilcox CM, Schwartz DA. Symptomatic CMV duodenitis. An important clinical problem in AIDS. J Clin Gastroenterol. 1992;14(4):293–7.
23. Kyriazis AP, Mitra SK. Multiple cytomegalovirus-related intestinal perforations in patients with acquired immunodeficiency syndrome. Report of two cases and review of the literature. Arch Pathol Lab Med. 1992;116(5):495–9.
24. Bartlett JG. Medical management of HIV infection. Glenview: Physicians and Scientist Publishing Co., Inc.; 1996.
25. Leder K, Weller PF. Epidemiology, clinical manifestations, and diagnosis of cryptosporidiosis [Internet]. 2017 [Updated 2017 Sep 18; cited 2018 Jan 25]. Available from: https://www.uptodate.com/contents/epidemiology-clinical-manifestations-and-diagnosis-of-cryptosporidiosis.
26. Cacciarelli AG, Naddaf SY, El-Zeftawy HA, Aziz M, Omar WS, Kumar M, et al. Acute cholecystitis in AIDS patients: correlation of Tc-99m hepatobiliary scintigraphy with histopathologic laboratory findings and CD4 counts. Clin Nucl Med. 1998;23(2):226–8.
27. Wu CM, Davis F, Fishman EK. Radiologic evaluation of the acute abdomen in the patient with acquired immunodeficiency syndrome (AIDS): the role of CT scanning. Semin Ultrasound CT MR. 1998;19(2):190–9.
28. Heise W, Arasteh K, Mostertz P, Skorde J, Schmidt W, Obst C, et al. Malignant gastrointestinal lymphomas in patients with AIDS. Digestion. 1997;58(3):218–24.
29. Wyatt SH, Fishman EK. The acute abdomen in individuals with AIDS. Radiol Clin N Am. 1994;32(5):1023–43.
30. Yee J, Wall SD. Gastrointestinal manifestations of AIDS. Gastroenterol Clin N Am. 1995;24(2):413–34.

What Is the Accuracy of the Physical Exam in Intra-abdominal Emergencies? Does Administration of Pain Medication Alter the Accuracy of the Physical Examination?

2

John C. Beauchamp and Jonathan Giordano

Pearls and Pitfalls
- Understanding the abdominal embryologic origins and their innervation can provide guidance on cause of pain.
- Physical exam findings should guide your workup but have limitations that clinicians should be aware of.
- A high index of suspicion for intra-abdominal pathology should be maintained for generalized abdominal pain especially in high-risk patients.

Patients presenting with complaints of abdominal pain comprise 5–10% of all emergency department (ED) visits in the United States [1–4]. It can be associated with significant morbidity and mortality. While it is important to remember that not all abdominal pain is originating from within the abdominal cavity, the physical examination of the abdomen is a vital component of the patient's assessment, guiding the emergency provider's (EP) cost-effective use of diagnostic resources. This chapter will focus on discussing its utility and application in the patient with abdominal pain.

Patients' abdominal pain presentation is a complex interaction of embryology and innervation. Abdominal visceral pain arises from smooth muscle stretching, followed by activation of nocireceptors on abdominal viscera. The embryonic gut develops as midline organs with bilateral splanchnic innervation, resulting in inconsistent, poorly localized midline pain, associated with nausea, vomiting, pallor, and sweating. Pain localized in the epigastric region is most specific for diseases of foregut structures: stomach, pancreas, liver, and proximal duodenum. Periumbilical pain has been found to be 99% specific for disease processes involving the midgut region, including the distal

small bowel, proximal third of the large colon, and appendix. Suprapubic pain is associated with hindgut organs: distal aspect of the large colon and bladder [2, 3]. Conversely, somatic pain with nocireceptors in the skin, muscles, and bones can be accurately localized by palpation and exacerbated by jarring or deep breaths [5].

But the perception of pain is not static. As acute inflammation and tissue injury progress, several pathways begin to intersect. As Smith outlined in 1967, rapid onset, severe visceral pain may "spill over" at the spinal cord level producing somatic pain [5]. In addition, "peripheral sensitization" occurs as advancing tissue injury recruits adjacent somatic nerves, producing localized pain and tenderness. Clinically, this intersection is reflected in the classic presentation of appendicitis, which begins as visceral, midline, periumbilical pain and progresses to localized right lower quadrant pain and tenderness on physical exam.

What Is the Accuracy of the Physical Exam in Intra-abdominal Emergencies?

Inspection

Inspection is an important initial component of the physical exam as it allows the EP to identify surgical scars, rashes, signs of liver disease, and possible intra-abdominal hemorrhage. Abdominal inspection findings such as surgical scars (possible SBO lead points), dermatomal rash (herpes zoster), caput medusa (liver), Grey Turner's sign (flank ecchymosis indicating retroperitoneal bleeding), and Cullen's sign (blue-colored periumbilical area indicating intraperitoneal bleeding) help to direct further workup [6].

Auscultation

The overall utility of abdominal auscultation is limited. In one study, researchers recorded bowel sounds of 98 patients; of which, 35 had a final diagnosis of bowel obstruction after

J. C. Beauchamp · J. Giordano (✉)
Department of Emergency Medicine, McGovern Medical School at The University of Texas Health Science Center at Houston (UTHealth), Houston, TX, USA
e-mail: Jonathan.a.Giordano@uth.tmc.edu

© Springer Nature Switzerland AG 2019
A. Graham, D. J. Carlberg (eds.), *Gastrointestinal Emergencies*, https://doi.org/10.1007/978-3-319-98343-1_2

laparotomy. Fifty-three physicians were asked to classify bowel sounds as abnormal or normal. While there was no significant difference between senior and junior physicians, neither group could accurately classify bowel sounds as abnormal in patients with bowel obstruction compared to patients without bowel obstruction (sensitivity 42%, specificity 78%) [7].

Percussion

When compared to bedside ultrasound, percussion has limited utility in the modern emergency department. One study found percussion and palpation unreliable and inaccurate in diagnosing hepatomegaly when compared to bedside US [8]. However, percussion can help to differentiate between drum-like tympany and shifting dullness, suggesting either large bowel free air due to obstruction or ascites [6].

Palpation

While an integral component of the physical examination, the accuracy for identifying common life-threatening abdominal pathology is variable.

For instance, a positive Murphy's sign (pain sufficient to cause an abrupt halt in inspiration during palpation of the right upper quadrant) is taught to be pathognomonic of gallbladder disease. While it has been found to be the strongest positive predictor of acute cholecystitis [3], a recent meta-analysis demonstrated it only has a sensitivity of 65% and specificity of 87% [4, 9–11].

In the case of right lower quadrant pain, there are several maneuvers that are thought to guide clinicians to the diagnosis of appendicitis, including the psoas, obturator, and Rovsing's signs. The psoas sign (pain with passive hip extension) has a sensitivity of 16% and specificity of 95% for appendicitis [12]. It can also be positive with pyelonephritis, pancreatitis, or psoas abscess [3, 4]. The obturator sign (positive if there is pain with internal rotation of the right hip while the hip and knee are both held in flexion to 90 degrees) is thought to have a sensitivity and specificity comparable to that of the psoas sign as they both indicate irritation of the underlying muscle by an inflamed appendix [12]. Rovsing's sign (pain is present in the RLQ when the emergency provider applies pressure to the LLQ) has reported sensitivities of 22–68% and specificities of 75–86% for appendicitis [3, 4, 9]. In limited studies, positive findings in any of the above three examinations have a low sensitivity but relatively high specificity (85–95%) [2, 9]. In comparison, computed tomography imaging with intravenous contrast following positive RLQ findings has a diagnostic accuracy of 98% [11].

Patients found to have generalized abdominal pain upon examination present a diagnostic challenge. It is difficult to narrow the differential diagnosis with precision given nonfocal physical exam findings. In this patient population, initial history and physical examination may be of utmost impor-

tance. A patient complaining of excruciating abdominal pain out of proportion to physical examination should raise concern for acute mesenteric ischemia. In several studies 95% of patients with acute mesenteric ischemia presented with severe generalized abdominal pain [13]. Abdominal aortic aneurysms can also present with generalized abdominal pain with the most common physical exam finding being a pulsatile mass. This important finding, with the aid of bedside ultrasound, can lead to expedited care in an unstable patient [2, 3].

Clinical Assessment Accuracy

When evaluating patients with left lower quadrant pain for diverticulitis, the American Society of Colon and Rectal Surgeons' (ASCRS) clinical guidelines (2014) state "the diagnosis of acute diverticulitis can often be made following a focused history and physical examination, especially in patients with recurrent diverticulitis whose diagnosis has been previously confirmed" [14]. However, studies on the accuracy of clinical diagnosis reflect high misdiagnosis rates of 34–67% [15].

When evaluating patients with right lower pain for appendicitis, a 2004 meta-analysis found that physical exam findings alone are not sufficiently accurate to diagnose acute appendicitis but should rather be used in concert with history and laboratory values to establish a predictive value [16].

When evaluating patients with suspected small bowel obstructions, physical exam findings are insufficient to determine the severity of the obstruction and whether concurrent bowel strangulation or ischemia is present. In addition to clinical presentation, physical exam, and labs, imaging is usually necessary to determine the severity of obstruction and need for acute surgical intervention [17].

Serial Examination

While risk literature and clinical dogma emphasizes the importance of serial examinations, published research to guide clinicians in terms of best practice in acute non-traumatic abdominal pain is lacking. There is limited current data, but one study from 1991 by Graff et al. found an increased ability to identify those patients with and without appendicitis after a short-term (approximately 10 h) observation period, suggesting a benefit of repeat abdominal exams in this specific population [18].

Does Administration of Pain Medication Alter the Accuracy of the Physical Examination?

Traditionally clinicians have avoided the use of analgesia in patients with abdominal pain until complete evaluation has been performed. It has been suggested that the use of opioid analgesics may mask significant findings during physical examination [14, 19, 20]. A randomized, prospective, placebo-controlled study published in the 1990s established that physical examination does change after administration of analgesics with the hypothesis being that early pain control allows the patient to relax which reduces guarding and allows localized tenderness to be better appreciated on examination, but there was no difference in final dispositions [19]. More recently, a review was published through the Cochrane Database that showed similar findings – the use of opioid analgesics in early management of abdominal pain does not increase the risk of diagnostic error or risk of errors in management [7, 20]. Administering pain medications in patients with acute abdominal pain is safe and does not impair clinically important diagnostic accuracy [21].

Summary

The physical exam is a critical portion of the initial evaluation of patients presenting with abdominal pain as the exam helps to narrow the differential and focus further laboratory testing and imaging. Studies have found that physical exam findings alone are insufficient to properly diagnose and treat disease processes such as appendicitis and small bowel obstructions. However, when the physical exam is combined with history, laboratory values, and imaging studies, an appropriate ED disposition can be established [22].

Suggested Resources

- CanadiEM. CRACKCast E027 – Abdominal pain. https://canadiem.org/crackcast-e027-abdominal-pain/#comments.
- EM Basic. Abdominal pain. (Podcast). 2011. http://embasic.org/abdominal-pain/
- LifeintheFastLane. Clinical examination. https://lifeinthefastlane.com/education/signs/.
- MedicalEd.org. Abdominal examination (Podcast). http://www.medicaled.org/abdominal-examination.html.
- Tintinalli JE, et al. Chap. 71: Acute abdominal pain. In: Tintinalli's emergency medicine: a comprehensive study guide. 8th ed: McGraw-Hill's AccessMedicine; 2016.
- University of Leicester. Abdominal examination – Demonstration (video). 2012. https://www.youtube.com/watch?v=nKYIcshakf4.
- Walls RM, Hockberger RS, Gausche-Hill M. Rosen's. Chap. 24: Abdominal pain. In: Emergency medicine: concepts and clinical practice. 9th ed. Philadelphia: Elseiver; 2018.

References

1. Mattson B, Dulaimy K. The 4 quadrants: acute pathology in the abdomen and current imaging guidelines. Semin Ultrasound CT MR. 2017;38(4):414–23.
2. McNamara R, Dean AJ. Approach to acute abdominal pain. Emerg Med Clin North Am. 2011;29(2):159–73.
3. Natesan S, Lee J, Volkamer H, et al. Evidence-based medicine approach to abdominal pain. Emerg Med Clin North Am. 2016;34(2):165–90.
4. Cartwright SL, Knudson MP. Evaluation of acute abdominal pain in adults. Am Fam Physician. 2008;77(7):971–8.
5. Sherman R. Abdominal Pain. In: Walker HK, Hall WD, Hurst JW, editors. Clinical methods: the history, physical, and laboratory examinations. 3rd ed. Boston: Butterworths; 1990. Chapter 86.
6. Macaluso CR, McNamara RM. Evaluation and management of acute abdominal pain in the emergency department. Int J Gen Med. 2012;5:789–97.
7. Breum Birger M, Bo R, Thomas K, Nordentoft T. Accuracy of abdominal auscultation for bowel obstruction. World J Gastroenterol. 2015;21(34):10018–24.
8. Joshi R, Singh A, Jajoo N, Pai M, Kalantri SP. Accuracy and reliability of palpation and percussion for detecting hepatomegaly: a rural hospital-based study. Indian J Gastroenterol. 2004;23(5):171–4.
9. Moll van Charante E, de Jongh TO. Physical examination of patients with acute abdominal pain. Ned tijdschr Geneeskd. 2011;155:A2658.
10. Mills LD, Mills T, Foster B. Association of clinical and laboratory variables with ultrasound findings in right upper quadrant abdominal pain. South Med J. 2005;98(2):155–61.
11. Avegno J, Carlisle M. Evaluating the patient with right upper quadrant abdominal pain. Emerg Med Clin North Am. 2016;34(2):211–28.
12. Wagner James M, McKinney W, Paul C, John L. Does this patient have appendicitis? JAMA. 1996;276:1589–94.
13. Bala M, Kashuk J, Moore EE, et al. Acute mesenteric ischemia: guidelines of the world Society of Emergency Surgery. World J Emerg Surg. 2017;12:38.
14. Feingold D, Steele S, Lee S, Kaiser A, Boushey R, Buie D, Rafferty J. Practice parameters for the treatment of sigmoid diverticulitis. Dis Colon Rectum. 2014;57:284–94.
15. Toorenvliet BR, Bakker RF, Breslau PJ, et al. Colonic diverticulitis: a prospective analysis of diagnostic accuracy and clinical decision making. Color Dis. 2009;12:179–187.
16. Andersson RE. Meta-analysis of the clinical and laboratory diagnosis of appendicitis. Br J Surg. 2004;91:28–37.
17. Paulson Erik K, Thompson WM. Review of small-bowel obstruction: the diagnosis and when to worry. Radiology. 2015;275(2):332–42.
18. Graff L, Radford MJ, Werne C. Probability of appendicitis before and after observation. Ann Emerg Med. 1991;20(5):503–7.
19. LoVecchio F, Oster N, Sturmann K, Nelson LS, et al. The use of analgesics in patients with acute abdominal pain. J Emerg Med. 1997;15(6):775–9.
20. Manterola C, Vial M, Moraga J, Astudillo P. Analgesia in patients with acute abdominal pain. Cochrane Database Syst Rev. 2011;1:CD005660.
21. Gallagher EJ, et al. Randomized clinical trial of morphine in acute abdominal pain. Ann Emerg Med. 2006;48(2):150–60.
22. Onur OE, et al. Outpatient follow-up or "Active clinical observation" in patients with nonspecific abdominal pain in the Emergency Department. A randomized clinical trial. Minerva Chir. 2008;63(1):9–15.

The Utility of Laboratory Data: What to Consider and How to Interpret in Common Abdominal Diseases

Bradley J. Serack and Samuel D. Luber

Pearls and Pitfalls
- Laboratory testing should not take the place of an appropriately gathered history of present illness and physical examination.
- The adept clinician understands that laboratory testing does not always offer adequate likelihood ratios to definitively rule in or rule out disease.
- Consider the use of tests which will change disposition or treatment plan, i.e., gathering tests to round out completion of a validated clinical prediction rule.
- A persistently elevated serum lactate level is an independent predictor of in-hospital mortality in a wide range of disease states, including intra-abdominal emergencies, and can significantly change disposition.
- In the consideration of acute appendicitis, there may be a role for combined complete blood count (CBC) and C-reactive protein (CRP) testing in identifying low-risk patients that can be safely discharged.
- Be cognizant of "extra-abdominal" sources of abdominal pain when determining which diagnostic studies to order, including the utilization of troponins (acute coronary syndrome), finger stick (diabetic ketoacidosis), and D-dimer (pulmonary embolism) in the appropriate context.

The Utility of Laboratory Data: How to Interpret the Data

The evaluation of undifferentiated abdominal pain in the emergency department is often augmented by the collection of laboratory data. An understanding of what tests will best complement the data gathered in the history of present illness (HPI) and physical examination can expedite an appropriate and timely diagnosis. The routine gathering of "abdominal labs" in the pursuit of a diagnosis is not supported by the literature, and failure to follow up abnormal tests accounts for a significant percentage of clinical error [1]. As such, laboratory studies can complement a carefully gathered HPI and physical exam and should be meticulously followed up.

Biliary Disease

Biliary disease is an important consideration in undifferentiated right upper quadrant (RUQ) pain. When cholelithiasis is present, no studies to date have demonstrated pathognomonic laboratory findings, and laboratory studies in biliary colic are often normal. Similarly, in acute cholecystitis, no laboratory tests are capable of independently establishing or excluding the diagnosis [2]. A complete blood count (CBC) is often obtained to evaluate the white blood cell (WBC) count. One recent meta-analysis showed pooled sensitivity of the presence of leukocytosis at only 63% [2]. Alkaline phosphatase (ALP) and total bilirubin levels may help evaluate for common bile duct obstruction which often mandates intervention via an endoscopic retrograde cholangiopancreatography (ERCP). However, normal ALP and bilirubin levels can be found in a large percentage of patients with common bile duct stones, with one study showing 48% of patients with stones to have normal levels of both [3]. Of note, though non-specific, elevation of total bilirubin in the right context may herald more serious disease, such as gangrenous cholecystitis [4].

B. J. Serack · S. D. Luber (✉)
Department of Emergency Medicine, McGovern Medical School at The University of Texas Health Science Center at Houston (UTHealth), Houston, TX, USA
e-mail: bserack@email.arizona.edu;
Samuel.D.Luber@uth.tmc.edu

© Springer Nature Switzerland AG 2019
A. Graham, D. J. Carlberg (eds.), *Gastrointestinal Emergencies*, https://doi.org/10.1007/978-3-319-98343-1_3

Pancreatitis

Based on a multitude of studies and meta-analyses, lipase and amylase testing, while potentially useful in the diagnosis of acute pancreatitis, can be problematic. Most guidelines now recommend the use of lipase over amylase, as lipase is more specific to pancreatic function, remains elevated in serum longer than amylase, and provides a higher sensitivity (64–100% vs. 45–87%, respectively) in diagnosing acute pancreatitis [5]. Both tests can be elevated by extra-pancreatic processes, such as diabetes mellitus, and there is no definitive laboratory test which confirms the diagnosis. In patients with strongly suspected pancreatitis, clinicians may order labs to risk stratify patients using scoring systems, such as the admission Bedside Index for Severity in Acute Pancreatitis (BISAP) score. A recent study has shown that the BISAP score may outperform the admission Ranson criteria in predicting mortality in acute pancreatitis, but both have limited applicability in the acute care setting [6].

Appendicitis

Based on the best available studies, no single laboratory test can sufficiently rule in or out the presence of acute appendicitis [7, 8]. Several studies and meta-analyses have demonstrated that leukocytosis does not have the sensitivity or specificity to rule in or out acute appendicitis [9, 10]. In pediatric patients, a recent meta-analysis demonstrated a sensitivity of 88% and specificity of 56% for WBC counts of 10,000/mm³ or greater [7]. There may be a role for combining the CBC with inflammatory markers. One study demonstrated the role of combined CBC/CRP testing in pediatric patients, with the combination of a WBC count of 12,000/mm³ or more and a CRP of at least 3 yielding a positive likelihood ratio of 4.36 for the presence of acute appendicitis [8]. In patients with a low pretest probability of disease, the combination of a normal WBC count and non-elevated CRP may be sufficient to exclude the diagnosis. It has been shown in at least one recent study that CRP may be used in the diagnosis of complicated acute appendicitis, as CRP is expected to rise as inflammation of the appendix progresses [11].

Gastrointestinal Bleeding (GI)

Type and screen in anticipation of transfusing packed red blood cells (RBCs) or even fresh frozen plasma (FFP) is an important consideration in the potential GI bleed patient. A CBC can hold significant diagnostic value, as studies have shown that a restrictive transfusion approach leads to fewer transfusions, a lower incidence of re-bleeding, and an overall decreased mortality [12]. However, caution should be taken when interpreting a CBC, as acute bleeding may not be reflected with the hemoglobin/hematocrit ratio at the time of presentation. For upper GI bleeds, laboratory data can be used for scoring systems such as the Glasgow-Blatchford Score, which has shown to be useful in predicting 30-day mortality [13].

Refining the Laboratory Evaluation of Abdominal Pain

- Troponin in a patient with upper abdominal pain and risk factors for acute coronary syndrome.
- Finger stick blood glucose in a diabetic patient with generalized abdominal pain to screen diabetic ketoacidosis.
- D-dimer if upper quadrant abdominal pain and respiratory symptoms, in patient with risk factors for thromboembolic disease.
- Serum lactate levels can be particularly important in altering patient disposition. In a wide range of disease states, including in the patient with undifferentiated abdominal pain, persistently elevated serum lactate levels are an independent predictor of in-hospital mortality [14].

Suggested Resource

- Medford-Davis L, Park E, Shlamovitz G, Suliburk J, Meyer A, Singh H. Diagnostic errors related to acute abdominal pain in the emergency department. Emerg Med J. 2015;33(4):253–9.

References

1. Medford-Davis L, Park E, Shlamovitz G, Suliburk J, Meyer A, Singh H. Diagnostic errors related to acute abdominal pain in the emergency department. Emerg Med J. 2015;33(4):253–9.
2. Trowbridge R, Rutkowski N, Shojania K. Does this patient have acute cholecystitis? JAMA. 2003;289(1):80–6.
3. Videhult P, Sandblom G, Rudberg C, Rasmussen I. Are liver function tests, pancreatitis and cholecystitis predictors of common bile duct stones? Results of a prospective, population-based, cohort study of 1171 patients undergoing cholecystectomy. HPB. 2011;13(8):519–27.
4. Bourikian S, Anand R, Aboutanos M, Wolfe L, Ferrada P. Risk factors for acute gangrenous cholecystitis in emergency general surgery patients. Am J Surg. 2015;210(4):730–3.
5. Ismail O, Bhayana V. Lipase or amylase for the diagnosis of acute pancreatitis? Clin Biochem. 2017;50(18):1275–80.

6. Yang L, Liu J, Xing Y, Du L, Chen J, Liu X, et al. Comparison of BISAP, Ranson, MCTSI, and APACHE II in predicting severity and prognoses of hyperlipidemic acute pancreatitis in Chinese patients. Gastroenterol Res Pract. 2016;2016:1–7.

7. Benabbas R, Hanna M, Shah J, Sinert R. Diagnostic accuracy of history, physical examination, laboratory tests, and point-of-care ultrasound for pediatric acute appendicitis in the emergency department: a systematic review and meta-analysis. Acad Emerg Med. 2017;24(5):523–51.

8. Kwan K, Nager A. Diagnosing pediatric appendicitis: usefulness of laboratory markers. Am J Emerg Med. 2010;28(9):1009–15.

9. Mandeville K, Pottker T, Bulloch B, Liu J. Using appendicitis scores in the pediatric ED. Am J Emerg Med. 2011;29(9):972–7.

10. Bachur RG, Callahan MJ, Monuteaux MC, Rangel SJ. Integration of ultrasound findings and a clinical score in the diagnostic evaluation of pediatric appendicitis. J Pediatr. 2015;166(5):1134–9.

11. Monsalve S, Ellwanger A, Montedonico S. White blood cell count and C-reactive protein together remain useful for diagnosis and staging of acute appendicitis in children. South African Med J. 2017;107(9):773.

12. Villanueva C, Colomo A, Bosch A, Concepcion M, Hernanadez-Gea V, Aracil C, et al. Transfusion strategies for acute upper gastro-intestinal bleeding. N Engl J Med. 2013;368(1):11–21.

13. Tang Y, Shen J, Zhang F, Zhou X, Tang Z, You T. Comparison of four scoring systems used to predict mortality in patients with acute upper gastrointestinal bleeding in the emergency room. Am J Emerg Med. 2017;356:i6432.

14. Suarez-de-la-Rica A, Maseda E, Anillo V, Tamayo E, García-Bernedo C, Ramasco F, et al. Biomarkers (procalcitonin, C reactive protein, and lactate) as predictors of mortality in surgical patients with complicated intra-abdominal infection. Surg Infect. 2015;16(3):346–51.

What Imaging Strategies Are Effective for Rapid and Accurate Diagnosis of Abdominal Pain Etiologies?

4

Lindley E. Folkerson and Adeola A. Kosoko

Pearls and Pitfalls
- Specific imaging often is necessary to supplement a patient's physical exam findings to identify the cause of pain.
- Inappropriate imaging can cause a delay in appropriate interventions.
- Bedside ultrasound has become a rapid diagnostic modality that can be utilized at bedside by trained emergency providers.

Abdominal pain is a common complaint for patients who present in the emergency department (ED) [1–4]. Non-traumatic abdominal pain can be a symptom of a serious disease and should be approached in a systematic manner. Significant advances in technology and diagnostic studies in the acute care setting are now available, and it is important to have a clear understanding of which imaging modality will expedite patients' care and help establish an accurate diagnosis [4, 5].

General Imaging Approach

Though abdominal radiographs were once a mainstay for evaluation of acute abdominal pain, recently they have been displaced by computed tomography (CT) and ultrasound [6]. Several studies have shown that overall, CT imaging leads to the highest diagnostic accuracy (sensitivity 89% compared to ultrasound at 70%) [7]. However, ultrasound can also be a useful diagnostic tool in the acute care setting. In fact, a study from the *British Medical Journal* demonstrated that ultrasound followed by CT imaging in only those with negative or inconclusive ultrasound studies was an effective approach to distinguish urgent from nonurgent causes of abdominal pain. In this study, only 6% of urgent cases were missed, and there was a significant reduction in CT utilization [7].

A special population to note is the elderly patient (older than 75 years of age) presenting to the ED with acute abdominal pain. They can often be a diagnostic challenge due to multiple underlying comorbidities and atypical presentations. Many of these patients will require a CT scan to delineate the cause of their pain. While a CT scan with intravenous (IV) contrast is standard for abdominal pain, in the elderly population, the diagnostic accuracy and general management is often maintained without the use of IV contrast [8].

Focused Imaging Approach

A focused imaging approach based on the location of abdominal pain is often an effective strategy for diagnosis, reducing the need for excess CT imaging. Right upper quadrant (RUQ) pain generally derives from a hepatobiliary source, while epigastric and left upper quadrant (LUQ) most commonly are gastric, pancreatic, or associated with other etiologies. Lower abdominal pain, both on the right and left side, is associated most commonly with intestinal or genitourinary problems.

Right Upper Quadrant (RUQ) Pain

The differential diagnosis of right upper quadrant pain includes cholelithiasis, acute cholecystitis, common bile duct etiologies (e.g., dilation or choledocholithiasis), liver abnormalities (e.g., tumors, abscesses, cholestasis, hepatomegaly), and right kidney disorders. Ultrasound has emerged as the imaging modality of choice for most causes of RUQ pain and is the initial diagnostic choice to evaluate the liver as a cause of pain [9, 10].

L. E. Folkerson · A. A. Kosoko (✉)
Department of Emergency Medicine, McGovern Medical School at The University of Texas Health Science Center at Houston (UTHealth), Houston, TX, USA

© Springer Nature Switzerland AG 2019
A. Graham, D. J. Carlberg (eds.), *Gastrointestinal Emergencies*, https://doi.org/10.1007/978-3-319-98343-1_4

Gallbladder disease is one of the most common causes of RUQ pain in the United States and accounts for approximately 20 million cases per year [1, 4, 11, 12]. Ultrasound has become an indispensable tool in the ED, allowing rapid bedside evaluation [4–7, 9]. In select undifferentiated patients presenting with acute abdominal pain, CT imaging has shown good diagnostic accuracy. According to the American College of Radiology Appropriateness Criteria, US is considered the most appropriate modality for patients suspected of having acute cholecystitis [10]. It has also been shown that gallstones can be detected using bedside ultrasound with a sensitivity of 94%, a positive predictive value (PPV) of 99%, a specificity of 99%, and a negative predictive value (NPV) of 73% [4, 6, 12].

Epigastric Pain

Common differential diagnoses include gastritis, acute pancreatitis, peptic ulcer disease, atypical acute coronary syndrome, perforated peptic ulcer, and ruptured abdominal aortic aneurysm (AAA) [1, 3, 4]. The diagnosis of gastritis or peptic ulcer disease (PUD) typically does not require imaging. These maladies of the intestinal lining often are made clinically and confirmed with outpatient specialty tests. If PUD progression to perforation of the stomach or proximal intestine is suspected, an upright chest x-ray can reveal free intraperitoneal air under the diaphragm. Unfortunately, the sensitivity of upright plain abdominal radiographs alone varies, and up to 40% of free air may be overlooked [1–4, 13, 14]. Identification and localization of a perforated viscus is achieved best with computer tomography (CT) imaging [4, 14]. In severe cases of acute pancreatitis, CT imaging is recommended to evaluate for complications such as pseudocysts, abscesses, or necrosis [1, 3–5]. In patients with a suspected AAA, bedside ultrasound may assist the clinician in rapidly risk stratifying patients with epigastric pain radiating to the back or hemodynamic instability. A systematic review published in 2013 found that bedside aortic ultrasound performed by a trained EP has a sensitivity of 99% and a specificity of 98% in identifying a AAA, thus expediting a very time-sensitive diagnosis [3–5, 15].

Right Lower Quadrant (RLQ) Pain

RLQ pain has a broad differential diagnosis, including appendicitis, inflammatory bowel disease, colitis, bowel obstruction, right renal colic, and gynecological disorders. Acute appendicitis is the most common cause of RLQ pain, and in many studies, a CT scan with IV contrast has been found to be the imaging modality of choice to diagnose acute appendicitis accurately with a sensitivity of 91% and specificity of 90% [1, 4, 16]. In pediatric and pregnant patients with a presenting complaint of RLQ pain, ultrasound is the imaging modality of choice, followed by MRI if ultrasound results are equivocal to avoid radiation exposure [4, 17]. For other intestinal etiologies that cause RLQ pain, i.e., inflammatory bowel diseases, colitis, or bowel obstruction, CT imaging has been found to be the most useful [1–5, 10, 13] The physician should be concerned about an intrinsic gynecological problem as the cause of abdominal pain in a female with RLQ pain, especially in the case of a normal CT scan. Studies have shown that the use of transabdominal pelvic ultrasound to diagnose ovarian torsion has a specificity of 93% and positive predictive value of 87% [1, 4, 18].

Left Lower Quadrant (LLQ) Pain

Causes of LLQ pain in adults are similar to those that cause RLQ pain. The most common cause of LLQ pain is acute sigmoid diverticulitis [1, 4, 19]. CT imaging with IV contrast has been found to be the modality of choice to detect acute diverticulitis and its complications (abscess formation, fistula formation) with a sensitivity of 99–100% and specificity of 91–97% [4, 10, 19]. Further, the use of oral and rectal contrast has been reported to increase the accuracy of diagnosing diverticulitis to almost 100% but may lead to delayed diagnosis and long ED stays compared to IV contrast alone [20]. In patients who present with complaints of left (or right) flank pain that radiates to the groin, one should strongly consider renal colic. A study in 2001 found that a non-contrast CT scan was associated with less time in the ED with the same diagnostic accuracy as the traditional intravenous urography [21]. A con-contrast CT is the modality of choice to evaluate renal or ureteral colic, while renal ultrasound is preferred when acute pyelonephritis is suspected or in the patient with classic renal colic symptoms and a prior history of kidney stones [1, 4, 21]. For young patients with few comorbidities, classic symptoms and prior history of ureterolithiasis, ultrasound or close outpatient follow-up may be sufficient.

Left Upper Quadrant (LUQ) Pain

LUQ pain is the least specific of all abdominal pain complaints and is less likely to be associated with a diagnostic concern for classic intra-abdominal emergencies considered in other abdominal locations. Differential diagnoses for LUQ pain can include splenic injury, such as infarction or malignancy, gastric ulcer, gastritis, pyelonephritis, constipation, pancreatitis, or even diabetic ketoacidosis [1, 3–5]. For non-traumatic splenic etiologies, such as infarction or malignancy that leads to splenomegaly, a CT scan with IV contrast is the study of choice. Other more frequent causes of LUQ pain overlap with those of RUQ and epigastric pain.

Summary

In summary, non-traumatic abdominal pain is a common reason for patients to present in the ED. A systematic approach in evaluating the patient and an understanding of diagnostic imaging recommendations can lead to a timely diagnosis of intra-abdominal emergencies and allow the EP to make favorable interventions.

Suggested Resources
- Cline DM. Chap. 35: Acute abdominal pain. In: Tintinalli's emergency medicine manual. 7th ed. China: McGraw-Hill; 2012. p. 189–92.
- Donaldson R, Swartz J, Bookatz A, Khan AS, et al. Abdominal pain [internet]. 2017 [cited 2017 Sept 21]. Available from: https://wikem.org/wiki/Abdominal_pain.
- Nickson C. Abdominal Pain [internet]. 2017 [cited 2017 Sep 21]. Available from: https://lifeinthefast-lane.com/resources/abdominal-pain-ddx/.

References

1. Mattson B, Dulaimy K. The 4 quadrants: acute pathology in the abdomen and current imaging guidelines. Semin Ultrasound CT MR. 2017;38(4):414–23.
2. Hastings RS, Powers RD. Abdominal pain in the ED: a 35-year retrospective. Am J Emerg Med. 2011;29(7):711–6.
3. McNamara R, Dean AJ. Approach to acute abdominal pain. Emerg Med Clin North Am. 2011;29(2):159–73.
4. Natesan S, Lee J, Volkamer H, Thoureen T. Evidence-based medicine approach to abdominal pain. Emerg Med Clin North Am. 2016;34(2):165–90.
5. Nagurney JT, Brown DF, Chang Y, Sane S, Wang AC, Weiner JB. Use of diagnostic testing in the emergency department for patients presenting with non-traumatic abdominal pain. J Emerg Med. 2003;25(4):363–71.
6. Gans SL, Pols MA, Stoker J, Boermeester MA. Experts steering group. Guideline for the diagnostic pathway in patients with acute abdominal pain. Dig Surg. 2015;32(1):23–31.
7. Lameris W, van Randen A, van Es HW, van Heesewijk JP, van Ramshorst B, Bouma WH, et al. Imaging strategies for detection of urgent conditions in patients with acute abdominal pain: diagnostic accuracy study. BMJ. 2009;338:b2431.
8. Millet I, Sebbane M, Molinari N, Pages-Bouic E, Curros-Doyon F, Riou B, et al. Systematic unenhanced CT for acute abdominal symptoms in the elderly patients improves both emergency department diagnosis and prompt clinical management. Eur Radiol. 2017;27(2):868–77.
9. Bektas F, Eken C, Soyuncu S, Kusoglu L, Cete Y. Contribution of goal-directed ultrasonography to clinical decision-making for emergency physicians. Emerg Med J. 2009;26(3):169–72.
10. Stoker J, van Randen A, Lameris W, Boermeester MA. Imaging patients with acute abdominal pain. Radiology. 2009;253(1): 31–46.
11. Summers SM, Scruggs W, Menchine MD, Lahham S, Anderson C, Amr O, et al. A prospective evaluation of emergency department bedside ultrasonography for the detection of acute cholecystitis. Ann Emerg Med. 2010;56(2):114–22.
12. Kendall JL, Shimp RJ. Performance and interpretation of focused right upper quadrant ultrasound by emergency physicians. J Emerg Med. 2001;21(7):7–13.
13. Taylor MR, Lalani N. Adult small bowel obstruction. Acad Emerg Med. 2013;20(6):528–44.
14. Smith JE, Hall EJ. The use of plain abdominal x-rays in the emergency department. Emerg Med J. 2009;26(3):160–3.
15. Rubano E, Mehta N, Caputo W, Paladino L, Sinert R. Systematic review: emergency department bedside ultrasonography for diagnosing a suspected abdominal aortic aneurysm. Acad Emerg Med. 2013;20(2):128–38.
16. Rao PM, Rhea JT, Novelline RA, Mostafavi AA, McCabe CJ. Effect of computed tomography of the appendix on treatment of patients and use of hospital resources. N Engl J Med. 1998;338(3): 141–6.
17. Tremblay E, Therasse E, Thomassin-Naggara I, Trop I. Quality initiatives: guidelines for use of medical imaging during pregnancy and lactation. Radiographics. 2012;32(3):897–911.
18. Graif M, Itzchak Y. Sonographic evaluation of ovarian torsion in childhood and adolescence. AJR Am J Roentgenol. 1988;150(3):647–9.
19. Destigter KK, Keating DP. Imaging update: acute colonic diverticulitis. Clin Colon Rectal Surg. 2009;22(3):147–55.
20. Anderson SW, Soto JA. Multi-detector row CT of acute non-traumatic abdominal pain: contrast and protocol considerations. Radiol Clin N Am. 2012;50(1):137–47.
21. Rekant EM, Gibert CL, Counselman FL. Emergency department time for evaluation of patient discharged with a diagnosis of renal colic: unenhanced helical computed tomography versus intravenous urography. J Emerg Med. 2001;21(4):371–4.

Evaluation of Acute Abdominal Pain with Computed Tomography

Zachary Repanshek and Evan Kingsley

Pearls and Pitfalls
- Contrast reactions occur infrequently, and serious, life-threatening reactions are extremely rare.
- Evidence has challenged the clinical relevance of contrast-induced nephropathy.
- The risks and benefits of contrast should be considered when choosing whether to utilize a contrast-enhanced CT.
- Oral contrast should not routinely be used in abdominal computed tomography.

In 2014, approximately 6% of all patients presenting to United States emergency departments had computed tomography (CT) of their abdomen and pelvis. Abdominal pain was the most common presenting complaint, making up nearly 8% of all visits [1]. History, physical, and laboratory evaluation are often not enough to rule out or diagnose a dangerous etiology of abdominal pain. Therefore, patients presenting with focal abdominal pain or concern for a surgical cause of pain must be considered for imaging.

General Considerations

CT is the imaging test of choice for most acute abdominal pain (with exception of abdominal aortic aneurysm, acute cholecystitis, or gonadal pathology, in which ultrasound is first

Z. Repanshek (✉)
Lewis Katz School of Medicine, Temple University Hospital, Philadelphia, PA, USA
e-mail: Zachary.repanshek2@tuhs.temple.edu

E. Kingsley
Department of Emergency Medicine, Temple University Hospital, Philadelphia, PA, USA
e-mail: Evan.Kingsley@tuhs.temple.edu

line). It has a high sensitivity and specificity for many serious causes of abdominal pain including appendicitis, obstruction, perforation, diverticulitis, and bowel ischemia. However, the use of CT must be weighed against risk of radiation exposure especially in younger patients [2, 3]. Clinicians must also weigh benefits and drawbacks of contrast-enhanced CT.

Intravenous (IV) contrast is beneficial for its opacification of vascular structures and solid abdominal and pelvic organs. IV contrast in abdominal imaging is recommended for nearly all indications, with the notable exception of renal colic evaluation [4–7]. There are two primary barriers to patients receiving IV contrast in the emergency department: concern for an allergic-type contrast reaction and contrast-induced nephropathy. The decision to utilize IV contrast requires a risk-benefit analysis by the ordering physician, which requires a reasonable understanding of the risks of each of these entities.

Allergic-Type Contrast Reactions

Contrast reactions are not IgE mediated and therefore not true allergic reactions. The significance is that a patient may have a contrast reaction on their first exposure to iodinated contrast, as no sensitization is required. Likewise, a patient who has had a previous contract reaction may not have subsequent reactions. While it is recognized that a previous contrast reaction is a risk factor for future reactions, this rate of recurrence may be lower than expected. One study found in patients with a reported history of contrast reaction, only 7.4% had another adverse reaction when given IV contrast. Very few (0.02%) of these reactions were anaphylactoid and none were fatal [8].

Physicians may overestimate the incidence of contrast reactions. Historical studies which were performed using high-osmolar contrast agents, as compared to the low- and iso-osmolar agents used in current practice, may overinflate the suspected risk of reactions. Studies using these modern contrast agents have shown overall reaction rates of 0.6–1.5%, with very few (0.03–0.05%) of these being anaphylactoid or life-threatening [8–11]. Another study of the incidence of allergic-like contrast reactions specifically in the emergency department found an overall adverse reaction rate of 0.2% with no serious reactions [11].

Shellfish and "Iodine" Allergies

It is worth addressing a long-standing myth that someone with a reported shellfish allergy is unable to receive IV contrast. Allergies to shellfish do not increase the risk of contrast reaction over any other allergy. There is also the concern of patients reporting an "iodine allergy." Iodine is not an allergen, as it is found intrinsically in the human body as well as in table salt [7, 12].

Contrast-Induced Nephropathy

Contrast-induced nephropathy is typically defined as signs of acute kidney injury (AKI) within 48 h of contrast administration and has been called the third most common cause of in-hospital AKI [13, 14]. More recent evidence has shown a lack of association between contrast use and AKI [15–19]. While not definitive, the discrepancy between previous and current evidence may be that in instances where contrast was attributed causation for AKI, other coexisting factors, such as underlying illness, nephrotoxic drugs, and hypovolemia, may have contributed. Recent studies have likely been more regimented about controlling for these cofounders.

American College of Radiology (ACR) guidelines state that assessment of renal function prior to contrast use may be warranted in patients who are of age greater than 60, have history of renal disease, have history of hypertension requiring treatment, have history of diabetes mellitus, or are currently using metformin. For all other patients, a baseline serum creatinine measurement is not required prior to contrast administration. For patients who do have an assessment of renal function, the ACR recommends a threshold of eGFR <30 for risk of nephropathy [7].

Value of Oral Contrast

Oral contrast has not been shown to significantly improve the accuracy of CT in diagnosing the vast majority of acute abdominopelvic abnormalities in the emergency department [20]. Studies of emergency departments after the elimination of the routine use of oral contrast showed decrease in wait times, an average of 97 min in one study, without an increase in bouncebacks or missed findings [21, 22]. With the exception of inflammatory bowel disease and patients post-gastric bypass, the ACR does not strongly recommend the use of oral contrast in any of the indications for acute abdominal imaging [5, 6, 20]. There have been many studies that do not show a benefit in the use of oral contrast in the evaluation of appendicitis [23–26], and the ACR recommends against the use of oral contrast when evaluating for bowel obstruction [6, 7]. Oral contrast should not routinely be used in the CT evaluation of abdominal pain in the emergency department.

Suggested Resource

- ACR Manual on Contrast Media. https://www.acr.org/~/media/ACR/Documents/PDF/QualitySafety/Resources/Contrast-Manual/Contrast_Media.pdf.

References

1. National Hospital Ambulatory Medical Care Survey: 2014 Emergency Department. Atlanta, GA: U.S. Department of Health and Human Services, Centers for Disease Control and Prevention, National Center for Health Statistics; 2017. Available at: https://www.cdc.gov/nchs/data/nhamcs/web_tables/2014_ed_web_tables.pdf.
2. Gans S, Pols M, Stoker J, Boermeester M. Guideline for the diagnostic pathway in patients with acute abdominal pain. Dig Surg. 2015;32:23–31.
3. Stoker J, Randen A, Lameris W, Boermeester M. Imaging patients with acute abdominal pain. Radiology. 2009;253(1):31–46.
4. Rawson JV, Pelletier AL. When to order a contrast-enhanced CT. Am Fam Physician. 2013;88(5):312–6.
5. Broder JS, Hamedani AG, Liu SW, Emerman CL. Emergency department contrast practices for abdominal/pelvic computed tomography-a national survey and comparison with the American college of radiology appropriateness criteria(®). J Emerg Med. 2013;44(2):423–33.
6. ACR Appropriateness Criteria. Reston, VA: American College of Radiology; 2017. Available at: https://www.acr.org/Quality-Safety/Appropriateness-Criteria.
7. American College of Radiology. ACR manual on contrast media. Version 10.3. Reston, VA: American College of Radiology; 2017.
8. Kopp AF, Mortele KJ, Cho YD, Palkowitsch P, Bettmann MA, Claussen CD. Prevalence of acute reactions to iopromide: postmarketing surveillance study of 74,717 patients. Acta Radiol. 2008;49(8):902–11.
9. Häussler MD. Safety and patient comfort with iodixanol: a postmarketing surveillance study in 9515 patients undergoing diagnostic CT examinations. Acta Radiol. 2010;51(8):924–33.
10. Wang CL, Cohan RH, Ellis JH, Caoili EM, Wang G, Francis IR. Frequency, outcome, and appropriateness of treatment of nonionic iodinated contrast media reactions. AJR Am J Roentgenol. 2008 Aug;191(2):409–15.
11. Gottumukkala RV, Glover M 4th, Yun BJ, Sonis JD, Kalra MK, Otrakji A, Raja AS, Prabhakar AM. Allergic-like contrast reactions in the ED: incidence, management,and impact on patient disposition. Am J Emerg Med. 2017;36(5):825–8.
12. Schabelman E, Witting M. The relationship of radiocontrast, iodine, and seafood allergies: a medical myth exposed. J Emerg Med. 2010;39(5):701–7.
13. Tublin ME, Murphy ME, Tessler FN. Current concepts in contrast media-induced nephropathy. AJR. 1998;171:933–9.

14. Wichmann JL, Katzberg RW, Litwin SE, Zwerner PL, De Cecco CN, Vogl TJ, Costello P, Schoepf UJ. Contrast-induced nephropathy. Circulation. 2015;132(20):1931–6.

15. McDonald JS, McDonald RJ, Comin J, et al. Frequency of acute kidney injury following intravenous contrast medium administration: a systematic review and meta-analysis. Radiology. 2013;267(1):119–28.

16. Davenport MS, Khalatbari S, Cohan RH, Dillman JR, Myles JD, Ellis JH. Contrast material-induced nephrotoxicity and intravenous low-osmolality iodinated contrast material: risk stratification by using estimated glomerular filtration rate. Radiology. 2013;268(3): 719–28.

17. McDonald JS, McDonald RJ, Carter RE, Katzberg RW, Kallmes DF, Williamson EE. Risk of intravenous contrast material-mediated acute kidney injury: a propensity score-matched study stratified by baseline-estimated glomerular filtration rate. Radiology. 2014;271(1):65–73.

18. Hinson JS, Ehmann MR, Fine DM, Fishman EK, Toerper MF, Rothman RE, Klein EY. Risk of acute kidney injury after intravenous contrast media administration. Ann Emerg Med. 2017;69(5):577–586.e4.

19. Aycock RD, Westafer LM, Boxen JL, Majlesi N, Schoenfeld EM, Bannuru RR. Acute kidney injury after computed tomography: a meta-analysis. Ann Emerg Med. 2017;71(1):44–53.e4.

20. Kielar AZ, Patlas MN, Katz DS. Oral contrast for CT in patients with acute non-traumatic abdominal and pelvic pain: what should be its current role? Emerg Radiol. 2016;23(5):477–81.

21. Razavi SA, Johnson JO, Kassin MT, Applegate KE. The impact of introducing a no oral contrast abdominopelvic CT examination (NOCAPE) pathway on radiology turn around times, emergency department length of stay, and patient safety. Emerg Radiol. 2014;21(6):605–13.

22. Levenson RB, Camacho MA, Horn E, Saghir A, McGillicuddy D, Sanchez LD. Eliminating routine oral contrast use for CT in the emergency department: impact on patient throughput and diagnosis. Emerg Radiol. 2012;19(6):513–7.

23. Anderson BA, Salem L, Flum DR. A systematic review of whether oral contrast is necessary for the computed tomography diagnosis of appendicitis in adults. Am J Surg. 2005;190(3):474–8.

24. Drake FT, Alfonso R, Bhargava P, Cuevas C, Dighe MK, Florence MG, Johnson MG, Jurkovich GJ, Steele SR, Symons RG, Thirlby RC, Flum DR, Writing Group for SCOAP-CERTAIN. Enteral contrast in the computed tomography diagnosis of appendicitis: comparative effectiveness in a prospective surgical cohort. Ann Surg. 2014;260(2):311–6.

25. Kepner AM, Bacasnot JV, Stahlman BA. Intravenous contrast alone vs intravenous and oral contrast computed tomography for the diagnosis of appendicitis in adult ED patients. Am J Emerg Med. 2012;30(9):1765–73.

26. Lakuri CA, Fraser JD, Aguayo P, Fike FB, Garey CL, Sharp SW, Ostlie DJ, St Peter SD. The lack of efficacy for oral contrast in the diagnosis of appendicitis by computed tomography. J Surg Res. 2011;170(1):100–3.

What Is My Patient's Risk of Cancer from Radiation Exposure with Computed Tomography of the Abdomen and Pelvis? What Do I Tell My Patient?

Angelina Vishnyakova and Charles Maddow

Pearls and Pitfalls

- Computed tomography exposes patients to ionizing radiation and can potentially result in an increased risk of developing cancers.
- Individual risks of radiation-induced cancer are low, but these small risks in the setting of exponentially increasing use of CT studies in a large population can translate into a substantial increase in the number of cancers with a considerable public health impact.
- The risk of radiation-induced cancer in the pediatric population is even higher than adults since pediatric patients are more sensitive to radiation, have a longer remaining life expectancy, and thus have more time for cancer to develop.
- It is important to consider various strategies to help reduce the number of radiation-induced cancers, such as (1) decreasing the number of unnecessarily performed CT studies and replace them with other diagnostic imaging options when practical and (2) using CT protocol based on patient size to prevent over exposure to unnecessarily high doses of radiation.

Since the invention and technological advancements of computed tomography (CT), CT has allowed physicians to noninvasively visualize the inside of the human body and help guide diagnosis and treatment of disease. Because of its speed, ease of access, and image quality, CT use has increased

A. Vishnyakova · C. Maddow (✉)
McGovern Medical School at the University of Texas Health Science Center at Houston, Department of Emergency Medicine, Houston, TX, USA
e-mail: Angelina.Vishnyakova@uth.tmc.edu;
Charles.Maddow@uth.tmc.edu

exponentially. From 1980 to 2005, the US population grew by approximately 50%, while the number of CT scans performed sky rocketed from 3 million to an estimated 60 million tests performed, resulting in a 600% increase in medical radiation exposure to the US population [1]. This may translate into an increased risk of cancer associated with exposure to ionizing radiation.

Sieverts vs Grays

It is important to understand the various terms that describe CT radiation dose delivery to the body. Absorbed dose is the radiation absorbed per unit mass and is measured in grays (Gy) or milligrays (mGy). One gray is equal to "1 joule of radiation energy absorbed per kilogram" [2]. Since not all radiation produces equal effects in humans, the absorbed dose is multiplied by a radiation weighting factor to give the dose equivalent. This measurement is expressed in sieverts (Sv) or millisieverts (mSv) and is used to compare the amount of energy absorbed from different types of radiation. For example, x-rays or gamma-rays have a weighting factor of 1.0. Therefore one gray equals 1 sievert [3]. As radiation is not uniformly absorbed and different radiographic studies expose different areas of the body to varying amounts of radiation, the concept of effective dose was created to allow "for a rough comparison between different CT scenarios" [2]. Thus, effective dose, expressed in sieverts, is "designed to be proportional to a generic estimate of the overall harm to the patient caused by radiation" for a standardized patient [2].

Radiation from CT Exposure

Abdominopelvic CT exposes patients to approximately 10–20 mSv depending on the type of study, institutional protocols, and use of contrast (e.g., traditional study ~10–15 mSv, dissection protocol ~24 mSv, multiphase ~30 mSv) [4]. CT exposes patients to significantly larger radiation doses than conventional "plain film" x-rays. For example, an abdominal radiograph results in a dose of about 0.25 mSV, which is over 50 times less than the corresponding dose from abdominal CT radiation exposure [5], and an abdominopelvic CT scan is approximately equal to that of 100–250 chest x-rays depending on patient size, sex, and scanner calibration [2, 5].

Lifetime Attributable Risk (LAR)

The Biological Effects of Ionizing Radiation (BEIR) report is a landmark study providing the most widely accepted models evaluating radiation exposure and the resultant cancer risk. Using the epidemiological data of survivors of the atomic bombings of Japan in 1945 alongside an unexposed cohort, the lifetime attributable risk to various doses of ionizing radiation can be calculated. The lifetime attributable risk is the additional risk of cancer above baseline cancer risk. In the United States, approximately 38% of the population will be diagnosed with cancer during their lifetime. According to the BEIR VII report, one resultant radiation-induced cancer with a 50% mortality rate will occur per 1000 patients exposed to a 10-mSv effective dose, such as one abdominopelvic CT scan [6, 7].

Smith-Bindman et al. [4] expanded on these risk models established by the BEIR report in order to calculate the LAR of various types of abdominopelvic CT scans. Across four sites in the San Francisco Bay area, the study calculated the effective dose (mSv) for four different types of abdominopelvic CT: no contrast, with contrast, multiphase scan, and aneurysm/dissection protocoled scans. The results demonstrated a huge variability in effective radiation doses received by patients, with median values ranging from 15 mSv without contrast to 31 mSv in multiphase scans. Combining the median radiation exposure with the applied effective doses, the estimated number of patients undergoing a routine abdominopelvic CT with contrast differs by age and sex: 470 CTs for a 20-year-old female, 620 CTs for a 20-year-old male, 930 CTs for a 40-year-old female, 1002 CTs for a 40-year-old male, and ~1360 CTs for 60-year-old patients. In a clinical context, a 20-year-old female receiving a multiphase scan is exposed to an effective dose of about 31 mSv. This corresponds to a LAR of four cancers per 1000 patients. In other words, there is a 0.004% increased risk of developing a radiation-induced cancer above the baseline risk for this particular patient.

From a population health perspective, Berrington de González et al. [8] also used these risk models from the BEIR report and combined them with estimates of CT scan frequencies in the United States to project radiation-induced cancer risk. They estimated that about 57 million scans were performed in 2007 in the United States (excluding scans associated with preexisting cancer and scans performed in the last 5 years of life). Using the LAR of radiation-induced cancer and mortality rates determined by the BEIR report,

they estimated that 29,000 future cancers and 14,500 cancer-related deaths could occur from exposure to CT in 2007. Based on these projections, it could be expected that 2% of the 1.4 million annually diagnosed cancers in the United States could be related to CT radiation exposures.

Risk of Radiation-Induced Cancer in the Pediatric Population

The risk of radiation-induced cancer in the pediatric population is even higher than adults since pediatric patients are more sensitive to radiation and have a longer life expectancy. Miglioretti et al. [9] estimated that as a result of 4 million pediatric CT scans performed annually in the United States, it is projected that 4870 future radiation-induced cancers will arise. This retrospective study evaluated pediatric scanning practices of six health care systems and calculated ranges of effective doses from a variety of scanners. These results were applied to the estimated 4 million pediatric CT scans performed nationally to obtain lifetime attributable cancer risks in the pediatric population. They found that cancer risks were highest in the abdominopelvic studies and projected 1 radiation-induced cancer from every 300–390 abdominopelvic scans in females and 670–760 abdominopelvic scans in males. When comparing these values to the previously mentioned study by Smith-Bindman [4] on the lifetime attributable risk of abdominopelvic CT with contrast, one can see that pediatric risk of radiation-induced cancer, particularly in females, is generally higher than in the adult population.

Applying the Data to Individual Patients

It is important to remember that even though the data reported by BEIR and other studies can be used to estimate the risk of cancer mortality, there is an uncertainty factor of two to three for a standard adult patient. That is, these approximations can either be two to three times higher or lower than estimated given that each patient drastically differs from another when considering age, size, and gender [3]. Thus, effective dose can be convenient in evaluating health risks of a variety of radiologic studies performed on a standard patient, but it is not especially applicable in determining the excess relative risk in the individual patient.

One way to help patients place these risks in perspective is by comparing CT effective doses with natural or societal effective doses (Table 6.1) [3, 5]. For example, the general population will be exposed to a baseline natural radiation effective dose of about three to four mSv per year compared to an effective dose of 10 mSv from an abdominopelvic CT [3, 5]. Another proposed method is to compare the additional risk of death from cancer associated with CT radiation exposure

Table 6.1 Average low-dose radiation exposures

Exposure	Radiation dose (mSv)
Adult abdominal computed tomography	10
Flight – New York to London, round-trip	0.1
Background natural radiation exposure	3–4 per year
Radiation worker exposure limit	20 per year
International space station exposure	170 per year

Refs. [3, 5]
Adapted from Brenner et al. [5]. Ref. [3]. With permission from the National Academy of Sciences. Copyright (2003) National Academy of Sciences, U.S.A.
Legend: *mSv* = millisieverts

with the risk of death associated with common activities that are largely considered acceptable [3]. For instance, there is a minimal risk of death (4×10^{-6}) when flying approximately 7200 km (4500 mi) compared to a very low risk of death (1×10^{-4}) for a CT scan of the abdomen and pelvis [3]. In the end, it is important for the physician to convey that despite the small increased risk of radiation-induced cancer, the benefits of a medically necessary CT scan far outweigh the risks since it can provide significant diagnostic value.

What Do I Tell My Patient?

How much do emergency medicine physicians know about radiation doses/risk and what do they tell their patients? Lee et al. [10] recently conducted a survey of 45 emergency medicine physicians in a US academic medical center to determine awareness of radiation dose of abdominopelvic CT scans, lifetime cancer risk from exposure, and if this information was outlined to their patients. They found that in this particular group, 73% of ED physicians underestimated radiation doses, 91% believed there to be no lifetime increased risk of cancer, and only 22% of these physicians outlined the risks and benefits of the CT scan to the patient. A similar study performed by Puri et al. [1] found that only approximately 18% of emergency medicine providers surveyed had accurate knowledge of lifetime attributable cancer risk associated with abdominopelvic CT scans. This demonstrates how important it is that emergency medicine providers are educated about diagnostic imaging radiation doses and lifetime cancer risks in order to be able to have informative discussions with patients about associated risks and benefits.

Summary

Individual risks of radiation-induced cancer are very low, but these small risks in the setting of exponentially increasing use of CT studies in a large population can translate into a substantial increase in the number of cancers and a considerable public health issue in the future. Therefore, it is important to consider various strategies to help reduce the number of radiation-induced cancer such as (1) decreasing the number of unnecessarily performed CT studies and replace them with other diagnostic imaging options when practical and (2) using CT protocols based on patient size to prevent overexposure to unnecessarily high doses of radiation.

References

1. Puri S, Hu R, Quazi RR, Voci S, Veazie P, Block R. Physicians' and midlevel providers' awareness of lifetime radiation–attributable Cancer risk associated with commonly performed CT studies: relationship to practice behavior. Am J Roentgenol. 2012;199:1328–36.
2. Brenner DJ, Hall EJ. Computed tomography — an increasing source of radiation exposure. N Engl J Med. 2007;357:2277–84.
3. Verdun FR, Bochud F, Gundinchet F, Aroua A, Schnyder P, Meuli R. Quality initiatives radiation risk: what you should know to tell your patient. Radiographics. 2008;28:1807–16.
4. Smith-Bindman R, Lipson J, Marcus R, Kim K, Mahesh M, Gould R, et al. Radiation dose associated with common computed tomography examinations and the associated lifetime attributable risk of cancer. Arch Intern Med. 2009;169:2078–86.
5. Brenner DJ, Doll R, Goodhead DT, Hall EJ, Land CE, Little JB, et al. Cancer risks attributable to low doses of ionizing radiation: assessing what we really know. Proc Natl Acad Sci. 2003;100:13761–6.
6. Committee to Assess Health Risks from Exposure to Low Levels of Ionizing Radiation; Board on Radiation Effects Research; Division on Earth and Life Studies; National Research Council. Health risks from exposure to low levels of ionizing radiation: BEIR VII Phase 2. Washington, D.C.: National Academies Press; 2006.
7. Griffey RT, Sodickson A. Cumulative radiation exposure and cancer risk estimates in emergency department patients undergoing repeat or multiple CT. Am J Roentgenol. 2009;192:887–92.
8. Gonzalez ABD, Mahesh M, Kim K-P. Projected cancer risks from computed tomographic scans performed in the United States in 2007. Arch Intern Med. 2010;169:2071–7.
9. Miglioretti DL, Johnson E, Williams A, Greenlee RT, Weinmann S, Solberg LI, et al. The use of computed tomography in pediatrics and the associated radiation exposure and estimated Cancer risk. JAMA Pediatr. 2013;167:700–7.
10. Lee CI, Haims AH, Monico EP, Brink JA, Forman HP. Diagnostic CT scans: assessment of patient, physician, and radiologist awareness of radiation dose and possible risks. Radiology. 2004;231:393–8.

Who Should Be Admitted? Who Can Be Discharged? What Should Be Included in the Discharge Planning?

Basil Z. Khalaf and Kimberly A. Chambers

Pearls and Pitfalls
- Patients who need an in-hospital intervention, such as surgery or resuscitation, or who are at high risk for decompensation should admitted or placed in observation.
- For some disease processes, such as pancreatitis, the etiology and the patient's severity of illness will determine whether a patient can be safely managed as an outpatient.

Abdominal pain accounts for approximately 7 million emergency department visits annually [1]. Despite advances in abdominal imaging and diagnostic testing, many patients are discharged with a diagnosis of undifferentiated abdominal pain. In one retrospective study of 1000 consecutive patients presenting with non-traumatic abdominal pain, 21% were diagnosed with undifferentiated abdominal pain [2].

Disposition for patients with abdominal pain can be a high-risk decision. For some diagnoses, scoring systems and clinical guidelines provide guidance by assessing a patient's illness severity and predicting prognosis [3–7]. These can guide clinicians toward admission or discharge. For those who are stable for outpatient management, discharge instructions should contain disease-specific return precautions when possible (Table 7.1).

Safe discharge planning includes several components.

- A repeat abdominal examination that is improving and reassuring or addresses any abnormal findings should be documented.
- An oral intake (PO) challenge can help clinicians increase the likelihood that discharged patients will be able to stay hydrated at home.
- Follow-up is critical and specific instructions, including with whom and in what time frame should be included in the discharge instructions. For undifferentiated abdominal pain in patients without established medical care, it may be reasonable to ask patients to return to the emergency department in 24–48 h for repeat evaluation.
- At time of discharge, vital signs, laboratory values, and imaging results should be reviewed for discrepancies and any issues addressed in the documentation.

High-risk patients include those at extremes of age, immunocompromised patients, and those with significant comorbidities, such as liver cirrhosis. Neonates are generally excluded from conservative management protocols [8]. Geriatric patients have a higher mortality rate compared to younger adults. For example, the overall incidence of appendicitis is lower in elderly patients, but their mortality is 4–8 times higher, accounting for up to half of all deaths from appendicitis [9]. A study of adult ED patients who returned within 72 h of discharge and were admitted to the ICU found that abdominal pain patients with a malignancy or cirrhosis had the highest mortality [10].

B. Z. Khalaf · K. A. Chambers (✉)
Department of Emergency Medicine, McGovern Medical School at The University of Texas Health Science Center at Houston (UTHealth), Houston, TX, USA
e-mail: Basil.Z.Khalaf@uth.tmc.edu;
Kimberly.A.Chambers@uth.tmc.edu

© Springer Nature Switzerland AG 2019
A. Graham, D. J. Carlberg (eds.), *Gastrointestinal Emergencies*, https://doi.org/10.1007/978-3-319-98343-1_7

Table 7.1 Patients who may be safely discharged

Diagnosis	Scoring system/criteria necessary for safe discharge	Discharge pearls

Abdominal pain of unknown etiology	For discharge, the patient must
	  Have no signs or symptoms consistent with sepsis or shock (Table 7.2)
	  Tolerate oral intake
	  Have a negative diagnostic work-up, including imaging or consultation if patient's signs and symptoms were suggestive of surgical disease; a single symptom or physical exam finding often lacks adequate sensitivity and specificity to predict surgical disease [11], and clinical decision tools may not be superior to clinical judgment [12]
		Advise patients to return if:
		  Abdominal pain does not resolve within 24 h
		  Abdominal pain migrates to the right lower quadrant
		  They develop a fever >100.4
		  They develop weakness, nausea and vomiting, jaundice, dizziness, or fainting
		  They develop blood in their stool or urine or cannot urinate

Cholelithiasis	To consider discharge, the patient must have:
	  No signs of acute cholecystitis
	  Normal vital signs
	  Normal labs, including lipase
	  A common bile duct that is not dilated
	  Ability to tolerate oral intake
		Advise patients to:
		  Eat a low-fat diet
		  Return to the ED if they develop pain in RUQ lasting longer than 2 h, have abdominal pain for more than 5 h, develop fevers or chills, persistent nausea and vomiting, jaundice, dark urine, or light colored stools
		  Follow up with general surgery for elective cholecystectomy

Peptic ulcer disease	When discharged, the patient should not have:
	  Bleeding
	  Perforation
	  Obstruction
		Advise patients to:
		  Refrain from nonsteroidal anti-inflammatory use
		  Test for and, if present, treated for *Helicobacter pylori*
		  Consider acid suppression therapy
		  Return to the ED if they develop a recurrence or worsening of pain, fever, or evidence of GI bleeding
		  Follow-up with a primary doctor or GI specialist for further assessment and prescription of maintenance therapy with a proton pump inhibit or histamine 2-receptor blocker to prevent ulcer relapse

Uncomplicated diverticulitis (Absence of sepsis, peritonitis, fistula, or obstruction)	CT confirmed, uncomplicated diverticulitis
	Mild to moderate signs and symptoms
	No associated abdominal distention
	No vomiting, able to tolerate fluids and take medications
	Able to control pain with oral medications
	Able to follow up with physician in 2–3 days
	Able to care for self at home
		Advise patients to return if:
		  Abdominal pain does not resolve or worsens despite therapy
		  Fever >100.4 develops
		  They develop blood in their stool, vomiting or signs of obstruction, dizziness, or weakness

GI bleeding	*The Glasgow-Blatchford Bleeding Score (4)* is a well-validated scoring system to identify patients who are likely to need a transfusion or intervention. It incorporates lab values (hemoglobin, BUN), gender, physiologic response to bleeding (heart rate, systolic blood pressure, recent syncope), and the presence of hepatic disease and melena. Patients with scores <1 can likely be safely discharged
	The *AIMS65 Score (5)* is a simpler system that was derived from a large patient population. The score ranges from 0 to 5 based on five criteria formulated as yes/no questions, where every yes answer is worth 1 point
	  Factors included in the score are albumin <3 g/dL, INR > 1.5, alteration in mental status, SBP $\leq$ 90 mm Hg, age $\geq$ 65
	  A score of 0 has an in-hospital mortality risk of 0.3%; a score of 5 has an in-hospital mortality of ~25%
		Advise patients to:
		  Discontinue agents (such as nonsteroidal anti-inflammatories) that will contribute to ulceration or bleeding
		  Return for syncope, shortness of breath, dizziness, generalized weakness, palpitations, chest pain, increased or continued bleeding, vomiting blood, or abdominal pain

Table 7.1 (continued)

Diagnosis	Scoring system/criteria necessary for safe discharge	Discharge pearls
Pancreatitis	Harmless acute pancreatitis score (HAPS) was developed to identify low-risk patients who are unlikely to have a severe clinical course. Non-severe course is predicted by the presence of three clinical parameters: no rebound or guarding on physical examination, normal creatinine, and normal hematocrit (6) The *American College of Gastroenterology* provides additional risk factors for a severe course, including obesity (body mass index >30 kg/m²), elevated creatinine, and additional lab and imaging findings. Cholecystectomy is recommended during the index visit for patients with gallstone pancreatitis since ~18% will have a second event within 90 days (7)	Advise patients: Abdominal pain should improve within the next 72 h They need to remain well hydrated They should return if they develop new or worsening symptoms; if they have persistent pain, weakness, and nausea and vomiting despite taking medications; if their skin becomes jaundiced; and if they start feeling faint or dizzy and develop a blood glucose level greater than 300 or a fever of greater than 100.4
Pediatric gastroenteritis	To be considered for conservative ED therapy and discharge, the patient must: Not be severely dehydrated Not be a neonate Be tolerating oral intake	Advise parents to return if the child develops: Fever, abdominal pain, or intractable or bilious vomiting

Table 7.2 The systemic inflammatory response syndrome (SIRS)

Temperature > 38° C or < 36° C
Heart rate > 90 beats/minute
Respiratory rate > 20 breaths/minute or $PaCO_2$ < 32 torr
WBC count >12,000 cells/mm³, <4000 cells/mm³, or > 10% immature (bands) forms

Suggested Resources

- American College of Gastroenterology – Clinical Guidelines. http://gi.org/clinical-guidelines/.
- https://sinaiem.org/safe-discharge-for-undifferentiated-abdominal-pain/.

References

1. Bhuiya F, Pitts SR, LF MC. Emergency department visits for chest pain and abdominal pain: United States, 1999–2008. NCHS data brief, no 43. Hyattsville: National Center for Health Statistics; 2010.
2. Hastings R, Powers R. Abdominal pain in the ED: a 35 year retrospective. Am J Emerg Med. 2011;29:711–6.
3. Satoh K, Yoshino J, Akamatsu T, et al. Evidence-based clinical practice guidelines for peptic ulcer disease 2015. J Gastroenterol. 2016;51(3):177–94.
4. Blatchford O, Murray WR, Blatchford M. A risk score to predict need for treatment for upper-gastrointestinal hemorrhage. Lancet. 2000;356(9238):1318–21.
5. Satlzman RJ, Tabak YP, Hyett BH, Sun X, Travis AC, Johannes RS. A simple risk score accurately predicts in-hospital mortality, length of stay, and cost in acute upper GI bleeding. Gastrointest Endosc. 2011;74(6):1215–24.
6. Oskarsson V, Mehrabi M, Orsini N, Hammarqvist F, Segersvard R, Andren-Sandberg A, et al. Validation of the harmless acute pancreatitis score in predicting nonsevere course of acute pancreatitis. Pancreatology. 2011;11(5):464–8.
7. Tenner S, Baillie J, DeWitt J, Vege SS. Management of acute pancreatitis. Am J Gastroenterol. 2013;108:1400–15.
8. Bahm A, Freedman SB, Guan J, Guttman A. Evaluating the impact of clinical decision tools in pediatric acute gastroenteritis: a population-based cohort study. Acad Emerg Med. 2016;23(5):599–609.
9. Spangler R, Pham TV, Khoujah D, Martinez JP. Abdominal emergencies in the geriatric pateint. Int J of Emerg Med. 2014;7:43.
10. Tsai IT, Sun CK, Chang CS, Lee KH, Liang CY, Hsu CW. Characteristics and outcomes of patients with emergency department revisits within 72 hours and subsequent admission to the intensive care unit. Tzu Chi Medical Journal. 2016;28(4):151–6.
11. Macaluso CR, McNamara RM. Evaluation and management of acute abdominal pain in the emergency department. Int J Gen Med. 2012;5:789–97.
12. Lui JL, Wyatt JC, Deeks JJ, Clamp S, Keen J, Verde P, et al. Systematic reviews of clinical decision tools for acute abdominal pain. Health Technol Assess. 2006;10(47):1–167.

Consultant Corner: General Approach to Abdominal Pain

Hani Zamil

Pearls and pitfalls in the evaluation of acute abdominal pain

- Abdominal pain should undergo prompt evaluation with the goal of diagnosing the underlying cause of pain. When the cause is not clear and the patient has concerning signs or symptoms, the patient should be observed closely, and a consultation with a gastroenterologist should be sought.
- Proper diagnosis of abdominal pain requires familiarity of the abdominal pain syndromes and various clinical presentations.
- Certain "special populations" like immunocompromised, elderly, and pregnant patients can have unusual presentations of abdominal pain.
- A high index of suspension is needed for diagnosis of vascular causes of abdominal pain.

Introduction

Hani Zamil, MD, CMQ, is an Assistant Professor of Medicine and Gastroenterology at the McGovern Medical School, UT Health. Dr. Zamil is the Director of the Gastrointestinal Physiology and Motility lab at Memorial Hermann – Texas Medical Center and the Medical Quality Officer for the division of gastroenterology. Dr. Zamil is trained in advanced endoscopy, GI motility, and celiac disease and sees a variety of conditions in a major tertiary referral center as well as a busy general county hospital.

H. Zamil
McGovern Medical School, UT Health, Houston, TX, USA
e-mail: Hani.A.Zamil@uth.tmc.edu

Answers to Key Clinical Questions

When do you recommend consultation with a gastroenterologist for acute abdominal pain and in what time frame?

Abdominal pain due to bowel perforation or ischemic bowel can have devastating outcomes without a prompt, early diagnosis. Therefore, a gastroenterologist and/or a general surgeon should be consulted within 6 h from onset of pain. Additionally, patients with no clear etiology of their symptoms and a concerning exam (even when testing has been negative) should have consultation with a gastroenterologist or surgeon. The patient should be evaluated by a gastroenterologist and/or surgeon when the pain is associated with bleeding; when there is evidence of a perforated viscous or bowel obstruction, a hepatobiliary etiology (e.g., jaundice, ascites, or acute pancreatitis); and when endoscopy is indicated in the acute phase (e.g., bleeding peptic ulcer or sigmoid volvulus).

In patients whose pain is resolved in the ED or when a nonurgent cause is identified, a planned 2-week follow-up is reasonable. If a cause is identified and treated in the ED (such as peptic disorders, constipation, or gastroenteritis), the patient should be seen in follow-up within 7–10 days.

What pearls can you offer emergency care providers when evaluating a patient with generalized abdominal pain?

- Proper diagnosis of abdominal pain requires a practitioner to be familiar with patterns of abdominal pain. For example, pain originating from biliary disease can present with upper abdominal pain and shoulder pain and can be associated with acute constitutional symptoms like fever and jaundice. If there are signs of peritonitis, then a perforated viscous should be suspected. Pain from ischemia of the gut requires a high index of suspension to ensure early diagnosis.

- A practitioner should be familiar with classic and common pathologies. For example, pain from pancreatitis is usually localized and severe, while pain from dyspepsia can be more vague and generalized.
- Patients who are immunocompromised can present with vague and poorly localized pain with pathologies that are expected to present with more specific symptoms in patients with intact immune systems.
- Pregnancy temporarily changes the anatomy and can displace abdominal organs; therefore, a practitioner must be familiar with evaluation of abdominal pain in pregnancy. For example, acute appendicitis can present with right upper quadrant pain rather than lower abdominal pain.

What are the "rules of the road" when managing a patient with generalized abdominal pain?

- A careful, chronological history is important. In the vast majority of cases, an accurate diagnosis can be achieved from history if you are familiar with abdominal pain syndromes and attentive when listening to the patient.
- Context is important. Ask which symptoms started first, what are the exacerbating factors, in what setting did the pain begin, and how the pain has progressed.
- Carefully observe the patients before you touch them. Note their posture and general appearance. A patient with peritonitis will lay still in bed, while a patient passing a kidney stone will be restless and constantly changing position.
- Examination of the abdomen should always include a search for the presence of enlarged lymph nodes (including supraclavicular enlarged lymph nodes which suggest abdominal malignancy).
- Do not defer the anorectal and groin/genital exam.
- Remember that general concepts may not apply in the immunocompromised or pregnant patient.

What are the "red flags" and how to avoid common diagnostic errors?

- Exam finding suggestive of peritonitis suggests a serious intra-abdominal event like a perforated viscous.
- Severe abdominal pain inconsistent of physical findings suggests early acute bowel ischemia. Ischemia of the bowel can present in three distinctive syndromes: chronic intestinal ischemia (postprandial pain associated with weight loss due to fear of eating usually in an elderly patient), acute intestinal ischemia (acute- and abrupt-onset severe abdominal pain with minimal physical signs until late in the presentation when there is

bowel infarction and peritonitis), and ischemic colitis (acute-onset abdominal pain followed by watery diarrhea and subsequent hematochezia).
- Create a differential diagnosis based on your evaluation, then support your findings with testing, and do not shotgun testing.
- Tailor your imaging or endoscopy testing based on your findings. Peptic ulcer disease is best diagnosed by endoscopy, while bowel obstruction or biliary stones disease is best diagnosed by imaging.
- Beware of the limitations of imaging. An abdominal or chest radiograph can miss signs of free air if not done in the proper position (PA and lateral) and if the imaged field does not cover areas under the diaphragm. Plain radiographs can miss serious pathologies like bowel ischemia and bowel inflammation.

Do all patients with acute abdominal pain require laboratory data? What laboratory data is most helpful when determining urgent versus nonurgent causes of acute abdominal pain?

Not all patients with abdominal pain require laboratory testing in the acute setting, assuming they are hemodynamically stable and have a benign history and physical exam. The CBC can be used to evaluate for anemia, lipase for pancreatitis, and LFTs for biliary disease (but can be normal with cholecystitis). Elevated lactic acid should raise suspicion for ischemic colitis; however, it may be elevated in shock states or simply with dehydration. No single test can determine urgent vs. nonurgent causes of acute abdominal pain.

Suggested Resources

- Feldman M, Friedman LS, Brandt LJ. Sleisenger and Fordtran's gastrointestinal and liver disease: pathophysiology/diagnosis/management. 10th ed. Philadelphia: Saunders/Elsevier; 2016. Vol 2 (xxxi, 2369, 89 pages)
- Cartwright SL, Knudson MP. Evaluation of acute abdominal pain in adults. Am Fam Physician. 2008;77(7):971–8.
- Cartwright SL, Knudson MP. Diagnostic imaging of acute abdominal pain in adults. Am Fam Physician. 2015;91(7):452–9.
- McKean J, Ronan-Bentle S. Abdominal Pain in the Immunocompromised Patient-Human Immunodeficiency Virus, Transplant, Cancer. Emerg Med Clin North Am. 2016;4(2):377–86.

Part II

Gastrointestinal Bleeding

How Can I Tell If My Patient Has a Gastrointestinal Bleed? Is It an Upper Gastrointestinal Bleed (UGIB) or Lower Gastrointestinal Bleed (LGIB)?

Ainsley Adams and Andrew C. Meltzer

Pearls and Pitfalls
- Gastrointestinal (GI) bleeding typically presents with hematemesis, coffee-ground emesis, hematochezia, melena, or unexplained anemia.
- Physical exam and occult blood tests can assist with localization of the source of GI bleeding.
- An upper GI bleed is likely if there is a history of melena, melenic stool on exam, nasogastric lavage with blood or coffee grounds, or a serum urea nitrogen-to-creatinine ratio of more than 30.
- Direct visualization with endoscopy can definitively determine the bleeding source.

Does My Patient Have a Gastrointestinal Bleed?

Gastrointestinal bleeding is a common diagnosis in the United States, accounting for approximately 1 million hospitalizations annually [1]. The diagnosis can be confirmed with a clinical presentation consistent with gastrointestinal bleeding and supporting laboratory data or ancillary tests/procedures. In the acute care setting, clinicians are focused on identifying overt or acute gastrointestinal bleeding rather than occult (chronic) GI bleeding. Occult GIB is defined by the American Gastroenterological Association (AGA) as a positive fecal occult blood test without evidence of visible blood loss or symptoms of anemia [2]. While a stool occult blood test may be used to confirm the presence of blood in the stool, false-positive occult blood tests can occur with red meat, turnips, horseradish, and vitamin C consumption [3]. It is worth noting that while oral iron supplements may cause stools to appear similar to melena, iron supplementation does not cause false-positive stool occult blood results [4].

The classic presentation of an upper gastrointestinal bleed (UGIB) is hematemesis, coffee-ground emesis, and melena (observed or on examination). For a lower GI bleed (LGIB), the classic presentation includes bright red blood per rectum or maroon blood in the stool. Several conditions and medications may mimic these findings (Table 9.1). For instance, nosebleeds, intraoral bleeding, tonsillar bleeding, and some foods such as beets have been mistaken as hematemesis. Bismuth-containing medications such as Pepto-Bismol may mimic melena. Vaginal bleeding or hematuria may be confused by patients for bright red blood per rectum [5]. As well, not all patients with a GIB will present classically. Symptoms suggestive of decreased oxygen carrying capacity (e.g., weakness, light-headedness, chest pain, syncope, palpitations, fatigue, dyspnea on exertion) especially in the context of risk factors for gastrointestinal bleeding (Table 9.2) and anemia may be the clinical presentation of an acute gastrointestinal hemorrhage. Vital sign abnormalities alone may be the only indication of blood loss. Supine tachycardia is one of the most sensitive, early vital sign abnormalities associated with acute bleeding [1].

Table 9.1 Mimics of gastrointestinal bleeding

Mimics for hematemesis	Nosebleeds, tonsillar bleeding, red drinks, and food
Mimics for melena	Bismuth medications such as Pepto-Bismol™
Mimics for bright red blood	Red food, vaginal bleeding, gross hematuria
False-positive occult blood test	Red meat, turnips, horseradish, vitamin C

Ref. [5]

A. Adams, MD · A. C. Meltzer, MD, MS (✉)
Department of Emergency Medicine, George Washington University School of Medicine & Health Sciences, Washington, DC, USA
e-mail: ainsleyadams@gwu.edu; ameltzer@mfa.gwu.edu

© Springer Nature Switzerland AG 2019
A. Graham, D. J. Carlberg (eds.), *Gastrointestinal Emergencies*, https://doi.org/10.1007/978-3-319-98343-1_9

Table 9.2 Risk factors of gastrointestinal bleeding

Upper gastrointestinal bleed	Lower gastrointestinal bleed
Smoking	Advanced age
Alcohol consumption	Male sex
Advanced age	Antiplatelet use
Previous history of UGIB	Nonsteroidal anti-inflammatory
Helicobacter pylori	medications
Nonsteroidal anti-	Anticoagulation
inflammatory drugs	Comorbidities: HIV, diverticular
Antiplatelet	disease, gastrointestinal cancer,
Anticoagulants	inflammatory bowel disease,
Steroids	angiodysplasia
Selective serotonin inhibitors	Polyps
(twofold increase in UGIB	
with SSRI) [18]	
Comorbidities: cancer,	
cirrhosis, esophageal varices,	
peptic ulcer disease, gastritis	

Ref. [1]

Is It an UGIB or LGIB?

Gastrointestinal bleeding describes bleeding originating anywhere in the gastrointestinal tract. Clinicians further delineate GIB as upper and lower because they have unique diagnostic and treatment considerations.

Upper Gastrointestinal Bleed

An UGIB is a hemorrhage above the ligament of Treitz, a suspensory muscle of the duodenum, and in effect represents the portion of the GI tract that can be evaluated with an upper endoscopy (e.g., EGD). The annual incidence of acute UGIB in the United States is estimated to be 50–160 cases per 100,000 [6]. The most common cause of UGIB remains peptic ulcer disease which accounts for up to 67% of UGIB cases [7] (Table 9.3). Variceal hemorrhage usually occurs in patients with portal hypertension and is always considered high-risk for re-bleeding and mortality. Variceal bleeding should be suspected in any patient with known liver disease, liver cirrhosis, or stigmata of portal hypertension. As part of the natural course of an UGIB, 80% of the non-variceal hemorrhages resolve spontaneously, while 10% lead to death [8].

Clinical findings associated with upper GI bleeds include melena, nasogastric (NG) aspiration of frank blood or "coffee grounds" appearing blood, and a ratio of serum urea nitrogen to creatinine greater than 30. Based on a study of approximately 1800 patients, the risk of upper GI bleed increased with a patient history of melena (likelihood ratio (LR), 5.1–5.9), melenic stool on exam (LR, 25), NG lavage with blood or coffee grounds (LR, 9.6), and a serum urea nitrogen-to-creatinine ratio of more than 30 (LR, 7.5) [9]. In the same analysis, the presence of blood clots in the stool decreased the likelihood of upper GI bleed (LR, 0.05) [9].

Table 9.3 Causes of gastrointestinal bleeding

Upper GI bleed	Lower GI bleed
Peptic ulcer disease	Diverticular disease
Gastritis	AVM
Esophagogastric varices/portal	Angiodysplasia
hypertension	Neoplasm
Mallory- Weiss	Hemorrhoids
Gastric cancer	Anal fissures
Aortoenteric fistula	Inflammatory bowel disease
	Aortoenteric fistula
	Colitis (ischemic, infectious,
	inflammatory)

Melena is blood in the stool which has become black, sticky, and tar-like after exposure to the low pH in the stomach. In one study, melena alone was reported to have an 80% sensitivity in predicting an upper GI source [10]. However, melena does not determine the severity of bleeding as only 50 ml of blood in the stomach is required to turn stools black [11]. While bright red blood per rectum (BRBPR) is most commonly seen in LGIB, brisk upper gastrointestinal bleeding should be considered in patients with BRBPR who appear unstable or when there is a suspicion for a highly unstable etiology, such as varices or aortoenteric fistulas. Other factors associated with *severe* upper GI bleeding include bright red blood on nasogastric aspiration, tachycardia, and hemoglobin level less than 8 g/dL [9].

Lower Gastrointestinal Bleed

Lower gastrointestinal bleeding (LGIB) originates below the ligament of Treitz (e.g., distal small bowel, colon, rectum, and anus) and accounts for 20% of GIB cases [12]. The prevalence of lower GI bleed is directly associated with advanced age. One study found that age < 50 years was 92% specific for an upper GI source and not LGIB, with a positive likelihood ratio of 3.5 [13]. The most common sources of lower GI bleeding are diverticular disease (26%), benign anorectal disorders (17%), colitis (14%), and hemorrhoids (12%) [14] (Table 9.3). Painless severe bleeding with clots is often seen with diverticular disease. Bloody diarrhea often occurs with ischemic and infectious colitis.

In general, a fecal occult blood test does not add much value to diagnosis. A positive fecal occult test result had 24% sensitivity and 89% specificity for predicting lower gastrointestinal tract lesions on colonoscopy and no significant correlation with upper gastrointestinal tract lesions on endoscopy [15]. However, for diagnosis of subtle GI bleeding or to confirm what is seen on direct visualization, a fecal occult blood test may be helpful. The most commonly used fecal occult blood test is the guaiac stool detector which traditionally requires blood loss of at least 2–10 ml per day to turn positive (blue) [16].

After diagnosing a lower GI bleed, risk assessment is helpful to direct management. Strate et al. identified seven factors that correlated with severe lower GI bleeding: heart rate > 100 beats/min, systolic blood pressure < 115 mmHg, syncope, non-tender abdominal exam, rectal bleeding within the first 4 h of evaluation, use of aspirin, and > 2 comorbid illnesses. In patients with more than three of the seven factors, the likelihood of severe LGIB was 80% [17]. For patients with abnormal vital signs or a decrease in hemoglobin by 2 g/ dL, more urgent intervention should be considered including interventional radiography or general surgery [18].

Suggested Resources

- PODCAST. https://www.stitcher.com/podcast/emergency-medicine-cases/e/51768269.
- Srygley FD, Gerardo CJ, Tran T, Fisher DA. Does this patient have a severe upper gastrointestinal bleed? JAMA. 2012;307(10):1072. https://doi.org/10.1001/jama.2012.253.

References

1. Nable J, Graham A. Gastrointestinal bleeding. Emerg Med Clin. 2016;34(2):309–25.
2. American Gastroenterological Association. (n.d.). Retrieved from http://www.gastro.org/.
3. Jaffe RM, Kasten B, Young DS, MacLowry JD. False-negative stool occult blood tests caused by ingestion of ascorbic acid (Vitamin C). Ann Intern Med. 1975;83(6):824. https://doi.org/10.7326/0003-4819-83-6-824.
4. Kulbaski MJ, Goold SD, Tecce MA, Friedenheim RE, Palarski JD, Brancati FL. Oral iron and the Hemoccult test: a controversy on the teaching wards. N Engl J Med. 1989;320(22):1500.
5. Goralnick E, Meguerdichian D. Gastrointestinal bleeding. In: Walls RM, Hockberger RS, Gausche-Hill M, editors. Rosen's emergency medicine: concepts and clinical practice. 9th ed. Philadelphia: Elsevier; 2014.
6. Rotondano G. Epidemiology and diagnosis of acute nonvariceal upper gastrointestinal bleeding. Gastroenterol Clin N Am. 2014;43(4):643–63.
7. Khamaysi I, Gralnek IM. Acute upper gastrointestinal bleeding (UGIB) – initial evaluation and management. Best Pract Res Clin Gastroenterol. 2013;27(5):633–8.
8. Sugawa C, Steffes CP, Nakamura R, et al. Upper GI bleeding in an urban hospital. Etiology, recurrence, and prognosis. Ann Surg. 1990;212(4):521–6-7.
9. Srygley FD, Gerardo CJ, Tran T, Fisher DA. Does this patient have a severe upper gastrointestinal bleed? JAMA. 2012;307(10):1072.
10. Witting MD, Magder L, Heins AE, et al. ED predictors of upper gastrointestinal tract bleeding in patients without hematemesis. Am J Emerg Med. 2006;24(3):280–5.
11. Schiff L, Stevens RJ, Goodman S, Garber E, Lublin A. Observations on the oral administration of citrated blood in man - I. the effects on the blood urea nitrogen. Am J Dig Dis. 1939;6(9):597–602.
12. Strate L, Gralnek I. ACG Clinical Guideline: management of patients with acute lower gastrointestinal bleeding. Am J Gastroenterol. 2016;111(5):755. Advance Online Publication
13. El-Kersh K, Chaddha U, Siddhartha R, Saad M, Guardiola J, Cavallazzi R. Predictive role of admission lactate level in critically ill patients with acute upper gastrointestinal bleeding. J Emerg Med. 2015;49(3):318–25.
14. Oakland K, Guy R, Uberoi R, et al. Acute lower GI bleeding in the UK: patient characteristics, interventions and outcomes in the first nationwide audit. Gut. 2017; https://doi.org/10.1136/gutjnl-2016-313428.
15. Chiang T-H, Lee Y-C, Tu C-H, Chiu H-M, Wu M-S. Performance of the immunochemical fecal occult blood test in predicting lesions in the lower gastrointestinal tract. CMAJ. 2011;183(13):1474–81.
16. Rockey DC. Occult gastrointestinal bleeding. Gastroenterol Clin North Am. 2005;34(4):699–718. https://www.sciencedirect.com/science/article/pii/S0889855305000816?via%3Dihub.
17. Strate L, Ayanian J, Kotler G, Syngal S. Risk factors for mortality in lower intestinal bleeding. Clin Gastroenterol Hepatol. 2008;6(9):1004–10.
18. Jiang HY, Chen HZ, Hu X, Yu Z, Yang W, Deng M, Zhang Y, Ruan B. Use of selective serotonin reuptake inhibitors and risk of upper gastrointestinal bleeding: a systematic review and meta-analysis. Clin Gastroenterol Hep. 2015;13:42–50.

What Is the Best Risk Stratification Tool for a Patient with a Suspected Upper GI Bleed?

Ainsley Adams and Andrew C. Meltzer

Pearls and Pitfalls
- Clinical decision tools are important to estimate disease severity in patients with suspected upper GI bleeding in order to plan endoscopy, determine the need for the intensive care unit, and communicate with consultants.
- Lactate level on admission and lactate clearance after resuscitation are useful in predicting patient outcomes.
- There are three relevant clinical decision scores that rely on pre-endoscopic data to risk stratify patients in the ED.
- The Glasgow-Blatchford Score is the only tool that has been validated to safely discharge patients.

Table 10.1 Glasgow-Blatchford Score [5]

Risk marker	Score value
BUN (mmol/L)	
6.5–8.0	2
8.0–10.0	3
10.0–25.0	4
≥25.0	6
Hemoglobin (g/L) for men	
120–130	1
100–120	3
<100	6
Hemoglobin (g/L) for women	
100–120	1
≤100	6
SBP (mmHg)	
100–109	1
90–99	2
<90	3
Other markers	
Pulse≥100 BPM	1
Melena	1
Syncope	2
Hepatic disease	2
Cardiac failure	2

Adapted from Blatchford et al. [5] with automatic permission from Elsevier through the STM signatory guidelines

Estimating severity of bleeding and predicting the clinical course at initial presentation is important in early management and resource utilization. Lacking the ability to directly visualize the bleeding source, clinical decision tools may help emergency medicine providers anticipate which patients will require aggressive resuscitation and higher levels of care. Three clinical decision rules, the clinical Rockall score (CRS), the Glasgow-Blatchford Score (GBS), and the AIMS65 score, incorporate vital signs, initial examination, lab values, and comorbidities to risk stratify patients prior to endoscopy [1–8] (Tables 10.1 and 10.2).

The Rockall score was the earliest attempt at creating a clinical decision rule for upper GI bleeding and is the most well-known [2, 3]. While the initial Rockall score incorpo-rated endoscopic data, the score has been modified into the *clinical* Rockall score (CRS), which only includes data available prior to endoscopy. The CRS (also called the pre-endoscopic Rockall score) incorporates only clinical data available immediately at presentation, such as systolic blood pressure, pulse, patient age, and comorbidities. It has been shown to predict the risk of further bleeding and death in patients hospitalized with UGIB [4].

The GBS was derived to predict the need for intervention (transfusion, endoscopic interventions, or surgical therapy). The initial study by Blatchford derived the score from 1748 patients in Scotland to identify risk factors associated with

A. Adams · A. C. Meltzer (✉)
Department of Emergency Medicine, George Washington University School of Medicine & Health Sciences, Washington, DC, USA
e-mail: ainsleyadams@gwu.edu; ameltzer@mfa.gwu.edu

© Springer Nature Switzerland AG 2019
A. Graham, D. J. Carlberg (eds.), *Gastrointestinal Emergencies*, https://doi.org/10.1007/978-3-319-98343-1_10

Table 10.2 Clinical Rockall score [2]

Variable	Score			
	0	1	2	3
Age	<60	60–79	≥80	
Shock	No shock	SBP ≥ 100 Pulse≥100	Hypotension	
Comorbidity	No major		Cardiac failure, ischemic heart disease, major comorbidities	Renal failure, liver failure, disseminated malignancy
Diagnosis	Mallory-Weiss tear, no lesion identified and no stigmata	All other diagnoses	Malignancy upper GI tract	

Reproduced from Rockall et al. [2] with permission from the BMJ group

rebleeding or death [5]. In a prospective study of 676 ED patients with UGIB, Blatchford scores of 0 were not admitted. Sixteen percent had a GBS score of zero, and none of these patients required endoscopic interventions or died prior to outpatient follow-up [9]. As a result of this study, very low-risk patients with Blatchford scores of 0 may be discharged from the emergency department without inpatient endoscopy. This follow-up study was undertaken at four hospitals in the UK. Limitations to the GBS include the low adoption by US physicians and the low specificity of the test [10, 11].

The third score, the AIMS65, has been derived and validated in a large group of patients to predict in-hospital mortality and the need for ICU admission [12]. AIMS65 gives one point if albumin <3 g/dL (30 g/L), INR >1.5, alteration in mental status, systolic blood pressure equal to or less than 90 mmHg, or age >65 years; Scores of 0 or 2 are associated with in-hospital mortality rates of 0.3% and 1.2% respectively while scores of 4 or 5 are associated with mortality rates of 16.5% and 24.5% respectively [12]. The study used a CareFusion Inc. database of more than 29,000 patients across 187 US hospitals to examine the relationship between several demographic and clinical data points with mortality. Comparison studies suggest that it may be more accurate at predicting in-hospital mortality than either GBS or CRS [1, 9, 13].

A limitation of all of the clinical decision rules is that endoscopy is often still desired by physicians and patients regardless of the risk score [14]. In addition, both scores may be less accurate in patients who are less likely to become tachycardic in response to blood loss, such as the elderly or patients who are taking a beta-blocker [14].

Regardless of the score used, ICU admission and urgent endoscopy should be considered for all patients with suspected varices, on anticoagulation, with significant comorbidities, with abnormal vital signs, or with significant anemia [15]. Although lactate is not a part of the GBS, AIMS65, or CRS, early data suggests that elevated lactate is a sensitive but nonspecific predictor of in-hospital mortality for patients with upper GI bleeds [16, 17]. One study that examined 6 years of retrospective data from 1644 patients in an urban tertiary referral ED found that those with an ED lactate

greater than 4 mmol/L had a 6.4-fold increased chance of in-hospital mortality, even when controlling for other factors [17]. This suggests that an elevated early lactate is an important prognostic indicator. In addition, reduced lactate clearance may be associated with active bleeding, while improved lactate clearance may indicate that bleeding has stopped [18]. Further studies are needed to validate these results.

Suggested Resources
- Emergency medicine cases: GI bleed emergencies. https://emergencymedicinecases.com/gi-bleed-emergencies-part-2/.
- Loren Laine MD, Dennis M, Jensen MD. Management of patients with ulcer bleeding. Am J Gastroenterol. 2012;107:345–60.

References

1. Robertson M, Majumdar A, Boyapati R, et al. Risk stratification in acute upper GI bleeding: comparison of the AIMS65 score with the Glasgow-Blatchford and Rockall scoring systems. Gastrointest Endosc. 2016;83(6):1151–60.
2. Rockall TA, Logan RF, Devlin HB, Northfield TC. Risk assessment after acute upper gastrointestinal haemorrhage. Gut. 1996;38(3):316–21.
3. Vreeburg EM, Terwee CB, Snel P, et al. Validation of the Rockall risk scoring system in upper gastrointestinal bleeding. Gut. 1999;44(3):331–5.
4. Tham TCK, James C, Kelly M. Predicting outcome of acute non-variceal upper gastrointestinal haemorrhage without endoscopy using the clinical Rockall score. Postgrad Med J. 2006;82(973):757–9.
5. Blatchford O, Murray WR, Blatchford M. A risk score to predict need for treatment for upper-gastrointestinal haemorrhage. Lancet (London, England). 2000;356(9238):1318–21.
6. Gralnek IM, Dulai GS. Incremental value of upper endoscopy for triage of patients with acute non-variceal upper-GI hemorrhage. Gastrointest Endosc. 2004;60(1):9–14.
7. Schiefer M, Aquarius M, Leffers P, et al. Predictive validity of the Glasgow Blatchford Bleeding Score in an unselected emergency department population in continental Europe. Eur J Gastroenterol Hepatol. 2012;1(4):382–7.

8. Gralnek IM. Outpatient management of "low-risk" nonvariceal upper GI hemorrhage. Are we ready to put evidence into practice? Gastrointest Endosc. 2002;55(1):131–4. https://doi.org/10.1067/mge.2002.120661.

9. Stanley AJ, Laine L, Dalton HR, et al. Comparison of risk scoring systems for patients presenting with upper gastrointestinal bleeding: international multicentre prospective study. BMJ. 2017;356:i6432.

10. Bryant RV, Kuo P, Williamson K, et al. Performance of the Glasgow-Blatchford score in predicting clinical outcomes and intervention in hospitalized patients with upper GI bleeding. Gastrointest Endosc. 2013;78(4):576–83.

11. Meltzer AC, Pinchbeck C, Burnett S, et al. Emergency physicians accurately interpret video capsule endoscopy findings in suspected upper gastrointestinal hemorrhage: a video survey. Lewis L, ed. Acad Emerg Med. 2013;20(7):711–715.

12. Saltzman JR, Tabak YP, Hyett BH, Sun X, Travis AC, Johannes RS. A simple risk score accurately predicts in-hospital mortality, length of stay, and cost in acute upper GI bleeding. Gastrointest Endosc. 2011;74(6):1215–24.

13. Yaka E, Yılmaz S, Özgür Doğan N, Pekdemir M. Comparison of the Glasgow-Blatchford and AIMS65 scoring systems for risk strat-ification in upper gastrointestinal bleeding in the emergency depart-ment. Mark Courtney D, ed. Acad Emerg Med. 2015;22(1):22–30. doi:https://doi.org/10.1111/acem.12554.

14. Meltzer AC, Burnett S, Pinchbeck C, et al. Pre-endoscopic Rockall and Blatchford scores to identify which emergency department patients with suspected gastrointestinal bleed do not need endo-scopic hemostasis. J Emerg Med. 2013;44(6):1083–7.

15. Westhoff JL, Holt KR. Gastrointestinal bleeding: an evidence-based ED approach to risk stratification. Emerg Med Pract. 2004;6(3):1–20.

16. El-Kersh K, Chaddha U, Sinha RS, Saad M, Guardiola J, Cavallazzi R. Predictive role of admission lactate level in critically ill patients with acute upper gastrointestinal bleeding. J Emerg Med. 2015;49(3):318–25.

17. Shah A, Chisolm-Straker M, Alexander A, Rattu M, Dikdan S, Manini AF. Prognostic use of lactate to predict inpatient mor-tality in acute gastrointestinal hemorrhage. Am J Emerg Med. 2014;32(7):752–5.

18. Wada T, Hagiwara A, Uemura T, Yahagi N, Kimura A. Early lactate clearance for predicting active bleeding in critically ill patients with acute upper gastrointestinal bleeding: a retrospective study. Intern Emerg Med. 2016;11(5):737–43.

Diagnostic Testing for Patients with Gastrointestinal Hemorrhage

11

Ainsley Adams and Andrew C. Meltzer

Pearls and Pitfalls
- Patients admitted with a suspected upper GI bleed should have an endoscopy performed within 24 h.
- Patients admitted with a lower GI bleeding may receive a delayed sigmoidoscopy or colonoscopy if stable. If continuous bleeding is evident, surgery or interventional radiography consultation may be required.
- Video capsule endoscopy has shown potential to risk stratify patients in the ED.

All patients evaluated in the emergency department (ED) with a concern for a significant GI bleed require a thorough history, physical exam, complete blood count, blood urea nitrogen, liver function tests, coagulation studies, type and screen, and lactate. Resuscitation is the first priority of the emergency clinician, but the history, physical exam, and laboratory data will allow early risk stratification either as part of an unstructured gestalt or a formal clinical decision score. Following risk stratification, further diagnostic testing needs to be considered. In this chapter, we will discuss those additional tests.

Upper Endoscopy

Patients with a concern for upper GI bleed should be admitted for endoscopic evaluation within 24 h [1]. In patients with hemodynamic instability or active bloody hematemesis, immediate endoscopy or within 12 hours is recommended

A. Adams, MD · A. C. Meltzer, MD, MS (✉)
Department of Emergency Medicine, George Washington University School of Medicine & Health Sciences, Washington, DC, USA
e-mail: ainsleyadams@gwu.edu; ameltzer@mfa.gwu.edu

[2]. Prior to endoscopy, intravenous proton pump inhibitors and pro-motility agents can be initiated in the ED [3]. Hemostatic control via endoscopy is achieved by one of several options including vasoconstrictive medication, thermal cauterization, and vascular clips.

Colonoscopy

Patients suspected of having an active lower GI bleed often determined by a drop in hemoglobin, abnormal vital signs, or evidence of continuous bleeding should be admitted for evaluation. Risk factors for more severe disease include anticoagulation, comorbidities, and advanced age. Unfortunately, in cases of brisk or acute bleeding, a colonoscopy may not be able to visualize the source. In addition, colonoscopy is more technically difficult in the emergency setting due to the lack of bowel prep. For this reason, patients with acute lower gastrointestinal bleeding that need urgent evaluation may benefit from an interventional radiology evaluation or surgery consultation [4].

Angiography

Brisk lower GI bleeding is usually handled in the interventional suite with selective embolization, while less severe bleeding may initially be evaluated and treated with colonoscopy after an 8–12-hour bowel prep [5]. Embolization has replaced local vasoconstrictive therapy as the catheter-based treatment of choice [5]. Interventional radiology procedures typically follow a CT angiogram which is used to identify the source of bleeding and detect active extravasation into the bowel. Occasionally, an interventional radiologist will be willing to perform a similar embolization for refractory upper GI bleeding or perform an emergency transjugular portosystemic shunt (TIPS) for refractory variceal bleeding [6].

CT Angiography

When performing a CT angiogram for bleeding, oral contrast is typically not used because it may obscure active extravasation of blood into the GI tract. In addition, both arterial and portal-venous phase imaging may be used to discover the source of acute GI bleeding. Since bleeding may be intermittent, the absence of active bleeding on CT angiogram does not always mean that bleeding has permanently stopped but may represent a momentary cessation [7].

Laparotomy

In severe cases of GI bleeding, surgery may be the only method to control brisk GI bleeding. The successful use of endoscopy and embolization procedures has made emergency surgical treatment, such as non-resective surgery, Billroth I, Billroth II, and gastric wedge resection, extremely rare [8].

Bleeding Scan

Scintigraphy, or radioactive tagged red blood cell scans, can identify slow bleeding that is unable to be directly visualized on colonoscopy or seen with angiography. A radioactive tracer, most often technetium-99 m (Tc-99 m), is injected intravenously, and serial images are taken, allowing providers to identify blood present in the gastrointestinal tract. Scintigraphy is most useful after endoscopy or colonoscopy has failed to visualize the bleeding source. There is currently no defined role for a bleeding scan in the emergency evaluation of GIB. The study is noninvasive, and a bleeding scan can image over a prolonged period of time, thus detecting intermittent bleeding [9]. Studies in dog models suggest that Tc-99 m scans are able to detect GI bleeding at rates as slow as 0.04 ml/min [9]. The main limitation of RBC nuclear imaging is it may give an imprecise anatomic location of bleeding.

Video Capsule Endoscopy

A novel approach to risk stratify upper GI hemorrhages in the ED is to use video capsule endoscopy to directly visualize the bleeding. In three ED-based studies, video capsule endoscopy demonstrated good patient tolerance and good sensitivity for detecting acute upper GI hemorrhage [10–12]. Potential advantages of video capsule endoscopy include improved patient tolerance as compared to nasogastric aspiration, point of care results obtained without a specialist at the bedside, and decreased hospitalization rates. Potential barriers to adoption include the cost of the equipment, the need to train emergency department physicians to interpret the videos, the need to create a secure means to transmit images to on-call GI specialists, and the increased ED length of stay of video capsule endoscopy utilization. Further studies will be needed to confirm the sensitivity of this test in multiple settings and as a means to guide clinical decisions compared to current standard of care.

Blakemore Tube

The Sengstaken-Blakemore and Minnesota tubes are nonsurgical approaches to temporarily treat active variceal hemorrhage. The enduring image of the Blakemore tube is the football helmet with the proximal end of the tube attached to the facemask to secure positioning. The tube works by inflating a balloon inside the esophagus and proximal stomach to tamponade varices. The Blakemore tube is considered an eleventh-hour effort to temporarily control bleeding in a critically ill patient. A few limited studies have demonstrated moderate effectiveness of the Blakemore tube in controlling bleeding prior to definitive care such as transjugular intrahepatic portosystemic shunt or sclerotherapy [13].

Suggested Resources
- Barkun AN, Bardou M, Kuipers EJ, et al. International consensus recommendations on the management of patients with nonvariceal upper gastrointestinal bleeding. Ann Intern Med. 2010;152(2):101. https://doi.org/10.7326/0003-4819-152-2-201001190-00009.
- Bethea ED, Travis AC, Saltzman JR. Initial assessment and management of patients with nonvariceal upper gastrointestinal bleeding. J Clin Gastroenterol. 14:1. https://doi.org/10.1097/MCG.0000000000000194.
- EMRAP HD. Placement of a blakemore tube for bleeding varices.
- Laine L, Jensen DM. Management of patients with ulcer bleeding. Am J Gastroenterol. 2012;107(3):345–60. https://doi.org/10.1038/ajg.2011.480.
- LITFL. EBM Upper GI Haemorrhage.

References

1. Barkun AN, Bardou M, Kuipers EJ, et al. International consensus recommendations on the management of patients with nonvariceal upper gastrointestinal bleeding. Ann Intern Med. 2010;152(2):101.
2. Laine L, Jensen DM. Management of patients with ulcer bleeding. Am J Gastroenterol. 2012;107(3):345–60.
3. Bethea ED, Travis AC, Saltzman JR. Initial assessment and management of patients with nonvariceal upper gastrointestinal bleeding. J Clin Gastroenterol. 2014;1(10):823–9.

4. Strate LL, Gralnek IM. ACG clinical guideline: management of patients with acute lower gastrointestinal bleeding. Am J Gastroenterol. 2016;111(4):459–74.
5. Speir EJ, Ermentrout RM, Martin JG. Management of acute lower gastrointestinal bleeding. Tech Vasc Interv Radiol. 2017;20(4):258–62.
6. Copeland A, Kapoor B, Sands M. Transjugular intrahepatic portosystemic shunt: indications, contraindications, and patient workup. Semin Intervent Radiol. 2014;31(3):235–42.
7. Sos TA, Lee JG, Wixson D, Sniderman KW. Intermittent bleeding from minute to minute in acute massive gastrointestinal hemorrhage: arteriographic demonstration. AJR Am J Roentgenol. 1978;131(6):1015–7.
8. Czymek R, Großmann A, Roblick U, et al. Surgical management of acute upper gastrointestinal bleeding:still a major challenge. Hepatogastroenterology [Internet]. 2012;59(115):768–73. Available from: http://www.ncbi.nlm.nih.gov/pubmed/22469719
9. Zuckier LS. Acute gastrointestinal bleeding. Semin Nucl Med. 2003;33(4):297–311.
10. Chandran S, Testro A, Urquhart P, et al. Risk stratification of upper GI bleeding with an esophageal capsule. Gastrointest Endosc. 2013;77(6):891–8.
11. Sung JJY, Tang RSY, Ching JYL, Rainer TH, Lau JYW. Use of capsule endoscopy in the emergency department as a triage of patients with GI bleeding. Gastrointest Endosc. 2016;84(6):907–13.
12. Meltzer AC, Ali MA, Kresiberg RB, et al. Video capsule endoscopy in the emergency department: a prospective study of acute upper gastrointestinal hemorrhage. Ann Emerg Med. 2013;61(4):438–443.e1.
13. Jaramillo JL, de la Mata M, Mino G, Costan G, Gomez-Camacho F. Somatostatin versus Sengstaken balloon tamponade for primary haemostasia of bleeding esophageal varices: a randomized pilot study. J Hepatol. 1991;12(1):100–5.

Is NG Aspiration Sensitive and Specific to Detect Upper GI Bleeding?

12

Ainsley Adams and Andrew C. Meltzer

Pearls and Pitfalls
- Nasogastric lavage (NGL) in the emergency department has a low sensitivity but high specificity for localizing upper gastrointestinal (GI) bleeds.
- Nasogastric tube placement is one of the most uncomfortable procedures performed in the emergency department.
- Nasogastric aspiration may improve visualization for endoscopy, but similar results may be achieved with pro-motility agents.

What Is the Usefulness of Nasogastric Aspiration (NGA) in Localizing the Source of Bleeding?

Nasogastric (NG) aspiration has been routinely used for diagnosis and risk stratification of suspected upper GI hemorrhage. In distinguishing between UGIB and LGIB, NGA has a low sensitivity (44%) but high specificity (95%) [1]. In a systematic review by Srygley et al. of 1776 patients studying predictors of UGIB versus LGIB, nasogastric aspiration with frank blood or coffee grounds had a positive likelihood ratio of 9.6 (4.0–23, 95% CI). Nasogastric aspiration without evidence of blood corresponded with a decreased likelihood of UGIB (LR 0.58, 0.49–0.70 95% CI) [2]. It is worth noting that in this analysis, melena (observed or confirmed with rectal examination) with a LR of 25 (4–174, 95% CI) was more predictive of UGIB compared to a positive NGA [2]. In a retrospective cohort study of 220 patients admitted for gastrointestinal bleeding without hematemesis, a positive NGA had a positive predictive value of 92% (79–97%), a LR of 11

A. Adams, MD · A. C. Meltzer, MD, MS (✉)
Department of Emergency Medicine, George Washington
University School of Medicine & Health Sciences,
Washington, DC, USA
e-mail: ainsleyadams@gwu.edu; ameltzer@mfa.gwu.edu

(4–30), and accurately predicted the source of bleeding in 66% of patients. The authors concluded that "in patients without hematemesis, a positive nasogastric aspiration seen in 23% (of patients), indicates probable upper gastrointestinal tract bleeding (LR+ 11), but a negative nasogastric aspiration, seen in 72% (of patients), provides little information (LR- 0.6)." [3].

The accuracy of NGA is also controversial. The false-negative rate of NGA in diagnosing UGIB has been reported as high as 20% in the literature [4–6]. A possible limitation of NGA is the placement of the nasogastric tube which often does not pass through the pylorus and may miss bleeding in the proximal duodenum [2]. False positives can occur from epistaxis caused by tube insertion [6].

Can Nasogastric Aspiration or Lavage Identify High-Risk Patients in Need of Endoscopy and Does It Impact Patient Outcomes?

A positive NGA correlates with lesions on endoscopy with a sensitivity of 45% and specificity of 72–76% [3, 5]. In a study of 520 patients with NGA prior to endoscopy, a bloody nasogastric aspirate was strongly associated with high-risk lesions (OR 4.82) compared to coffee ground aspirate (OR 2.8) [5]. These high-risk lesions often require endoscopic hemostasis, and by extension, NGA/NGL has been used to predict the likelihood that a patient with an UGIB will require endoscopic hemostasis. In a recent study of 613 patients with an UGIB of which 329 required endoscopic hemostasis, a bloody nasogastric aspirate (adjusted OR 6.8) and hemoglobin less than 8.6 g/dL (adjusted OR 1.8) were independent predictors of patients requiring endoscopic hemostasis [7].

It is less clear if NGL predicts GIB severity or impacts patient outcomes. Early studies reported that NGL was predictive of active bleeding and poor outcomes [8]. When evaluating clinical scoring systems such as the clinical Rockall score and Glasgow-Blatchford score (GBS), the GBS detected significant UGIB with a sensitivity of 98.3%. The addition of NGL data only increased the sensitivity to 99.6%, thus not adding significantly to clinical scoring systems in predicting patients who will have a complicated course and likely require transfusion and endoscopy [9]. NG aspiration has also been shown to have no effect on clinical outcomes such as mortality (OR 0.84), surgery (OR 1.5), length of hospital stay (7.3 vs 8.1 days), or transfusion requirements (3.2 units vs 3.0 units). However, NG aspiration was associated with a decreased time to endoscopy [8].

Does Nasogastric Lavage Improve Visualization for Endoscopy?

Some gastroenterologists advocate for NGL prior to endoscopy to improve visualization of gastric mucosa. Studies have found that NGL and specifically NGL in combination with erythromycin, a pro-motility agent, is associated with improved endoscopic visualization [9]. In a head-to-head study of NGL alone, erythromycin alone, or a combination of NGL and erythromycin, there was no significant difference in clinician satisfaction with stomach visualization between the groups. There were also no significant differences between the groups in duration of procedure, re-bleeding, need for second endoscopy, transfusion requirements, or mortality [10]. Thus intravenous erythromycin and other pro-motility medications such as metoclopramide provide similar visualization as NGL without the procedural risks or patient discomfort [11].

Expert Recommendations

The European Society of Gastrointestinal Endoscopy (ESGE) Guideline:

"ESGE does not recommend the routine use of nasogastric or orogastric aspiration/lavage in patients presenting with acute UGIH (strong recommendation, moderate quality evidence)." [1]

Our opinion: NGA does assist clinicians in discriminating between an UGIB source versus a LGIB as well as identifying patients with a higher likelihood of a high risk lesion on endoscopy but the procedural risk, significant patient discomfort with NGT placement, and lack of proven benefit to patient outcomes does not warrant the routine use of NGA or NGL in the evaluation of suspected UGIB patients.

Suggested Resources
- Academic Life in Emergency Medicine: NG lavage – indicated or outdated?. https://www.aliem.com/2013/04/ng-lavage-indicated-or-outdated/.
- Emergency Medicine Cases: gastrointestinal bleed emergencies. https://emergencymedicinecases.com/gi-bleed-emergencies-part-1/.
- EMJ Club Emergency Medicine Podcast, Washington University School of Medicine in St Louis: NG lavage for GI bleed. https://www.aliem.com/2013/04/ng-lavage-indicated-or-outdated/.
- Pallin DJ, Saltzman JR. Is nasogastric lavage in patients with acute upper GI bleeding indicated or antiquated? Gastrointest Endosc. 2011;74:981.

References

1. Gralnek I, Dumonceau J, Kuipers E, et al. Diagnosis and management of nonvariceal upper gastrointestinal hemorrhage: European Society of Gastrointestinal Endoscopy (ESGE) guideline. Endoscopy. 2015;47:a1–a46.
2. Srygley F, Gerardo C, Tran T, Fisher D. Does this patient have a severe upper gastrointestinal bleed? JAMA. 2012;307(10):1072–9.
3. Witting MD, Magder L, Heins AE, Mattu A, Granja CA, Baumgarten M. Usefulness and validity of diagnostic nasogastric aspiration in patients without hematemesis. Ann Emerg Med. 2004;43(4):525–32.
4. Ahmad S, Le V, Kaitha S, Morton J, Ali T. Nasogastric tube feedings and gastric residual volume: a regional survey. South Med J. 2012;105(8):394–8.
5. Aljebreen AM, Fallone CA, Barkun AN. For the RUGBE investigators. Nasogastric aspirate predicts high-risk endoscopic lesions in patients with acute upper-GI bleeding. Gastrointest Endosc. 2004;59(2):172–8.
6. Cuellar RE, Gavaler JS, Alexander JA, et al. Gastrointestinal tract hemorrhage. Arch Intern Med. 1990;150(7):1381.
7. Kim S, Kim K, et al. Predictors for the need for endoscopic therapy in patients with presumed acute upper gastrointestinal bleeding. Korean J Intern Med. 2017.; Publication Date (Web): 2017 December 15 (Original Article)
8. Huang E, Karsan S, Kanwal F, Singh I, Makhani M, Spiegel B. Impact of nasogastric lavage on outcomes in acute GI bleeding. Gastrointest Endosc. 2011;74(5):971–80.
9. Hassan K, Srygley F, Chiu S, Chow S, Fisher D. Clinical performance of prediction rules and nasogastric lavage for the evaluation of upper gastrointestinal bleeding: a retrospective observational study. Gastroenterol Res Pract. 2017;2017:3171697.
10. Pateron D, Vicaut E, Debuc E, et al. Erythromycin infusion or gastric lavage for upper gastrointestinal bleeding: a multicenter randomized controlled trial. Ann Emerg Med. 2011;57(6):582–9. https://doi.org/10.1016/j.annemergmed.2011.01.001.
11. Singer AJ, Richman PB, Kowalska A, Thode HC. Comparison of patient and practitioner assessments of pain from commonly performed emergency department procedures. Ann Emerg Med. 1999;33(6):652–8.

What Is the Optimal Timing of Endoscopy?

13

Kathleen Ogle and Andrew C. Meltzer

Pearls and Pitfalls
- The optimal timing of an upper endoscopy in patients with an upper GI bleed requires balancing the need for resuscitation and the need for definitive hemostasis.

Table 13.1 Optimal timing of endoscopy and lowest mortality [7]

Optimal timing of endoscopy and lowest mortality (12,500 patients)	
Hemodynamically stable and ASA 1–2:	0–36 h
Hemodynamically stable and ASA 3–5:	12–36 h
Hemodynamically unstable and ASA 1–5:	6–24 h

The optimal timing of an upper endoscopy for a patient with upper GI bleeding is controversial. In general, emergency medicine clinicians and gastroenterologists must work together to weigh the safety, cost, and availability of emergent or early endoscopy versus next-day endoscopy for admitted patients. With no high-quality randomized controlled studies to answer this question, evidence is based on retrospective reviews and observational studies. Adding complexity to this issue is that the term "early" refers to different time frames throughout the literature, including less than 6 hours, 12 hours, or 24 hours [1].

Current specialty guidelines by the American Society of Gastrointestinal Endoscopy (ASGE) and the European Society of Gastrointestinal Endoscopy (ESGE) recommend further workup for all GIB patients within 24 hours except those with the lowest risk [1]. In this time frame, endoscopy has been shown to be safe for all risk groups and has been associated with reduced hospital length of stay and decreased transfusion requirements [2–5].

An early endoscopy may reduce mortality in the critically ill patients from GIB. In patients with a Glasgow Blatchford Score (GBS) greater than 12, endoscopy performed within 12 hours from presentation was associated with a reduction

in all-cause mortality [6]. In another study of 10,000 patients, decreased mortality was associated with early endoscopy for patients who were unstable and had significant comorbidities [7]. In this study, patients with high acuity and high American Society of Anesthesia scores (e.g., a marker of health status) appeared to benefit from endoscopy performed within 6–24 hours from presentation. The observation that the optimal time window appeared to be after 6 hours suggests endoscopy is ideally performed after a brief period of resuscitation in this subset of patients (Table 13.1).

Summary

In general, for stable patients with non-variceal hemorrhage, delaying endoscopy is unlikely to be associated with increased mortality but may be associated with a longer length of stay, increased cost, and more blood transfusions. For unstable patients and patients with significant comorbidities, the timing of endoscopy requires a collaborative discussion between the emergency medicine providers who lead the resuscitative efforts and the gastroenterologists who lead the hemostatic efforts. Urgent endoscopy may be considered in patients who are hemodynamically unstable, anticoagulated, or with persistent bloody emesis.

© Springer Nature Switzerland AG 2019
A. Graham, D. J. Carlberg (eds.), *Gastrointestinal Emergencies*, https://doi.org/10.1007/978-3-319-98343-1_13

References

1. British Society of Gastroenterology Endoscopy Committee. Nonvariceal upper gastrointestinal haemorrhage: guidelines. Gut. 2002;51(Suppl 4):iv1–6.
2. Lin HJ, Wang K, Perng CL, et al. Early or delayed endoscopy for patients with peptic ulcer bleeding. A prospective randomized study. J Clin Gastroenterol. 1996;22(4):267–71.
3. Kumar NL, Cohen AJ, Nayor J, Claggett BL, Saltzman JR. Timing of upper endoscopy influences outcomes in patients with acute nonvariceal upper GI bleeding. Gastrointest Endosc. 2017;85(5):945–952.e1.
4. Kumar NL, Travis AC, Saltzman JR. Initial management and timing of endoscopy in nonvariceal upper GI bleeding. Gastrointest Endosc. 2016;84(1):10–7.
5. Sarin N, Monga N, Adams PC. Time to endoscopy and outcomes in upper gastrointestinal bleeding. Can J Gastroenterol. 2009;23(7):489–93.
6. Lim LG, Ho KY, Chan YH, et al. Urgent endoscopy is associated with lower mortality in high-risk but not low-risk nonvariceal upper gastrointestinal bleeding. Endoscopy. 2011;43(4):300–6.
7. Laursen SB, Leontiadis GI, Stanley AJ, Møller MH, Hansen JM, Schaffalitzky de Muckadell OB. Relationship between timing of endoscopy and mortality in patients with peptic ulcer bleeding: a nationwide cohort study. Gastrointest Endosc. 2017;85(5):936–944.e3.

Further Reading

Barkun A. What is the ideal timing for endoscopy in acute upper gastrointestinal bleeding? Endosc Int Open. 2017;5(5):E387–8.

What Medications Are Helpful in Treating a GIB?

14

Anita Kumar, Maxine Le Saux, and Andrew C. Meltzer

Pearls and Pitfalls
- Proton-pump inhibitors can downstage the grade of a bleeding peptic ulcer.
- Tranexamic acid may be a helpful adjunct for patients with uncontrolled bleeding.
- Octreotide decreases portal pressures thereby reducing bleeding in variceal hemorrhage.
- Metoclopramide and erythromycin may improve visualization during endoscopy.
- Antibiotics should be used in cirrhotic patients with ascites and GI bleeding.

Proton-Pump Inhibitors

Proton-pump inhibitors (PPIs) are the cornerstone of pharmacological management in patients with an upper gastrointestinal (GI) bleed. Proton-pump inhibitors work by suppressing gastric acid production at the parietal cells. The recommended dose of the IV PPI pantoprazole is 80 mg bolus followed by 8 mg/hour infusion [1].

Initiating PPIs prior to endoscopy lessens the stigmata of recent hemorrhage and reduces the risk of further bleeding [1]. Intravenous PPI treatment has not been shown to reduce mortality or rebleeding [2]. Other pre-endoscopic

A. Kumar, MD
George Washington University School of Medicine & Health Sciences, Department of Medicine, Division of Gastroenterology, Washington, DC, USA
e-mail: akumar@mfa.gwu.edu

M. Le Saux · A. C. Meltzer, MD, MS (✉)
Department of Emergency Medicine, George Washington University School of Medicine & Health Sciences, Washington, DC, USA
e-mail: ameltzer@mfa.gwu.edu

medications, such as histamine H2 antagonists, are not recommended for patients with acute bleeding ulcers.

Octreotide

If a variceal hemorrhage is suspected, octreotide, a somatostatin analog, should be started and continued for 3–5 days after confirmation of diagnosis [3]. The usual dosage of octreotide is a 50 mcg IV bolus followed by a continuous infusion of 50 mcg/hour. Octreotide reduces bleeding but has an uncertain effect on mortality. As a first-line therapy, somatostatin analogues are as effective as emergency sclerotherapy [4].

In non-variceal hemorrhage, no definitive studies have demonstrated a benefit from octreotide in terms of need for endoscopic therapy or mortality. Similar to PPIs, octreotide should not be a substitute for an emergent EGD but can be considered prior to EGD in a patient with either variceal or non-variceal hemorrhage [5].

Vasopressin

Vasopressin promotes splanchnic vasoconstriction. Current evidence is insufficient to recommend vasopressin in professional organization guidelines. Terlipressin has been shown to be helpful in patients with end-stage renal disease (ESRD) by stimulating the release of von Willebrand factor [6, 7].

Erythromycin and Metoclopramide

Prokinetic drugs such as erythromycin or metoclopramide given prior to endoscopy improve visualization during endoscopy [8]. Pre-procedural erythromycin is associated with an increased incidence of an empty stomach during

© Springer Nature Switzerland AG 2019
A. Graham, D. J. Carlberg (eds.), *Gastrointestinal Emergencies*, https://doi.org/10.1007/978-3-319-98343-1_14

endoscopy, a decreased need for a second look endoscopy, as well as a decreased need for blood transfusion and a shorter length of hospital stay [9].

Tranexamic Acid

Tranexamic acid (TXA) is an antifibrinolytic agent. This drug reduces the breakdown of fibrin; fibrin provides the framework for the formation of a blood clot, which is needed to stop bleeding. TXA has been shown to improve outcomes in postpartum hemorrhage and trauma. Tranexamic acid may also improve outcomes in upper gastrointestinal bleeding. In a Cochrane review of over 1700 patients in 8 studies, there was a reduction in mortality compared to placebo in patients with upper GI bleeding, citing a relative risk of 0.6 (95% CI: 0.42–0.87.) [10].

Antibiotics

In addition to vasogenic and pro-motility drugs, short-term antibiotic prophylaxis should be started in the emergency room for patients with known cirrhosis and any type of GI bleeding. Recommended antibiotics for most patients include ciprofloxacin 400 mg IV daily or ceftriaxone 1 g/day IV [3]. Antibiotic prophylaxis with norfloxacin 400 mg orally twice daily may reduce mortality and bacterial infection in cirrhotic inpatients with gastrointestinal bleeding [3].

Summary

Recommended in Non-Variceal GIB Patients:
- Metoclopramide or erythromycin to improve EGD visualization
- Protonix 80 mg IV then 8 mg/hour infusion

Recommended in Patients with Variceal Bleeding:
- TXA if there is evidence of coagulopathy and/or the patient has cirrhosis (as these patients have excess fibrinolysis)

- Broad-spectrum antibiotics
- Octreotide – 50 mcg IV bolus followed by a continuous infusion 50 mcg/hour

Suggested Resource
- https://emergencymedicinecases.com/gi-bleed-emergencies-part-1/.The NNT. Prophylactic Antibiotics for Cirrhotics with Upper GI Bleed.The NNT. Somatostatin Analogues (Octreotide) for Acute Variceal Bleeding.

References

1. Laine L, Jensen DM. Management of patients with ulcer bleeding. Am J Gastroenterol. 2012;107(3):345–60.
2. Sreedharan A, Martin J, Leontiadis GI, et al. Proton pump inhibitor treatment initiated prior to endoscopic diagnosis in upper gastrointestinal bleeding. Cochrane Database Syst Rev. 2010;7:CD005415.
3. Garcia-Tsao G, Bosch J. Management of varices and variceal hemorrhage in cirrhosis. N Engl J Med [Internet]. 2010;362(9):823–32. Available from:. https://doi.org/10.1056/NEJMra0901512.
4. Jaramillo JL, de la Mata M, Miño G, Cóstan G, Gomez-Camacho F. Somatostatin versus Sengstaken balloon tamponade for primary haemostasia of bleeding esophageal varices: a randomized pilot study. J Hepatol. 1991;12(1):100–5.
5. Ahmad S, Le V, Kaitha S, Morton J, Ali T. Nasogastric tube feedings and gastric residual volume: a regional survey. South Med J. 2012;105(8):394–8.
6. Cremers I, Ribeiro S. Management of variceal and nonvariceal upper gastrointestinal bleeding in patients with cirrhosis. Therap Adv Gastroenterol. 2014;7(5):206–16.
7. Ioannou GN, Doust J, Rockey DC. Terlipressin for acute esophageal variceal hemorrhage [Internet]. In: Cochrane Database of Systematic Reviews. 2003. Available from: https://doi.org/10.1002/14651858.CD002147.
8. Barkun AN, Bardou M, Kuipers EJ, et al. International consensus recommendations on the management of patients with nonvariceal upper gastrointestinal bleeding. Ann Intern Med. 2010;152(2):101.
9. Bai Y, Guo JF, Li ZS. Meta-analysis: erythromycin before endoscopy for acute upper gastrointestinal bleeding. Aliment Pharmacol Ther. 2011;34(2):166–71.
10. Bennett C, Klingenberg S, Langholz E, Gluud L. Tranexamic acid for upper gastrointestinal bleeding. Cochrane Database of Syst Rev. 2014;11:CD006640.

What Is the Optimal Resuscitation of the Patient with a Gastrointestinal Bleed?

15

Kathleen Ogle and Andrew C. Meltzer

Pearls and Pitfalls
- Resuscitation including airway support, volume management, and increasing oxygen-carrying capacity to limit end-organ injury is the priority when treating a gastrointestinal (GI) hemorrhage.
- Early risk stratification to assess for likely the need for transfusion or surgery as well as risk of rebleeding will help clinicians identify the subset of patients most likely to benefit from aggressive resuscitation and close observation.
- Improved survival has been shown to be associated with a "restrictive strategy" of blood transfusion for hemoglobin levels <7 gm/L.

As with all critically ill patients, early assessment begins with the *A*, *B*, *C*s: airway, breathing, and circulation. Once hemodynamic stability has been established, a thorough history and secondary survey should be conducted with specific questions regarding prior episodes of bleeding, including the amount of blood and color of the blood. However, it should be noted that a patient's assessment of blood loss is frequently inaccurate [1]. Comorbidities such as congestive heart failure, renal disease, liver disease, or vascular disease increase overall mortality risk and help determine the source of bleeding. Recent vascular surgery raises the risk for an aorto-enteric fistula, a particularly severe cause of upper GI hemorrhage [2]. Finally, medications such as steroids, non-steroidal anti-inflammatory drugs, and anticoagulants also increase the risk of bleeding. Patients should be examined for signs of liver failure that might indicate that the bleed is a variceal source. Stigmata of liver disease include vascular collaterals (caput medusa), ascites, asterixis, gynecomastia, hepatomegaly, jaundice, scleral icterus, vascular spiders (spider telangiectasias, spider angiomata), and splenomegaly.

Airway and Breathing

In the setting of GI hemorrhage, airway control is especially important because aspiration of vomited blood is associated with significant morbidity and mortality [3]. The placement of an advanced airway may be indicated in cases of profuse vomiting or altered mental status. Rapid sequence intubation, a method of intubation that quickly induces unconsciousness and paralysis, is the ideal method to perform endotracheal intubation because the reduced time under sedation prior to intubation is associated with a reduced risk of aspiration.

Intubating patients who are actively vomiting blood can be difficult to accomplish. There are several options to help maximize the chance of success per expert opinion. One method to increase first-pass success in the hematemesis patient was described by Dr. Scott Weingart. Dr. Weingart recommends that the clinician first insert a Salem sump or nasogastric tube to aspirate the stomach contents. Second, intubate the patient with head-of-bed at 45 degrees to keep the gastric contents from moving up the esophagus. Third, use paralytic agents in order to optimize first-pass success [6].

Another method of airway management in the actively vomiting GI bleed patient described in the literature is the SALAD (suction-assisted laryngoscopy airway decontamination) method. This technique requires a continuous suction catheter to be inserted into the patient's esophagus, where it will remain through the rest of the intubation attempt. The suction catheter may collect the vomit that will otherwise fill the mouth and obscure the view [9].

K. Ogle · A. C. Meltzer (✉)
Department of Emergency Medicine, George Washington University School of Medicine & Health Sciences, Washington, DC, USA
e-mail: kogle@mfa.gwu.edu; ameltzer@mfa.gwu.edu

© Springer Nature Switzerland AG 2019
A. Graham, D. J. Carlberg (eds.), *Gastrointestinal Emergencies*, https://doi.org/10.1007/978-3-319-98343-1_15

Circulation

Circulatory or hemodynamic status is assessed with blood pressure, heart rate, and signs of end-organ hypoperfusion, such as altered mental status, increased capillary refill, decreased urine output, and elevated lactate. Emergency department providers should consider that elderly patients and patients on hypertensive medications may not become tachycardic in response to volume loss. An abnormal change in vital signs measured while the patient is in a lying, sitting, and standing position ("orthostatics") will support the presence of volume loss and augment the information gathered from standard vital signs; however, orthostatics are only sensitive for large blood loss (630–1100 ml) [7]. Potential volume loss should be addressed with two large-bore (16 g or 18 g) intravenous angio-catheters to enable fluid resuscitation and targeted blood transfusion.

Crystalloid Fluids

The initial fluid replacement is typically crystalloid, and a complete blood count, metabolic panel, coagulation panel, and type and screen should be ordered with initial intravenous access. However, in patients with signs of hypovolemia and GI bleeding, transfusion should be started early on in resuscitative efforts. For a patient who recently lost a large volume of the blood and has signs of hypovolemia, the hemoglobin will not reflect the actual blood loss. Two units of packed red blood cells are typically given early in the resuscitation. For patients who are actively bleeding and appear to have signs of hypovolemic shock, a massive transfusion protocol similar to that developed in military and trauma research should be initiated [8]. A massive transfusion protocol typically involves a 1:1:1 transfusion of red blood cells, fresh frozen plasma, and platelets [9].

Restrictive Versus Liberal Transfusion

Once a patient is no longer actively extravasating and blood pressure stabilizes, there is evidence that less aggressive transfusion strategies provide a mortality benefit for many patients with acute bleeding. The physiological explanation is that aggressive blood transfusion leads to an increase in portal hypertension and a subsequent increase in bleeding [4]. A randomized controlled study of 921 patients compared the efficacy and safety of using a restrictive approach versus a liberal

approach to blood transfusion [5]. The restrictive group, in whom transfusion occurred if hemoglobin was within a 7.0–9.0 g/dL range, required less total transfusions (51% vs. 14%, $p < 0.05$), demonstrated less rebleeding (16% vs. 10%, $P < 0.05$), and had lower mortality (5% vs. 9%, $p < 0.05$) than the liberal transfusion group, in whom transfusion was initiated if hemoglobin was within a 9.0–11.0 g/dL range [5].

The established quality indicators for early management of GI hemorrhage revolve around rapid diagnosis, risk stratification, and early management. Effective pre-endoscopic treatment may improve survivability of the critically ill patient and improve resource allocation for all patients. Early management prior to the definitive endoscopy is essential to improving outcomes for patients with GI bleeding.

> **Suggested Resource**
> - https://lifeinthefastlane.com/ccc/suction-assisted-laryngoscopy-airway-decontamination-salad/.

References

1. Oliwa N, Mort TC. Is a rapid sequence intubation always indicated for emergency airway management of the upper GI bleeding patient? Crit Care Med. 2005;33:A97.
2. Strote J, Mayo M, Townes D. ED patient estimation of blood loss. Am J Emerg Med. 2009;27(6):709–11.
3. Rubin M, Hussain SA, Shalomov A, Cortes RA, Smith MS, Kim SH. Live view video capsule endoscopy enables risk stratification of patients with acute upper GI bleeding in the emergency room: a pilot study. Dig Dis Sci. 2011;56(3):786–91.
4. Hébert PC, Wells G, Blajchman MA, et al. A multicenter, randomized, controlled clinical trial of transfusion requirements in critical care. N Engl J Med. 1999;340(6):409–17.
5. Villanueva C, Colomo A, Bosch A, et al. Transfusion strategies for acute upper gastrointestinal bleeding. N Engl J Med. 2013;368(1):11–21.
6. Weingart S. EMCrit Podcast 5 – Intubating the Critical GI Bleeder. EMCrit Blog. Published on June 21, 2009. Accessed on 10 May 2018. Available at: https://emcrit.org/emcrit/intubating-gi-bleeds/.
7. McGee S, et al. The rational clinical examination. Is this patient hypovolemic. JAMA. 1999;281(11):1022–9.
8. DuCanto J, Serrano KD, Thompson RJ. Novel airway training tool that simulates vomiting: suction-assisted laryngoscopy assisted decontamination (SALAD) system. West J Emerg Med. 2017;18(1):117–20. https://doi.org/10.5811/westjem.2016.9.30891.
9. Borgman MA, Spinella PC, Perkins JG, Grathwohl KW, Repine T, Beekley AC, Sebesta J, et al. The ratio of blood products transfused affects mortality in patients receiving massive transfusions at a combat support hospital. J Trauma. 2007;63:805–13.

Reversing Coagulopathy in Patients with Suspected GI Bleed

16

Kathleen Ogle and Andrew C. Meltzer

Pearls and Pitfalls
- Oral vitamin K reversal takes approximately 24 h; parenteral vitamin K reversal occurs after 4–6 h.
- Transfuse platelets in patients taking antiplatelet therapy or with thrombocytopenia, platelet count <50,000.
- PCC may be the preferred choice for patients with active bleeding who have an INR > 2.0 and are candidates for urgent surgery or endoscopy.
- Only one DOAC, dabigatran, currently has a specific reversal agent to stop bleeding.
- Severe bleeding in patients taking DOAC may also be improved with hemodialysis.

Patients who present to the ED with an upper GI hemorrhage, while anticoagulated, are in urgent need of reversal to stop the bleeding. Endoscopic intervention is less likely to be successful in patients for whom the INR is greater than 2.5 [1]. The major risk of anticoagulation reversal is thromboembolic complications which occur 1–5% of the time. Unfortunately, oral vitamin K reversal takes approximately 24 h, and parenteral vitamin K reversal occurs 4–6 h after initiation of treatment [2]. Fresh frozen plasma (FFP) does reverse the effects of warfarin almost immediately; however, its use is limited by the fact that FFP must be thawed prior to administration. FPP also carries the risk of transmission of disease and risk of volume overload in patients with congestive heart failure or renal disease.

Prothrombin complex concentrate (PCC) is generally preferred to FFP. PCC contains the vitamin K-dependent coagulation factors II, VII, IX, and X that are deficient in patients on warfarin therapy. PCC may be the preferred choice for patients with active bleeding who have an INR > 2.0 and are candidates for urgent surgery [3, 4]. The most serious adverse outcome associated with PCC is also thromboembolic events, albeit a rare event [1, 5, 6]. Cost of PCC is a limiting factor at some centers. PCC (Kcentra) is the four-factor prothrombin complex concentrate approved by the FDA and is significantly more expensive than FFP, leading some institutions to adopt the less expensive product. Another limitation of PCC is that it lacks fibrinogen which is required to maintain clotting. For patients with massive hemorrhage, fibrinogen can be supplemented by FFP or cryoprecipitate. Following normalization of the INR with PCC or FFP, vitamin K should be administered to maintain reversal of anticoagulation. PCC can be dosed at a standard dose of 1500 units for adult patients or weight based at 25 units/kilogram.

Direct oral anticoagulants (DOACs) have becoming more common due to their stable pharmacokinetics compared to warfarin. Examples of DOAC medications include apixaban (Eliquis), dabigatran (Pradaxa), rivaroxaban (Xarelto), and edoxaban (Savaysa). Both dabigatran, a direct thrombin inhibitor, and rivaroxaban, a direct factor Xa inhibitor, may be used to treat thromboembolic disease and can be dosed without regular blood monitoring. DOACs tend to have no response to protamine or vitamin K [7]. In addition, there is no standardized way to measure the anticoagulant effect of most DOACs [1]. Some studies are exploring the use of thromboelastography as a guide to measuring anticoagulant effect [8, 9].

In patients who present with GI bleeding and are taking DOACs, PCCs may be effective for reversal. There is limited evidence that PCC improves outcomes in patients with active hemorrhage. PCCs may also be used for reversal in patients who have taken edoxaban and rivaroxaban, according to evidence published in 2011 and 2015, respectively [10, 11].

Idarucizumab is the only agent to have received FDA approval for reversal of the DOAC, dabigatran. Idarucizumab is a monoclonal antibody that binds dabigatran, with about

K. Ogle, MD · A. C. Meltzer, MD, MS (✉)
Department of Emergency Medicine, George Washington University School of Medicine & Health Sciences, Washington, DC, USA
e-mail: kogle@mfa.gwu.edu; ameltzer@mfa.gwu.edu

© Springer Nature Switzerland AG 2019
A. Graham, D. J. Carlberg (eds.), *Gastrointestinal Emergencies*, https://doi.org/10.1007/978-3-319-98343-1_16

350 times the avidity with which dabigatran binds to thrombin, and completely reverses the anticoagulant effect of dabigatran within minutes [12]. Several new reversal agents for DOACs are under development [5].

Suggested Resources
- EMCRIT: New reversal agents for new antico-agulants. https://emcrit.org/emcrit/new-reversals-agents-for-new-anticoagulants/.
- HIPPOED: Massive GI Bleed. https://www.hip-poed.com/em/ercast/episode/massivegibleed/may2018massive.
- Samuelson BT, Cuker A. Measurement and reversal of the direct oral anticoagulants. Blood Rev. 2017;31(1): 77–84.

References

1. Gralnek I, Dumonceau J-M, Kuipers E, et al. Diagnosis and management of nonvariceal upper gastrointestinal hemorrhage: European Society of Gastrointestinal Endoscopy (ESGE) guide-line. Endoscopy. 2015;47(10):a1–46.
2. Pollack CV. Managing bleeding in anticoagulated patients in the emergency care setting. J Emerg Med. 2013;45(3):467–77.
3. Lankiewicz MW, Hays J, Friedman KD, Tinkoff G, Blatt PM. Urgent reversal of warfarin with prothrombin complex con-centrate. J Thromb Haemost. 2006;4(5):967–70.
4. Hickey M, Gatien M, Taljaard M, Aujnarain A, Giulivi A, Perry JJ. Outcomes of urgent warfarin reversal with frozen plasma versus prothrombin complex concentrate in the emergency department. Circulation. 2013;128(4):360–4.
5. Dentali F, Marchesi C, Pierfranceschi MG, et al. Safety of prothrombin complex concentrates for rapid anticoagula-tion reversal of vitamin K antagonists. Thromb Haemost. 2011;106(3):429–38.
6. Radaelli F, Dentali F, Repici A, et al. Management of anticoagula-tion in patients with acute gastrointestinal bleeding. Dig Liver Dis. 2015;47(8):621–7.
7. Johansen M, Wikkelsø A, Lunde J, Wetterslev J, Afshari A. Prothrombin complex concentrate for reversal of vitamin K antagonist treatment in bleeding and non-bleeding patients. Cochrane Database Syst Rev. 2015;7:CD010555.
8. Dias JD, Norem K, Doorneweerd DD, Thurer RL, Popovsky MA, Omert LA. Use of thromboelastography (TEG) for detection of new oral anticoagulants. Arch Pathol Lab Med. 2015;139(5): 665–73.
9. Samuelson BT, Cuker A. Measurement and reversal of the direct oral anticoagulants. Blood Rev. 2017;31(1):77–84. https://doi.org/10.1016/j.blre.2016.08.006.
10. Zahir H, Brown KS, Vandell AG, et al. Edoxaban effects on bleed-ing following punch biopsy and reversal by a 4-factor prothrombin complex concentrate. Circulation. 2015;131(1):82–90.
11. Eerenberg ES, Kamphuisen PW, Sijpkens MK, Meijers JC, Buller HR, Levi M. Reversal of rivaroxaban and dabigatran by pro-thrombin complex concentrate: a randomized, placebo-controlled, crossover study in healthy subjects. Circulation. 2011;124(14): 1573–9.
12. Pollack CV, Reilly PA, Eikelboom J, et al. Idarucizumab for Dabigatran Reversal. N Engl J Med. 2015;373(6):511–20.

When to Suspect an Aortoenteric Fistulae

17

Anita Kumar, Maxine Le Saux, and Andrew C. Meltzer

Pearls and Pitfalls
- Aortoenteric fistulas are rare but life-threatening.
- This condition is often preceded by a "herald bleed."
- In patients with a history of prior abdominal aortic surgery, providers should consider aortoenteric fistulas as a cause of GI bleeding.
- CT angiography can diagnose aortoenteric fistulas.

Aortoenteric fistulas are rare but have a high mortality. Mortality ranges from 33% to 43%, and advanced age is a predictor of increased mortality [1, 2]. There are two types of aortoenteric fistulas, primary and secondary. About 10% of primary aortoenteric fistulas present with the classical triad of gastrointestinal bleeding, abdominal pain, and a pulsating mass [3]. Primary aortoenteric fistulas are caused by arteriosclerosis, aortic aneurysms, or aortic infections. Secondary aortoenteric fistulas are a complication of an aortic repair with a synthetic graft. Occasionally, an aortoenteric fistula can develop due to a retained esophageal foreign body [4].

A. Kumar, MD
George Washington University School of Medicine & Health Sciences, Department of Medicine, Division of Gastroenterology, Washington, DC, USA
e-mail: abkumar@mfa.gwu.edu

M. Le Saux · A. C. Meltzer, MD, MS (✉)
Department of Emergency Medicine, George Washington University School of Medicine & Health Sciences, Washington, DC, USA
e-mail: mlesaux@mfa.gwu.edu; ameltzer@mfa.gwu.edu

What Is a Herald Bleed?

A herald bleed refers to a minor intermittent GI bleed that precedes massive hemorrhage from an aortoenteric fistula. In 50% of aortoenteric fistula cases, patients present initially with a herald bleed. Primary fistulas are more likely than secondary aortoenteric fistulas to present with repetitive gastrointestinal bleeds such as herald bleeds as opposed to an initial massive hemorrhage [3, 5].

How Do We Diagnose an Aortoenteric Fistula?

Multiple case reports have described the challenges of diagnosing an aortoenteric fistula and the life-threatening nature of the disease [3]. Due to its low incidence, diagnosis is often delayed. Patients are often misdiagnosed with more common causes of GI bleeding or flank pain [6]. A history of prior aortic surgery and GI bleeding, particularly severe GI bleedings with no source of bleeding found on endoscopy, should raise suspicion for an aortoenteric fistula [3]. Since most aortoenteric fistulas occur at the level of the distal duodenum or the jejunum, they are beyond the reach of a standard upper endoscope.

When there is clinical suspicion, diagnosis is typically made by performing a CT scan with intravenous contrast [7]. CT scans are reported to have a high specificity but moderate sensitivity for aortoenteric fistulas [8]. The presence of intravascular contrast material in the GI tract is highly specific. In addition, the presence of periaortic ectopic gas in the context of GI blood loss is highly specific for aortoenteric fistula. Following diagnosis, an emergent surgical consultation is required for repair which can increase survival rates.

© Springer Nature Switzerland AG 2019
A. Graham, D. J. Carlberg (eds.), *Gastrointestinal Emergencies*, https://doi.org/10.1007/978-3-319-98343-1_17

Suggested Resources
- Aortoenteric fistula: Recognition and management – UpToDate.
- https://coreem.net/core/abdominal-aortic-aneurysm/.
- Primary Aortoduodenal Fistula: First you Should Suspect it – NCBI – NIH.

References

1. Batt M, Jean-Baptiste E, O'Connor S, et al. Early and late results of contemporary management of 37 secondary Aortoenteric fistulae. Eur J Vasc Endovasc Surg. 2011;41(6):748–57.
2. Busuttil SJ, Goldstone J. Diagnosis and management of aortoenteric fistulas. Semin Vasc Surg. 2001;14(4):302–11.
3. Saers SJF, Scheltinga MRM. Primary aortoenteric fistula. Br J Surg. 2005;92(2):143–52.
4. Zhang X, Liu J, Li J, et al. Diagnosis and treatment of 32 cases with aortoesophageal fistula due to esophageal foreign body. Laryngoscope. 2011;121(2):267–72.
5. Deijen CL, Smulders YM, Coveliers HME, Wisselink W, Rauwerda JA, Hoksbergen AWJ. The importance of early diagnosis and treatment of patients with aortoenteric fistulas presenting with herald bleeds. Ann Vasc Surg. 2016;36:28–34.
6. Simó Alari F, Molina González E, Gutierrez I, Ahamdanech-Idrissi A. Secondary aortoduodenal fistula and the unrecognised herald bleed. BMJ Case Rep. 2017;2017:bcr-2017–220186.
7. Sipe A, McWilliams SR, Saling L, Raptis C, Mellnick V, Bhalla S. The red connection: a review of aortic and arterial fistulae with an emphasis on CT findings. Emerg Radiol. 2017;24(1):73–80.
8. Hughes FM, Kavanagh D, Barry M, Owens A, MacErlaine DP, Malone DE. Aortoenteric fistula: a diagnostic dilemma. Abdom Imaging. 2007;32(3):398–402.

18

End-Stage Liver Disease and Variceal Bleeding

Autumn Graham and Andrew C. Meltzer

Pearls and Pitfalls
- By the time patients have ascites associated with their liver dysfunction, 60% have varices on EGD.
- Nasogastric tube placement is likely safe in patients with varices, but risks and benefits should be carefully weighed and discussed with patient.
- Risk factors associated with early re-bleeding and poor outcomes include severe initial bleeding as defined by a hemoglobin less than 8 g/dL, gastric variceal bleeding, thrombocytopenia, encephalopathy, alcohol-related cirrhosis, large varices, and active bleeding during endoscopy.
- Antibiotics have a proven benefit in variceal bleeding with decreased morbidity and mortality.

Cirrhosis occurs when damage to the liver results in scar tissue (hepatic fibrosis), affecting liver function. Cirrhosis is the third leading cause of death in patients between the ages of 45 years and 64 years, with a median survival of 9–12 years after diagnosis. In the United States, end-stage liver disease is most often due to hepatitis C infections [1]. Gastrointestinal bleeding in patients with cirrhosis is common and carries a high mortality rate of approximately 15–30% [2–4].

A. Graham
Department of Emergency Medicine, MedStar Washington Hospital Center, MedStar Georgetown University Hospital, Washington, DC, USA

A. C. Meltzer (✉)
Department of Emergency Medicine, George Washington University School of Medicine & Health Sciences, Washington, DC, USA
e-mail: ameltzer@mfa.gwu.edu

When Should I Suspect Esophagogastric Varices in a Patient with a History of Liver Disease?

Portal hypertension is defined as a hepatic venous pressure gradient greater than 5 mmHg and occurs due to increased structural resistance and decreased endogenous nitric oxide production [5]. Esophagogastric varices develop when the hepatic venous pressure gradient (HPVG) rises above 10 mmHg.

By the time cirrhosis is diagnosed or suspected based on stigmata of chronic liver disease (e.g., spider angiomas, jaundice, pruritis, palmar erythema) and laboratory abnormalities, approximately 30–40% of patients will have varices [3]. The American College of Gastroenterology (ACG) recommends screening esophagogastroduodenoscopy (EGD) at time of cirrhosis diagnosis; thus, many patients with a diagnosis of cirrhosis will know if they have varices [5]. Of those without varices at the time of diagnosis, another 10–15% will develop varices each year [3]. By the time patients have ascites associated with their liver dysfunction, 60% have varices on EGD [3]. In advanced disease (e.g., Child-Pugh C), 85% of patients have varices [5, 6].

Once varices are present, portal hypertension causes them to grow in size by approximately 7% each year [4]. The size of varices directly correlates with the risk of bleeding: 1–2% without varices, 5% with small varices, and 15% with medium or large (>5 mm) varices [3, 5]. When patients present with gastrointestinal bleeding and have a history of varices, 70% of cases are due to ruptured esophageal varices, usually at the GE junction [3, 5].

Can I Place a Nasogastric Tube (NGT) in Patients with Esophagogastric Varices?

Traditional dogma would suggest that blind placement of nasogastric tubes for nasogastric aspiration (NGA) or nasogastric lavage (NGL) is unsafe in the advanced liver disease patient with varices. Unfortunately, there is little literature published on this topic. In a couple small retrospective series (~100 patients total) of liver transplantation candidates with varices who had NGT placement, there were no incidents of gastrointestinal bleeding due to the procedure. Many of these patients were noted to have medium to large varices, prior variceal bleeding, and significant coagulopathies [7, 8]. Despite its probable safety, the decision to place an NGT for aspiration or lavage requires a careful assessment of the potential risks (e.g., bleeding, pain, aspiration, unclear prognostic and outcome value) and benefits (e.g., localization of bleed and assessment of active bleeding) of the procedure.

Which Clinical Prognosis Score Is Best in Patients with Esophageal Varices?

While both the clinical Rockall score and Glasgow Blatchford score (GBS) take into account the increased risk in patients with liver disease, neither was developed specifically to predict prognosis in variceal bleeding. In 1 study of 178 patients with cirrhosis and variceal hemorrhaging, the overall mortality was 16% at 6 weeks, with deaths due to uncontrolled bleeding (31%), liver failure (28%), or sepsis with multiorgan failure (41%). In this study, MELD (see Table 18.1) outperformed Child-Pugh (see Table 18.2) in discriminating patients at high risk of death at 6 weeks after a variceal bleeding episode [9]. In

Table 18.1 MELD score (model for end-stage liver disease)

If unknown score: (initial score)
MELD(i) = 0.957 × ln(Cr) + 0.378 × ln(bilirubin) + 1.120 × ln(INR) + 0.643
If known score:
MELD = MELD(i) + 1.32 × (137 − Na) − [0.033 × MELD(i) × (137 − Na)]
Helpful hints:
All values in US units (Cr and bilirubin in mg/dL, Na in mEq/L, and INR unitless).
If bilirubin, Cr, or INR is <1.0, use 1.0
If any of the following is true, use Cr 4.0:
Cr >4.0
≥2 dialysis treatments within the prior 7 days
24 h of continuous veno-venous hemodialysis (CVVHD) within the prior 7 days
If Na <125 mmol/L, use 125. If Na >137 mmol/L, use 137
MAX MELD SCORE = 40

Interpretation: Prediction of 6-week mortality	
MELD >19	20% mortality rate at 6 weeks
MELD <11	5% mortality rate at 6 weeks

Reverter et al. [9]

Table 18.2 Child-Pugh score

	1 point	2 point	3 point
Serum albumin	> 35 g/dL	28–35 g/dL	< 28 g/dL
Total bilirubin	< 34 umol/L	34–50 umol/L	> 50 umol/L
PT INR	< 1.7	1.71–2.3	> 2.3
Ascites	None	Mild	Moderate to severe
Hepatic encephalopathy	None	Grades I–II Suppressed with medication	Grades III–IV Refractory

Interpretation of Child-Pugh score and mortality rate, not specifically related to variceal bleeding

Child-Pugh class A (5–6 points)	100% 1 year survival
Child-Pugh class B (7–9 points)	80% 1 year survival
Child-Pugh class C (10–15 points)	45% 1 year survival

another small study of 47 patients that compared MELD, Child-Pugh, and GBS, GBS was superior to Child-Pugh and MELD scores for predicting 1 week mortality, but the MELD score was superior at predicting 6-week mortality [10].

Given the high risk of significant bleeding and coagulopathy associated with advanced liver disease, the ACG recommends patients with variceal bleeding be admitted to intensive care units for close observation and balanced resuscitation [5]. Risk factors associated with early re-bleeding and poor outcomes include severe initial bleeding as defined by a hemoglobin less than 8 g/dL, gastric variceal bleeding, thrombocytopenia, encephalopathy, alcohol-related cirrhosis, large varices, and active bleeding during endoscopy [4].

What Pharmacologic Treatments Are Beneficial for Variceal Bleeding?

Antibiotics have a proven benefit in variceal bleeding with decreased morbidity and mortality. Vasoactive medications such as terlipressin (not available in US), octreotide, and somatostatin have all been studied and found to have varied levels of benefit in variceal bleeding. In a meta-analysis of 30 trials, vasoactive agents were associated with lower 1-week mortality, improved hemostasis, lower transfusion requirements, and shorter hospitalization stays. The risk of adverse events with these treatments is unclear. It is worth noting that in this analysis, there was no difference in mortality or re-bleeding between vasoactive agents [11].

Antibiotics

Concomitant infections are found in 30–40% of patients with variceal bleeding and are associated with increased morbidity and mortality [4]. In a study of patients with advanced cirrhosis (Child B/C) and GI hemorrhage, IV ceftriaxone (1 g/day) was more effective than oral norfloxacin in preventing bacterial infections [12]. In uncomplicated patients, fluoroquinolones (e.g., norfloxacin, ciprofloxacin) are appropriate [4].

Octreotide

In a Cochrane review of 21 studies, somatostatin and somatostatin analogues (e.g., octreotide) were associated with decreased blood transfusions (~1/2 unit per patient) but no statistically significant effect on mortality. Risk of re-bleeding was not significantly different in high-quality studies, but a more substantial decrease in re-bleeding was observed in those studies with a higher risk of bias [13]. Most octreotide regimens used a dose of 50 mcg IV bolus followed by 50 mcg/hour infusion for 5 days [13].

What Are the Keys to Resuscitation of the Patient with Variceal Bleeding?

- Airway management is critical given hepatic encephalopathy is commonly associated with gastrointestinal bleeding in cirrhotic patients, decreasing patients' ability to protect their airway.
- Volume resuscitation with blood products is a delicate balance of maintaining oxygen carrying capacity to decrease end organ injury without over-resuscitating. Over-resuscitation has been shown to worsen portal hypertension, increase re-bleeding rates, and increase mortality. In a sub-analysis of hemodynamically stable, GIB patients with cirrhosis in the Villanueva study, patients in the restrictive transfusion group were found to have lower rates of re-bleeding and death [14]. A goal hemoglobin of 8 g/dL is recommended by the ACG based on experimental studies [5].
- Aggressive resuscitation with isotonic fluids such as normal saline should be used cautiously as it may worsen ascites and extravascular fluid accumulation.
- Consideration of fresh frozen plasma (FFP) if active bleeding and INR >1.5, platelet transfusion for platelets $<50 \times 10^9$/L, or cryoprecipitate if fibrinogen <1.5 is

important but has to be weighed against contributing to portal hypertension and risk of re-bleeding [4, 6].

- Sengstaken-Blakemore/Minnesota tube placement may be employed as a bridging procedure to endoscopy.

What Is TIPS Procedure and What Should I Know About It?

Transjugular intrahepatic portosystemic shunt or TIPS procedure is a rescue therapy to prevent variceal re-bleeding when endoscopy and pharmacological treatments have failed. Interventional radiology creates an alternate circulation pathway between the inflow portal vein and outflow hepatic vein, thus decreasing the effective vascular resistance of the liver. A patient with a Child-Pugh class C is likely to have a hepatic vein pressure gradient >20 mmHg and more likely to fail standard therapy; those patients may benefit from an early TIPS procedure [4]. However, TIPS has not been shown to improve survival and is associated with an increased risk of encephalopathy [3].

Suggested Resources

- EMCRIT – Blakemore Tube Placement for Massive Upper GI Hemorrhage. 2013. https://emcrit.org/emcrit/blakemore-tube-placement/.
- EMCRIT – PulmCrit Wee: Ultrasound guided blakemore tube placement. 2016. https://emcrit.org/pulmcrit/pulmcrit-wee-ultrasound-guided-blakemore-tube-placement/.
- Emergency Medical Minute: Variceal Upper GI Bleed. https://emergencymedicalminute.com/podcast-27-variceal-upper-gi-bleed/.
- Life in the Fast Lane – Sengstaken-Blakemore and Minnesota Tubes. 2016. https://lifeinthefastlane.com/ccc/sengstaken-blakemore-and-minnesota-tubes/.
- Pulmcrit: Coagulopathy management in the bleeding cirrhotic. https://emcrit.org/pulmcrit/coagulopathy-bleeding-cirrhotic-inr/.

References

1. Kamath P, Shah V. Overview of cirrhosis. Chap 74: Sleisenger and Fordtran's gastrointestinal and liver disease. 1254–1260.e1.
2. Nable J, Graham A. Gastrointestinal bleeding. Emerg Med Clin. 2016;34(2):309–25.

3. Turan F, Casu S, Hernandez-Gea V, Garcia-Pagan J. Variceal and other portal hypertension related bleeding. Best Prac Res Clin Gastro. 2013;27:649–64.

4. Satapathy S, Sanyal A. Non-endoscopic management strategies for acute esophagogastric variceal bleeding. Gastroenterol Clin N Am. 2014;43(4):819–33.

5. Garcia-Tsao G, Sanyal A, Grace N, Carey W. Practice guidelines Committee of the American Association for the Study of liver diseases and the practice parameters Committee of the American College of Gastroenterology. Practice guidelines: Prevention and management of gastroesophageal varices and variceal hemorrhage in cirrhosis. Am J Gastroenterol. 2007;102:2086–102.

6. Haq I, Tripathi D. Recent advances in the management of variceal bleeding. Gastroenterology Rep. 2017;5(2):113–26.

7. Lopez-Torres A, Waye JD. The safety of intubation in patients with esophageal varices. Am J Dig Dis. 1973;18(12):1032–4.

8. Ritter D, Rettke S, Hughes R, Burritt M, Sterioff S, Ilstrup D. Placement of nasogastric tubes and esophageal stethoscopes in patients with documented esophageal varices. Anesth Analg. 1988;67:283–5.

9. Reverter E, Tandon P, Augustin S, Turon F, Casu S, et al. A MELD – based model to determine risk of mortality among patients with acute variceal bleeding. Gastroenterology. 2014;146:412–9.

10. Iino C, Shimoyama T, Igarashi T, Aihara T, Ishii K, Sakamoto J, Tono H, Fukuda S. Usefulness of the Glasgow Blatchford score to predict 1 week mortality in patients with esophageal variceal bleeding. Eur J Gastroenterol Hepatol. 2017;29(5):547–51.

11. Wells M, Chande N, Adams P, et al. Meta-analysis: vasoactive medications for the management of acute variceal bleeds. Aliment Pharmacol Ther. 2012;35:1267–78.

12. Fernandez J, Ruiz DA, Gomez C, Durandez R, Serradilla R, Guarner C, Planas R, Arroyo V, Navasa M. Norfloxacin vs ceftriaxone in the prophylaxis of infections in patients with advanced cirrhosis and hemorrhage. Gastroenterology. 2006;131:1049–56.

13. Gotzsche P, Hrobjartsson A. Somatostatin analogues for acute bleeding oesophageal varices. Cochrane Database Syst Rev. 2008;3:CD000193.

14. Villanueva C, Colomo A, Bosch A, et al. Transfusion strategies for acute upper gastrointestinal bleeding. N Engl J Med. 2013;368:11–21.

M. Aamir Ali

Pearls and Pitfalls
- The two determinants for an urgent gastroenterology consultation for a patient with gastrointestinal bleeding are a high suspicion for variceal bleeding and active upper gastrointestinal bleeding.
- Not all hematochezia is from lower GI bleeding.
- Transfusion with packed red blood cells should be initiated when the hemoglobin level falls below 7 g/deciliter; in patients with known cardiovascular disease, transfusion should be initiated at hemoglobin levels below 8 g/ deciliter or when symptoms develop.
- Given the low risk of short-term PPI use, this benefit warrants pre-endoscopic initiation of PPIs.

Introduction

M. Aamir Ali, M.D., specializes in gastroenterology and liver diseases. His clinical interests include colon cancer screening, gastroesophageal reflux disease, inflammatory bowel disease, and liver diseases. In addition to completing a residency in gastroenterology, Dr. Ali completed a postdoctoral fellowship in Gastrointestinal Motility at the Johns Hopkins University. He has published multiple abstracts, papers, and textbook chapters. Dr. Ali is board-certified in gastroenterology and liver diseases as well as internal medicine.

M. A. Ali
Division of Gastroenterology, George Washington University, Washington, DC, USA
e-mail: aali@mfa.gwu.edu

Answers to Key Clinical Questions

1. When do you recommend the ED consult with a gastroenterologist for upper GI hemorrhage, and when would you like to be called?

The two determinants of an urgent gastroenterology consultation for a patient with gastrointestinal bleeding are (1) a high suspicion for variceal bleeding and (2) active upper gastrointestinal bleeding.

(1) Variceal bleeding is suspected based on the following elements:

(a) History – history of cirrhosis, alcohol abuse, chronic viral hepatitis, or familial liver disease
(b) Physical findings – ascites, spider angiomas, gynecomastia, palmar erythema, caput medusae, and asterixis
(c) Laboratory evaluation – elevated transaminases, an elevated prothrombin time, or decreased albumin

(2) Active upper gastrointestinal bleeding is suspected in the setting of hematemesis and hemodynamic instability. Tachycardia, hypotension, syncope, orthostatic hypotension, and failure of these parameters to improve after volume resuscitation or blood transfusion are suggestive of active bleeding.

2. What pearls can you offer emergency care providers when evaluating patients with a suspected gastrointestinal hemorrhage?

Not all hematochezia is from lower GI bleeding. Approximately 15% of patients presenting with hematochezia have an upper GI source of bleeding. The rate of bleeding from an upper GI tract source has to be brisk to result in hematochezia; therefore, an upper GI source should be considered in any hemodynamically unstable patients presenting with hematochezia.

3. What is the role of nasogastric aspirate?

The nasogastric aspirate offers diagnostic information while clearing blood and clots from the stomach to reduce the likelihood of aspiration and to improve endoscopic visualization. Nasogastric aspiration has a high positive predictive value for active bleeding when the nasogastric aspirate expresses frank blood. However, the nasogastric aspirate is negative in up to 16% of patients having an active UGIB. While the presence of bile in the aspirate makes a false negative less likely, a negative nasogastric aspirate does not rule out an upper GI bleed source in a patient with other clinical indicators.

4. What concepts do you think are key to diagnose and manage patients with a suspected gastrointestinal hemorrhage?

Blood transfusion: In a hemodynamically stable patient who presents with GI bleeding, transfusion with packed red blood cells should be initiated when the hemoglobin level falls below 7 g/deciliter. In patients with known cardiovascular disease, transfusion should be initiated at hemoglobin levels below 8 g/ deciliter or when symptoms develop. These criteria do not apply to the hemodynamically unstable patient, as the delay in equilibration could result in the hemoglobin remaining falsely elevated despite a significant blood loss.

Proton pump inhibitors: A meta-analysis of randomized trials of PPI therapy in patients with upper gastrointestinal bleeding showed no significant difference in rates of re-bleeding, surgery, or death. However, PPI administration does reduce the likelihood of finding the types of high-risk lesions on endoscopy that would necessitate endoscopic hemostasis. Given the low risk of short-term PPI use, this benefit warrants pre-endoscopic initiation of PPIs.

5. What complications are you concerned for when deciding to do an emergency endoscopy?

As hypotension and hypoxemia can complicate sedation in an inadequately resuscitated patient, endoscopy should ideally be deferred until the patient has received sufficient intravenous fluids and, if necessary, blood products, to achieve hemodynamic stability. In addition, aspiration of blood or blood clots can occur during emergent endoscopy. Nasogastric lavage and a single dose of 250 mg IV erythromycin reduce the clot burden in the stomach. Pre-procedural endotracheal intubation to protect the airway during the procedure should be considered before emergent endoscopy.

6. How do you decide if an endoscopy should happen immediately or can wait until the next day?

Upper GI bleeding suspected to be from a variceal source warrants emergent upper endoscopy. Other high-risk features that warrant upper endoscopy within 12 h include bloody nasogastric aspirate that does not clear with lavage, as well as hypotension and tachycardia that do not respond to volume resuscitation.

Part III

Abdominal Aortic Aneurysm and Aortic Dissection

What Clinical Factors Should Arouse Suspicion for Abdominal Aortic Aneurysm?

20

Cullen Clark and Joseph P. Martinez

Pearls and Pitfalls
- The majority of abdominal aortic aneurysms (AAAs) are asymptomatic until rupture.
- An AAA that is symptomatic should be treated as an impending rupture until proven otherwise. These patients have the potential to become unstable quickly and need emergent imaging and evaluation by a vascular surgeon.
- The symptoms of a posterolateral AAA rupture can resolve before reaching emergency care but are likely to be followed by severe hemorrhage.
- Abdominal palpation has low sensitivity for detecting a pulsatile mass in AAA, and sensitivity is even lower for ruptured AAA.
- Fistula formation should be considered in patients who have had AAA repair and present with gastrointestinal hemorrhage or new-onset congestive heart failure.

Abdominal aortic aneurysm (AAA) is a serious degenerative vascular disease that affects approximately 8% of the US population [1]. An AAA is a localized dilation of the abdominal portion of the aorta, between the diaphragm and the aortic bifurcation [2–4]. Early suspicion based on history and physical examination, later confirmed with imaging, can facilitate treatment and monitoring to prevent rupture [3].

The majority of AAAs are asymptomatic until rupture, a catastrophic event that is often fatal [2, 3, 5–9]. The mortality rate for ruptured AAA is 65–85%, with many patients dying before reaching a hospital [2, 5]. The in-hospital mortality is ~ 50% [10], and even after emergent surgical intervention, the mortality is still 27–41% [1]. Identification and repair of symptomatic AAA prior to frank rupture can reduce in-hospital and operative mortality to 1–4% [1].

The classic presentation of ruptured AAA includes the triad of rapid-onset mid-abdominal or flank pain, hypotension, and pulsatile abdominal mass. Unfortunately, one, two, or all three of the symptoms are absent in the majority of patients with rupture [2, 5, 7, 9, 11, 12].

The location of the rupture will often dictate the presentation of the patient. A rupture into the peritoneal cavity often causes rapid exsanguination and death prior to reaching the hospital [2, 9]. A rupture into the retroperitoneal space may tamponade before extensive blood loss occurs, allowing the patient time to seek medical care. It is important to note that in the case of retroperitoneal rupture, the initial hemorrhage is consistently followed by a second, catastrophic hemorrhage that is fatal if not aggressively treated [2].

The pain associated with rupture is often sudden-onset mid-abdominal, flank, or back pain that can radiate to the buttock, groin, leg, or scrotum. Initial symptoms of rupture can also include syncope or presyncope [9], acute lumbar pain [2], hematuria, and hematochezia [6]. Unfortunately, the location, quality, or nature of the pain does not have sufficient sensitivity or specificity to diagnose AAA [11].

A handful of aspects in a patient's history can raise suspicion for AAA rupture in the correct clinical setting. The biggest predisposing factors for AAA rupture are aortic diameter above 5.5 cm in men, aortic diameter above 5 cm in women, and rate of growth exceeding 0.5 cm during a 6-month period [2, 6, 7, 10]. Current smoking increases the risk of AAA formation and doubles the rate of rupture compared to nonsmokers. Patients presenting with rupture are more likely to be older and nonwhite. They are also more likely to have renal insufficiency, poorly controlled hypertension, and a family history of AAA in a first-degree relative [2, 4, 6, 7, 10, 12, 13]. Chronic kidney disease causes aortic wall thinning, so

C. Clark (✉)
Emergency Medicine/Pediatrics Resident, Louisiana State University Health Sciences Center – New Orleans, New Orleans, LA, USA

J. P. Martinez
University of Maryland School of Medicine, Baltimore, MD, USA
e-mail: jmartinez@som.umaryland.edu

© Springer Nature Switzerland AG 2019
A. Graham, D. J. Carlberg (eds.), *Gastrointestinal Emergencies*, https://doi.org/10.1007/978-3-319-98343-1_20

these patients are more likely to develop AAA, and they rupture at a smaller diameter [10, 13]. Although AAA is more common in males, the rate of rupture is four times higher in females [10]. Connective tissue disorders such as Marfan and Ehlers-Danlos syndromes put patients at higher risk for AAA formation and rupture [12].

A thorough physical exam may help elicit other signs suggestive of AAA. Bimanual abdominal palpation for a pulsatile mass has notoriously poor sensitivity to detect AAA or rupture [2, 6, 7, 10, 12]. Sensitivity of palpation increases with the size of the AAA but decreases as BMI increases. False positives can occur in thin patients and those with tortuous aortas [2, 5]. Other potential physical exam findings include [5, 7, 12]:

- Bruising over the trunk or flanks (Grey Turner sign)
- Signs of hypoperfusion: pulse deficits in the lower extremities, cyanosis (blue toe syndrome), and focal necrosis of the foot (trash foot)
- Scrotal ecchymosis (scrotal sign of Bryant)
- Weakness, spasticity, and hyperreflexia if the rupture compromises the radicular arteries from the aorta to the spinal cord
- Abdominal bruit, potentially indicating either rupture or aortocaval fistula

Aortocaval fistula is a communication between the aorta and inferior vena cava (IVC) that can result from an AAA putting prolonged direct pressure on the IVC. Although rare, an aortocaval fistula can lead to rapid decompensation. Patients present with lower extremity edema, dyspnea, and other signs of high-output congestive heart failure. Patients often have continuous machine-like murmurs (similar to classic patent ductus arteriosus murmurs) auscultated in the upper abdomen [2].

Aortoenteric fistula, shown in Fig. 20.1, is another rare but dangerous manifestation of AAA rupture. This can occur either as a primary aortoenteric fistula, where a native AAA erodes into the gastrointestinal tract or, more commonly, as a secondary aortoenteric fistula where a communication develops at the site of a previously repaired AAA. This fistula most commonly occurs in the duodenum and causes hemorrhage into the gastrointestinal tract. Risk factors include previous AAA repair with mesh. Aortoenteric fistulas caused by mesh implants can occur years after the initial implantation. Patients present with gastrointestinal bleeding, which can be self-limited in some cases. This falsely reassuring "sentinel bleed" is always followed closely by massive gastrointestinal hemorrhage [12, 14].

A clinically apparent or symptomatic AAA is at high risk for rupture and requires emergent evaluation by a vascular surgeon. Any suspicion of rupture raised by history and physical exam should be explored with emergent imaging and consultation with a vascular specialist.

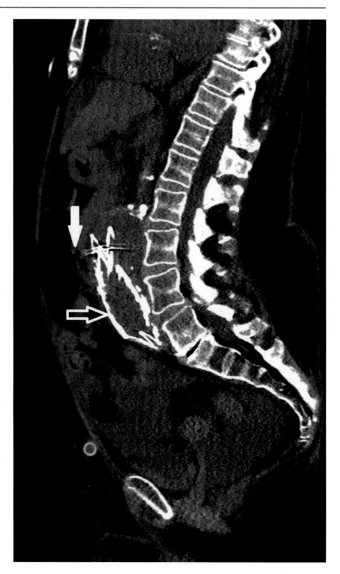

Fig. 20.1 Non-contrast sagittal CT image of the aorta showing previous endovascular AAA repair (open arrow) with gas surrounding the graft (closed arrow) at the site of abnormal connection to the gastrointestinal tract

Suggested Resources
- Abdominal Aortic Aneurysm. Core EM. https://coreem.net/core/abdominal-aortic-aneurysm.
- Abdominal Aortic Aneurysm: Clinical Highlights/Updates. emDocs. March 2015. https://www.emdocs.net/abdominal-aortic-aneurysm-clinical-highlights-updates.

References

1. Dua A, Kuy SR, Lee CJ, Upchurch GR, Desai SS. Epidemiology of aortic aneurysm repair in the United States from 2000 to 2010. J Vasc Surg. 2014;59:1512–7.

2. Sakalihasan N, Limet R, Defawe OD. Abdominal aortic aneurysm. Lancet. 2005;365:1577–89.

3. Savolainen H, Novak J, Dick F, et al. Prevention of rupture of abdominal aortic aneurysm. Scand J Surg. 2010;99:217–20.

4. Wanahainen A, Björck M, Boman K, Rutegård J, Bergqvist D. Influence of diagnostic criteria on the prevalence of abdominal aortic aneurysm. J Vasc Surg. 2001;34:229–35.

5. Karkos CD, Mukhopadhyay U, Papakostas I, Ghosh J, Thompson GJL, Hughes R. Abdominal aortic aneurysm: the role of clinical examination and opportunistic detection. Eur J Vasc Endovasc Surg. 2000;19:299–303.

6. Kent KC. Abdominal aortic aneurysms. N Engl J Med. 2014;371:2101–8.

7. Aggarwal S, Qamar A, Sharma V, Sharma A. Abdominal aortic aneurysm: a comprehensive review. Exp Clin Cardiol. 2011;16(1):11–5.

8. Sweeting MJ, Thompson SG, Brown LC, Powell JT. Meta-analysis of individual patient data to examine factors affecting growth and rupture of small abdominal aortic aneurysms. Br J Surg. 2012;99:655–65.

9. Long B, Koyfman A. Vascular causes of Syncope: an emergency medicine review. J Emerg Med. 2017;53(3):1–11.

10. Schmitz-Rixen T, Keese M, Hakimi M, Peters A, Böckler D. Ruptured abdominal aortic aneurysm - epidemiology, predisposing factors, and biology. Langenbeck's Arch Surg. 2016;401:275–88.

11. Azhar BA, Patel SR, et al. Misdiagnosis of ruptured abdominal aortic aneurysm: systematic review and meta-analysis. J Endovasc Ther. 2014;21:568–75.

12. Reed KC, Curtis LA. Aortic emergencies – part II: abdominal aneurysms and aortic trauma. Emerg Med Pract. 2006;8(3):1–20.

13. Chun KC, Teng KY, Chavez LA, Van Spyk EN, et al. Risk factors associated with the diagnosis of abdominal aortic aneurysm in patients screened at a regional Veterans Affairs health care system. Ann Vasc Surg. 2014;28:87–92.

14. Vitturi BK, Frias A, Sementilli R, Racy MCJ, Caffaro RA, Pozzan G. Mycotic aneurysm with aortoduodenal fistula. Autops Case Rep. 2017;7(2):27–34.

What Is the Ideal Imaging Strategy for Diagnosing AAA, Abdominal Aortic Dissection, and Aortic Rupture?

Bennett A. Myers

Pearls and Pitfalls

- Diagnostic studies should not delay operative management when there is a strong clinical suspicion for aortic rupture, especially if patients are hemodynamically unstable and have a previous diagnosis of aortic aneurysm and/or dissection.
- Bedside ultrasound, done by an experienced emergency clinician, allows for rapid and accurate diagnosis of abdominal aortic aneurysm with high sensitivity and specificity.
- Computed tomography imaging is the preferred modality for operative planning in aortic disease.
- Bedside ultrasound is limited in diagnosing a ruptured aorta, as it may show intraperitoneal hemorrhage but does not show rupture into the retroperitoneum, which is more common.

Sir William Osler once said, "There is no disease more conducive to clinical humility than aneurysm of the aorta" [1]. Aortic pathologies, including aneurysm and dissection, present with a myriad of different symptoms and are often found incidentally or with routine screening [1, 2]. While a large abdominal aortic aneurysm can occasionally be diagnosed on physical exam alone, confirmation with diagnostic imaging is still required. The emergency provider has multiple sensitive and specific imaging modalities to aid in the diagnosis of aortic disease, each with different advantages and disadvantages. Table 21.1 shows sensitivities and specificities of different imaging modalities for aortic aneurysm and dissection.

Table 21.1 Sensitivities and specificities of different imaging modalities in the diagnosis of aortic aneurysm and dissection

Imaging modality	Sensitivity		Specificity	
	Aneurysm	Dissection	Aneurysm	Dissection
X-ray	50% [3]	n/a	100% [3]	n/a
Ultrasound	81% [4]	67–80% [5]	91.1% [4]	99–100% [5]
Computed tomography	84.3% [4]	95–100% [6, 7]	98.4% [4]	95–99% [6, 7]
Magnetic resonance imaging	95.8% [4]	95–98% [6]	98.5% [4]	94–98% [6]

Table 21.2 Abdominal aortic aneurysm size, expansion rate, rupture risk, and recommended time for re-imaging

Aortic diameter	Average annual expansion rate [2]	Annual risk of rupture [1]	Absolute lifetime risk of rupture [2]	Time interval between re-imaging [9]	
<4 cm	1–4 mm	<2%		3.5–4.4 cm	1 year
4–5 cm	3–5 mm	1–5%		4.5–5.4 cm	6 months
5–6 cm	3–5 mm	3–15%	5 cm– 20%	>5.5 cm	
6–7 cm	7–8 mm	10–20%	6 cm– 40%	No repeat imaging, surgical repair indicated	
>7 cm	7–8 mm	20–50%	7 cm– 50%		

Abdominal Aortic Aneurysm

An arterial aneurysm is typically defined as a vessel with an increase in size over 50% of the normal vessel caliber. For an abdominal aortic aneurysm (AAA), the generally accepted diagnostic criterion is an aortic outer wall diameter of 3.0 centimeters or more [2, 8]. Accurately diagnosing the caliber of the aneurysm is important to management. The larger the aneurysm, the greater the risk for rupture [1, 2, 9]. Table 21.2 shows AAA size and associated management.

B. A. Myers
Department of Emergency Medicine, University of Maryland School of Medicine, Baltimore, MD, USA
e-mail: Bennett.Myers@som.umaryland.edu

© Springer Nature Switzerland AG 2019
A. Graham, D. J. Carlberg (eds.), *Gastrointestinal Emergencies*, https://doi.org/10.1007/978-3-319-98343-1_21

Ultrasound

Due to its high mortality risk, screening for AAA by abdominal ultrasound (US) is recommended in the outpatient setting [1, 9–11]. The United States Preventive Services Task Force recommends screening only in men over age 65 who have ever smoked. The Society for Vascular Surgery has broader guidelines including screening all men over age 65, men over age 55 with a family history of AAA, and women over age 65 who have smoked or who have a family history of AAA [9, 11].

Point-of-care US in the emergency setting has facilitated rapid bedside diagnosis of AAA. US is a zero-radiation, low-cost, and accurate imaging modality [1, 2, 13, 8–12]. A systemic review by Rubano et al., in 2013, showed that emergency clinicians performing bedside US to detect AAA have a pooled sensitivity of 99% and specificity of 98% [13]. Limitations include operator dependence, body habitus, and bowel gas [1, 3, 14]. Some sources suggest that any patient presenting to the emergency department over age of 50 with abdominal, back, or flank pain should have an US for AAA [1].

Figure 21.1a shows a large AAA imaged with US.

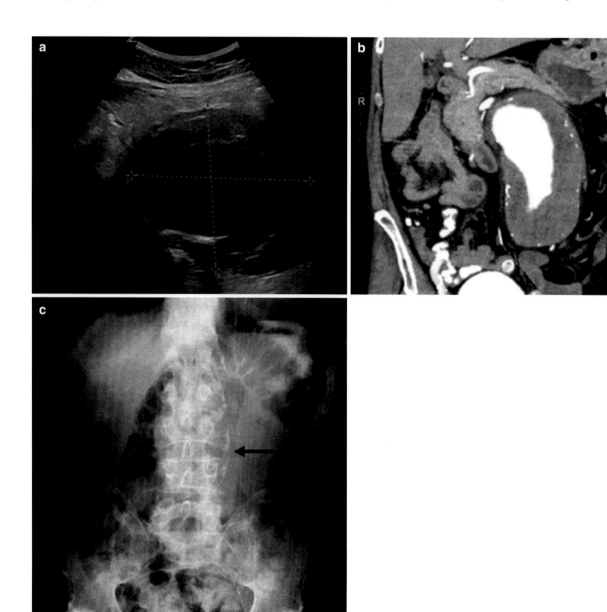

Fig. 21.1 Abdominal aortic aneurysm. (**a**) Transverse ultrasound view of an abdominal aortic aneurysm with intramural hematoma. (**b**) Coronal CT angiography depicting an abdominal aortic aneurysm. (**c**) Plain radiograph with an arrow depicting the calcified edge of an abdominal aortic aneurysm

Computed Tomography

Since the development of the less invasive endovascular aneurysm repair (EVAR), many surgeons prefer to evaluate AAA with computed tomography (CT) to assist with operative planning [10, 12, 14]. As such, even if US is used to diagnose AAA rapidly, a CT is frequently ordered subsequently to assess whether the AAA is amenable to EVAR and provide measurements needed for operative planning. CT shows aneurysm size and intramural thrombus, and it may show a dissection flap [8, 12]. The optimal CT modality is CT angiography (CTA). This allows precise measurements of the AAA, shows involvement of other arterial branches off the aorta, and develops three-dimensional reconstructions that can aid in surgical planning [8, 12–15].

CTA can find complications of a previously repaired AAA, including infection and leak [8, 12].

Figure 21.1b shows a coronal CTA image of a large AAA.

The major disadvantages of CT and CTA are radiation exposure, IV contrast allergy, contrast-induced thyrotoxicosis, and potential contrast-induced nephrotoxicity [8, 12, 15].

Magnetic Resonance Imaging

Due to the length of time needed for a scan, costliness, and limited availability, magnetic resonance imaging (MRI) has limited utility in the emergency setting and should be considered only in a stable patient with contraindication to CT contrast who is being considered for possible EVAR and not open repair [8, 12, 15]. Imaging is not needed for preoperative planning for an open repair but is indicated for EVAR, which has become the preferred repair method due to reduced perioperative mortality [9]. MR angiography (MRA) is preferred over normal MRI for the same reasons CTA is preferred [8, 12, 15]. Scanning with gadolinium is preferred, but an MRI or MRA can be performed without gadolinium when contraindicated [8, 12, 15]. Not all institutions have the capability to perform and interpret MRA without gadolinium.

Angiography

Traditional angiography, also known as digital subtraction angiography, has been mostly replaced by CTA/MRA. Angiography requires the availability of trained staff and can be considered on the rare occasion when contraindications to both CTA and MRA exist. Angiography may underestimate the size of an AAA, as it cannot distinguish the true size of the vessel if there is mural thrombus [8].

Plain Radiography

A large, calcified AAA can occasionally be seen as a thin line of calcification on plain radiographs of the abdomen or lumbar spine, as shown in Fig. 21.1c. While this is a poor imaging modality to evaluate for an AAA, practitioners should be aware of this abnormality, especially in elderly patients with nonspecific abdominal/back/flank symptoms. If an AAA is discovered on plain film, additional imaging is indicated [3].

Abdominal Aortic Dissection

The generally accepted classification system for aortic dissection is the Stanford system. A Stanford type A dissection includes the ascending aorta and/or the aortic arch and may extend into the descending aorta, whereas a type B dissection only includes the descending aorta, starting below the left subclavian artery. An abdominal aortic dissection could either be type A or type B. If a dissection is found with isolated abdominal imaging, further imaging of the chest should be pursued to determine the extent of spread [6, 7, 16].

Ultrasound

While most of the studies on diagnosing dissection by ultrasound are focused on the thoracic aorta, an intimal tear can be seen on abdominal ultrasound. Only case series have been published, with abdominal aortic ultrasound showing a sensitivity of 67–80% and a specificity of 99–100%. A negative ultrasound does not rule out abdominal aortic dissection [5, 17]. If an abdominal aortic dissection is found on ultrasound, especially in a hemodynamically unstable patient, a rapid bedside echocardiogram should be performed to assess for pericardial effusion, which would suggest retrograde extension of a type A dissection, potentially causing cardiac tamponade [6, 7].

Computed Tomography

Similar to AAA, an abdominal aortic dissection is best evaluated with CTA.

There is limited utility of non-contrast CT: it can evaluate for intramural hematoma, a variant of an aortic dissection where there is hemorrhage and hematoma contained in the medial layer of the blood vessel wall with no extension into the aortic lumen.

CTA is the gold standard because it evaluates the full extent of the dissection and determines true and false luminal sizes. It evaluates for the involvement of branches arising from the aorta and for areas of poor perfusion. Sensitivity of CTA for dissection is 100% and specificity is 98% [6, 7, 16, 18].

Figure 21.2 shows CTA images of an aortic dissection.

Information provided by CTA helps optimize presurgical assessment for open versus endovascular repair [6, 7, 16]. Images should ideally be obtained from the thoracic inlet through the pelvis. Again, the major disadvantages of CT/CTA are radiation exposure, IV contrast allergy, contrast-induced thyrotoxicosis, and the potential for contrast-induced nephrotoxicity [6, 7, 16]. The risks of these disadvantages generally pale in comparison to the risks of aortic dissection. When there is a strong suspicion for aortic dissection, patients should undergo CTA imaging immediately.

Magnetic Resonance Imaging

In patients with contraindications to CT/CTA, MRI/MRA may be considered. The main disadvantages of MRI include the length of time needed to perform the scan and lack of availability [6, 7, 16]. The black blood MRA imaging sequence does not need contrast and makes blood appear dark by removing pulsation artifact. This allows for visualization of a dissection flap and better visualization of the blood vessel wall [6]. MRA produces a three-dimensional reconstruction of a dissection, which, as stated before, is helpful in preoperative planning. MRA with contrast is preferred because it obtains the most diagnostic data [7, 16].

Angiography

With the availability of CTA and MRA, angiography is rarely performed for the diagnosis of aortic dissection. While angiography can diagnose the location of a dissection and its spread to various branches of the aorta, a thrombosed false lumen or intramural hematoma can lead to incomplete evaluation and false-negative results. Angiography requires availability of a trained provider and support team, and it is much more invasive than CTA/MRA [7].

Aortic Rupture

Missed aortic rupture carries a mortality of up to 90% [10, 14]. As such, diagnostic studies should not delay operative management if there is a strong clinical suspicion for aortic rupture, especially if the patient is hemodynamically unstable and has a previous diagnosis of aortic aneurysm and/or dissection.

Point-of-care ultrasound is beneficial as it may quickly confirm the diagnosis of aortic rupture. As little as 100 milliliters of intraperitoneal hemorrhage can be detected by bedside ultrasound [19]. In an unstable patient with intraperitoneal fluid and AAA/abdominal aortic dissection on ultrasound, rapid surgical consultation is indicated. Ultrasound is limited by its inability to evaluate the retroperitoneum, the most common site of aortic rupture [14, 20–22].

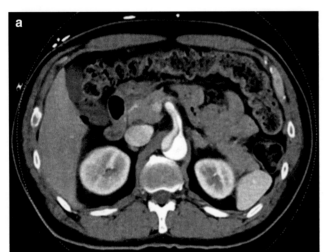

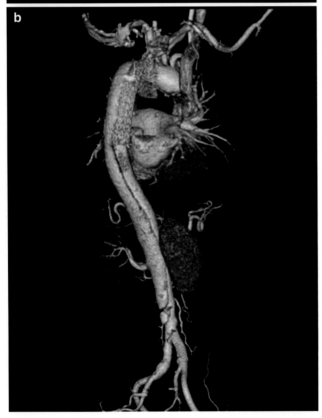

Fig. 21.2 CTA of an aortic dissection. (**a**) Abdominal aortic dissection visualized in an axial image. (**b**) Three-dimensional reconstruction of an aortic dissection. Note that the patient has received previous aortic and iliac artery repair

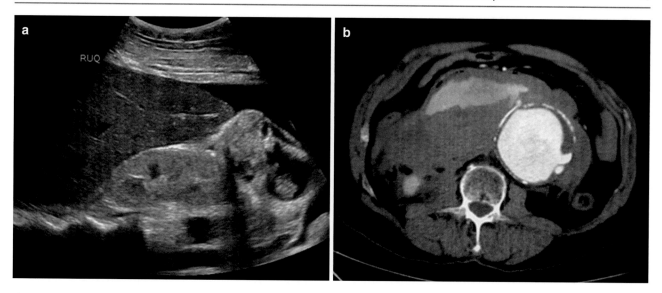

Fig. 21.3 Aortic rupture. (**a**) Right upper quadrant ultrasound showing free intraperitoneal fluid. (**b**) CTA of a ruptured abdominal aortic aneurysm with intraperitoneal hemorrhage

Figure 21.3a shows an abdominal ultrasound with intraperitoneal hemorrhage in a patient with aortic rupture.

Even in a hemodynamically stable patient with suspected aortic rupture, CTA poses risks because it forces the patient to leave the closely monitored acute care setting. A rapid CTA can be considered, generally in conjunction with surgical consultation. The CTA shows the location of rupture, including intraperitoneal, retroperitoneal, aortoenteric, and aortocaval [20–22].

Figure 21.3b shows a CTA with intraperitoneal aortic rupture.

There is no role for MRI or traditional angiography in suspected aortic rupture.

Suggested Resources
- Bedside ultrasound of the abdominal aorta. ACEP Now. May 2010; http://www.acepnow.com/article/bedside-ultrasound-abdominal-aorta/3/?singlepage=1
- Hiratzka LF, Bakris GL, Beckman JA, Bersin RM, Carr VF, Casey J, Donald E, et al. ACCF/ AHA/ AATS/ ACR/ ASA/ SCA/ SCAI/ SIR/ STS/ SVM guidelines for the diagnosis and management of patients with thoracic aortic disease. J Am Coll Cardiol. 2010;55:e27–e129.
- Reis SP, Majdalany BS, AF AR, Collins JD, Francois CJ, Ganguli S, et al. Appropriate use criteria: ACR appropriateness criteria® pulsatile abdominal mass, suspected abdominal aortic aneurysm. J Am Coll Radiol. 2017;14(5S): S258–65.

References

1. Reardon RF, Clinton ME, Madore F, Cook TP. Abdominal aortic aneurysm. In: Ma OJ, Mateer JR, Reardon RF, Joing SA, editors. Ma & Mateer's emergency ultrasound. 3rd ed. New York (NY): McGraw Hill; 2014. p. 225–45.
2. Keisler B, Carter C. Abdominal aortic aneurysm. Am Fam Physician. 2015;91(8):538–43.
3. Silverstein MD, Pitts SR, Chaikof EL, Ballard DJ. Abdominal aortic aneurysm (AAA): cost-effectiveness of screening, surveillance of intermediate-sized AAA, and management of symptomatic AAA. BAYLOR UNIV MED CENT PROC 2005. 2005;18(4):345–67.
4. Alamoudi AO, Haque S, Srinivasan S, Mital DP, (2015) Diagnostic efficacy value in terms of sensitivity and specificity of imaging modalities in detecting the abdominal aortic aneurysm: a systematic review. International Journal of Medical Engineering and Informatics 7 (1):15.
5. Fojtik JP, Costantino TG, Dean AJ. The diagnosis of aortic dissection by emergency medicine ultrasound. J Emerg Med. 2007;32(2):191–6.
6. Baliga RR, Nienaber CA, Bossone E, Oh JK, Isselbacher EM, Sechtem U, et al. The role of imaging in aortic dissection and related syndromes. JACC Cardiovasc Imaging. 2014;7(4):406–24.
7. Hiratzka LF, Bakris GL, Beckman JA, Bersin RM, Carr VF, Casey J, Donald E, et al. Practice guideline: full text: 2010 ACCF/AHA/AATS/ACR/ASA/SCA/SCAI/SIR/STS/SVM guidelines for the diagnosis and management of patients with thoracic aortic disease. J Am Coll Cardiol. 2010;55:e27–e129.
8. Reis SP, Majdalany BS, AbuRahma AF, Collins JD, Francois CJ, Ganguli S, et al. Appropriate use criteria: ACR appropriateness criteria® pulsatile abdominal mass suspected abdominal aortic aneurysm. J Am Coll Radiol. 2017;14(5S):S258–65.
9. Chaikof EL, Brewster DC, Dalman RL, Makaroun MS, Illig KA, Sicard GA, et al. SVS practice guidelines: SVS practice guidelines for the care of patients with an abdominal aortic aneurysm: executive summary. J Vasc Surg. 2009;50:880–96.
10. Kent KC. Clinical practice. Abdominal aortic aneurysms. N Engl J Med. 2014;371(22):2101–8.

11. Guirguis-Blake J, Beil TL, Sun X, Senger CA, Whitlock EP. Primary care screening for abdominal aortic aneurysm: a systematic evidence review for the U.S. Preventive Services Task Force. Jan 2014.

12. Hong H, Yang Y, Liu B, Cai W. Imaging of abdominal aortic aneurysm: the present and the future. Curr Vasc Pharmacol. 2010;8(6):808–19.

13. Rubano E, Mehta N, Caputo W, Paladino L, Sinert R, Carpenter C. Systematic review: emergency department bedside ultrasonography for diagnosing suspected abdominal aortic aneurysm. Acad Emerg Med. 2013;20(2):128–38.

14. Singh M, Koyfman A, Martinez JP. Abdominal vascular catastrophes. Emerg Med Clin North Am. 2016;34:327–39.

15. Hirsch AT, Haskal ZJ, Hertzer NR, Bakal CW, Creager MA, Halperin JL, et al. ACC/AHA practice guideline: ACC/AHA 2005 guidelines for the management of patients with peripheral arterial disease (lower extremity, renal, mesenteric, and abdominal aortic): executive summary a collaborative report from the American Association for Vascular Surgery/Society for Vascular Surgery, AAVS/SVS when guideline initiated, now merged into SVSSociety for Cardiovascular Angiography and Interventions, Society for Vascular Medicine and Biology, Society of Interventional Radiology, and the ACC/AHA task force on practice guidelines (writing committee to develop guidelines for the management of patients with peripheral arterial disease). Endorsed by the American Association of Cardiovascular and Pulmonary Rehabilitation; National Heart, Lung, and Blood Institute; Society for Vascular Nursing; TransAtlantic Inter-Society Consensus; and Vascular Disease Foundation. J Am Coll Cardiol. 2006;47:1239–312.

16. Thrumurthy SG, Karthikesalingam A, Patterson BO, Holt PJE, Thompson MM. The diagnosis and management of aortic dissection. BMJ (Overseas & Retired Doctors Edition). 2012;344(7839):37–42.

17. Williams J, Heiner JD, Perreault MD, McArthur TJ. Aortic dissection diagnosed by ultrasound. West J Emerg Med. 2010;11(1):98–9. 2010(1):98.

18. Mussa FF, Horton JD, Moridzadeh R, Nicholson J, Trimarchi S, Eagle KA. Acute aortic dissection and intramural hematoma: a systematic review. JAMA. 2016;316(7):754–63.

19. Paajanen H, Lahti P, Nordback I. Sensitivity of transabdominal ultrasonography in detection of intraperitoneal fluid in humans. Eur Radiol. 1999;9(7):1423–5.

20. Vu K, Kaitoukov Y, Morin-Roy F, Kauffmann C, Giroux M, Thérasse E, et al. Rupture signs on computed tomography, treatment, and outcome of abdominal aortic aneurysms. Insights Imaging. 2014;5(3):281–93.

21. Rakita D, Newatia A, Hines JJ, Siegel DN, Friedman B. Spectrum of CT findings in rupture and impending rupture of abdominal aortic aneurysms. Radiographics. 2007;27(2):497–507.

22. Kumar Y, Hooda K, Li S, Goyal P, Gupta N, Adeb M. Abdominal aortic aneurysm: pictorial review of common appearances and complications. Ann Transl Med. 2017;5(12):256.

Which Patients Can Be Treated Medically, and Who Needs Surgical Intervention?

22

Brit Long and Alex Koyfman

Abdominal aortic aneurysm (AAA), defined by aortic diameter greater than 3 cm, is potentially life-threatening. Rupture of an AAA is associated with significant mortality, approaching 100% without repair. When rupture occurs, 50% of patients will reach the hospital alive, and of these patients, 30–50% die during admission [1–5].

Which Abdominal Aortic Aneurysm Patients Need Surgical Intervention?

The patient's hemodynamic status guides management. Patients with ruptured AAA and patients with known AAA who present hemodynamically unstable with signs of rupture (abdominal pain, flank pain, back pain, pulsatile mass, limb ischemia) require immediate IV access and operative management. Patients who are hemodynamically stable but with symptoms potentially related to the AAA require emergent evaluation. If symptoms are due to AAA, urgent repair (open or endovascular aneurysm repair (EVAR)) is recommended. EVAR should be conducted if possible, though open repair may be needed [3–6].

Patients without symptoms may undergo elective repair, which is the most effective treatment to prevent rupture. Elective repair is recommended with aneurysm diameter greater than 5.5 cm [4, 5]. Several meta-analyses have found no mortality benefit to repairing AAAs between 4 and 5.5 cm [7–10]. However, patient age, gender, comorbidities, and rate of AAA growth are important factors for consideration. If patients do not meet criteria for elective repair, medical management includes treating risk factors that contribute to AAA expansion [4–6].

AAAs that enlarge >0.5 cm in 6 months or > 1 cm in 12 months have a higher risk of rupture. AAAs in the setting of other arterial disease, such as peripheral artery disease or aneurysm in the iliac, femoral, or popliteal artery, may also require repair before 5.5 cm [4, 5, 8]. Age must be considered, as an older patient with a short life expectancy and/or frailty may warrant observation, rather than surgery. Women have a higher rate of rupture compared to men with AAAs of the same size. Elective repair is associated with an increased risk of mortality in women, which must be balanced with the greater risk of rupture. For women with low risk of perioperative morbidity and mortality, elective repair for AAA > 5.0 cm may be an option [4, 5, 7, 9].

What Are the Surgical Options?

Open repair and EVAR are the two primary options for repair. Over 80% of patients in the United States undergo EVAR. The mortality rate for open repair is ~ 5%, while mortality with EVAR is 0.5–2%. Trials comparing open

B. Long (✉)
Brooke Army Medical Center, Department of Emergency Medicine, Fort Sam Houston, San Antonio, TX, USA

A. Koyfman
The University of Texas Southwestern Medical Center, Department of Emergency Medicine, Dallas, TX, USA

© Springer Nature Switzerland AG 2019
A. Graham, D. J. Carlberg (eds.), *Gastrointestinal Emergencies*, https://doi.org/10.1007/978-3-319-98343-1_22

repair to EVAR find improved short-term mortality with EVAR, but no difference in long-term outcomes. Pooled analysis suggests a 69% reduction in perioperative mortality with EVAR [4–6, 11]. The DREAM, EVAR 1, OVER, and ACE trials have evaluated outcomes at different time periods. They suggest EVAR has a greater reduction in short-term mortality but no long-term mortality benefit when compared to open repair due to increased need for reintervention with EVAR [10–16]. Open surgical repair may be better for younger patients (< 60 years) with greater life expectancy (> 10 years), though this is controversial. EVAR is likely better for all other patients [4–6].

Complications of repair vary by the specific technique. Open repair is associated with abdominal wall hernia, para-anastomotic aneurysm, renal injury, colonic ischemia, sexual dysfunction, graft infection, and aortoenteric fistula. EVAR is associated with limb occlusion, endoleak, device migration, aneurysm rupture post EVAR, buttock claudication, and sexual dysfunction. These complications occur more frequently with emergent ruptured AAA repair [4–6].

Who Can Be Treated Medically?

Medical management is warranted for most patients with AAA < 5.5 cm [4–6, 9]. AAAs naturally progress in size. Medical management does not prevent rupture but addresses modifiable risk factors for AAA and cardiovascular disease. Cardiovascular risk reduction includes smoking cessation, which is the most important modifiable risk factor. Regular exercise is vital. Aspirin and statin therapy are recommended, as AAA is considered a coronary risk equivalent. Hypertension should be treated, though no specific therapy alters the natural history of AAA [9, 10, 12]. Statins, beta blockers, and angiotensin-converting enzyme inhibitors are ineffective in reducing AAA progression. Antibiotics and anti-inflammatory agents do not limit progression either [7–9].

> **Suggested Resources**
> - Abdominal Aortic Aneurysm (AAA). Life in the fast lane. Dec 2015; https://lifeinthefastlane.com/ccc/abdominal-aortic-aneurysm-aaa/
> - Abdominal aortic aneurysm: clinical highlights/updates. emDocs. March 2015; http://www.emdocs.net/abdominal-aortic-aneurysm-clinical-highlights-updates/
> - Abdominal Aortic Aneurysm. CORE EM. Aug 2016; https://coreem.net/core/abdominal-aortic-aneurysm/

References

1. Bown MJ, Sutton AJ, Bell PR, Sayers RD. A meta-analysis of 50 years of ruptured abdominal aortic aneurysm repair. Br J Surg. 2002;89:714.
2. Hoornweg LL, Storm-Versloot MN, Ubbink DT, et al. Meta analysis on mortality of ruptured abdominal aortic aneurysms. Eur J Vasc Endovasc Surg. 2008;35:558.
3. Johnston KW, Rutherford RB, Tilson MD, et al. Suggested standards for reporting on arterial aneurysms. Subcommittee on Reporting Standards for Arterial Aneurysms, Ad Hoc Committee on Reporting Standards, Society for Vascular Surgery and North American Chapter, International Society for Cardiovascular Surgery. J Vasc Surg. 1991;13:452.
4. Hirsch AT, Haskal ZJ, Hertzer NR, et al. ACC/AHA 2005 practice guidelines for the management of patients with peripheral arterial disease (lower extremity, renal, mesenteric, and abdominal aortic): a collaborative report from the American Association for Vascular Surgery/Society for Vascular Surgery, Society for Cardiovascular Angiography and Interventions, Society for Vascular Medicine and Biology, Society of Interventional Radiology, and the ACC/AHA Task Force on Practice Guidelines (writing committee to develop guidelines for the management of patients with peripheral arterial disease): endorsed by the American Association of Cardiovascular and Pulmonary Rehabilitation; National Heart, Lung, and Blood Institute; Society for Vascular Nursing; TransAtlantic Inter-Society Consensus; and Vascular Disease Foundation. Circulation. 2006;113:e463.
5. Chaikof EL, Brewster DC, Dalman RL, et al. SVS practice guidelines for the care of patients with an abdominal aortic aneurysm: executive summary. J Vasc Surg. 2009;50:880.
6. Golledge J, Norman PE. Current status of medical management of abdominal aortic aneurysm. Atherosclerosis. 2011;217:57–63.
7. Mortality results for randomised controlled trial of early elective surgery or ultrasonographic surveillance for small abdominal aortic aneurysms. The UK small aneurysm trial participants. Lancet. 1998;352(9141):1649–55.
8. Lo RC, Lu B, Fokkema MT, et al. Relative importance of aneurysm diameter and body size for predicting abdominal aortic aneurysm rupture in men and women. J Vasc Surg. 2014;59:1209.
9. Baxter BT, Terrin MC, Dalman RL. Medical management of small abdominal aortic aneurysms. Circulation. 2008;117:1883.
10. Chagpar RB, Harris JR, Lawlor DK, et al. Early mortality following endovascular versus open repair of ruptured abdominal aortic aneurysms. Vasc Endovasc Surg. 2010;44:645.
11. Paravastu SC, Jayarajasingam R, Cottam R, et al. Endovascular repair of abdominal aortic aneurysm. Cochrane Database Syst Rev. 2014;1:CD004178.
12. Lederle FA, Johnson GR, Wilson SE, et al. The aneurysm detection and management study screening program: validation cohort and final results. Aneurysm detection and management veterans affairs cooperative study investigators. Arch Intern Med. 2000;160:1425.
13. Prinssen M, Verhoeven EL, Buth J, et al. A randomized trial comparing conventional and endovascular repair of abdominal aortic aneurysms. N Engl J Med. 2004;351:1607.
14. EVAR trial participants. Endovascular aneurysm repair versus open repair in patients with abdominal aortic aneurysm (EVAR trial 1): randomised controlled trial. Lancet. 2005;365:2179.
15. Becquemin JP, Pillet JC, Lescalie F, et al. A randomized controlled trial of endovascular aneurysm repair versus open surgery for abdominal aortic aneurysms in low- to moderate-risk patients. J Vasc Surg. 2011;53:1167.
16. Lederle FA, Freischlag JA, Kyriakides TC, et al. Long-term comparison of endovascular and open repair of abdominal aortic aneurysm. N Engl J Med. 2012;367:1988.

What Is the Role of Hypotensive Resuscitation/Damage Control Resuscitation in Ruptured AAAs?

23

Lindsay A. Weiner and Daniel B. Gingold

Pearls and Pitfalls
- Aggressive fluid resuscitation of the ruptured abdominal aortic aneurysm patient may produce the "lethal triad" of hypothermia, coagulopathy, and acidosis.
- Increased systolic blood pressure may contribute to clot dislodgement in ruptured AAA and worsen bleeding.
- Larger volumes of fluid administration are independently associated with increased mortality in retrospective studies.
- Permissive hypotension involves restricting fluid administration with a goal systolic blood pressure (SBP) of 50–100 mm Hg. The optimal target SBP is unclear.
- Limiting early large-volume fluid resuscitation and allowing permissive hypotension until after surgery may improve mortality.

Abdominal aortic aneurysm (AAA) rupture is frequently fatal, with mortality ranging from 53% to 93% [1]. Definitive treatment requires either endovascular repair or open surgery. Important predictors of death after rupture include advanced age, acidosis, loss of consciousness, renal insufficiency, and preoperative shock [2]. While preoperative shock is associated with increased mortality, the benefits of raising the systolic blood pressure to improve organ perfusion should be balanced against the risks of worsening hemorrhage. A normotensive resuscitation strategy, which involves rapid and aggressive fluid replacement, targets a systolic blood pressure (SBP) > 100 mmHg. An alternative method is controlled (or permissive) hypotension, which targets a SBP between 50 and 100 mmHg.

Evidence has shown that the vigorous fluid administration required for normotensive resuscitation may exacerbate bleeding [3]. Large-volume resuscitation in ruptured AAA patients may cause the "lethal triad" of dilutional and consumptive coagulopathy, hypothermia, and acidosis [1, 4]. Additionally, increased arterial blood pressure may disrupt a newly created clot [4]. A retrospective analysis of 154 patients with ruptured AAA demonstrated that an infusion of 3.5 L of fluid prior to repair was associated with an odds ratio (OR) of 3.54 for death. Decreased SBP was not independently associated with mortality in this study [5]. Another retrospective study in which patients undergoing permissive hypotension received a median of ~ 0.9 L of intravenous fluid per hour showed that each additional liter per hour was associated with an OR of 1.57 for death within 30 days [6]. Higher volumes of both colloid and crystalloid fluid administration were independently associated with mortality in an adjusted regression analysis. This evidence indicates that the volume of infused fluid may have more impact on mortality than SBP and suggests that limiting significant volume resuscitation until after operative repair may improve outcomes.

Currently, no prospective randomized trials compare permissive hypotension to aggressive resuscitation in patients with ruptured AAA. However, previous literature has noted that patients can maintain a SBP of 50–70 mmHg for short periods of time and that this pressure range helps limit internal bleeding and loss of clotting factors and platelets [4, 7]. The concept of permissive hypotension has long been used in trauma patients and has been extrapolated to patients with ruptured abdominal aneurysms with success, resulting in this strategy being included in AAA management protocols [8].

Van der Vliet et al. first investigated permissive hypotension in a case series of patients with ruptured AAA and determined it was feasible to limit prehospital fluid administration to 500 mL and to maintain the SBP between 50 and 100 mmHg until operative intervention [7]. A systematic review in 2014 concluded that permissive hypotension with delayed volume resuscitation is beneficial, though an ideal target SBP for elderly patients is not known [9]. A retrospec-

L. A. Weiner · D. B. Gingold (✉)
University of Maryland School of Medicine, Department of Emergency Medicine, Baltimore, MD, USA
e-mail: lweiner@som.umaryland.edu; dgingold@som.umaryland.edu

© Springer Nature Switzerland AG 2019
A. Graham, D. J. Carlberg (eds.), *Gastrointestinal Emergencies*, https://doi.org/10.1007/978-3-319-98343-1_23

tive study of a hospital that implemented damage control resuscitation and damage control operative techniques found a modest mortality decrease despite the fact that these patients had higher intraoperative blood loss and required increased plasma transfusion compared to patients receiving standard treatment [10]. These data have led to widespread use of permissive hypotension. The European Society for Vascular Surgery rated its recommendation to maintain SBP at 50–100 mmHg in patients with ruptured AAA as level 4, grade C, due to low-quality evidence [3].

The IMPROVE trial randomized patients with ruptured AAA to open or endovascular repair and found that 30-day mortality was higher among ruptured AAA patients whose lowest SBP was less than 70 mmHg [11]. The 30-day mortality rate was 51% vs. 34.1% in patients with a higher SBP nadir [11]. However, patients with the lowest blood pressures also received the most fluid prior to operative repair. It is difficult to tease out whether lesion severity dictates blood pressure, fluid requirement, and mortality, or whether increased fluid administration increases mortality independent of lesion severity or comorbidities.

Patients with ruptured abdominal aneurysms are more likely to be older with atherosclerotic disease; therefore, lower SBPs potentially induce renal injury and/or myocardial infarction [1].

Randomized clinical trials are necessary to provide higher-quality evidence to support the use of permissive hypotension in those with ruptured AAA. Further study should seek to optimize blood pressure goals; characterize risks of adverse effects such as cerebral, gut, limb, or myocardial ischemia; and investigate whether there is an age cutoff in which permissive hypotension is less likely to be beneficial.

While data quality is poor, permissive hypotension is a reasonable approach to the patient with ruptured AAA. Recent retrospective data has found independent associations between larger volume fluid administration and mortality after adjusting for key confounders. Because the lowest SBPs are associated with higher mortality, maintaining a systolic blood pressure between 70 and 100 mmHg is reasonable. However, some would argue for maintaining the lowest blood pressure possible without inducing end-organ ischemia, regardless of blood pressure measurement [4]. Resuscitating to a SBP > 100 mmHg should be avoided. Fluid administration to increase SBP above this level is likely harmful. Vasopressor use is discouraged as it may worsen bleeding and induce end-organ ischemia. Clinicians should routinely monitor patients for signs of impaired end-organ perfusion such as altered mental status, ischemic ECG changes, and elevated creatinine. The presence of any of these could result in consideration of raising the blood pressure goal. Crystalloids and colloids can both be used in moderation to treat severe hypotension in ruptured AAA, although evidence and experience with trauma patients suggest colloids may be more beneficial. A mixture of blood products approximating whole blood may be optimal. Early definitive surgical management may allow aggressive resuscitation to be delayed until after operative repair and optimize outcomes for patients with this deadly disease.

Suggested Resources
- Hamilton H, Constantinou J, Ivancev K. The role of permissive hypotension in the management of ruptured abdominal aortic aneurysms. J Cardiovasc Surg. 2014;55:151–9.
- Moreno DH, Cacione DG, Baptista-Silva JC. Controlled hypotension versus normotensive resuscitation strategy for people with ruptured abdominal aortic aneurysm. Cochrane Database Syst Rev. 2016;13(5):CD011664.

References

1. Moreno DH, Cacione DG, Baptista-Silva JCC. Controlled hypotension versus normotensive resuscitation strategy for people with ruptured abdominal aortic aneurysm. Cochrane Database Syst Rev. 2016;2016(5):1–16.
2. Kurc E, Sanioglu S, Ozgen A, Aka SA, Yekeler I. Preoperative risk factors for in-hospital mortality and validity of the Glasgow aneurysm score and Hardman index in patients with ruptured abdominal aortic aneurysm. Vascular. 2012 Jun;20(3):150–5.
3. Moll FL, Powell JT, Fraedrich G, Verzini F, Haulon S, Waltham M, et al. Management of abdominal aortic aneurysms clinical practice guidelines of the European society for vascular surgery. Eur J Vasc Endovasc Surg. 2011;41(Suppl 1):S1–S58.
4. Roberts K, Revell M, Youssef H, Bradbury AW, Adam DJ. Hypotensive resuscitation in patients with ruptured abdominal aortic aneurysm. Eur J Vasc Endovasc Surg. 2006;31(4):339–44.
5. Hardman DTA, Fisher CM, Patel MI, Neale M, Chambers J, Lane R, et al. Ruptured abdominal aortic aneurysms: who should be offered surgery? J Vasc Surg. 1996;23(1):123–9.
6. Dick F, Erdoes G, Opfermann P, Eberle B, Schmidli J, von Allmen RS. Delayed volume resuscitation during initial management of ruptured abdominal aortic aneurysm. J Vasc Surg. 2013;57(4):943–50.
7. van der Vliet JA, van Aalst DL, Schultze Kool LJ, Wever JJ, Blankensteijn JD. Hypotensive hemostatis (permissive hypotension) for ruptured abdominal aortic aneurysm: are we really in control? Vascular. 2007 Jul;15(4):197–200.
8. Park BD, Azefor N, Huang C-C, Ricotta JJ. Trends in treatment of ruptured abdominal aortic aneurysm: impact of endovascular repair and implications for future care. J Am Coll Surg. 2013;216(4):745–54.
9. Hamilton H, Constantinou J, Ivancev K. The role of permissive hypotension in the management of ruptured abdominal aortic aneurysms. J Cardiovasc Surg. 2014 Apr;55(2):151–9.
10. Tadlock MD, Sise MJ, Riccoboni ST, Sise CB, Sack DI, Sise RG, et al. Damage control in the management of ruptured abdominal aortic aneurysm: preliminary results. Vasc Endovasc Surg. 2010;44(8):638–44.
11. Powell JT. Observations from the IMPROVE trial concerning the clinical care of patients with ruptured abdominal aortic aneurysm. Br J Surg. 2014;101(3):216–24.

My Patient's Aorta Was Repaired. What Complications Arise from AAA Repair? When Should I Be Concerned About Recurrence?

Anne Walker and Sara Manning

Pearls and Pitfalls
- Computed tomography (CT) angiography is the initial study of choice for most complications related to abdominal aortic aneurysm (AAA) repair.
- Triple-phase CT is indicated when evaluating for endoleak.
- Fever and a history of AAA repair should raise suspicion for graft infection.
- Aortoenteric fistula may present with nonspecific symptoms. A history of bloody stools is not always present.
- Early vascular surgery consultation is important when a postoperative complication is suspected.

Improved imaging, including more widespread use of ultrasound, has led to earlier identification of abdominal aortic aneurysms (AAAs), closer monitoring, and ultimately an increase in operative interventions. While there is no identified mortality difference between open and endovascular repair, the decreased hospital length of stay, lower risk of renal, cardiac and infectious complications, and lower likelihood of early repeat operative intervention have caused a shift favoring the endovascular approach [1, 2].

The strongest predictor of morbidity and mortality following AAA repair is pre-existing cardiovascular and pulmonary disease [3, 4]. Independent of operative approach, the most common factors associated with readmission to the hospital are prolonged initial length of stay and discharge to a rehabilitation facility [5].

What Complications Arise from Open AAA Repair?

After open repair, the most frequent reasons for readmission are wound infection followed by bowel obstruction. Other complications include aortoenteric fistula, ischemic colitis, graft infection, and renal failure.

Aortoenteric fistula (AEF) is the most catastrophic complication of AAA repair with a mortality rate approaching 50% [6]. Adhesions can develop anywhere that the gastrointestinal (GI) tract comes into contact with the graft, and these adhesions may lead to graft erosion into the bowel. The most common location for an AEF is the duodenum. Patients often present at least 1–2 months post-op with nausea, vomiting, abdominal pain, hematemesis, or hematochezia [3]. An obvious GI bleed or history of hematochezia is not always identified. However, any patient with a known AAA or previous AAA repair that presents with GI bleeding should be evaluated emergently for AEF. The best emergent test for AEF is computed tomography angiography (CTA), shown in Fig. 24.1 [6].

Ischemic colitis is more common in patients who have undergone colon resection prior to open repair, as colon resection may cause a reduced collateral blood supply [3]. Ischemic colitis typically presents with abdominal pain and diarrhea, which may or may not be bloody.

The incidence of prosthetic graft infection is 1–4% after open surgical repair [7].

Renal failure occurs in ~ 2% of elective cases and in up to 20% of emergent cases after AAA rupture. Clamping superior to the renal vessels, hypotension, and intraoperative contrast administration contribute [8].

A. Walker (✉)
University of Maryland Medical Center, Baltimore, MD, USA
e-mail: awalker@som.umaryland.edu

S. Manning
Department of Emergency Medicine, University of Maryland
School of Medicine, Baltimore, MD, USA
e-mail: smanning@som.umaryland.edu

© Springer Nature Switzerland AG 2019
A. Graham, D. J. Carlberg (eds.), *Gastrointestinal Emergencies*, https://doi.org/10.1007/978-3-319-98343-1_24

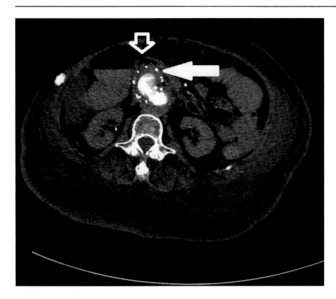

Fig. 24.1 Axial CT angiography showing previous endovascular AAA repair (*filled arrow*) with gas adjacent to the graft material (*open arrow*) at the site of an aortoenteric fistula

What Complications Arise from Endovascular AAA Repair?

After endovascular aneurysm repair (EVAR), the most frequent reasons for readmission are complications related to the graft [5]. Post-endovascular repair complications include organ ischemia, graft infection, and AEF.

Ischemia can present early due to graft kinking or late due to graft migration [9]. Case reports describe testicular, spinal, and lower extremity ischemia [9–11].

Large arterial embolization from the graft can present with sudden lower extremity weakness, numbness, or pulselessness [6]. Diagnosis requires CTA and can be augmented by duplex ultrasound if the administration of contrast is contraindicated. The patient should be placed on anticoagulation and vascular surgery consulted for consideration of thrombectomy or vascular bypass [6].

Graft infections can occur due to contamination at time of placement, but most are due to hematogenous spread. Most graft infections are caused by *Staphylococcus aureus* [6]. Infection should be suspected in any patient with a history of EVAR presenting with fever. Patients with graft infections can also present with nonspecific symptoms such as back pain, flank pain, and weight loss. Acute evaluation should include CTA and vascular surgery consultation. Sensitivity and specificity of CTA for graft infection have been estimated at 60% and 100%, respectively [12]. A CTA may show either air or evidence of inflammatory

changes around the graft site. If suspicion is high, a negative CTA should not be considered definitive. Cultures should be drawn and broad-spectrum antibiotics administered. Definitive diagnosis is only made by direct tissue sampling [12].

Although less common in EVAR than in open repair, AEF is still catastrophic and should be considered in any patient with evidence of GI bleed and history of AAA repair.

When Should I Be Concerned About Recurrence?

The risk of recurrence is an important difference between open and endovascular approaches. Because an open repair removes the diseased segment, risk of recurrence is eliminated. The risk of recurrence after endovascular approach is significant. Studies estimate the risk around 1% per year, with endoleaks significantly increasing this risk [13]. As such, long-term surveillance imaging is recommended after endovascular repair. An endoleak occurs when there is persistent bloodflow outside the lumen of the graft (but still within the aneurysm treated by the graft). Endoleaks are classified into five subtypes, shown in Table 24.1. Type I leaks can lead to rapid aneurysm enlargement and rupture. These require emergent operative intervention. Type II leaks result from the presence of collateral vessels supplying the aneurysmal sac. Although they can self-resolve, the continued pressure applied to the aneurysm sac can lead to aneurysm progression and ultimate rupture. Type II leaks should prompt urgent vascular surgery consultation. Types III and IV involve leaks around overlapping graft segments or through the graft material itself [6, 13]. Type V leaks are poorly understood theoretical phenomena in which pressure may be transmitted through the graft. A suspected or known endoleak is best evaluated with a triple-phase CT which evaluates the vasculature at three different time points after IV contrast administration.

Table 24.1 Endoleak classification

Leak type	Definition
Type I	Ineffective graft seal at either the proximal or distal end resulting in persistent filling
Type II	Backflow from branch vessels such as the IMA or lumbar arteries
Type III	Leak through the graft via a tear or ineffective seal in graft overlap sites
Type IV	Leak through porous graft material
Type V	Persistent enlargement of the aneurysmal sac with no identifiable leak, caused by "endopressure"

Suggested Resources

- emDOCS: abdominal vascular graft complications. June 2016; http://www.emdocs.net/abdominal-vascular-graft-complications/
- Slama R, Long B, Koyfman A. The emergency medicine approach to abdominal vascular graft complications. Am J Emerg Med. 2016;34(10): 2014–7.

References

1. Chandra V, Trang K, Virgin-Downey W, et al. Management and outcomes of symptomatic abdominal aortic aneurysms during the past 20 years. J Vasc Surg. 2017;66:1679–85. epub ahead of print. PMID: 28619644.
2. Gupta PK, Brahmbhatt R, Kempe K, et al. Thirty-day outcomes after fenestrated endovascular repair are superior to open repair of abdominal aortic aneurysms involving visceral vessels. J Vasc Surg. 2017;66:1653–8. epub ahead of print. PMID: 28711400.
3. Aggarwal S, Qamar A, Sharma V, Sharma A. Abdominal aortic aneurysm: a comprehensive review. Exp Clin Cardiol. 2011;16(1):11–5. Spring.
4. Healy GM, Redmond CE, Gray S, et al. Midterm analysis of survival and cause of death following endovascular abdominal aortic aneurysm repair. Vasc Endovasc Surg. 2017;51(5):274–81.
5. Greenblatt DY, Greenberg CC, Kind AJ, et al. Causes and implications of readmission after abdominal aortic aneurysm repair. Ann Surg. 2012;256(4):595–605.
6. Slama R, Long B, Koyfman A. The emergency medicine approach to abdominal vascular graft complications. Am J Emerg Med. 2016;34(10):2014–7.
7. Hausegger KA, Schedlbauer P, Deutschmann HA, et al. Complications in endoluminal repair of abdominal aortic aneurysms. Eur J Radiol. 2001;32:22–33.
8. Humphreys WV, Byrne J, James W. Elective abdominal aortic aneurysm operations – the results of a single surgeon series of 243 consecutive operations from a district general hospital. Ann R Coll Surg Engl. 2000;82:64–8.
9. Behrendt CA, Dayama A, Debus ES, et al. Lower extremity ischemia after abdominal aortic aneurysm repair. Ann Vasc Surg. 2017;45:206–12. epub ahead of print.
10. Thomas E, Parra BL, Patel S. Post-endovascular aneurysm repair (EVAR) testicular ischemia: a rare complication. Urol Case Rep. 2017;8(14):35–7.
11. Ke C, Feng Y, Chang C, et al. Extensive spinal cord ischemia following endovascular repair of an infrarenal abdominal aortic aneurysm: a rare complication. J Anesth. 2013;27(6):956–9.
12. Candell L, Tucker L, Goodney P, et al. Early and delayed rupture after endovascular abdominal aortic aneurysm repair in a 10-year multicenter registry. J Vasc Surg. 2014;6(5):1146–53.
13. Antoniou G, Georgiadis G, Antoniou S, et al. Late rupture of abdominal aortic aneurysm after previous endovascular repair: a systematic review and meta-analysis. J Endovasc Ther. 2015;22(5):734–44.

The Asymptomatic AAA: When to Be Concerned and What to Tell Your Patient?

25

Mark E. Sutherland and Joseph P. Martinez

Pearls and Pitfalls

- Abdominal aortic aneurysm (AAA) maximal diameter (> 5.5 cm in men, > 5.0 cm in women) and rate of expansion (> 0.5 cm per 6 months) are the best predictors of rupture risk.
- Mortality from AAA rupture is ~ 80%. Appropriate surveillance and elective repair if indicated are essential for mitigating this risk.
- Female gender, active smoking, COPD, and uncontrolled hypertension increase the risk of expansion and rupture.
- AAAs are associated with other abdominopelvic and lower extremity aneurysms, and patients with AAA should have femoral, popliteal, and pedal pulses closely examined.
- While ultrasound is a highly sensitive and specific screening test, patients who are at risk for AAA rupture should receive computed tomography angiography of the abdomen and pelvis either emergently or on an outpatient basis, as well as vascular surgery and primary care referrals.

The growing use of point of care ultrasound in the acute care setting and the rising utilization of advanced imaging have led to an increase in a variety of incidental findings, including asymptomatic abdominal aortic aneurysms (AAAs) [1–3]. Reviews of abdominal ultrasounds, computed tomography (CT) scans, and magnetic resonance imaging

M. E. Sutherland (✉)
University of Maryland Medical Center, Departments of Emergency Medicine, Internal Medicine, and Critical Care, Baltimore, MD, USA
e-mail: msutherland@som.umaryland.edu

J. P. Martinez
University of Maryland School of Medicine, Baltimore, MD, USA
e-mail: jmartinez@som.umaryland.edu

(MRI) scans have found AAAs as frequently as 1–2% of the time [1–3]. Asymptomatic AAAs can also be identified on physical exam, although abdominal exam is not sensitive for AAA [4]. When AAAs rupture, the pre-hospital mortality is greater than 50%, and of those who reach the operating room for emergent repair, the mortality is approximately 50%, emphasizing the devastating consequences of AAA rupture [5–7]. The emergency provider can play a pivotal role in the long-term outcome of a patient with an asymptomatic AAA by educating him or her on the importance of this finding and referring for proper monitoring and aneurysm management [8, 9].

The provider must first confirm that the patient is truly asymptomatic and that there is no evidence of active aneurysmal rupture. Although the triad of hypotension, back or flank pain, and a pulsatile mass is concerning, the absence of one or more of these findings does not rule out ruptured AAA, as only 25–50% of patients present with all three [4, 10]. If there is concern for active rupture, emergent surgical consultation and, if clinically feasible, CT angiography of the abdomen/pelvis should be obtained immediately [11]. Fig. 25.1 shows a CT of an AAA with evidence of rupture.

Because AAA is associated with other abdominopelvic and lower extremity vascular malformations, the femoral, popliteal, and pedal pulses should be closely examined and evaluated with imaging if there is concern for distal involvement [12].

In the instance of a truly asymptomatic, non-ruptured AAA, it is important for the acute care provider to risk stratify the patient to ensure an appropriate timeline for follow-up. All patients with AAA, which is defined as aortic diameter > 1.5 times normal at the renal arteries or > 3 cm [13, 14], are appropriate for referral to vascular surgery for further surveillance, but patients at high risk of rupture should be referred more urgently. Occasionally these patients may require evaluation while still in the acute care setting if there are significant barriers to outpatient follow-up. The most significant risk factors for rupture are large size and rapid expansion of the maximal diameter of the aneurysm [15].

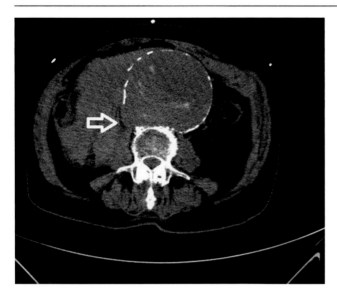

Fig. 25.1 Axial CT demonstrating an extremely large AAA with evidence of acute rupture (*arrow*)

and educated about the signs and symptoms of AAA rupture. Strict return precautions should be given. Because of the devastating consequences of AAA rupture, it is essential that emergency providers link patients with appropriate follow-up and provide counseling. Special attention should be paid to patients with larger aneurysms, AAAs known to be rapidly expanding, or other risk factors for rupture.

Suggested Resources

- Abdominal Aortic Aneurysm. American academy of family physicians. 1 Apr 2006. Available at: http://www.aafp.org/afp/2006/0401/p1198.html
- Abdominal Aortic Aneurysm. Core EM. 17 Aug 2016. Available at: https://coreem.net/core/abdominal-aortic-aneurysm/
- Abdominal Aortic Aneurysm. Wiki EM. 5 May 2017. Available at: http://wikem.org/wiki/Abdominal_aortic_aneurysm

---

Other risk factors for rupture include female gender, active smoking, COPD, and uncontrolled hypertension [4]. The timing of elective AAA repair is a highly individualized decision based on patient values, age, comorbid conditions, and other factors [16], but most US and international guidelines recommend repair of aneurysms larger than 5.5 cm in men, 5.0 cm in women, and those that grow by more than 0.5 cm in a 6-month span [2, 4, 17, 18]. Patients with any of these findings should be evaluated by vascular surgery on an urgent basis to discuss elective repair. In the absence of active rupture or other complications, it is appropriate for this consultation to be performed in the outpatient setting.

AAAs are significantly more common in patients of advanced age and with multiple comorbidities, including coronary artery disease [19]. As a result, these patients also benefit from referral to primary care, as these comorbidities need to be optimized prior to elective repair, and patients who would otherwise be suboptimal surgical candidates can be considered for repair when conditions such as hypertension, diabetes, smoking, angina, and COPD are appropriately addressed [5, 7, 20]. There is weak evidence that pharmacotherapy with angiotensin-converting enzyme inhibitors [21], angiotensin receptor blockers [4], beta-blockers [22], and/or statins [4] may slow aneurysm expansion and thus limit rupture risk. These benefits accrue over long spans of time and are likely appropriate to defer to primary care or vascular surgery. In patients who are known to have hypertension and are on anti-hypertensive medications, assessment of barriers to medication adherence and restarting self-discontinued therapies may be appropriate, as blood pressure control is one of the aims of outpatient therapy to reduce risk of AAA rupture. Patients should be counseled on smoking cessation

References

1. van Walraven C, Wong J, Morant K, et al. The influence of incidental abdominal aortic aneurysm monitoring on patient outcomes. J Vasc Surg. 2011;54(5):1290–1297.e2. https://doi.org/10.1016/j.jvs.2011.05.045.
2. van Walraven C, Wong J, Morant K, Jennings A, Jetty P, Forster AJ. Incidence, follow-up, and outcomes of incidental abdominal aortic aneurysms. J Vasc Surg. 2010;52(2):282–289.e2. https://doi.org/10.1016/j.jvs.2010.03.006.
3. Gordon JRS, Wahls T, Carlos RC, Pipinos II, Rosenthal GE, Cram P. Failure to recognize newly identified aortic dilations in a health care system with an advanced electronic medical record. Ann Intern Med. 2009;151(1):21–7. W5, http://www.ncbi.nlm.nih.gov/pubmed/19581643. Accessed 2 Aug 2017.
4. Chaikof EL, Brewster DC, Dalman RL, et al. The care of patients with an abdominal aortic aneurysm: the Society for Vascular Surgery practice guidelines. J Vasc Surg. 2009;50(4 SUPPL):S2–S49. https://doi.org/10.1016/j.jvs.2009.07.002.
5. Katz DJ, Stanley JC, Zelenock GB. Operative mortality rates for intact and ruptured abdominal aortic aneurysms in Michigan: an eleven-year statewide experience. J Vasc Surg. 1994;19(5):804–15. http://www.ncbi.nlm.nih.gov/pubmed/8170034. Accessed 31 July 2017.
6. Steyerberg EW, Kievit J, de Mol Van Otterloo JC, van Bockel JH, Eijkemans MJ, Habbema JD. Perioperative mortality of elective abdominal aortic aneurysm surgery. A clinical prediction rule based on literature and individual patient data. Arch Intern Med. 1995;155(18):1998–2004. http://www.ncbi.nlm.nih.gov/pubmed/7575054. Accessed 31 July 2017.
7. Cosford PA, Leng GC, Thomas J. Screening for abdominal aortic aneurysm. In: Cosford PA, editor. Cochrane database of systematic reviews. Chichester, UK: John Wiley & Sons, Ltd; 2007. p. CD002945. https://doi.org/10.1002/14651858.CD002945.pub2.
8. Screening for abdominal aortic aneurysm: U.S. Preventive Services Task Force recommendation statement. I National Guideline Clearinghouse. https://www.guideline.gov/summaries/summary/48460/

screening-for-abdominal-aortic-aneurysm-us-preventive-services-task-force-recommendation-statement?q=abdominal+aortic+aneurysm. Accessed 31 July 2017.

9. Thompson SG, Ashton HA, Gao L, Scott RAP. Multicentre Aneurysm Screening Study Group. Screening men for abdominal aortic aneurysm: 10 year mortality and cost effectiveness results from the randomised multicentre aneurysm screening study. BMJ. 2009;338:b2307. http://www.ncbi.nlm.nih.gov/pubmed/19553269. Accessed 2 Aug 2017.

10. Assar AN, Zarins CK. Ruptured abdominal aortic aneurysm: a surgical emergency with many clinical presentations. Postgrad Med J. 2009;85(1003):268–73. https://doi.org/10.1136/pgmj.2008.074666.

11. ACR Appropriateness Criteria® abdominal aortic aneurysm: interventional planning and follow-up. | National Guideline Clearinghouse. https://www.guideline.gov/summaries/summary/43867/acr-appropriateness-criteria%2D%2Dabdominal-aortic-aneurysm-interventional-planning-and-followup?q=abdominal+aortic+aneurysm. Accessed 31 July 2017.

12. Diwan A, Sarkar R, Stanley JC, Zelenock GB, Wakefield TW. Incidence of femoral and popliteal artery aneurysms in patients with abdominal aortic aneurysms. J Vasc Surg. 2000;31(5):863–9. https://doi.org/10.1067/mva.2000.105955.

13. Lederle FA, Simel DL. The rational clinical examination. Does this patient have abdominal aortic aneurysm? JAMA. 1999;281(1):77–82. http://www.ncbi.nlm.nih.gov/pubmed/9892455. Accessed 31 July 2017.

14. Aggarwal S, Qamar A, Sharma V, Sharma A. Abdominal aortic aneurysm: a comprehensive review. Exp Clin Cardiol. 2011;16(1):11–5. http://www.ncbi.nlm.nih.gov/pubmed/21523201. Accessed 13 Nov 2017.

15. Brown LC, Powell JT. Risk factors for aneurysm rupture in patients kept under ultrasound surveillance. UK small aneurysm trial participants. Ann Surg. 1999;230(3):289–96. http://www.ncbi.nlm.nih.gov/pubmed/10493476. Accessed 31 July 2017.

16. Knops AM, Goossens A, Ubbink DT, et al. A decision aid regarding treatment options for patients with an asymptomatic abdominal aortic aneurysm: a randomised clinical trial. Eur J Vasc Endovasc Surg. 2014;48(3):276–83. https://doi.org/10.1016/j.ejvs.2014.04.016.

17. Brewster DC, Cronenwett JL, Hallett JW, Johnston KW, Krupski WC, Matsumura JS. Guidelines for the treatment of abdominal aortic aneurysms: report of a subcommittee of the Joint Council of the American Association for Vascular Surgery and Society for Vascular Surgery. J Vasc Surg. 2003;37(5):1106–17. https://doi.org/10.1067/mva.2003.363.

18. Guidelines for Management of Patients with Abdominal Aortic Aneurysm: OneSearch - One search box for articles, books and more…. http://eds.a.ebscohost.com/eds/detail/detail?vid=1&sid=1116af19-181a-40ce-8522-7734fee73635%40sessionmgr4008&bdata=JnNpdGU9ZWRzLWxpdmU%3D#AN=edsdoj.6cdaa33ee4ef4e9cbabfede6f7132a0b&db=edsdoj. Accessed 31 July 2017.

19. Rodin MB, Daviglus ML, Wong GC, et al. Middle age cardiovascular risk factors and abdominal aortic aneurysm in older age. Hypertension. 2003;42(1):61–8. https://doi.org/10.1161/01.HYP.0000078829.02288.98.

20. McFalls EO, Ward HB, Moritz TE, et al. Coronary-artery revascularization before elective major vascular surgery. N Engl J Med. 2004;351(27):2795–804. https://doi.org/10.1056/NEJMoa041905.

21. Debus ES, Grundmann RT. Abdominal Aortic Aneurysm (AAA). In: Evidence-based therapy in vascular surgery. Cham: Springer International Publishing; 2017. p. 69–95. https://doi.org/10.1007/978-3-319-47148-8_4.

22. Poldermans D, Boersma E, Bax JJ, et al. The effect of bisoprolol on perioperative mortality and myocardial infarction in high-risk patients undergoing vascular surgery. Dutch echocardiographic cardiac risk evaluation applying stress echocardiography study group. N Engl J Med. 1999;341(24):1789–94. https://doi.org/10.1056/NEJM199912093412402.

26

Consultant Corner: Abdominal Aortic Aneurysm and Aortic Dissection

Shahab Toursavadakohi and Joseph P. Martinez

Pearls and Pitfalls
- Emergency providers should have contact information readily available for vascular surgery teams that can be rapidly mobilized in the event of an aortic catastrophe. Protocols should be in place to treat these cases similar to brain attack teams or ST-elevation myocardial infarction teams.
- Popliteal and/or femoral artery aneurysms have a strong association with abdominal aortic aneurysms.
- In cases of ruptured AAA or suspected rupture, permissive hypertension should be pursued with titration of blood pressure according to the patient's mental status.

Introduction

Dr. Toursavadkohi is Assistant Professor in the Department of Surgery, Division of Vascular Surgery at the University Maryland School of Medicine. He is also director of the aortic program at the University Maryland Medical Center.

S. Toursavadakohi
Department of Surgery, Division of Vascular Surgery,
University of Maryland School of Medicine, Baltimore, MD, USA

Aortic Center, University of Maryland Medical Center,
Baltimore, MD, USA
e-mail: stoursavadkohi@smail.umaryland.edu

J. P. Martinez (✉)
University of Maryland School of Medicine, Baltimore, MD, USA
e-mail: Jmartinez@som.umaryland.edu

Answers to Key Clinical Questions

When do you recommend consultation with a surgeon and in what time frame?
Expert consultation should be pursued with great urgency in cases of suspected aortic catastrophes. All emergency providers should have contact information readily available for their vascular surgery team and have protocols in place similar to those used for suspected brain attacks or suspected myocardial infarctions. This allows for streamlined care without unnecessary delays when these patients arrive for emergency care.

What pearls can you offer emergency care providers when evaluating patients with suspected abdominal aortic aneurysms or dissections?
The mortality rate is directly related to how quickly the patient is diagnosed and transferred to a center that can provide appropriate care. Delays in workup of suspected aortic catastrophes should be minimized.

What concepts do you think are key to diagnosis and management of this patient population?
It is important to consider these diagnoses in patients with risk factors, including a family history of aortic disease.

Management of known or suspected aortic rupture should include permissive hypotension.

What clinical factors should arouse my suspicion for abdominal aortic aneurysm?
The classic triad includes abdominal or flank pain, palpable mass, and hypotension. This is rarely seen in clinical medicine. Family history plays an important role in this disease process. Providers should be highly suspicious for abdominal aortic aneurysm (AAA) in patients that have a first-degree relative (parent or sibling) with a history of AAA.

In addition, peripheral aneurysms, such as popliteal or femoral artery aneurysms, are highly associated with AAA. If the patient has a unilateral popliteal aneurysm, he or she has approximately a 30% chance of having an AAA. The patient with bilateral popliteal aneurysms has an approximately 70% chance of having an AAA. Femoral artery aneurysms are even more closely associated. If the patient has a femoral artery aneurysm, he or she has ~ 90% chance of having an AAA [1, 2]. Patients with abdominal and or back pain should have careful examinations of peripheral pulses, as any suspicion of femoral or popliteal aneurysm would increase the level of suspicion for AAA.

What is the ideal imaging strategy for diagnosing AAA, abdominal aortic dissection, and aortic rupture?

This is an area that has really evolved over the last 20 years. Previously, traditional angiography was pursued frequently. However, with the evolution of multidetector computed tomography (CT), CT angiography has become the first-line test for patients with suspected AAA or aortic dissection. It is typically readily available in most emergency settings and has high sensitivity and specificity for these conditions.

Which patients can be treated medically and who needs surgical intervention?

Asymptomatic aneurysms that are less than 5 cm in women or 5.5 cm in men should be treated medically. This typically includes blood pressure control and statin medication. Statin medication does not reduce growth but impacts overall cardiovascular health, which is one of the leading causes of death in patients with AAA. Multiple other medications have been investigated as possibly being utilized to decrease AAA expansion. While they have shown encouraging results in small studies [3], larger randomized controlled trials are needed before they are ready for widespread use.

If an AAA exhibits rapid growth or reaches 5.5 cm in a man or 5 cm in a woman, surgical repair should be considered.

What is the role of hypotensive resuscitation in ruptured AAA?

Permissive hypotension is absolutely crucial in cases of known or suspected aortic rupture. My preferred approach is that emergency providers should have blood ready but hold off on transfusion if the patient is not exhibiting signs of end-organ damage. The most critical sign is altered mental status. If the patient is mentating appropriately, I recommend holding off on transfusion, even when these patients are hypotensive. If the blood pressure drops and the patient becomes altered, blood transfusion should be initiated and continue until the blood pressure improves enough that the patient's mental status clears. At this point the transfusion can be stopped.

My patient's aorta was repaired. What complications arise from AAA repair? When should I be concerned about recurrence?

The major complication from EVAR is endoleak. This is seen in approximately 20% of cases. Any patient who has had endovascular repair and presents with any symptoms concerning for aortic pathology (including abdominal pain, flank pain, hypotension, and/or limb ischemia) should be emergently evaluated for endoleak. AAA recurrence after EVAR is more common than after open repair. Recurrence is usually screened for with surveillance at 1, 3, 6, and 12 months. If these initial screens are negative, then yearly surveillance is recommended.

With open repair, recurrence is minimal and usually occurs at a distant site, rather than at the site of initial repair. Other complications of open repair include aortoenteric fistula, hernia, lower extremity ischemia, and bowel ischemia.

Suggested Resources
- Kent KC. Abdominal aortic aneurysms. N Engl J Med. 2014;371:2101–8.
- LeFevre ML. Screening for abdominal aortic aneurysm: U.S. preventive services task force recommendation statement. Ann Intern Med. 2014;161(4):281–90.

References

1. Whitehouse WM Jr, Wakefield TW, Graham LM, et al. Limb-threatening potential of arteriosclerotic popliteal artery aneurysms. Surgery. 1983;93:694.
2. Graham LM, Zelenock GB, Whitehouse WM Jr, et al. Clinical significance of arteriosclerotic femoral artery aneurysms. Arch Surg. 1980;115:502.
3. Mosorin M, Juvonen J, Biancari F, et al. Use of doxycycline to decrease the growth rate of abdominal aortic aneurysms: a randomized, double-blind, placebo-controlled pilot study. J Vasc Surg. 2001;34(4):606–10.

Part IV

Mesenteric Ischemia

What Clinical Features Lead to the Diagnosis of Acute Mesenteric Ischemia?

27

Susan Owens and Sarah Ronan-Bentle

Pearls and Pitfalls
- Mesenteric ischemic presents with nonspecific exam findings in early stages; thus, clinicians must maintain a high vigilance.
- In the early stages of acute mesenteric ischemia both symptoms and exam findings are vague and nonspecific thus clinicians must maintain high degree of vigilance for chronicity of symptoms and risk factors for thrombi/emboli.
- There are four main types of mesenteric ischemia though early on their clinical features and physical exam findings are very similar.
- Delay to diagnosis leads to greater tissue loss, increased morbidity, and increased mortality. This is an easy diagnosis to miss until it is too late.
- There is no defining symptom or exam finding that clinches the diagnosis of acute mesenteric ischemia.
- Although this disease primarily affects the elderly, mesenteric venous thrombosis affects young people and can have significant morbidity associated.

In 1926, A.J. Cokkinis described mesenteric ischemia as "the diagnosis is impossible, the prognosis hopeless, and the treatment useless." Today, acute mesenteric ischemia remains a complex disease process that is both difficult to diagnose and difficult to treat. Acute mesenteric ischemia (AMI) remains a rare diagnosis with an incidence of 10 per 100,000 adults and represents less than 1 in every 1000 hospital admissions [1, 2]. AMI is a surgical emergency; despite advances in diagnostic technology, primarily the development of the multi-slice CT scanner, and new surgi-

cal techniques, mortality remains high at 30–90% [3]. Unfortunately AMI shares many clinical features with other etiologies of the acute abdomen, often delaying diagnosis unless there is a high index of suspicion when reviewing history and exam findings. Herein is a review of the historical and clinical features that can be helpful to increase suspicion for AMI.

What Clinical Features Lead to the Diagnosis of Acute Mesenteric Ischemia?

Classic Presentation

Classically, the AMI patient is an elderly white female in her 60–70s presenting with abdominal pain out of proportion to exam findings and history of cardiovascular disease [1]. Patients may present with a spectrum of additional symptoms, including nausea, vomiting, and forceful evacuation of bowels that progresses to fever, bloody diarrhea, and hemodynamic instability once transmural infarction of the bowel occurs [4]. Classic exam findings include "pain out of proportion to exam," referring to a lack of reproducible localizable abdominal tenderness during palpation, and epigastric bruit. While these exam findings are characteristic of AMI, they are dependent on the degree of bowel infarction and will progress to peritoneal abdominal pain only once transmural infarction has occurred [5].

In one systematic review by Cudnick et al. (2013) of 1970 patients diagnosed with acute mesenteric ischemia, the prevalence of risk factors and physical exam findings suggestive of AMI was summarized. Atrial fibrillation, a history of abdominal pain, and diffuse abdominal tenderness were frequently reported [6].

S. Owens · S. Ronan-Bentle (✉)
University of Cincinnati College of Medicine, Department of Emergency Medicine, Cincinnati, OH, USA
e-mail: owens2sn@ucmail.uc.edu; ronanse@uc.edu

© Springer Nature Switzerland AG 2019
A. Graham, D. J. Carlberg (eds.), *Gastrointestinal Emergencies*, https://doi.org/10.1007/978-3-319-98343-1_27

Refining Your Diagnostic Gestalt by Underlying Etiology

There a four common types of AMI that relate to the mechanism of bowel insult and can be differentiated early based on patient history and presenting symptoms (Table 27.1). These primary four mechanisms are arterial embolism, arterial thrombosis, non-occlusive mesenteric ischemia, and mesenteric venous thrombosis. Regardless of mechanism, all typically effect the superior mesenteric artery resulting in gut ischemia. [3] (Table 27.2).

Arterial embolism is the most common pathophysiology resulting in AMI and accounts for 40–50% of cases. It often originates from a cardiac source and the patient may have a past medical history of atrial fibrillation, valvular disorder, recent myocardial ischemia, or any pathology that predisposes the patient to mural thrombosis. One-third of patients have had a preceding arterial occlusive event, and these patients typically do not have a history of chronic mesenteric ischemia [7]. Notably, chronic atrial fibrillation managed with appropriate anticoagulation does not decrease risk of arterial embolic pathophysiology [8]. Patients describe an abrupt onset of abdominal pain with rapid worsening, associated with vomiting and forceful diarrhea. Symptom acuity is related to a lack of collateral circulation in the splanchnic vasculature. Exam will likely reveal diffuse abdominal tenderness and other findings consistent with peritonitis. Survival is approximately 50% when diagnosis is made within 24 h of presentation and sharply declines thereafter [2].

Table 27.1 Characteristics of acute mesenteric ischemia based on etiology

Type of acute mesenteric ischemia	Common historical factors	Signs and symptoms
Arterial embolism	Elderly female, history of cardiac arrhythmia, or valvular disease	Abrupt onset of pain associated with vomiting and diarrhea, abdominal pain out of proportion to exam, vistal sign instability
Arterial thrombosis	History of chronic mesenteric ischemia, chronic intermittent abdominal pain associated with meals, weight loss, diarrhea	Severe abdominal pain, gastrointestinal bleeding, vital sign instability
Non-obstructive mesenteric ischemia	Severely ill patient in ICU, low cardiac output state, patients on hemodialysis	Vital sign instability, severe abdominal pain
Mesenteric venous thrombosis	20–40 yo, recent abdominal trauma, chronic inflammatory abdominal disease, hypercoagulability	Subacute abdominal pain worst in bilateral lower quadrants

Table 27.2 Prevalence ranges of historical features, signs, and symptoms in AMI

		Sensitivity range
Risk factors	Atrial fibrillation	7.7–79%
	Coronary artery disease (CAD)	13–75%
	Heart failure	5.6–58%
	Hypercoagulable state	2.4–29%
	Valvulopathy	3.3–11%
Historical features	Acute abdominal pain	60–100%
	Nausea/vomiting	39–93%
	Diarrhea	18–48%
	Rectal bleeding	12–48%
Physical examination findings	Pain out of proportion	45–54%
	Diffuse tenderness	54–90%
	Peritoneal signs	13–65%
	Tachycardia	31%
	Distention	18–54%
	Hypotension	5.2–54%
	Guaiac positive stool	5.9–23%

Adapted from Cudnick et al. [6] with permission from John Wiley and Sons

Arterial thrombosis accounts for 25–30% of AMI cases and is often superimposed on pre-existing severe systemic atherosclerotic disease. In many cases, these patients have been diagnosed with or have symptoms consistent with chronic mesenteric ischemia (up to 73%) preceding their acute presentation [9]. Symptom onset tends to be insidious as the splanchnic vasculature has had ample time to form collaterals. Intestinal injury tends to be more extensive and devastating due to proximal nature of the occlusion. Mortality for arterial thrombosis AMI is greatest with a 90% mortality rate across several studies [3]. Symptoms typically are described as a chronic phase of intermittent abdominal pain, weight loss, and diarrhea, followed by an acute episode of severe abdominal pain associated with diarrhea, hemodynamic instability, or gastrointestinal bleeding [2, 8]. Physical exam findings in arterial thrombotic disease are similar to findings in arterial embolism.

Non-occlusive mesenteric ischemia (NOMI) is an etiology of AMI that is seen primarily in critically ill patients resulting from prolonged visceral arterial vasoconstriction and accounts for 20% of the disease burden [6]. These patients are typically severely ill, intubated, or altered such that they are unable to complain of abdominal pain and their exam is limited. Certain medications, such as digitalis, dopamine, and ergot derivatives, as well as cocaine, have been shown to cause NOMI [10]. Past medical history is the largest clue to this pathology and typically includes diagnoses that predispose the patient to low cardiac output such as congestive heart failure, aortic insufficiency, recent cardiovascular surgery, as well as a history of diffuse severe atherosclerotic disease. NOMI has also been well described in hemodialysis patients; thus, clinicians need to maintain a high suspicion in patients presenting with abdominal pain during or immediately after dialysis [3]. NOMI is similar to the concept of demand ischemia in cardiovascular disease during severe systemic illness or during resuscitative efforts which cause physiologic changes resulting in bowel injury.

The least common cause of AMI is mesenteric venous thrombosis (MVT), accounting for just 5–15% of cases, though mortality remains high at 20–50% [3, 5]. Disease occurs when clot forms in the venous arcades and propagates to occlude the intramural vessels resulting in hemorrhagic bowel infarction. Ninety percent of patients with MVT have at least one of the following three risk factors: (1) hypercoagulability (e.g., thrombophilia, oral contraceptive use, neoplasm), (2) recent abdominal trauma, and/or (3) local inflammation (e.g., pancreatitis, diverticulitis, etc.) [8]. Approximately 50% of patients will have a personal or family history of pulmonary or deep venous thromboembolism. While AMI is typically a disease of the elderly, MVT predominantly affects patients between the ages of 20 and 40 years without atherosclerotic disease history [11]. These patients often have subacute or late presentations with vague diffuse abdominal pain, anorexia, and diarrhea without preceding prodromal symptoms [5]. On exam, abdominal tenderness frequently localizes to bilateral lower quadrants. Exam findings may also include signs of portal hypertension (e.g., caput medusa, ascites, and hemorrhoids) if the inciting clot occurred well before symptom presentation [12].

Summary

Regardless of etiology, the final common pathway includes bowel infarction though distribution of clot burden determines extent of intestinal damage. MVT is the least likely to present in extremis given the extent of disease required to cause infarction, though all four pathologies can present with Klass' classic description of severe abdominal pain, bloody stool, and relatively normal physical exam [8]. History is the key to recognizing AMI as a cause of the patient's pain and determining the etiology of AMI.

Suggested Resources
- EMRap C3 elderly abdominal pain Jan 2017.
- Herbert M, Swadron S, Spangler M, Mason J. C3-elderly abdominal pain. Jan 2017; [cited 31 Jan 2018]. In: EM:RAP [Internet]. Available from: https://www.emrap.org/episode/c3elderly/introduction.

References

1. Crawford RS, Harris DG, Klyushnenkova EN, Tesoriero RB, Rabin J, Chen H, Diaz JJ. A statewide analysis of the incidence and outcomes of acute mesenteric ischemia in Maryland from 2009 to 2013. Front Surg. 2016;3:22.
2. Wyers MC. Acute mesenteric ischemia: diagnostic approach and surgical treatment. Semin Vasc Surg. 2010;23(1):9–20.
3. Herbert GS, Steele SR. Acute and chronic mesenteric ischemia. Surg Clin North Am. 2007;87(5):1115–34. ix.
4. Tilsed JV, Casamassima A, Kurihara H, Mariani D, Martinez I, Pereira J, et al. ESTES guidelines: acute mesenteric ischaemia. Eur J Trauma Emerg Surg. 2016;42(2):253–70.
5. Clair DG, Beach JM. Mesenteric Ischemia. N Engl J Med. 2016;374(10):959–68.
6. Cudnick M, Darbha S, Jones J, Macedo J, Stockton S, Hiestand B. The diagnosis of acute mesenteric ischemia: a systematic review and meta-analysis. Acad Emerg Med. 2013;20(11):1088–99.
7. Oldenburg WA, Lau LL, Rodenberg TJ, Edmonds HJ, Burger CD. Acute mesenteric ischemia: a clinical review. Arch Intern Med. 2004;164(10):1054–62.
8. Paterno F, Longo WE. The etiology and pathogenesis of vascular disorders of the intestine. Radiol Clin N Am. 2008;46(5):877–85.
9. Acosta S. Epidemiology of mesenteric vascular disease: clinical implications. Semin Vasc Surg. 2010;23(1):4–8.
10. Walker TG. Mesenteric ischemia. Semin Intervent Radiol. 2009;26(3):175–83.
11. Spangler R, Van Pham T, Khoujah D, Martinez JP. Abdominal emergencies in the geriatric patient. Int J Emerg Med. 2014;7:43. https://doi.org/10.1186/s12245-014-0043-2.
12. Karkkainen JM, Acosta S. Acute mesenteric ischemia (part I) - incidence, etiologies, and how to improve early diagnosis. Best Pract Res Clin Gastroenterol. 2017;31(1):15–25.

What Is the Most Sensitive and Specific Laboratory Test(s) for the Detection of Acute Mesenteric Ischemia? What Is the Utility of Lactate? Are There Other Laboratory Tests Which Are Helpful in Making the Diagnosis?

28

Courtney H. McKee and Sarah Ronan-Bentle

Pearls and Pitfalls
- No one laboratory test is sufficient to exclude or confirm the diagnosis of AMI.
- Elevated serum lactate level correlates with mortality and irreversible intestinal ischemia, and may be a marker of late disease, but is not diagnostic.
- D-lactate, D-dimer, I-FAPB, and other novel biomarkers may have a role in the early diagnosis of AMI, but further research is required to assess their role.

Unfortunately, there is no single biomarker that is adequate to diagnose acute mesenteric ischemia (AMI) [1–3]. No test has adequate specificity and sensitivity to give a definitive diagnosis, particularly early in the disease process, when prompt recognition and treatment have the opportunity to affect mortality. However, despite small cohorts and heterogeneity in the literature, there are laboratory tests that are helpful adjuncts for diagnosis and new biomarkers that show promise in assisting in the early detection of AMI.

Elevated serum lactate levels are nearly ubiquitous in confirmed cases of AMI, as is an elevated white blood cell count. Both were elevated in > 90% of patients with AMI [4, 5]. Serum lactate is felt to be, unfortunately, a late marker of disease and correlates with both irreversible transmural bowel ischemia as well as mortality [6, 7]. An initial lactate level > 2 mmol/L and maximum lactate level were both associated with increased risk of death, with an OR 3.4 and 2.2, respectively, in one study [6]. However, when assessed for diagnostic power, lactate was found to have a pooled specificity of 86% and sensitivity of only 40% [8]. Alone, an elevated lactate is insufficient to diagnose AMI and may not detect early disease.

The stereoisomer D-lactate has been proposed as an earlier indicator of intestinal ischemia, reflecting bacterial translocation indicative of mucosal ischemia. However, this has not borne out in pooled data, which demonstrated poor sensitivity and specificity, 71% and 74%, respectively [9]. Additionally, measurement of D-lactate may not be feasible at all institutions. In the future, it may have a role in diagnosis and as a marker to guide management, but currently it is not a viable option as an isolated diagnostic tool.

D-dimer has been investigated due to the contribution of thrombosis in the pathophysiology of AMI. Powell et al. found that an elevated D-dimer had an 80% sensitivity and 60% specificity in their cohort [1]. However, pooled data revealed the sensitivity and specificity of D-dimer to be 96% and 40%, respectively [8]. D-dimer also does not have utility in predicting bowel ischemia [10]. A negative D-dimer may be reassuring if suspicion for AMI is very low; however, the D-dimer may not be elevated early in AMI and should not be used to definitively rule out the diagnosis [11].

Elevations in troponin I (TnI) in AMI patients have been noted. Acosta et al. found that in a review of 55 patients with AMI, 28 also underwent TnI testing. Of those patients, 64% were found to have a positive TnI without concurrent ECG changes or objective evidence of cardiac ischemia. Patients with acute embolic superior mesenteric artery (SMA) occlusion were more likely to undergo TnI testing, and of these patients, 47% were found to have a positive TnI [12]. The authors suggest that this may reflect global increased oxygen demand in the critically ill patient, as well as the catecholamine surge and associated tachycardia associated with acute SMA occlusion. It is important to note that elevations of TnI have been shown to predict higher mortality in elderly patients [13]. TnI may emerge as an adjunctive laboratory marker in the patient with AMI and if positive may suggest an embolic arterial occlusion to providers, but its utility as a diagnostic tool will require further study.

C. H. McKee · S. Ronan-Bentle (✉)
University of Cincinnati College of Medicine, Department of Emergency Medicine, Cincinnati, OH, USA
e-mail: mckeech@ucmail.uc.edu; ronanse@uc.edu

© Springer Nature Switzerland AG 2019
A. Graham, D. J. Carlberg (eds.), *Gastrointestinal Emergencies*, https://doi.org/10.1007/978-3-319-98343-1_28

A number of novel biomarkers have been proposed for the diagnosis of AMI, including intestinal fatty acid-binding protein (I-FABP), cobalt albumin-binding assay (CABA), and α-GST (α-glutathione S-transferase) [9, 14–16]. Ultimately, I-FABP has emerged with promising results. I-FABP is a marker of intestinal mucosal damage, of which one form is excreted in the urine. This is unique among most intestine-specific biomarkers. Most are cleared through the liver and difficult to detect systemically [14]. In one study, I-FABP had a promising sensitivity of 90% and specificity of 89%, though this was not borne out in pooled data [15]. Treskes et al. found a pooled sensitivity and specificity of 75–79% and 79–91% [9]. These experimental biomarkers, in particular I-FABP, will require further research to elucidate, and then validate, their role in diagnosing AMI.

Summary

While no single laboratory test can diagnose AMI, practitioners must recognize that elevated serum lactate levels are a common but likely late finding in AMI and correlate with poor outcomes as well as mortality. Additionally, D-dimer, TnI, and novel biomarkers may be useful in the early diagnosis of AMI, but their diagnostic applicability is not clear at this time.

Suggested Resources

- Bala M, Kashuk J, Moore E, Kluger Y, Biffl W, Gomes C, et al. Acute mesenteric ischemia: guidelines of the World Society of Emergency Surgery. World J Emerg Surg. 2017;12(38).
- Lee A, Aldeen A. Focus on: acute mesenteric ischemia ACEP News. March 2011.

References

1. Powell A, Armstrong P. Plasma biomarkers for early diagnosis of acute intestinal ischemia. Semin Vasc Surg. 2014;27(3):170–5.
2. Evennett N, Petrov M, Mittal A, Windsor J. Systematic review and pooled estimates for the diagnostic accuracy of serological markers for intestinal ischemia. World J Surg. 2007;33(7):1374.
3. Bala M, Kashuk J, Moore E, Kluger Y, Biffl W, Gomes C, et al. Acute mesenteric ischemia: guidelines of the World Society of Emergency Surgery. World J Emerg Surg. 2017;12(38). https://doi:10.1186/s13017-017-0150-5
4. Kougias P, Lau D, El Sayed HF, Zhou W, Huynh TT, Lin PH. Determinants of mortality and treatment outcome following surgical interventions for acute mesenteric ischemia. J Vasc Surg. 2007;46(3):467–74.
5. Ritz J, Germer C, Buhr HJ. Prognostic factors for mesenteric infarction: multivariate analysis of 187 patients with regard to patient age. Ann Vasc Surg. 2005;19(3):328–34.
6. Arthurs ZM, Titus J, Bannazadeh M, Eagleton MJ, Srivastava S, Sarac TP, et al. A comparison of endovascular revascularization with traditional therapy for the treatment of acute mesenteric ischemia. J Vasc Surg. 2011;53(3):698–705.
7. Nuzzo A, Maggiori L, Ronot M, Becq M, Plessier A, Gault N, et al. Predictive factors of intestinal necrosis in acute mesenteric ischemia: prospective study from an intestinal stroke center. Am J Gastroenterol. 2017;112:597–605.
8. Cudnik MT, Darbha S, Jones J, Macedo J, Stockton SW, Hiestand BC. The diagnosis of acute mesenteric ischemia: a systematic review and meta-analysis; El Diagnóstico de Isquemia Mesentérica Aguda: Revisión Sistemática y Metanálisis. Acad Emerg Med. 2013;20(11):1087–100.
9. Treskes N, Persoon A, van Zanten A. Diagnostic accuracy of novel serological biomarkers to detect acute mesenteric ischemia: a systematic review and meta-analysis. Intern Emerg Med. 2017;12(6):821–36.
10. Chiu YH, Huang MK, How CK, Hsu TF, Chen JD, Chern CH, Yen DH, Huang CI. D-dimer in patients with suspected acute mesenteric ischemia. Am J Emerg Med. 2009;27:975–9.
11. Acosta S, Nilsson J. Current status on plasma biomarkers for acute mesenteric ischemia. J Thromb Thrombolysis. 2012;33(4):355–61.
12. Acosta S, Block T, Björnsson S, Resch T, Björck M, Nilsson T. Diagnostic pitfalls at admission in patients with acute superior mesenteric artery occlusion. J Emerg Med. 2012 Jun 1;42(6):635–41.
13. Zethelius B, Berglund L, Sundström J, Ingelsson E, Basu S, Larsson A, et al. Use of multiple biomarkers to improve the prediction of death from cardiovascular causes. N Engl J Med. 2008;358(20):2107–16.
14. Matsumoto S, Sekine K, Funaoka H, Yamazaki M, Shimizu M, Hayashida K, et al. Diagnostic performance of plasma biomarkers in patients with acute intestinal ischaemia. Br J Surg. 2014;101(3):232–8.
15. van den Heijkant T, Aerts B, Teijink J, Buurman W, Luyer M. Challenges in diagnosing mesenteric ischemia. World J Gastroenterol. 2013;19(9):1338–41.
16. Block T, Nilsson TK, Björck M, Acosta S. Diagnostic accuracy of plasma biomarkers for intestinal ischaemia. Scand J Clin Lab Invest. 2008;68(3):242–8.

What Is the Most Sensitive and Specific Imaging Study for the Detection of Acute Mesenteric Ischemia? Is MDCT the Gold Standard?

29

Courtney H. McKee and Sarah Ronan-Bentle

Pearls and Pitfalls
- Angiography was the previous gold standard for diagnosis of AMI, allowing immediate therapeutic intervention as well.
- CT angiography (CTA) is fast, accurate, sensitive, and specific for the diagnosis of AMI and should be considered the first-line test for AMI.
- Because of the significant morbidity and mortality associated with AMI, it is important to obtain a CTA, even in patients with renal insufficiency.

Rapid and accurate diagnosis of acute mesenteric ischemia (AMI) is crucial to minimize morbidity and mortality [1, 2]. The gold standard test for diagnosis of acute mesenteric ischemia (AMI) was previously formal angiography [3, 4]. Angiography is an attractive option because it provides the opportunity for diagnosis and immediate treatment of AMI [4–6].

Advances in multidetector computed tomography (MDCT) technology have allowed CTA to replace formal angiography as a first-line diagnostic test for AMI. There is a large and growing body of literature that strongly supports CTA as the first-line diagnostic test for AMI. CTA is a rapid, noninvasive, and accurate means of diagnosing AMI and is readily available to emergency department (ED) physicians. CTA has been found to have a 96% accuracy rate, with a pooled specificity of 93% and a pooled sensitivity of 96%, as well as excellent negative and positive predictive values [7–10]. Given the high morbidity and mortality associated with delayed diagnosis of AMI and CTA's excellent performance in detecting AMI, it is important to perform this test early, regardless of renal insufficiency [8, 10]. CTA is also able to detect irreversible bowel wall ischemia, which is useful in discussion with surgical colleagues [11].

Notably, the World Society of Emergency Surgery guidelines, published in 2017, made a 1A recommendation that any patient with suspicion for AMI undergoes a CTA as soon as possible [12]. Radiologists use a number of different criteria for diagnosis including evidence of arterial occlusion, bowel wall thickening, bowel dilatation, pneumatosis or portal air, fat stranding, perforation, and organ infarction [8].

Magnetic resonance angiography (MRA) with intravenous contrast is an alternate diagnostic tool for clinicians when suspicious for acute mesenteric ischemia. MRA is particularly strong when diagnosing proximal arterial occlusions and quantifying stenosis, though it may overestimate the degree of stenosis [13–16]. There is also no radiation or iodinated contrast exposure to the patient. However, MRI technology, while increasingly common, is still not ubiquitous among hospitals. Even if available, the increased time to perform the study confers a potential delay in both diagnosis and treatment of AMI. Furthermore, MRA does not reliably demonstrate bowel necrosis [17]. The American College of Radiology 2018 Appropriateness Criteria continues to recommend CTA over MRA. There may be situations where MRA is preferred: for improved vessel mapping or if CTA is absolutely contraindicated or unavailable and the time delay is not prohibitive [7].

Summary

Angiography will remain a relevant diagnostic and therapeutic tool in the management of AMI in specific patient populations. MRA is an additional diagnostic modality that should be used only in the appropriate clinical setting if there is a high concern for AMI. CTA is reliable, fast, and accurate, and provides critical information that assists clinicians in the diagnosis and management of AMI. CTA should be considered the first-line test for evaluation of AMI.

C. H. McKee · S. Ronan-Bentle (✉)
University of Cincinnati College of Medicine, Department of Emergency Medicine, Cincinnati, OH, USA
e-mail: mckeech@ucmail.uc.edu; ronanse@uc.edu

© Springer Nature Switzerland AG 2019
A. Graham, D. J. Carlberg (eds.), *Gastrointestinal Emergencies*, https://doi.org/10.1007/978-3-319-98343-1_29

Suggested Resource
- Lotterman S. Mesenteric ishcemia: a power review. Nov 2014; http://www.emdocs.net/mesenteric-ischemia-power-review/

References

1. Bradbury AW, Brittenden J, McBride K, Ruckley CV. Mesenteric ischaemia: a multidisciplinary approach. Br J Surg. 1995;82(11):1446–59.
2. Kassahun W, Schulz T, Richter O, Hauss J. Unchanged high mortality rates from acute occlusive intestinal ischemia: six year review. Langenbeck's Arch Surg. 2008;393(2):163–71.
3. Lock G. Acute intestinal ischaemia. Best Pract Res Clin Gastroenterol. 2001;15(1):83–98.
4. Cangemi JR. Intestinal ischemia in the elderly. Gastroenterol Clin N Am. 2009;38(3):527–40.
5. Acosta S, Wadman M, Syk I, Elmståhl S, Ekberg O. Epidemiology and prognostic factors in acute superior mesenteric artery occlusion. J Gastrointest Surg. 2010;14(4):628–35.
6. Wyers MC. Acute mesenteric ischemia: diagnostic approach and surgical treatment. Semin Vasc Surg. 2010;23(1):9–20.
7. Oliva I, Davarpanah A, Rybicki F, Desjardins B, Flamm S, Francois C, et al. ACR appropriateness criteria® imaging of mesenteric ischemia. Abdom Imaging. 2013;38(4):714–9.
8. Aschoff A, Stuber G, Becker B, Hoffmann M, Schmitz B, Schelzig H, et al. Evaluation of acute mesenteric ischemia: accuracy of biphasic mesenteric multi-detector CT angiography. Abdom Imaging. 2009;34(3):345–57.
9. Hagspiel K, Flors L, Hanley M, Norton P. Computed tomography angiography and magnetic resonance angiography imaging of the mesenteric vasculature. Tech Vasc Interv Radiol. 2015;18(1):2–13.
10. Menke J. Diagnostic accuracy of multidetector CT in acute mesenteric ischemia: systematic review and meta-analysis. Radiology. 2010;256(1):93–101.
11. Kirkpatrick I, Kroeker M, Greenberg H. Biphasic CT with mesenteric CT angiography in the evaluation of acute mesenteric ischemia: initial experience. Radiology. 2003;229(1):91–8.
12. Bala M, Kashuk J, Moore E, Kluger Y, Biffl W, Gomes C, et al. Acute mesenteric ischemia: guidelines of the World Society of Emergency Surgery. World J Emerg Surg. 2017;12(38). https://doi.org/10.1186/s13017-017-0150-5
13. Gaa J, Laub G, Edelman RR, Georgi M. First clinical results of ultrafast, contrast-enhanced 2-phase 3D-angiography of the abdomen. Röfo. 1998;169(2):135–9.
14. Gilfeather M, Holland GA, Siegelman ES, et al. Gadolinium-enhanced ultrafast three-dimensional spoiled gradient-echo MR imaging of the abdominal aorta and visceral and iliac vessels. Radiographics. 1997;17(2):423–32.
15. Holland GA, Dougherty L, Carpenter JP, et al. Breath-hold ultrafast three-dimensional gadolinium-enhanced MR angiography of the aorta and the renal and other visceral abdominal arteries. AJR Am J Roentgenol. 1996;166(4):971–81.
16. Meaney JF, Prince MR, Nostrant TT, Stanley JC. Gadolinium-enhanced MR angiography of visceral arteries in patients with suspected chronic mesenteric ischemia. J Magn Reson Imaging. 1997;7(1):171–6.
17. Shetty AS, Mellnick VM, Raptis C, Loch R, Owen J, Bhalla S. Limited utility of MRA for acute bowel ischemia after portal venous phase CT. Abdom Imaging. 2015;40(8):3020–8.

What Is the Utility of Clinical Scoring Systems for the Diagnosis/Prognosis of Mesenteric Ischemia?

30

Courtney H. McKee and Sarah Ronan-Bentle

Pearls and Pitfalls
- No validated scoring system exists for the diagnosis of AMI.
- Mortality has been correlated with a number of factors in patients with AMI.
- Delay in diagnosis of AMI > 24 h from onset of symptoms increased risk of mortality by 30% in one study.
- Elevated lactate, elevated shock index, and other indicators of decompensated illness correlate with mortality in AMI, which approaches 100% in severe illness.

There is no widely accepted diagnostic scoring system that has been validated for the diagnosis of acute mesenteric ischemia (AMI). However, a number of historical, exam, and laboratory values when interpreted in aggregate are suggestive of the diagnosis as well as the prognosis.

Diagnostic Predictors

Wang et al. are among the first to propose a diagnostic scoring system for AMI. Their model was built from a retrospective review of 106 patients, 42.5% of whom had confirmed mesenteric ischemia. Their scoring system awards points for leukocytosis, increased red cell distribution width, increased mean platelet volume, and elevated D-dimer, which when applied to their patient population had a sensitivity of 97.8%, specificity of 91.8%, positive predictive value of 91.8%, and negative predictive value of 98.2% [1]. However, in a letter to the editor, Safiri and Ayubi appropriately raise concerns

with Wang's methodology, including comments regarding their very wide confidence intervals, for example, an elevated white blood cell count had a 95% confidence interval of 1.10–235.34; other variables had similarly wide confidence intervals that ultimately may not be clinically meaningful [2]. This likely reflects limitations from a small data pool and implies potentially biased data [2]. Additionally, this model has yet to be prospectively validated. At this time, it is difficult to argue for the implementation of Wang's model in its current form. However, Wang's model may form an important starting point upon which other diagnostic tools can be built.

Cudnik et al. in a 2013 meta-analysis of current literature on AMI, eloquently describe the limitations in current literature. Studies are frequently small, retrospective, and lack adequate control populations to account for intrinsic bias [3]. Further study is required to articulate the most appropriate diagnostic model and validate it for clinical practice.

Prognostic Predictors

Certain clinical data has been well correlated with an increased mortality in AMI. These include elevated serum lactate levels, delay in diagnosis >24 h from onset of symptoms, associated sepsis, and the presence of bowel necrosis [4–7]. Symptoms >24 h prior to diagnosis in particular were noted to decrease survival 30% in one study [6]. Regarding risk factors, a number of vascular comorbidities, as expected, have been investigated, but only atrial fibrillation appears to be negatively correlated with mortality in one large study by Bhardari et al. They found that prior diagnosis of atrial fibrillation was independently correlated with increased mortality ($p < 0.001$), but anticoagulation at time of diagnosis correlated with fewer complications in patients who lived [8].

A few investigators have attempted to link physiologic data to prognosis. One team looked at the systemic organ failure assessment (SOFA) compared to the multiorgan dysfunction (MOD) score in ICU patients with AMI and found that

C. H. McKee · S. Ronan-Bentle (✉)
University of Cincinnati College of Medicine, Department of Emergency Medicine, Cincinnati, OH, USA
e-mail: mckeech@ucmail.uc.edu; ronanse@uc.edu

© Springer Nature Switzerland AG 2019
A. Graham, D. J. Carlberg (eds.), *Gastrointestinal Emergencies*, https://doi.org/10.1007/978-3-319-98343-1_30

higher scores, or greater than 13, were associated with 100% mortality in both groups and there was no significant difference between the two scores in terms of predicting outcome [9]. Haga et al. examined a cohort of 110 patients and found that shock index >0.7 and EKG abnormalities, i.e., atrial fibrillation or interval abnormalities, were acceptable approximations of mortality in this cohort. Elevated shock index had an impressive odds ratio of 11 ($p = 0.019$), while EKG abnormalities had an odds ratio of 1.7 ($p = 0.0022$) [10].

While not yet generalizable or validated, the data suggest that indicators of poor systemic function, such as elevated lactate, sepsis, elevated shock index, elevated SOFA, delay in diagnosis, and comorbidities such as atrial fibrillation all negatively impact mortality in patients with AMI. Further research is required to build models that can assist with diagnosis and prognostication in these patients who carry such a high risk of mortality already.

Suggested Resources

- Long B, Koyfman A. The dangerous miss: recognizing acute mesenteric ischemia. May 2016; http://epmonthly.com/article/the-dangerous-miss/.
- Onal M, Atahan K, Kamer E, Yaşa H, Tarcan E, Onal M. Prognostic factors for hospital mortality in patients with acute mesenteric ischemia who undergo intestinal resection due to necrosis. Ulus Travma Acil Cerrahi Derg. 2010;16:63–70.

References

1. Cudnik MT, Subrahmanyam D, Janice J, Julian M, Stockton SW, Hiestand BC. The diagnosis of acute mesenteric ischemia: a systematic review and meta-analysis. Acad Emerg Med. 2013;20(11):1087–100.
2. Safiri S, Ayubi E. A novel scoring system for diagnosing acute mesenteric ischemia in the emergency Ward: methodological issues. World J Surg. 2018;42(2):608.
3. Wang Z, Chen J, Liu J, Tian L. A novel scoring system for diagnosing acute mesenteric ischemia in the emergency ward. World J Surg. 2017;41(8):1966–74.
4. Arthurs ZM, Titus J, Bannazadeh M, Eagleton MJ, Srivastava S, Sarac TP, et al. A comparison of endovascular revascularization with traditional therapy for the treatment of acute mesenteric ischemia. Journal of Vascular Surgery. 2011;53(3):698–705.
5. Nuzzo A, Maggiori L, Ronot M, Becq M, Plessier A, Gault N, et al. Predictive factors of intestinal necrosis in acute mesenteric ischemia: prospective study from an intestinal stroke center. Am J Gastroenterol. 2017;112:597–605.
6. Kassahun W, Schulz T, Richter O, Hauss J. Unchanged high mortality rates from acute occlusive intestinal ischemia: six year review. Langenbeck's Arch Surg. 2008;393(2):163–71.
7. Unalp HR, Atahan K, Kamer E, Yasa H, Tarcan E, Onal MA. Prognostic factors for hospital mortality in patients with acute mesenteric ischemia who undergo intestinal resection due to necrosis. Ulus Travma Acil Cerrahi Derg. 2010 Jan;16(1):63–70.
8. Bhandari S, Dang G, Shahreyar M, Hanif A, Muppidi V, Bhatia A, et al. Predicting outcomes in patients with atrial fibrillation and acute mesenteric ischemia. J Patient Cent Res Rev. 2016;3(4):177–86.
9. Viswanathan R, Vivekanandan S, Ravi A. Analysis of incidence and the value of SOFA and MOD scoring in predicting the outcome in acute mesenteric ischemia. Int Surg J. 2015;2(4):480–6.
10. Haga Y, Odo M, Homma M, Komiya K, Takeda K, Koike S, et al. New prediction rule for mortality in acute mesenteric ischemia. Digestion. 2009;80(2):104–11.

Chronic Mesenteric Ischemia: What Clinical Features Lead to the Diagnosis of CMI? Can This Diagnosis Be Made in the Emergency Department? What Is the Appropriate Disposition?

31

Susan Owens and Sarah Ronan-Bentle

Pearls and Pitfalls
- Chronic mesenteric ischemia classically presents as postprandial abdominal pain in elderly patients with history of extensive atherosclerotic disease.
- Young female patients with chronic, intermittent abdominal pain and previous extensive negative work-up may have chronic mesenteric ischemia from vasculitis or rheumatologic disease.
- Physical exam and lab work are often nonspecific; this disease is often diagnosed by imaging when looking for more emergent causes of abdominal pain.
- Chronic mesenteric ischemia is rare and difficult to diagnose in the acute care setting due to lack of a long patient-physician relationship.
- Outpatient referral to vascular surgery for planned intervention is an appropriate disposition.

Chronic mesenteric ischemia (CMI), also referred to as intestinal angina, represents a spectrum of diseases related to the narrowing of the mesenteric vasculature most commonly caused by atherosclerosis. Thus, mesenteric occlusive disease is often found among the elderly, with radiographic evidence of mesenteric artery stenosis present in 18–67% of patients greater than 75 years of age. The diagnosis of CMI requires both radiographic evidence of stenosis coupled with abdominal symptoms [1]. Similar to acute mesenteric ischemia, the estimated incidence of CMI is less than 1 per 100,000 hospital admissions and less than 2% of all admissions for gastrointestinal conditions [2]. CMI is similar to cardiovascular or peripheral vascular disease, with progressive symptoms that ultimately present with acute vascular occlusion. Because the mesenteric vasculature is complex and well-collateralized, patients typically remain asymptomatic until multiple vessels are critically stenosed. Over 90% of patients have superior mesenteric artery involvement [3, 4].

What Clinical Features Lead to the Diagnosis of CMI?

The classic patient profile for CMI is a 70–80-year-old female with a history of heavy smoking. Past medical history likely includes other risk factors for atherosclerotic disease. In younger patients, CMI has been found in patients with suspected vasculitis, fibromuscular dysplasia, or median arcuate ligament compression. Median arcuate ligament syndrome and fibromuscular dysplasia with CMI are diagnosed in females aged 20–40 years who have undergone an extensive negative work-up for chronic intermittent abdominal pain associated with eating [5, 6]. Patients with fibromuscular dysplasia may also have hypertension diagnosed at a young age if there is renal vasculature involvement. Vasculitis resulting in mesenteric ischemia is most commonly associated with Takayasu arteritis, systemic lupus erythematosus, and polyarteritis nodosa [7].

The defining symptom of CMI is postprandial abdominal pain, which is present in over 90% of patients [1, 2]. Pain is described as dull, crampy, or colicky and begins 15–30 min after eating, persisting up to 5–6 h after finishing a meal. Postprandial pain is due to a significant increase in blood flow to the splanchnic vasculature. Splanchnic vasculature accounts for 10–20% of cardiac output prior to meals but increases to approximately 35% of cardiac output to meet the increased metabolic demand of the intestinal tissue [2]. Changes in blood flow are dependent on meal content, with the largest and longest postprandial blood flow peaks noted after meals with high fat content. Due to the nature of the pain, patients typically develop food aversion or may eat

S. Owens · S. Ronan-Bentle (✉)
University of Cincinnati College of Medicine, Department of Emergency Medicine, Cincinnati, OH, USA
e-mail: owens2sn@ucmail.uc.edu; ronanse@uc.edu

© Springer Nature Switzerland AG 2019
A. Graham, D. J. Carlberg (eds.), *Gastrointestinal Emergencies*, https://doi.org/10.1007/978-3-319-98343-1_31

several small meals throughout the day resulting in significant weight loss. Studies have documented up to a 15 kg weight loss in CMI patients, depending on length of symptoms and severity of disease [8]. Patients also have symptoms of gastrointestinal upset including bloating, nausea, vomiting, diarrhea, and/or constipation, these have been attributed to progressive mucosal ischemia. As the disease progresses pain duration lengthens and may become constant, diarrhea is more common, and patients present with more vague chief complaints such as fatigue [1].

Physical exam findings in CMI are nonspecific, making the diagnosis of CMI in the acute care setting difficult. Due to food aversion and significant weight loss, patients can appear cachectic with flat or scaphoid abdomens. Debus comments the patients "are easier to examine due to their chronically poor nutritional status" [3]. The abdominal exam often reveals non-focal tenderness that may be out of proportion to exam. Abdominal bruit was once thought to be a diagnostic criteria of CMI though has since been declared a nonspecific finding; while bruit absence does not rule out disease, its presence should raise suspicion for vascular pathology [2].

Can This Diagnosis Be Made in the Emergency Department?

The differential diagnosis for CMI is broad, and the final diagnosis is one of exclusion, particularly in the emergency department. Epigastric or right upper quadrant pain related to eating may prompt work-up for gallbladder disease, reflux, peptic ulcer disease, and pancreatitis. Chronic abdominal pain and nausea may spur work-ups for gastroparesis. The presence of diarrhea may prompt a work-up for irritable bowel syndrome or inflammatory bowel disease. Unexplained weight loss often results in an evaluation for malignancy. Symptoms have typically been present for several years, and patients may have undergone extensive testing including invasive procedures to further elucidate the diagnosis. One of the most helpful diagnostic tools to the emergency clinician is chart review; records may reveal extensive outpatient work-up or several visits to the emergency department for unexplainable abdominal pain. Due to difficulty in diagnosing CMI, review of patient records has shown the duration of complaints last 20–25 months prior to CMI diagnosis [1]. Studies further report that 25–84% of patients had documented symptoms of CMI for months to years prior to presenting with acute mesenteric ischemia [1].

While diagnosing CMI remains difficult, the diagnosis can be made with imaging modalities readily available in most emergency departments. Mesenteric contrast aortogram, a procedure similar to a heart catheterization, remains the gold standard for occlusive mesenteric vessel disease. However, this invasive procedure is done in the operating room by vascular surgery and is often timed with planned repair or intervention; thus, it is not a practical diagnostic tool in the emergency department. Computerized tomographic angiography (CTA) is associated with 95–100% sensitivity and specificity for mesenteric artery stenosis. CTA is readily available in most emergency departments and has become the recommended imaging modality for diagnosis because it provides information about etiology of disease and vasculature anatomy. Although CTA provides detailed information about mesenteric vasculature anatomy and stenosis, it does require a large contrast bolus; thus, CTA has limited utility in patients with renal insufficiency [2, 9]. Duplex ultrasonography has a sensitivity and specificity of 85–90% and is particularly useful for proximal lesions. Several patient factors limit applicability, including bowel gas, obesity, and heavily calcified vessels [9]. Magnetic resonance angiography (MRA) is a third imaging modality that can be used for diagnosis of CMI; notably, it has less radiation exposure, although MRA cannot be used in patients with renal insufficiency [1].

What Is the Appropriate Disposition?

Ultimately CMI is a disease requiring surgical intervention and requires referral to vascular surgery or interventional radiology [10]. Symptomatic patients are primarily managed surgically with either endovascular therapy or open reconstruction to prevent bowel infarction. Medical management is used only in patients that are poor surgical candidates. While awaiting surgical intervention, smoking cessation, bowel rest, vasodilators, and anticoagulation to prevent acute thrombosis may be used to ameliorate symptoms temporarily, but these interventions do not stop disease progression [11]. Patients exhibiting failure to thrive may warrant admission for initiation of total parenteral nutrition to improve nutritional status before intervention. Patients with abdominal pain at rest and imaging evidence of CMI typically require intervention within 24 h given high risk of bowel infarction [12]. Without symptoms at rest, patients can likely be discharged from the ED with follow-up with either vascular surgery or interventional radiology depending on institutional preference for planned intervention and perioperative optimization. Explaining to patients the urgency for follow-up and lifestyle modifications such as smoking cessation and low-fat diet is of great importance.

Suggested Resource

- Mastoraki A, Mastoraki S, Tziava E, Touloumi S, Krinos N, Danias N, Lazaris A, Arkadopoulos N. Mesenteric ischemia: pathogenesis and challenging diagnostic and therapeutic modalities. World J Gastrointest Pathophysiol. 2016;7(1):125–30.

References

1. Kolkman JJ, Geelkerken RH. Diagnosis and treatment of chronic mesenteric ischemia: an update. Best Pract Res Clin Gastroenterol. 2017;31(1):49–57.
2. Chandra A, Quinones-Baldrich WJ. Chronic mesenteric ischemia: how to select patients for invasive treatment. Semin Vasc Surg. 2010;23(1):21–8.
3. Debus ES, Muller-Hulsbeck S, Kolbel T, Larena-Avellaneda A. Intestinal ischemia. Int J Color Dis. 2011;26(9):1087–97.
4. Paterno F, Longo WE. The etiology and pathogenesis of vascular disorders of the intestine. Radiol Clin N Am. 2008;46(5):877–85.
5. Lainez R, Richardson W. Median arcuate ligament syndrome: a case report. Ochsner J. 2013;13(4):561–4.
6. Senadhi V. A rare cause of chronic mesenteric ischemia from fibromuscular dysplasia: a case report. J Med Case Rep. 2010;19(4):373.
7. Angle J, Nida B, Matsumoto A. Managing mesenteric vasculitis. Radiology. 2015;18(1):38–42.
8. Rheudasil JM, Stewart MT, Schellack JV, Smith RB III, Salam AA, Perdue GD. Surgical treatment of chronic mesenteric arterial insufficiency. J Vasc Surg. 1988;8(4):495–500.
9. Clair DG, Beach JM. Mesenteric ischemia. N Engl J Med. 2016;374(10):959–68.
10. Pecoraro F, Rancic Z, Lachat M, Mayer D, Amann-Vesti B, Pfammatter T, Bajardi G, Veith FJ. Chronic mesenteric ischemia: critical review and guidelines for management. Ann Vasc Surg. 2013;27(1):113–22.
11. Mastoraki A, Mastoraki S, Tziava E, Touloumi S, Krinos N, Danias N, et al. Mesenteric ischemia: pathogenesis and challenging diagnostic and therapeutic modalities. World J Gastrointest Pathophysiol. 2016;7(1):125–30.
12. Kolkman JJ, Mensink PB, van Petersen AS, Huisman AB, Geelkerken RH. Clinical approach to chronic gastrointestinal ischaemia: from 'intestinal angina' to the spectrum of chronic splanchnic disease. Scand J Gastroenterol Suppl. 2004;39(Suppl 241):9–16.

What Are the Goals of Resuscitation in the ED? What Intravenous Fluids Should Be Used? Are Vasopressors Beneficial or Harmful? Should Antibiotics Be Administered?

32

Sarah Ronan-Bentle

Pearls and Pitfalls
- Goals of resuscitation include preserving perfusion, minimizing ischemic tissue damage and preventing sepsis and multiorgan failure.
- Antibiotic coverage includes coverage for Gram-negative and anaerobic bacteria.
- There is no benefit to resuscitation with colloid fluids over crystalloid fluids.
- Vasopressors should be used with caution but if indicated, norepinephrine alone or in combination with dobutamine is recommended.

Goals of resuscitation for patients with confirmed or suspected acute mesenteric ischemia (AMI) are to preserve perfusion, minimize tissue ischemia, and prevent development of sepsis or multiorgan failure [1]. Endpoints of resuscitation include monitoring lactate levels for estimation of tissue perfusion. Hemodynamic monitoring provides additive information about volume status. Another important aspect of resuscitation is optimization of comorbid conditions which, in the setting of AMI, increase morbidity and mortality. Often these include cardiac conditions such as congestive heart failure or arrhythmias.

The splanchnic circulation is a large vascular system that receives approximately 20–25% of cardiac output and accounts for 25% of the total resting blood volume [1, 2]. With food ingestion, the splanchnic flow increases to meet the increased oxygen demand for digestion. Splanchnic vasoconstriction is modulated by catecholamines (e.g., norepinephrine, epinephrine), angiotensin II, and endothelin, while vasodilation is due to nitric oxide and prostaglandins [2]. The pathophysiology of splanchnic circulation is important because medications and interventions that are commonly administered in the acute care setting may exacerbate mesenteric ischemia. For instance, NSAIDs (nonsteroidal anti-inflammatory drugs) inhibit prostaglandins thus decreasing vasodilation and increasing susceptibility of GI mucosa in circulatory shock [2].

Due to extensive collateral blood flow, bowel tissue can tolerate up to 12 h of 75% decreased blood flow without irreversible injury [1]. Thus supporting collateral blood flow and maintaining as much mesenteric blood flow as possible are critical during the evaluation of suspected AMI and before definitive intervention to re-establish blood flow.

What Intravenous Fluids Should Be Used?

Because the downstream effects of ischemia include decreased oxygen delivery to hypo-perfused tissues resulting in lactate accumulation and acidemia, fluid resuscitation with crystalloid fluid should be initiated as soon as AMI is suspected. There is no benefit to resuscitation with colloid fluids over crystalloid fluids [3]. Hypovolemia in patients with AMI is common. In one animal study examining the effect of fluid resuscitation and antibiotics on survival in AMI, aggressive fluid resuscitation (> 300 mL per hour) and antibiotics both increased survival rates (40% and 80%, respectively) compared to controls [4]. However, aggressive intravascular volume repletion has to be balanced with increased vascular permeability and extravasation into extravascular spaces including the bowel wall with ensuing worsening ischemia [1].

Are Vasopressors Beneficial or Harmful?

Vasopressors must be used judiciously in patients with AMI. Splanchnic perfusion is decreased with the use of vasopressors. For instance, both norepinephrine and epinephrine have been shown to cause mesenteric steal

S. Ronan-Bentle
University of Cincinnati College of Medicine, Department of Emergency Medicine, Cincinnati, OH, USA
e-mail: ronanse@uc.edu

© Springer Nature Switzerland AG 2019
A. Graham, D. J. Carlberg (eds.), *Gastrointestinal Emergencies*, https://doi.org/10.1007/978-3-319-98343-1_32

syndrome, diversion of blood from the mesenteric circulation; high-dose vasopressin infusions decrease mesenteric and collateral blood flow but low dose as adjunct may be safe based on septic shock models; digitalis produces mesenteric vasoconstriction with proximal SMA stenosis [1].

Once a patient is euvolemic but cardiac output and tissue oxygen delivery is still inadequate, vasopressors are indicated. Because both epinephrine and phenylephrine cause severe splanchnic vasoconstriction, the pressor of choice in resuscitation of patients with AMI is norepinephrine [1, 2]. Addition of dobutamine which has been shown to increase hepato-splanchnic blood flow may further support blood pressure while maintaining splanchnic perfusion [5].

Adjunct low-dose vasopressin may also be beneficial. In one study of nonocclusive mesenteric ischemia due to vasodilatory shock after cardiopulmonary bypass, patients were titrated to maximal doses of norepinephrine. In 11 patients in whom the mean arterial pressure could not be maintained, vasopressin was given as an adjunct. After 2 days of treatment, the group of 11 patients who received both vasopressin and norepinephrine had improved intestinal perfusion and required significantly lower doses of norepinephrine than the control group (norepinephrine alone). All patients who received vasopressin survived, while 17 of the 67 patients in the norepinephrine alone group died in the hospital. The authors concluded that vasopressin administration during nonocclusive mesenteric ischemia treatment after cardiopulmonary bypass improved small intestine perfusion and was associated with improved hospital survival [6].

Should Antibiotics Be Administered?

Because of the high risk of intraabdominal infection among patients with AMI, early administration of broad-spectrum antibiotics is recommended [7]. Gut bacteria translocation and development of intraabdominal sepsis is common in acute mesenteric ischemia (AMI) and contributes to mortality. Antibiotic coverage should include both Gram-negative and anaerobic bacteria coverage. However, animal studies suggest that antibiotic coverage for anaerobes is more clinically important than Gram-negative bacteria. In a study comparing antibiotic regimens in rats after transection of the superior mesenteric artery, longer survival times were noted in animals who received either metronidazole alone or metronidazole plus gentamicin compared to rats who received gentamicin alone [8]. Given the high acuity and complex clinical management of AMI, we recommend broad-spectrum antibiotics that cover both anaerobes and Gram-negative bacteria.

What Adjunct Therapies May Be Considered or Should Be Avoided?

- In patients who have atrial fibrillation/flutter and AMI, cardiac glycosides (e.g., digoxin) should be avoided [9].
- Anticoagulation if mesenteric vein thrombosis and intra-arterial thrombolytics if superior mesenteric artery (SMA) embolic disease may be beneficial. Supporting literature for thrombolytics is limited and mostly consists of small series and case reports [10]. However, intra-arterial thrombolytics as an adjunct to thrombectomy or embolectomy as a combined management strategy with surgery has demonstrated success [11].

> **Suggested Resources**
> - NOW @NEJM: Mesenteric ischemia; https://blogs.nejm.org/now/index.php/mesenteric-ischemia/2016/03/11/
> - Vitin AA, Metzner JI. Anesthetic management of acute mesenteric ischemia in elderly patients. Anesthesiol Clin. 2009;27(3):551–67.

References

1. Vitin AA, Metzner JI. Anesthetic management of acute mesenteric ischemia in elderly patients. Anesthesiol Clin. 2009;27(3):551–67.
2. Kolkman J, Geelkerken R. Chapter 162: splanchnic ischemia. In: Textbook of critical care, vol. e2. New York: Elsevier; 2017. p. 1135–42.
3. Perel P, Roberts I, Ker K. Colloids versus crystalloids for fluid resuscitation in critically ill patients. Cochrane Database Syst Rev. 2013;2:CD000567. https://doi.org/10.1002/14651858.CD000567.pub6.
4. Jamieson W, Pliagus G, Marchuk S, et al. Effect of antibiotic and fluid resuscitation upon survival times in experimental intestinal ischemia. Surg Gynecol Obstet. 1988;167(2):103–8.
5. Lisbon A. Dopexamine, dobutamine, and dopamine increase splanchnic blood flow: what is the evidence? Chest. 2003;123(Suppl 5):460S–3S.
6. Bomberg H, Groesdonk HV, Raffel M, et al. Vasopressin as therapy during nonocclusive mesenteric ischemia. Ann Thorac Surg. 2016;102(3):813–9.
7. Bala M, Kashuk J, Moore EE, et al. Acute mesenteric ischemia: Guidelines of the world society of emergency surgery. World J Emerg Surg. 2017;12:38. –017–0150-5. eCollection 2017.
8. Plonka AJ, Schentag JJ, Messinger S, Adelman MH, Francis KL, Williams JS. Effects of enteral and intravenous antimicrobial treatment on survival following intestinal ischemia in rats. J Surg Res. 1989;46(3):216–20.
9. Tilsed JV, Casamassima A, Kurihara H, et al. ESTES guidelines: acute mesenteric ischaemia. Eur J Trauma Emerg Surg. 2016;42(2):253–70.
10. Schoots I, Levi M, Reekers J, Lameris J, van Gulik T. Thrombolytic therapy for acute superior mesenteric artery occlusion. J Vasc Interv Radiol. 2005;16(3):317–29.
11. Ieradi A, Tsetis D, Angileri S, et al. The role of endovascular therapy in acute mesenteric ischemia. Ann Gastroenterol. 2017;20(5):526–33.

Morbidity and Mortality of Acute Mesenteric Ischemia: How Can Emergency Medicine Clinicians Impact Outcomes?

33

Kelli L. Jarrell and Sarah Ronan-Bentle

Pearls and Pitfalls
- The key to improving outcomes for patient with acute mesenteric ischemia (AMI) is early recognition and diagnosis. The ED provider should maintain a high level of suspicion for this relatively uncommon but deadly diagnosis in elderly patients with abdominal pain and vascular or embolic risk factors.
- Early surgical consultation is crucial with high suspicion for AMI as patients with early revascularization have better outcomes.
- Emergency department resuscitation with fluids and treatment of sepsis with antibiotics can optimize patients for surgery.
- Patient factors, such as older age, longer duration of symptoms, and laboratory evidence of acute organ failure or end organ hypoperfusion, portend a worse prognosis.

Emergency medicine clinicians can improve morbidity and mortality in patients with acute mesenteric ischemia (AMI) with early recognition of the disease process, resuscitation of the patient prior to surgery, and early surgical consultation. Although mortality rates have declined for AMI over the past 50 years, they remain unacceptably high at 50–69% [1, 2]. Overall, 26% of the people admitted to the hospital with AMI will be alive 1 year later. Of the four types of AMI (e.g., venous thrombotic, nonocclusive venous events, arterial embolic, and arterial thrombotic), nonocclusive venous events have the lowest overall mortality rates. Acute mesenteric ischemia following cardiac surgery, although relatively uncommon, occurs more frequently in older, dehydrated patients with generalized atherosclerosis and is particularly deadly with a 70–100% mortality rate [1].

What Factors Affect the Morbidity and Mortality of Acute Mesenteric Ischemia (AMI)?

Because early diagnosis is critical to improving morbidity and mortality, the emergency medicine provider must maintain a high level of clinical suspicion, particularly in high-risk patient populations (e.g., the elderly and/or those with a medical history of atrial fibrillation). AMI is relatively uncommon with an incidence 0.09–0.2% of all surgical admissions, but its high mortality makes it a "can't miss" cause of abdominal pain and time-dependent diagnosis. The gut can survive a 75% reduction in blood flow for up to 12 h without significant injury; irreversible bowel damage occurs within 6 h of complete vascular occlusion [2].

Patient factors that predict a poor prognosis and increased mortality include older age, those with delayed presentation, peritonitis at presentation, and those who present with organ failure. In one study, in addition to older age, patients admitted from nursing homes, those with partial dependence on a secondary caregiver, and the existence of a pre-existing DNR order were all associated with mortality [3]. One Swedish study of 74 patients from 1987 to 1996 reported a 30-day survival of 81% for patients less than 71 years of age. This fell to 30% in patients who were 71–84 years of age. The survival rate for patients greater than age 84 years was 7%. They found corresponding increased rates of non-resectable gangrene with advancing age (9% in patients <71 years old, 45% in patients 71–84 years old, 79% in patients >84 years old) [4]. In a study of 72 patients over a 12-year period, the perioperative morbidity was 39% with a 30-day mortality rate of 31%. They found age greater than 70 and prolonged symptom duration to be independent predictors of mortality [5].

K. L. Jarrell · S. Ronan-Bentle (✉)
University of Cincinnati College of Medicine, Department of Emergency Medicine, Cincinnati, OH, USA
e-mail: kelli.jarrell@uc.edu; ronanse@uc.edu

© Springer Nature Switzerland AG 2019
A. Graham, D. J. Carlberg (eds.), *Gastrointestinal Emergencies*, https://doi.org/10.1007/978-3-319-98343-1_33

There are patient comorbidities that contribute to increased mortality. These include contaminated wounds prior to surgery, history of myocardial ischemia within 6 months, and history of chronic obstructive pulmonary disease (COPD) [1]. Another study from Turkey demonstrated that a history of diabetes mellitus, the use of digoxin for treatment of atrial fibrillation, and antiplatelet drugs were negative predictors of perioperative mortality [6]. The European Society for Trauma and Emergency Surgery (ESTES) and World Society of Emergency Surgeon (WSES) recommend against using digoxin for the acute treatment of atrial fibrillation in patients with acute mesenteric ischemia [1, 2, 6].

Patients presenting in a coma, those requiring mechanical ventilation, those in acute renal and liver failure, or those with preoperative sepsis tended to have worse outcomes. Those presenting with peritonitis tended to have high rates of bowel necrosis and worse prognosis overall. Specific laboratory abnormalities that are risk factors for mortality include renal failure and acidosis. These abnormalities resulting from shock and sepsis have been identified as independent risk factors of mortality [1, 2]. One study in China of patients diagnosed with AMI in the emergency department identified bandemia, elevated AST, and increased BUN as independent risk factors, in addition to old age and metabolic acidosis [7]. Interestingly, elevated lactate is a nonspecific marker, although it is classically taught as being associated with acute mesenteric ischemia. One study demonstrated that lactic acidosis develops late in the course of this disease process with extensive transmural infarction and tissue hypoperfusion due to sepsis. By this point, the mortality is near 75% [1].

How Can Emergency Medicine Clinicians Impact Outcomes?

Early recognition is paramount to improving mortality. The aforementioned Swedish study demonstrated that mortality was 10.6% for patients operated on within the first 24 h after onset of symptoms and was 72.9% if operated on after 24 h of symptoms. They also found that operation within 6 h of admission resulted in better survival compared with operations done after more than a 6 h delay [4]. Gut viability is believed to be 100% within first 12 h of ischemia. This drops to 54% between 12 and 24 h and to 18% beyond 24 h [1]. This should reinforce the importance of timely diagnosis of AMI in the ED and the avoidance of delays to diagnosis and surgical consultation, particularly in those patients in whom you have a high suspicion and/or those presenting with symptoms of longer duration.

Although there is no data to support or refute whether the reversal of laboratory abnormalities such as elevated lactate levels is associated with improvements in outcomes, the

ESTES and WSES both recommend resuscitating AMI patients with IV fluids and broad-spectrum antibiotics [1, 2]. These therapies can and certainly should begin in the emergency department. Another recommendation is that patients with AMI should be admitted to the ICU for further resuscitation when appropriate.

The management of venous acute mesenteric ischemia (VAMI) is different than the other types of AMI, as these patients should be anticoagulated as soon as the diagnosis is made and will require lifelong anticoagulation. Patients with ischemia related to venous thrombosis have the lowest mortality of all patients with acute mesenteric ischemia, with rates as low as 11–30% quoted in the literature [1]. In general with acute mesenteric ischemia, patients presenting earlier in their disease have better outcomes. Conversely, those with venous thrombosis who presented early in their disease course, within 3 days of onset of symptoms, had poorer outcomes. This group was also more likely to undergo laparotomy within 12 h of hospital admission (83% vs. 20%). It is hypothesized that this early presenting group had more rapid progression of their disease process which was why they had poorer outcomes and higher mortality overall [1].

Although decisions should be made in conjunction with surgical consultation, a certain subset of patients are unlikely to benefit from operative intervention, and emergency medicine clinicians may initiate goals of care discussions with the patient and available family members. Moribund patients with significant comorbidities and those who have a poor baseline performance status are unlikely to benefit from intervention. Avoiding operative intervention in these moribund patients is included in both the ESTES and WSES guidelines [1, 2]. These patients will likely still require admission for coordination of care and palliative management.

Summary

Despite the exceedingly high mortality rate, those patients with AMI that do survive to hospital discharge have relatively good outcomes with 84% alive at 1 year and 50–77% at 5 years. Most of the mortality in this cohort of patients was related to cardiovascular disease rather than recurrence of mesenteric ischemia or morbidity related to this disease process [1]. One study of 48 patients from 1963 to 2000 showed that overall late survival rates were 54% and 20% at 5 and 10 years, respectively. However, after the exclusion of perioperative deaths, the probability of long-term survival was 77% at 5 years and 29% at 10 years [8]. Once again, these survival rates should be viewed in the context of a patient population with significant cardiovascular comorbidities and advanced age. ED providers can help improve patient outcomes by with early recognition of this disease process and consultation with a surgeon early in order to maximize the opportunity for surgical intervention and the likelihood of survival to hospital discharge.

Suggested Resources

- Episode 42: Mesenteric ischemia and pancreatitis. Emergency medicine cases. https://emergencymed-icinecases.com/episode-42-mesenteric-ischemia-pancreatitis-3/
- Mesenteric Ischemia. Life in the fast lane. https://lifeinthefastlane.com/ccc/mesenteric-ischaemia/

References

1. Tilsed JV, Casamassima A, Kurihara H, Mariani D, Martinez I, Pereira J, et al. ESTES guidelines: acute mesenteric ischaemia. Eur J Trauma Emerg Surg. 2016 Apr;42(2):253–70.
2. Bala M, Kashuk J, Moore EE, Kluger Y, Biffl W, Gomes CA, et al. Acute mesenteric ischemia: guidelines of the World Society of Emergency Surgery. World J Emerg Surg. 2017;12:38. https://doi.org/10.1186/s13017-017-0150-5. eCollection 2017.
3. Gupta PK, Natarajan B, Gupta H, Fang X, Fitzgibbons RJ. Morbidity and mortality after bowel resection for acute mesenteric ischemia. Surgery. 2011;150(4):779–87.
4. Wadman M, Syk I, Elmstahl S. Survival after operations for ischaemic bowel disease. Eur J Surg. 2000;166(11):872–7.
5. Kougias P, Lau D, El Sayed HF, Zhou W, Huynh TT, Lin PH. Determinants of mortality and treatment outcome following surgical interventions for acute mesenteric ischemia. J Vasc Surg. 2007;46(3):467–74.
6. Alhan E, Usta A, Çekiç A, Saglam K, Türkyılmaz S, Cinel A. A study on 107 patients with acute mesenteric ischemia over 30 years. Int J Surg. 2012;10(9):510–3.
7. Huang H, Chang Y, Yen DH, Kao W, Chen J, Wang L, et al. Clinical Factors and Outcomes in Patients with Acute Mesenteric Ischemia in the Emergency Department. J Chin Med Assoc. 2005;68(7):299–306.
8. Cho J, Carr JA, Jacobsen G, Shepard AD, Nypaver TJ, Reddy DJ. Long-term outcome after mesenteric artery reconstruction: A 37-year experience. J Vasc Surg. 2002;35(3):453–60.

Consultant Corner: Acute Mesenteric Ischemia

34

Stephanie Streit and Sarah Ronan-Bentle

Answers to Key Clinical Questions

Pearls and Pitfalls
- Early recognition and consultation with a surgeon is imperative in preserving and restoring tissue perfusion and decreasing mortality.
- Multidetector CT is the standard imaging study for diagnosis of AMI.
- Resuscitation with balanced crystalloid intravenous fluids aids in prevention/correction of acidemia and swift transition to vasopressor therapy when needed for resultant sepsis.
- A hybrid surgical approach, utilizing endovascular interventions for the vascular lesion and open or laparoscopic bowel evaluation, should be the surgical standard of care.

Introduction

Dr. Stephanie Streit is board certified in general surgery and surgical critical care since 2015. She is currently practicing acute care surgery and critical care at the University Medical Center in Las Vegas, NV. She is a major in the US Air Force, currently stationed at Nellis Air Force Base.

1. When do you recommend consultation with a surgeon and in what time frame?

Mesenteric ischemia can be frightening and life threatening in all of its forms. It remains a relatively rare diagnosis, which can make it all the more daunting. As with many things in medicine, a thorough history and a sense of urgency are often the best tools in the toolbox. Just as time is myocardium in acute coronary syndrome, time is bowel and survival, in the setting of acute mesenteric ischemia (AMI). As soon as the diagnosis of AMI is considered, a surgeon should be involved in the patient's care. Knowing your institution's resources will determine whom to call and whether transferring the patient to another institution may be necessary. It is likely correct to start with your general surgeon, but vascular surgery and interventional radiology are often key consultants as well. The literature supports endovascular intervention on vascular lesions, even when bowel resection is also required; this "hybrid technique" should be the standard of care.

2. What pearls can you offer emergency care providers when evaluating patients with mesenteric ischemia?

The common denominator of mesenteric ischemia is decreased blood flow: decreased arterial inflow, venous obstruction stemming outflow, or a global low flow state related to shock. The end result of the loss of flow is progressive cell death, with the extent of tissue loss being determined by the degree of flow disruption and the duration of the low flow state that is unable to meet the metabolic demands of the tissue. The duration of symptoms, burden of clot, and presence or absence of collateral blood flow all determine the patient's tolerance for decreased flow to the bowel.

There are a few key clinical patterns which can raise clinical suspicions and accelerate workup in an emergency department. Each of the types of mesenteric ischemia has its classic history, but the majority of AMI cases are nonspecific

S. Streit
United States Air Force, Washington, DC, USA

Nellis Air Force Base, Las Vegas, NV, USA

University of Nevada Las Vegas, Las Vegas, NV, USA

S. Ronan-Bentle (✉)
University of Cincinnati College of Medicine, Department of Emergency Medicine, Cincinnati, OH, USA
e-mail: ronanse@uc.edu

© Springer Nature Switzerland AG 2019
A. Graham, D. J. Carlberg (eds.), *Gastrointestinal Emergencies*, https://doi.org/10.1007/978-3-319-98343-1_34

and overlap with a plethora of diagnoses on the differential. New onset atrial fibrillation or other cardiac dysthymia may create an embolus to the SMA. Smokers who suffer from other vascular diseases or who have recently lost weight may have a chronic SMA stenosis or thrombus that has now reached a critical level. Young women on hormonal birth control with a family history of blood clots may present with mesenteric venous thrombosis. Postoperative patients also make up a large portion of venous mesenteric ischemia. Low flow state mesenteric ischemia is not a common presentation in the emergency department apart from the profoundly ill, but it may accompany an exacerbation of systolic heart failure or cardiogenic shock.

In its early stages, AMI can and will present with relatively nonspecific symptoms and a benign abdominal exam. "Pain out of proportion to exam" often holds true prior to the point of bowel necrosis, but the pain is often vague and associated with other symptoms such as nausea, vomiting, and/or diarrhea. Excepting the minority of patients who present with peritoneal signs, the physical exam is widely variable based on the degree and location of occlusion within the mesenteric tree, as well as the presence or absence of chronic disease.

3. Is there a laboratory test that determines the diagnosis of AMI?

The liver's capacity to metabolize the portal venous contents often masks acidemia and other signs of cell death. As such, there is no single laboratory examination that can identify AMI. Rather, a constellation of inflammatory markers may suggest an ongoing ischemic process; this does not, however, have the capacity to distinguish AMI from other inflammatory or infectious gastrointestinal process.

4. How can emergency medicine provider's impact the outcome of patients with AMI?

More than any other practitioner, emergency medicine providers will be the ones to change the statistics on AMI. Earlier recognition and faster times to revascularization will be the only means of improving survival for patients with AMI.

- Hypotension and laboratory evaluation consistent with acidemia in patients with risk factors for AMI should increase the index of suspicion and prompt early surgical consultation even while resuscitation efforts are underway.
- Timing and protocoling of an imaging study can be discussed with the consulting surgeon. Because multidetector CT is widely available, it has become the imaging study standard for diagnosis of AMI. The ability to diagnose venous occlusion on CT is yet another advantage of the modality, presuming the study is protocoled in such a way that captures images with contrast in the venous

phase. The CTA appearance of the vasculature also influences both vascular and general surgeons' intervention algorithm. Surgeons will be influenced by the bowel wall appearance and CT signs of ischemia or necrosis in regard to preferred intervention (open or laparoscopic surgery, interventional radiology procedure).

5. What concepts do you think are key to the resuscitation of this patient population?

- Once mesenteric ischemia has been considered or identified, consultation with surgical colleagues is a top priority.
- An equal priority is restoration of blood pressure and systemic perfusion. In mild cases, this may be achieved with IV fluids alone. The choice of intravenous fluids should be tailored to the renal profile, but, in general, a balanced solution such as Plasma-Lyte A or Normosol is prefered. While not studied specifically for this indication, both are likely an improvement over normal saline given the tendency toward acidemia during the resuscitation of patients with mesenteric ischemia.
- If adequate blood pressure cannot be restored with fluids alone, vasopressors may be needed. Patients who are pressor-dependent likely have necrotic bowel which will not be affected by the relative impact of vasopressors on the splanchnic system. Norepinephrine is the vasopressor of choice, given that the hypotension most closely resembles a septic state.
- If no contraindication to anticoagulation exists, then systemic therapy with heparin may be warranted. This is particularly true if endovascular therapy is planned.
- Broad-spectrum antibiotics directed at gastrointestinal flora should be initiated if the CT shows evidence of bowel necrosis or if there are signs of systemic infection.

6. What complications are you concerned about in this patient population?

- Multisystem organ failure – Delay in diagnosis leads to worse outcomes of increased morbidity and mortality. Extended times of tissue necrosis, which occurs after 6–12 h of hypoperfusion, can create multisystem organ failure and remove surgical intervention as an option.
- Short gut syndrome (SGS) typically occurs when a patient is left with less than 100 cm of total bowel length without an ileocecal valve or less than 50 cm of small bowel length with an intact ileocecal valve. In adults with acute mesenteric ischemia, a large SMA clot may result in massive bowel loss and subsequent intestinal failure. SGS is associated with frequent, often debilitating, diarrhea, weakness, electrolyte imbalance, frequent

bouts of dehydration leading to renal injury, and a myriad of catheter-related complications as most people with SGS are TPN-dependent, at least for some period of time.

- Abdominal wall management and hernia – Patients requiring bowel resection for mesenteric ischemia are very often treated by damage control laparotomy or open abdomen technique. This is done primarily for two often concomitant reasons: (1) the patient is profoundly ill, and the operation is concluded in the timeliest fashion possible, and (2) a "second-look laparotomy" is strongly supported by the literature, particularly when the cause of ischemia isn't entirely clear. While damage control laparotomy is a highly useful and effective technique, patients whose abdomens are left open for any period of time have a higher rate of deep and superficial surgical site infections as well as abdominal wall hernia development.

- Bleeding and vascular complications – Open and endovascular interventions for mesenteric ischemia have associated complications. Open vascular repairs have a high primary and secondary patency rate. The surgical complication rate for open repairs, however, is higher and can be profound. While rare, vascular anastomotic leak (pseudoaneurysms) and blowouts are devastating events, often resulting in complex reoperations, prolonged critical illness or death. Endovascular repairs do have fewer short-term complications, but this likely represents selection bias as patients who can be treated without laparotomy have lower vascular burden and less bowel ischemia. There is a higher rate of re-intervention over time in those treated endovascularly, so it is important that these patients understand that risk and are followed closely.

7. Chronic mesenteric ischemia: can this diagnosis be made in the ED? If so, what clinical features lead to the diagnosis? What is the ED treatment? What is the appropriate disposition?

Chronic mesenteric ischemia (CMI) is a clinical diagnosis consisting of chronic abdominal pain, weight loss, and atherosclerotic disease of the mesenteric vessels. It occurs almost exclusively in smokers and people over the age of 60, and these patients may also suffer from other vascular disease burden such as claudication or angina. The pain that occurs with CMI is often epigastric or periumbilical. It is a vague pain that is most commonly brought on by eating. Patients who develop CMI slowly overtime often develop "food fear" as they know that eating will bring on their pain. As such, patients are often quite thin or have experienced significant weight loss, sometimes over a surprisingly short period of time.

The diagnosis of CMI can be difficult to make. When emergency clinicians see patients with abdominal pain (especially food fear) and weight loss but with a benign abdominal exam, CMI should be considered. A helical CT angiography will show calcifications in at least two of the three mesenteric vessels. Patients may also present with acute-on-chronic mesenteric ischemia, in which a chronic lesion has reached "critical stenosis" and bowel ischemia is starting to occur.

If there are bowel wall changes on CTA or the patient has a concerning abdominal exam or laboratory findings, then urgent surgical consultation should be pursued.

In the absence of these, then the CTA should be reviewed by a vascular surgeon or interventional radiologist. Whenever possible based on lesion characteristics, endovascular therapy should be the preferred intervention given the malnutrition and reduced healing capacity associated with CMI. Patients may require admission for dehydration, malnutrition, their overall vascular burden, or other complication of CMI. If the patient does not meet criteria for hospital admission, then short interval follow-up with a surgical provider should be ensured.

Suggested Resources
- Beaulieu RJ, et al. Comparison of open and endovascular treatment of acute mesenteric ischemia. J Vasc Surg. 2014;59(1):159–64.
- Pecoraro F, et al. Chronic mesenteric ischemia: critical review and guidelines for management. Ann Vasc Surg. 2013;27(1):113–22.
- Yang Z, et al. Management of acute mesenteric ischemia: a critical review and treatment algorithm. Vasc Endovascular Surg. 2016;50(3):183–92.

Part V

Abdominal Pain and Vomiting

When Should a Non-gastrointestinal Cause of Nausea and Vomiting Be Considered?

35

Kraftin E. Schreyer, Deena D. Wasserman, and Evan Kingsley

Pearls and Pitfalls
- Nausea and vomiting are nonspecific complaints, so associated symptoms should be used to help focus and narrow the differential diagnosis.
- The history and physical examination will reveal the diagnosis in the majority of cases.
- Directed laboratory testing and imaging is most useful when guided by the history and physical examination.

Nausea and vomiting are a common complaint seen in acute care settings, accounting for more than 1 million emergency department visits in 2014 [1]. Most patients have benign, self-limited causes and can be managed with supportive care [2, 3]. However, nausea and vomiting may be symptoms of serious disease processes, many of which are shown in Fig. 35.1. "Gastroenteritis mimics" in the Additional Reading section also reviews worrisome gastrointestinal and non-gastrointestinal causes of nausea and vomiting.

History and physical examination are the most important tools to evaluate for underlying causes of nausea and vomiting and should therefore guide further diagnostic testing. No randomized controlled trials compare evaluation strategies for nausea and vomiting. The approach discussed below is based on multiple review articles and expert consensus.

History

Determining the time course of symptoms plays an important role in evaluating potential causes of nausea and vomiting. Acute and chronic (>1 month) causes often have very different etiologies (Table 35.1). Sudden-onset nausea and vomiting are more likely related to infectious or toxic sources. They suggest a potential pathologic response to an underlying process. Insidious onset of symptoms over days or weeks points to metabolic or endocrine causes. Chronic symptoms are more likely to have an underlying functional gastrointestinal or psychiatric component [4].

Important historical factors include frequency, severity, content of the emesis (bloody, bilious, etc.), provoking factors (oral intake), sick contacts, travel, past medical history, previous abdominal surgeries, and medication or drug use [2–7]. Table 35.2 highlights medications that commonly cause vomiting, and Table 35.3 reviews common historical elements that may suggest specific diagnoses.

Symptoms associated with nausea and vomiting, along with past medical and social history, further narrow the differential diagnosis and guide additional investigation.

Headache and/or blurred vision suggest neurologic causes, as do slurred speech, ataxia, and vertigo, which may indicate posterior circulation stroke. Neurologic imaging should be considered in these patients and in patients who are at risk for intracranial pathology. High-risk patients include those with cancer that could metastasize to the brain and those with risk factors for intracranial hemorrhage, including hypertension, anticoagulation, and a history of aneurysm or polycystic kidney disease. Recent head injury may also warrant imaging, especially in the setting of anticoagulation.

Fever suggests potential gastrointestinal or non-gastrointestinal infection. Dysuria and flank pain with fever likely indicate pyelonephritis. Headache and stiff neck with fever suggest potential central nervous system infection.

Urinary or genital complaints should prompt evaluation of these respective organ systems. Potential sources include gonadal torsion and nephrolithiasis.

Confirmed or possible ingestion necessitates a toxicologic workup including aspirin and acetaminophen levels, electrocardiogram, and, if indicated, a urine toxicology screen.

A history of alcohol abuse could indicate pancreatitis or alcoholic ketoacidosis as the culprit, whereas a history of

K. E. Schreyer (✉) · D. D. Wasserman · E. Kingsley
Department of Emergency Medicine, Temple University Hospital, Philadelphia, PA, USA
e-mail: Kraftin.Schreyer@tuhs.temple.edu; Deena.Wasserman@tuhs.temple.edu; Evan.Kingsley@tuhs.temple.edu

© Springer Nature Switzerland AG 2019
A. Graham, D. J. Carlberg (eds.), *Gastrointestinal Emergencies*, https://doi.org/10.1007/978-3-319-98343-1_35

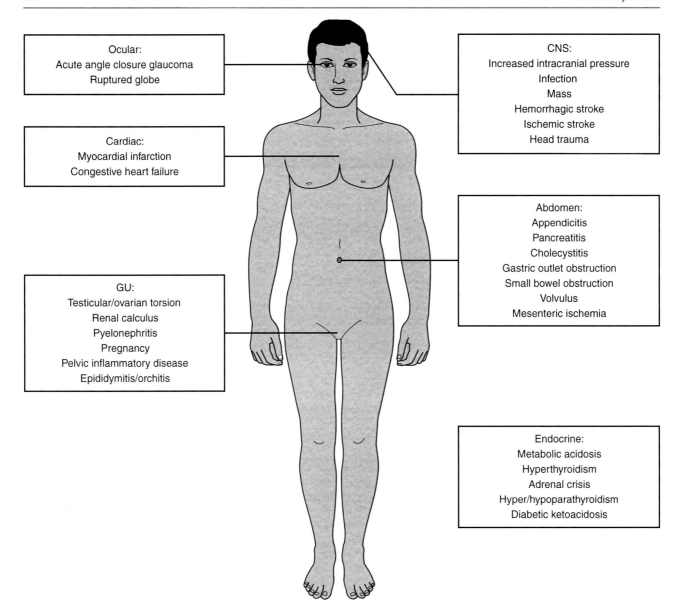

Fig. 35.1 Important causes of nausea and vomiting

Table 35.1 Acute vs chronic causes of nausea and vomiting

Acute		Chronic
Gastroenteritis	Withdrawal (opiate/ETOH)	Pregnancy
Foodborne illness	Pregnancy	Gastroesophageal reflux disease
Pancreatitis	Torsion (testicular/ovarian)	Peptic ulcer disease
Hepatitis	Myocardial infarction	Inflammatory bowel disease
Cholecystitis	Vertigo	Irritable bowel syndrome
Appendicitis	Thyrotoxicosis/thyroid storm	Gastroparesis
SBO	Hypercalcemia	Malignancy
Metabolic acidosis	Adrenal disease	Anorexia nervosa
Increased ICP	Pyelonephritis	Bulimia nervosa
Migraine headache	Angle closure glaucoma	Labyrinthine disorder (Meniere's disease)
Irritant ingestion	Medications	Cyclic vomiting syndrome
Overdose (ASA, ETOH)		Medications
		Marijuana

Table 35.2 Common medications causing nausea and vomiting

NSAIDs
Digoxin
Antiarrhythmics
Oral antidiabetics (metformin)
Antibiotics (erythromycin, bactrim)
Antivirals
Antiparkinson drugs
Antiepileptics
High-dose vitamins
Chemotherapy
Narcotics
Hormonal supplements

Table 35.3 Classic presentations

Acute onset	Cholecystitis, gastroenteritis, pancreatitis
Associated diarrhea, headache, myalgia	Gastroenteritis
Bilious emesis	Small bowel obstruction
Delayed vomiting (>1 h after a meal)	Gastric outlet obstruction, gastroparesis
Feculent emesis	Bowel obstruction
Insidious onset	Gastroesophageal reflux, medication, pregnancy
Projectile	Intracranial process
Regurgitation of undigested food	Achalasia, esophageal stricture, Zenker's diverticulum
Morning vomiting	Pregnancy, increased intracranial pressure, uremia

Tables created with information from sources [2–6]

marijuana use may suggest cannabinoid hyperemesis syndrome as the underlying cause. For more information on cannabinoid hyperemesis syndrome, please refer to Chap. 37 of this text [2, 8–10].

Nausea and vomiting can also be a presenting complaint in acute myocardial infarction, and this etiology should be considered in patients with cardiac risk factors, those with diaphoresis, epigastric discomfort, and/or chest discomfort.

Patients with known or suspected diabetes are at risk of developing diabetic ketoacidosis or hyperosmolar hyperglycemic syndrome.

Physical Examination

Abnormal vitals should be acknowledged and often merit further workup. Evaluation for dehydration (dry or tacky mucous membranes, poor skin turgor) may prompt aggressive fluid resuscitation. Abdominal tenderness, especially when focal, may prompt laboratory testing and/or imaging with ultrasound or computed tomography. Vomiting patients presenting with head trauma, visual symptoms, or imbalance require a thorough neurological, ocular, and otic examination. These patients potentially require neuroimaging, even when there is another potential cause of nausea and vomiting.

Diagnostic Testing

The history and physical exam guide diagnostic testing with two exceptions: women of child-bearing age should have pregnancy testing, and patients with a history of diabetes (or suspected undiagnosed diabetes) should have their blood glucose level checked. Blood glucose testing should be considered in younger patients with otherwise unexplained nausea and vomiting to evaluate for undiagnosed diabetes (potentially complicated by ketoacidosis).

Electrolytes and/or serum chemistry testing should be considered with evidence of dehydration on exam or a prolonged history of vomiting. Urine ketones may help determine severity of dehydration and may suggest alcoholic or diabetic ketoacidosis [2–7]. Additional laboratory workup, such as hepatic or pancreatic testing, is guided by the history and examination.

Likewise, imaging obtained should be based on the history and physical exam. A head CT should be considered if there is concern for an intracranial process, and abdominal imaging should be considered for patients with a concerning history and/or focal tenderness.

Electrocardiogram should be considered in appropriately selected patients with cardiac risk factors, including at-risk women and diabetics with nonspecific complaints, as these patients frequently have atypical presentations of acute coronary syndrome.

Approach

An approach to the undifferentiated patient with vomiting is shown in Fig. 35.2. Evaluation should begin with an assessment of acuity. Unstable patients should be resuscitated. Stable patients should have a thorough history and physical examination, followed by further workup if merited.

Fig. 35.2 Approach to the undifferentiated patient with nausea and vomiting

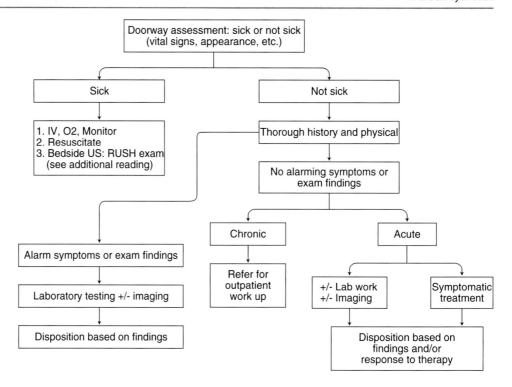

References

1. Agency for Healthcare Research and Quality: Healthcare Cost and Utilization Project. HCUPnet – Emergency Department National Statistics, 2014 National Diagnoses--ICD-9-CM Codes (ICD9), Principal Diagnosis: 787.01 Nausea With Vomiting (after Oct 1, 2009) [Internet]. 2017 [cited 16 Aug 2017]; Available from: https://hcupnet.ahrq.gov/#query/eyJEQVRBU0VUX1NPVVVJDRSI6WyJEU19ORURTIl0sIkFO-QUxZU0lTX1RZUEUiOlsiQVRfTSJdLCJZRUFSFSUyI6WyJZU-l8yMDE0Il0sIkNBVEVVHT1JJWkFUSU9OX1RZUEUiOlsiQ1Rf-SUNEOUQiXSwiQ1RfSUNEOUQiOlsiMTcyMDAiXX0=

2. Anderson WD, Strayer SM. Evaluation of nausea and vomiting: a case based approach. Am Fam Physician. 2013;88:371–9.

3. Harbord M. Nausea and vomiting. Medicine. 2009;37:115–8.

4. Scorza K, Williams A. Evaluation of nausea and vomiting. Am Fam Physician. 2007;76:76–84.

5. Hasler W, Chey W. Nausea and vomiting. Gastroenterology. 2003;125:1860–7.

6. Quigley E, Hasler W, Parkman H. AGA technical review on nausea and vomiting. Gastroenterology. 2001;120:263–86.

7. Metz A, Hebbard G. Evaluation of nausea and vomiting in adults: a diagnostic approach. Aust Fam Physician. 2007;36:688–92.

8. Batchelor J, McGuiness A. A meta-analysis of GCS 15 head injured patients with loss of consciousness or post-traumatic amnesia. Emerg Med J. 2002;19:515–9.

9. Hall J, Driscoll P. Nausea, vomiting and fever. Emerg Med J. 2005;22:200–4.

10. American Gastroenterological Association medical position statement. Nausea and vomiting. Gastroenterology. 2001;120:261–2.

Customizing Your Antiemetic: What Should You Consider?

36

James Murrett, Jennifer Repanshek, and Matthew Hinton

Pearls and Pitfalls

- Only about half of patients reporting nausea are treated for symptoms in the emergency department.
- Treating nausea and preventing emesis improve patient satisfaction, reduce distress, and improve the practice environment.
- Most head-to-head RCTs and meta-analyses have shown no single medication to be superior to other agents.
- Droperidol was shown to be superior in one small study but carries a black-box warning for QT interval prolongation.
- Ondansetron may have risk during the first trimester of pregnancy. Antiemetic selection during pregnancy can be challenging. Further research is required.

Providers encounter nausea and vomiting frequently in the acute care setting, either as a presenting complaint or accompanying another disease process. Treating these symptoms reduces suffering and distress and improves patient satisfaction [1]. It may also allow the patient to tolerate oral medications necessary to treat other conditions. A patient with active emesis or loud retching may adversely affect the practice environment for other nearby patients and providers. Antiemetics often fully meet patient expectations for improvement; they frequently allow patients to feel comfortable with discharge [1].

J. Murrett (✉) · J. Repanshek
Temple University Hospital, Philadelphia, PA, USA
e-mail: James.Murrett@tuhs.temple.edu; Jennifer.Fisher2@tuhs.temple.edu

M. Hinton
Department of Pharmacy, Temple University Hospital, Philadelphia, PA, USA
e-mail: Matthew.Hinton@tuhs.temple.edu

Factors in Antiemetic Selection

The choice of antiemetic can be complex, with a wide array of available medications. When selecting an antiemetic, the provider must consider the potential underlying cause that necessitates the medication in the first place. Nausea and vomiting may arise from a variety of processes. Gastrointestinal causes are common, but other causes include neurologic, psychologic, metabolic, toxicologic, and iatrogenic. The pathophysiology of nausea and vomiting is multimodal, through the activation of one of four major pathways. The medications that manage these symptoms act on these different pathways, allowing for a breadth of antiemetic options.

The route of administration is based on several factors. Oral agents are the simplest to administer. Some medications make orally dissolving formulations, so patients do not have to swallow pills. Some medications offer rectal formulations. Many patients requiring antiemetics will not tolerate oral medications and may require intravenous access for both antiemetics and fluid resuscitation. Intramuscular agents are typically more painful.

Patient age, weight, pregnancy status, and medication preference play roles in drug selection. Many providers fall into the practice pattern of having a first-line or "favorite" medication for all situations, and both providers and patients may have been exposed to marketing, affecting their choices and preferences. Finally, antiemetic medications have multiple side effects, and the choice of an agent may be dictated by comorbid conditions and/or the desire to avoid adverse reactions.

Pathophysiology of Vomiting

The vomiting center in the brain is located in the medulla oblongata. Four main pathways send signals to the vomiting center, and each is mediated by different neurotransmitters. There is a chemoreceptor trigger zone at the base of the skull that receives a variety of signals, including dopamine, serotonin, histamine, muscarine, and vasopressin. Toxins, metabolic abnormalities such as diabetic ketoacidosis, and medications may act on this center. Gastric inflammation and stretching of the gastrointestinal tract activate a vagal pathway via serotonin and dopamine. The vestibular center activates a pathway through histamine and muscarine. Finally, the cerebral cortex, which processes anxiety, fear, and foul odors, can activate vomiting.

Mechanisms of Action and Adverse Drug Reactions

Antiemetic medications come from multiple different classes, with varying effects and adverse reactions shown in Table 36.1.

The serotonin antagonists include ondansetron (Zofran) and granisetron (Kytril). Benzamides include metoclopramide (Reglan) and trimethobenzamide (Tigan). Phenothiazines include prochlorperazine (Compazine) and promethazine (Phenergan). Antihistamines such as diphenhydramine (Benadryl) and meclizine (Antivert) are also options. Other categories of medications shown to have antiemetic properties include antipsychotics such as haloperidol (Haldol) and droperidol (Inapsine), benzodiazepines, and corticosteroids.

Considering the source of nausea and vomiting can help providers select an appropriate agent. Ondansetron's serotoninergic effects treat nausea due to toxic, idiopathic, and metabolic causes, as well as gastric irritation and inflammation. Metoclopramide acts primarily on dopamine and may work well in patients presenting with vomiting secondary to headaches, gastrointestinal dysmotility, or other gastric causes. Haloperidol may work well for nausea and vomiting with cerebral cortex-associated causes. Similarly, benzodiazepines may work well as adjuvants to other medications and may manage symptoms caused by anxiety. Antihistamine and anticholinergic medications can be used for vestibular-related nausea, such as vertigo.

While these agents manage symptoms, they also have side effects. Some medications may cause mild sedation while others may cause agitation or restlessness (akathisia). Many medications may cause QT lengthening or non-specific repolarization abnormalities. For discussion on management of QT prolongation with antiemetic medications, please refer to Chap. 38 of this textbook. Extrapyramidal symptoms (EPS) may also occur: dystonia (spasms), parkinsonism (rigidity), bradykinesia (slowness), tardive dyskinesia (irregular spasms), and akathisia.

Ondansetron use in pregnancy was shown in some studies to be associated with increased fetal cardiac abnormalities [2]

Table 36.1 Antiemetics: mechanisms of action and adverse drug reactions

Medication/class	Common antiemetic doses in emergency medicine	Route of administration	Pregnancy class	Considerations and place in therapy
Antihistamines				
Diphenhydramine	25–50 mg q4–6 h PO 10–50 mg q2–4 h IV	PO, IV, IM	Category B	Anticholinergic effects (caution in elderly) Useful in cases of motion sickness/vertigo
Meclizine	12.5–25 mg 1 h before travel; repeat every 12–24 h prn	PO	Category B	
Benzamides				
Metoclopramide	10–20 mg q6h	PO, IV, IM	Category B	Potential for extrapyramidal symptoms
Trimethobenzamide	300 mg PO q6–8 h 200 mg IM q6–8 h	PO, IM	Not classified	Prokinetic effects useful in cases of gastroparesis
Butyrophenones				
Haloperidol	1–5 mg q12h	PO, IV, IM	Category C	May cause excess sedation
Droperidol	2.5 mg × 1, may give an additional 1.25 mg	IV, IM	Category C	12-lead EKG, cardiac monitoring may be considered due to QT prolonging potential
Corticosteroids				
Dexamethasone	Variable	PO, IV, IM	Category C	Adjunctive therapy or chemotherapy-induced nausea and vomiting
Phenothiazines				
Prochlorperazine	5–10 mg q4–6 h (max 40 mg/day)	PO, IV, IM, PR	Not classified	Useful in cases of motion sickness, vertigo, and migraine
Promethazine	12.5–25 mg q4–6 h	PO, IV, IM, PR	Category C	Potential for extrapyramidal symptoms May cause excess sedation
Serotonin antagonists				
Ondansetron (Zofran)	4–16 mg IV or PO	PO, IV, IM	Category B	Low doses well tolerated and efficacious in multiple etiologies QT-prolonging effects associated with higher doses and IV administration

PO, oral; *IM*, intramuscular; *IV*, intravenous; *PR*, rectal

and increased cleft palate [3], but other large studies have shown no correlation [4, 5]. Metoclopramide, like ondansetron, is listed as pregnancy category B. Studies have not shown an association between metoclopramide and adverse fetal outcomes, but metoclopramide risks maternal EPS while ondansetron does not [6]. The decision regarding antiemetic choice during pregnancy is challenging and will remain so until further studies bring better clarification to the issue. For discussion on management of hyperemesis gravidarum, including medication choice, please refer to Chap. 109 of this textbook.

Antiemetic Selection

Providers frequently undertreat nausea. One recent study noted that only half of emergency department patients with nausea were treated with an antiemetic [7]. However, the majority of patients with vomiting were treated with antiemetics [8, 9].

Antiemetics are effective at managing symptoms of nausea and vomiting; however, research has shown that placebos or IV fluids alone can also be effective [10]. Some randomized trials and meta-analyses comparing agents have shown no significant difference among medications or when medications were compared to placebo [11–13]. A large review comparing multiple trials of metoclopramide, ondansetron, prochlorperazine, promethazine, and droperidol showed no medication was significantly better than placebo. One small trial did show droperidol was superior to placebo [14]. While more commonly used in the past, droperidol use has become limited due to risk of QT prolongation. Most studies did not control for either administration of intravenous fluids or causes of nausea and vomiting.

Since many agents have been shown to have equal or non-inferior efficacy, the side effect profile for a medication may weigh most heavily in its selection or exclusion. For patients with long QT syndrome or at risk for repolarization abnormalities, providers should avoid serotonin antagonists and haloperidol. For patients on typical antipsychotics or with other risk factors, providers should avoid phenothiazines and benzamides, which may increase the risk of EPS. Many medications have sedative effects and should be used with caution in conjunction with other sedating agents. When treating pregnant patients, providers may consider using pyridoxine, antihistamines, or metoclopramide if they are concerned about risks with ondansetron.

In conclusion, the selection of an agent to treat nausea and vomiting remains complex but approachable. Symptoms often go undertreated but improve with most treatments. It is important to remain aware of medications side effects and how they apply to specific patient presentations. There is no "always right" answer when choosing an antiemetic, and certain agents may be more appropriate based on the suspected etiology of symptoms.

Suggested Resources

- Furyk JS, Meek RA, Egerton-Warburton D. Drugs for the treatment of nausea and vomiting in adults in the emergency department setting. Cochrane Database Syst Rev. 2015;9:CD010106.
- Pasternak B, Svanström H, Hviid A. Ondansetron in pregnancy and risk of adverse fetal outcomes. N Engl J Med. 2013;368:814–23.
- Singer AJ, Garra G, Thode HC. Oligoantiemesis or inadequate prescription of antiemetics in the emergency department: a local and national perspective. J Emerg Med. 2016;50:818–24.

References

1. Meek R, Graudins A, Anthony S. Antiemetic treatment in the emergency department: patient opinions and expectations. Emerg Med Australas. 2018;30:36–41.
2. Danielsson B, Wikner BN, Källén B. Use of ondansetron during pregnancy and congenital malformations in the infant. Reprod Toxicol. 2014;50:134–7.
3. Anderka M, Mitchell AA, Louik C, Werler MM, Hernández-Diaz S, Rasmussen SA. Medications used to treat nausea and vomiting of pregnancy and the risk of selected birth defects. Birth Defects Res A Clin Mol Teratol. 2012;94:22–30.
4. Pasternak B, Svanström H, Hviid A. Ondansetron in pregnancy and risk of adverse fetal outcomes. N Engl J Med. 2013;368:814–23.
5. Fejzo MS, MacGibbon KW, Mullin PM. Ondansetron in pregnancy and risk of adverse fetal outcomes in the United States. Reprod Toxicol. 2016;62:87–91.
6. Matok I, Gorodischer R, Koren G, Sheiner E, Wiznitzer A, Levy A. The safety of metoclopramide use in the first trimester of pregnancy. N Engl J Med. 2009;360:2528–35.
7. Furyk JS, Meek RA, Egerton-Warburton D, Vinson DR. Oligoevidence for antiemetic efficacy in the emergency department. Am J Emerg Med. 2017;35:921–2.
8. Mee MJ, Egerton-Warburton D, Meek R. Treatment and assessment of emergency department nausea and vomiting in Australasia: a survey of anti-emetic management. Emerg Med Australas. 2011;23:162–8.
9. Singer AJ, Garra G, Thode HC. Oligoantiemesis or inadequate prescription of antiemetics in the emergency department: a local and national perspective. J Emerg Med. 2016;50:818–24.
10. Furyk JS, Meek RA, Egerton-Warburton D. Drugs for the treatment of nausea and vomiting in adults in the emergency department setting. Cochrane Database Syst Rev. 2015;9:CD010106.
11. Braude D, Crandall C. Ondansetron versus promethazine to treat acute undifferentiated nausea in the emergency department: a randomized double-blind, noninferiority trial. Acad Emerg Med. 2008;15:209–15.
12. Patka J, Wu DT, Abraham P, Sobel RM. Randomized controlled trial of ondansetron vs. prochlorperazine in adults in the emergency department. West J Emerg Med. 2011;12:1–5.
13. Patanwala AE, Amini R, Hays D, Rosen P. Antiemetic therapy for nausea and vomiting in the emergency department. J Emerg Med. 2010;39:330–6.
14. Braude D, Soliz T, Crandall C, Hendey G, Andrews J, Weichenthal L. Antiemetics in the ED: a randomized controlled trial comparing 3 common agents. Am J Emerg Med. 2006;24:177–82.

What Is the Best Management of Cyclic Vomiting Syndrome and Cannabinoid Hyperemesis Syndrome?

37

F. James Squadrito and Clare Roepke

Pearls and Pitfalls
- Evidence for treatment of cyclic vomiting syndrome (CVS) and cannabis hyperemesis syndrome (CHS) in the acute setting is extremely limited.
- CVS and CHS are diagnoses of exclusion. If "red flags" are present, they may indicate more serious etiologies.
- Treatment of both entities focuses on symptomatic relief, and disposition should be based on the success or failure of achieving symptomatic relief in the acute care setting.
- Capsaicin is a noninvasive, low-risk treatment option for CHS, though evidence is limited.
- The only proven long-term treatment of CHS is cessation of cannabis use.
- CVS and CHS are poorly understood and may be overlapping entities; as such, a social history is imperative in diagnosis and treatment.

Cyclic vomiting syndrome (CVS) and cannabis hyperemesis syndrome (CHS) are both poorly understood functional gastrointestinal (GI) disorders characterized by acute episodes of severe nausea and vomiting, separated by asymptomatic periods of weeks to months. Although considered separate entities, there may be more overlap between the two than previously thought. In one survey of CVS patients, 81% reported frequent use of marijuana [1].

CVS and CHS are diagnoses of exclusion. A broad differential must be considered, and "red flags" that suggest more serious etiologies should be identified through history and physical exam (Table 37.1) [2].

Cyclic Vomiting Syndrome

Evaluation

Much of how providers manage adult CVS is based on the pediatric literature. In both children and adults, the acute care workup of cyclic vomiting depends on whether the patient has a known diagnosis of CVS. In the child with known CVS without "red flag" symptoms, a basic metabolic panel and an abdominal x-ray to evaluate for malrotation are recommended [3]. There are no established guidelines for diagnostic evaluation in adults; however, in the adult patient without red flag signs or symptoms with a known diagnosis of CVS who states he or she is experiencing a typical exacerbation, imaging and advanced testing may be deferred.

In both children and adults with cyclic vomiting symptoms but no prior CVS diagnosis, further investigation is warranted. No diagnostic markers have been identified for CVS. A basic metabolic panel, lipase, liver function panel, and urinalysis can assist in the evaluation for other conditions [4]. Ketones on a urinalysis and electrolyte abnormalities such as hypokalemia are often seen in patients with CVS [5]. That said, laboratory testing will frequently be normal, even during CVS flares. Imaging should be performed as indicated and may include neuroimaging, abdominal computed tomography, abdominal ultrasound, genitourinary

Table 37.1 Clinical "red flags" [2]

Symptoms suggesting concerning etiology
Severe headache
Focal neurologic deficit
Altered mental status
Focal abdominal pain
Weight loss
Progressive worsening of symptoms
New/different symptoms
Gastrointestinal bleeding
Prolonged episodes with a change in pattern

F. J. Squadrito (✉) · C. Roepke
Lewis Katz School of Medicine at Temple University Hospital, Philadelphia, PA, USA
e-mail: Francis.Squadrito2@tuhs.temple.edu; Clare.Roepke@tuhs.temple.edu

© Springer Nature Switzerland AG 2019
A. Graham, D. J. Carlberg (eds.), *Gastrointestinal Emergencies*, https://doi.org/10.1007/978-3-319-98343-1_37

ultrasound, and/or cholescintigraphy as indicated. Children should be spared ionizing radiation when possible [6].

Management

Dextrose-containing fluid (D10) is recommended for all pediatric patients, as dextrose can lead to rapid improvement of symptoms in acute attacks. In one study, dextrose and electrolyte-containing fluids alone helped in 43% of children [6]. Ondansetron is the antiemetic of choice in children, with a recommended dosing of 0.3–0.4 mg/kg with an upper limit of 16 mg/dose [5]. Combination therapy of dextrose infusion, high-dose 5-HT3 receptor antagonist antiemetics (ondansetron), and sedation appears to be the most efficacious supportive therapy in pediatric patients. In pediatric patients, promethazine, prochlorperazine, and metoclopramide are less effective than ondansetron and are not recommended [7].

Management recommendations for acute CVS flares in adults are based on a combination of case reports, anecdotal evidence, and expert opinion. No standard evidence-based regimens exist to manage adult CVS [6, 8]. Interventions focus on supportive care and include providing a less stimulating environment, fluid and electrolyte replacement, and use of antiemetics with or without sedation (benzodiazepines).

When managing the adult patient with CVS, following the pediatric algorithm is a reasonable approach. First-line interventions such as dextrose containing fluids and intravenous ondansetron administration are likely to be helpful in these patients. Prochlorperazine, promethazine, and metoclopramide are all reasonable second-line treatment options in these patients. QT interval prolongation with antiemetics must be considered, especially in higher-risk populations. See Chap. 38 of this text for more discussion of QT interval prolongation with antiemetics.

When disposition planning, supportive care is necessary until the emetic phase of CVS resolves. Resolution is defined as successfully resuming oral intake. Premature discharge from the acute care setting may result in repeated visits and patient dissatisfaction. Arranging outpatient gastroenterology follow-up may be beneficial.

Cannabis Hyperemesis Syndrome

CHS is poorly understood, but has a similar presentation to CVS. Recommendations are based only on case reports and anecdotal evidence, as there are no higher quality studies on CHS management [9]. Most available data is retrospective and does not control for concurrent interventions.

A good history is imperative in the diagnosis of CHS. Patients with CHS often vomit daily without intervals of normal health. This helps differentiate CHS from CVS. Patients often report daily cannabis use with symptom onset reliably following cannabis use. Patients frequently report repetitively utilizing bathing or hot showers to relieve symptoms. This is an important part of the patient history, as it may prove to be a sensitive predictor of CHS. A review of case reports showed that hot showers and bathing were universally effective at mitigating or abating CHS [10]. The reason for this effect remains poorly understood.

The most used medications for acute CHS symptoms are benzodiazepines, followed by haloperidol and capsaicin. One case series suggested that an initial dose of 5 mg or less of IV haloperidol can be effective [10]. Several case reports have suggested that patients with little or no relief from antiemetic administration may receive relief from application of topical capsaicin. There is no standardization of dosing or application method for capsaicin; however, capsaicin is both noninvasive and low risk [11].

The only proven long-term treatment of CHS is cessation of cannabis use [10]. A review of the available case reports and case series demonstrated that among 64 patients with documented cannabis cessation, 62 (96.8%) had complete resolution of symptoms. Furthermore, among 21 patients who did not abstain from cannabis use, none had symptom resolution [10]. Counseling cannabis cessation may be the acute care provider's best tool in combating repeat visits for CHS.

Suggested Resources
- Cannabis Hyperemesis Syndrome. EM:RAP. Aug 2011; https://www.emrap.org/episode/august2011/cannabis
- Cyclic vomiting: pearls and pitfalls. emDocs. Apr 2016;http://www.emdocs.net/cyclic-vomiting-syndrome-pearls-and-pitfalls/
- Therapeutic Showering. Life in the fastlane. Oct 2016; https://lifeinthefastlane.com/therapeutic-showering/

References

1. Venkatesan T, Sengupta J, Lodhi A, et al. An internet survey of marijuana and hot shower use in adults with cyclic vomiting syndrome (CVS). Exp Brain Res. 2014;232:2563–70.
2. Li BU, Misiewicz L. Cyclic vomiting syndrome: a brain-gut disorder. Gastroenterol Clin N Am. 2003;32:997–1019.
3. Olson AD, Li BU. The diagnostic evaluation of children with cyclic vomiting: a cost-effectiveness assessment. J Pediatr. 2002;141(5):724–8.

4. Venkatasubramani N, Venkatesan T, Li BU. Extreme emesis: cyclic vomiting syndrome. Pract Gastroenterol. 2007;31:21.

5. Fleisher DR. Management of cyclic vomiting syndrome. J Pediatr Gastroenterol Nutr. 1995;21:S52–6.

6. Li BU, Lefevre F, Chelimsky GG, et al. North American Society for Pediatric Gastroenterology, Hepatology, and Nutrition consensus statement on the diagnosis and management of cyclic vomiting syndrome. J Pediatr Gastroenterol Nutr. 2008;47:379–93.

7. Li BU, Balint J. Cyclic vomiting syndrome: evolution in our understanding of a brain-gut disorder. Adv Pediatr Infect Dis. 2000;47:117–60.

8. Pareek N, Fleisher DR, Abell T. Cyclic vomiting syndrome: what a gastroenterologist needs to know. Am J Gastroenterol. 2007;102:2832–40.

9. Richards RJ, Gordon BK, Danielson AR, Moulin AK. Pharmacologic treatment of cannabinoid hyperemesis syndrome: a systematic review. Pharmacotherapy. 2017;37:725–34.

10. Sorensen CJ, DeSanto K, Borgelt L, Phillips KT, Monte AA. Cannabinoid hyperemesis syndrome: diagnosis, pathophysiology, and treatment-a systematic review. J Med Toxicol. 2017;13:71–87.

11. Dezieck L, Hafez Z, Conicella A, Blohm E, O'Connor MJ, Schwarz ES, Mullins ME. Resolution of cannabis hyperemesis syndrome with topical capsaicin in the emergency department: a case series. Clin Toxicol (Phila). 2017;55:908–13.

When Should QT Prolongation Be Considered in Antiemetic Use?

38

Efrat Rosenzweig Kean, Matthew Hinton, and Clare Roepke

Pearls and Pitfalls

- QTc prolongation from routine doses of 4–8 mg of ondansetron is minimal and is unlikely to be clinically significant or cause a dangerous arrhythmia.
- A patient who receives a single dose of an antiemetic does not require routine screening electrolytes or an electrocardiogram (ECG).
- Patients receiving greater than 8 mg of ondansetron within 4 h and patients taking other QTc-prolonging agents should receive a screening ECG.
- Metoclopramide may be a safe alternative to 5-HT3 receptor antagonists in patients with underlying QTc prolongation, but it is not studied well enough to fully establish safety in this regard.
- Benzodiazepines are effective for nausea and vomiting and do not carry a significant risk of QTc prolongation.

Management of nausea and vomiting with antiemetics is a common occurrence in the acute care setting. Patients frequently receive 5-HT3 (serotonin), dopamine, or histamine receptor antagonists for treatment. These drugs are highly effective; [1] however, nearly all carry a potential side effect of QTc prolongation, which may lead to fatal arrhythmias including torsades de pointes (TdP). Ondansetron likely produces its QTc-prolonging effects through its interaction with rapidly acting potassium channels during myocardial depolarization. Several other common classes of medications potentiate these effects [2]. While some providers routinely screen vomiting patients for underlying QTc prolongation or electrolyte abnormalities prior to administration of antiemetic medications, others administer multiple doses of antiemetic medications without screening. Emerging evidence suggests that screening is unnecessary in most patients but may benefit patients with known risk factors for QTc prolongation. Table 38.1 depicts various antiemetics and their associations with QTc interval prolongation and cardiac arrhythmias.

Ondansetron

Ondansetron is the most commonly administered antiemetic in the US emergency departments [3]. While it carries an FDA warning for QTc prolongation, recent studies have found inconsistent evidence for this. A 2013 study of 100 pediatric patients given ondansetron showed no change in the QTc interval at peak effect and 1 h post-peak effect [4]. A more recent study in 22 adult patients showed a mean increase in QTc of 20 ms, with no adverse cardiac events reported [5]. The Federal Drug Administration (FDA)

E. R. Kean (✉)
Temple University Hospital, Philadelphia, PA, USA
e-mail: efrat.kean@tuhs.temple.edu

M. Hinton
Department of Pharmacy, Temple University Hospital, Philadelphia, PA, USA
e-mail: matthew.hinton@tuhs.temple.edu

C. Roepke
Lewis Katz School of Medicine at Temple University Hospital, Philadelphia, PA, USA
e-mail: clare.roepke@tuhs.temple.edu

Table 38.1 Common antiemetic agents and their risk of QTc prolongation

Antiemetic agent	Reported QTc prolongation	Reported clinically significant arrhythmias
Ondansetron	Drug-specific [1]	Yes [1]
Metoclopramide	Drug-specific [1]	Yes [1]
Promethazine	Drug-specific [1]	No
Prochlorperazine	Reported for other drugs in the same class [1]	No
Haloperidol	Yes [1]	Yes
Midazolam	No [1]	No
Lorazepam	No [1]	No

© Springer Nature Switzerland AG 2019
A. Graham, D. J. Carlberg (eds.), *Gastrointestinal Emergencies*, https://doi.org/10.1007/978-3-319-98343-1_38

recommends that no single intravenous (IV) dose exceed 16 mg, due to evidence that a dose of 32 mg caused a QTc increase of 20 ms. More typical 4 or 8 mg doses were demonstrated to cause more modest increases in QTc interval (6 ms) [6]. Overall, the evidence for QTc prolongation with typical doses of 4–8 mg appears to be mixed and inconclusive, suggesting that a routine screening ECG for patients receiving ondansetron in the acute care setting is unnecessary.

While some studies do show QTc prolongation associated with low doses of ondansetron and other 5-HT3 receptor blockers [7], newer literature suggests that this prolongation may not be clinically significant and is unlikely to be associated with cardiac arrhythmia in the absence of other risk factors. In a post-marketing analysis of single oral ondansetron doses, no cardiac arrhythmias were reported despite over 20 years of frequent use in both ambulatory and inpatient settings [8]. Some argue that this data can likely be extrapolated to single intravenous doses, as the pharmacokinetics is quite similar. There are a small number of cardiac arrhythmias reported in the literature, but the majority of these were associated with repeated intravenous administration, long-term use, concomitant use of other QTc-prolonging agents including chemotherapy drugs, or underlying electrolyte abnormalities. Similarly, a 2016 study evaluating the effect of ondansetron on pediatric intensive care unit patients showed a statistically significant increase in QTc to greater than 500 ms in 11% of patients; however, this increase was associated with underlying electrolyte abnormalities and/or organ failure. Ondansetron alone, in the absence of other risk factors, was less likely to cause significant QTc prolongation [9]. Another 2016 pediatric study retrospectively analyzed nearly 200,000 doses of ondansetron administered in the emergency department. The authors reported seven incidences of ventricular arrhythmias within 24 h of administration; all seven were associated with underlying major cardiac diagnoses or congenital conduction abnormalities [10].

Taken together, these studies suggest that, in the absence of other known causes of cardiac arrhythmia, including underlying cardiac conduction abnormality, electrolyte abnormality, or organ failure, cardiac arrhythmia associated with ondansetron is highly unlikely, and the typical doses of 4–8 mg of ondansetron are safe for the majority of patients. A screening ECG should be considered in patients with underlying congenital or acquired heart disease, as well as in patients with significant electrolyte abnormalities that may prolong the QTc, including hypokalemia, hypocalcemia, or hypomagnesemia [11]. Screening ECG should also be considered in those who are taking QTc-prolonging medications, including antiarrhythmic, antipsychotic, or antibiotic agents [12].

Metoclopramide

Metoclopramide has a different mechanism of action from the more commonly used 5-HT3 receptor antagonists, as it is a competitive antagonist of dopamine D1 and D2 receptors, in addition to having 5-HT3 antagonist activity at higher doses. There have been fewer studies examining its effects on the QTc interval. A small 2015 study comparing intravenous metoclopramide to intravenous haloperidol showed no effect on QTc with either drug [13]. However, there have been sporadic case reports of significant adverse cardiac events immediately after IV administration of metoclopramide, typically associated with underlying electrolyte abnormalities or organ dysfunction [14]. While some providers feel that metoclopramide is a safe alternative to ondansetron in higher-risk patients, more thorough studies are needed before a recommendation can be made.

Medications Without QTc Prolongation

Several 5-HT3 receptor antagonist medications have been shown not to carry a risk of QTc prolongation. FDA labeling suggests that, if available, palonosetron and granisetron are safe for patients with underlying long QTc or other risk factors for cardiac arrhythmias.

Trimethobenzamide is a D2 receptor antagonist without apparent 5-HT3 receptor antagonist effects that has not been shown to have any effect on QTc interval and is also safe for patients with congenital long QT syndromes or other risk factors [15]. These drugs are not likely to be available to most emergency providers, and they are not cost-effective.

Lorazepam and other benzodiazepines are more available and cost-effective alternatives to QTc-prolonging agents. They have been shown to be effective for preventing and treating nausea and vomiting [16], and they do not carry a significant risk of QTc prolongation [17]. If there is a contraindication to benzodiazepines or if patients require more than one agent to control symptoms, then patients who are felt to be high risk for developing an arrhythmia can receive low doses of more common antiemetics if they are appropriately screened with an ECG prior to administration and observed on a cardiac monitor following administration.

Conclusions

Ondansetron (and other 5-HT3 receptor antagonists) and metoclopramide are the most commonly administrated antiemetics in emergency settings. While ondansetron carries an FDA warning for prolonged QTc interval and cardiac arrhythmias at higher doses, the FDA has not provided recommendations for screening patients. Routine ECG and blood testing create delays in patient care, discomfort for patients, and the increased expense of potentially unnecessary investigations. A review of the literature shows that it is unclear whether ondansetron causes QTc prolongation at typical doses of 4–8 mg. Even if it does, this increase is highly unlikely to be clinically significant or result in cardiac arrhythmia. Patients with underlying congenital conduction delay, electrolyte abnormalities, or organ failure may be at a higher risk for developing QTc prolongation with repeated doses of antiemetics and may require more monitoring and screening. Patients who chronically use other QTc-prolonging agents, who are receiving multiple intravenous doses of antiemetics, or who have underlying conditions that increase their risk for fatal cardiac arrhythmias (such as cardiac or renal failure) should also be more closely monitored with a screening ECG and a period of cardiac monitoring. The vast majority of patients receiving a single dose of an oral or intravenous antiemetic in the emergency setting can do so without any screening or monitoring. If higher-risk patients are to be discharged with a prescription for multiple doses of an antiemetic, it would be preferable to use agents such as promethazine or prochlorperazine, which carry a risk of QTc prolongation but have not been associated with clinically significant cardiac toxicity.

Suggested Resources
- Episode 101: Puke- Antiemetics in adult emergency department patients. The Skeptic's guide to emergency medicine. Jan 2015; http://thesgem.com/2015/01/sgem101-puke-antiemetics-in-adult-emergency-department-patients/
- Freedman SB, et al. Ondansetron and the risk of cardiac arrhythmias: a systematic review and postmarketing analysis. Ann Emerg Med. 2014;64(1):19–25.
- Pharmacology pearls – antiemetics and the QTc. EM:RAP. Feb 2017; https://www.emrap.org/episode/badbleedsinthe/pharmacology

References

1. Cunningham RS. 5-HT3-receptor antagonists: a review of pharmacology and clinical efficacy. Oncol Nurs Forum. 1997;24(7 Suppl):33–40.
2. Pourmand A, Mazer-Amirshahi M, Chistov S, et al. Emergency department approach to QTc prolongation. Am J Emerg Med. 2017;35(12):1928–33.
3. Cohen IT. An overview of the clinical use of ondansetron in preschool age children. Ther Clin Risk Manag. 2007;3(2):333–9.
4. Krammes SK, Jacobs T, Clark JM, Lutes RE. Effect of intravenous ondansetron on the QT interval of patients' electrocardiograms. Pediatr Emerg Care. 2018;34:38–41.
5. Moffett PM, Cartwright L, Grossart EA, O'Keefe D, Kang CS. Intravenous ondansetron and the QT interval in adult emergency department patients: an observational study. Acad Emerg Med. 2016;23(1):102–5.
6. Center for Drug Evaluation and Research. Drug Safety and Availability – FDA Drug Safety Communication: New information regarding QT prolongation with ondansetron (Zofran) [Internet]. U S Food and Drug Administration Home Page. Center for Drug Evaluation and Research; 2012 [cited 26 Oct 2017]; Available from: https://www.fda.gov/Drugs/DrugSafety/ucm310190.htm
7. Hafermann MJ, Namdar R, Seibold GE, Page RL 2nd. Effect of intravenous ondansetron on QT interval prolongation in patients with cardiovascular disease and additional risk factors for torsades: a prospective, observational study. Drug Healthc Patient Saf. 2011;3:53–8. https://doi.org/10.2147/DHPS.S25623.
8. Freedman SB, Uleryk E, Rumantir M, Finkelstein Y. Ondansetron and the risk of cardiac arrhythmias: a systematic review and postmarketing analysis. Ann Emerg Med. 2014;64(1):19–25.e6.
9. Trivedi S, Schiltz B, Kanipakam R, Bos JM, Ackerman MJ, Ouellette Y. Effect of ondansetron on QT interval in patients cared for in the PICU. Pediatr Crit Care Med. 2016;17(7):e317–23.
10. Moeller JR, Gummin DD, Nelson TJ, Drendel AL, Shah BK, Berger S. Risk of ventricular arrhythmias and association with ondansetron. J Pediatr. 2016;179:118–123.e1.
11. Goy J-J, Stauffer J-C, Schlaepfer J, Christeler P, editors. Electrolyte disturbances and QT interval abnormalities. In: Electrocardiography (ECG) [Internet]: Bentham Science Publishers; 2013. p. 133–41. [cited 15 Nov 2017]. Available from: http://www.eurekaselect.com/node/112318.
12. Armahizer MJ, Seybert AL, Smithburger PL, Kane-Gill SL. Drug-drug interactions contributing to QT prolongation in cardiac intensive care units. J Crit Care. 2013;28(3):243–9.
13. Gaffigan ME, Bruner DI, Wason C, Pritchard A, Frumkin K. A randomized controlled trial of intravenous haloperidol vs intravenous metoclopramide for acute migraine therapy in the emergency department. J Emerg Med. 2015;49(3):326–34.
14. Barni S, Petrelli F, Cabiddu M. Cardiotoxicity of antiemetic drugs in oncology: An overview of the current state of the art. Crit Rev Oncol Hematol. 2016;102:125–34.
15. Smith HS, Cox LR, Smith BR. Dopamine receptor antagonists. Ann Palliat Med. 2012;1(2). [Internet]. [cited 1 Jan 2012]; Available from: http://apm.amegroups.com/article/view/1039
16. Malik IA, Khan WA, Qazilbash M, Ata E, Butt A, Khan MA. Clinical efficacy of lorazepam in prophylaxis of anticipatory, acute, and delayed nausea and vomiting induced by high doses of cisplatin. A prospective randomized trial. Am J Clin Oncol. 1995;18(2):170–5.
17. Goodnick PJ, Jerry J, Parra F. Psychotropic drugs and the ECG: focus on the QTc interval. Expert Opin Pharmacother. 2002;3(5):479–98.

Richard Wroblewski and Jennifer Repanshek

Pearls and Pitfalls
- Gastroparesis is a chronic illness causing vomiting and pain that can be a challenge to manage in the acute care setting.
- National opioid prescribing guidelines recommend avoiding narcotic pain medication in gastroparesis.
- Antipsychotics are an effective class of antiemetic with increasing evidence for use in acute exacerbations of gastroparesis.
- Low-dose ketamine, which has been used safely in acute pain management and reduces opioid use, has potential benefit in gastroparesis.

Gastroparesis is a chronic illness with a significant negative impact on a patient's quality of life. Patients tend to be older and female, with most cases secondary to diabetes; however, post-infectious and idiopathic causes are also documented. Patients tend to report chronic nausea and vomiting as their primary complaints, but a significant number live with chronic abdominal pain related to the delayed gastric emptying. Outpatient management includes pro-motility agents, antiemetics, pain medication, specialized diets, and, in some cases, implantable gastric pacemakers [1, 2].

Patients typically present for acute care with worsening of chronic symptoms: nausea, emesis, and abdominal pain. A study of 200,000 emergency department encounters for gastroparesis primarily demonstrated approximately 54% of patients required admission. The admission rate approaches 75% when gastroparesis is listed as either a primary or secondary condition [3].

Management of patients with acute exacerbations of gastroparesis can be challenging, especially from a pain control standpoint. Many patients receive outpatient opioid pain medications and often request them for acute exacerbations in the emergency department; however, new guidelines recommend against opioids as a first-line treatment and should be avoided in patients with chronic abdominal pain and gastroparesis [4]. Because they receive outpatient opioid management, patients may expect opioids when they present for acute care.

Few studies evaluate management options in patients with acute gastroparesis flares. The use of antipsychotics such as olanzapine, haloperidol, and mirtazapine for chronic nausea and vomiting has been well studied in the palliative care setting [5, 6], and recent studies have started to evaluate their utility for acute symptom management. In a retrospective case-matched review of 52 patients receiving 5 mg of intramuscular haloperidol for treatment of gastroparesis-related vomiting, haloperidol was associated with reduced opioid requirements and a lower admission rate [7]. Another small prospective study evaluated 5 mg of intramuscular haloperidol compared to placebo and showed that 1 h after administration, those who received haloperidol showed significant reductions in both nausea and pain [8]. Patients in both studies still received opioids for pain control, but the overall morphine equivalent used was lower in patients receiving haloperidol [7, 8].

Case reports have described other potential management options for acute gastroparesis flares. One described how phentolamine administration (0.5 mg/kg over 60 min) led to complete resolution of abdominal pain in a patient with a gastric stimulator for gastroparesis [9]. An outpatient case report described drastic symptom improvement after a patient took 15 mg of mirtazapine as an orally disintegrating tablet.

A recent review of 11 studies using low-dose ketamine (<1 mg/kg) showed that it was as effective as opioids for acute pain management. Ketamine also produced fewer adverse events and was effective in opioid tolerant patients [10]. Although ketamine use in gastroparesis has not been studied, it has been evaluated in chronic pain patients, including those with chronic abdominal pain [11]. Ketamine for analgesia can

R. Wroblewski (✉) · J. Repanshek
Temple University Hospital, Philadelphia, PA, USA
e-mail: Richard.Wroblewski@tuhs.temple.edu; Jennifer.Fisher2@tuhs.temple.edu

be administered as an intravenous push (IVP), an infusion, or a combination. Most studies showed that doses between 0.1 and 0.5 mg/kg IVP provided adequate pain relief [10]. One study showed significant pain relief with minimal adverse events using 15 mg ketamine IVP followed by 20 mg infused over 60 min [12]. Because of its utility for pain control in various circumstances, ketamine holds promise as a potential treatment for gastroparesis-related pain, but future studies are necessary to elucidate what specific role, if any, it will play.

Continued research on the optimal management of acute gastroparesis flares remains crucial as physicians look to reduce opioid use and find safer analgesic therapies.

Suggested Resources
- Bonus lecture: ketamine analgesia in the ED. EM:RAP Aug 2017; https://www.emrap.org/episode/ema-2017-8/lecture
- Low dose ketamine for acute pain in the ED: IV push vs short infusion. Rebel EM. Apr 2017; http://rebelem.com/low-dose-ketamine-for-acute-pain-in-the-ed-iv-push-vs-short-infusion
- Ramirez R, Stalcup P, Croft B, Darracq MA. Haloperidol undermining gastroparesis symptoms (HUGS) in the emergency department. Am J Emerg Med. 2017;35(8):1118–20.

References

1. Bharucha AE. Epidemiology and natural history of gastroparesis. Gastroenterol Clin N Am. 2015;44:9–19. https://doi.org/10.1016/j.gtc.2014.11.002.
2. Camilleri M, Parkman HP, Shafi MA, Abell TL, Gerson L. Clinical guideline: management of gastroparesis. Am J Gastroenterol. 2012;108:18–37. https://doi.org/10.1038/ajg.2012.373.
3. Bielefeldt K. Factors influencing admission and outcomes in gastroparesis. Neurogastroenterol Motil. 2013;25:389–98, e294. https://doi.org/10.1111/nmo.12079.
4. American Academy of Emergency Medicine. Model emergency department pain treatment guidelines [internet]. 2013 [updated 10 Mar 2013; cited 23 Mar 2018]; Available from http://www.aaem.org/publications/news-releases/model-emergency-department-pain-treatment-guidelines
5. Glare P, Miller J, Nikolova T, Tickoo R. Treating nausea and vomiting in palliative care: a review. Clin Interv Aging. 2011;6:243–59. https://doi.org/10.2147/CIA.S13109.
6. Kim S, Shin I, Kim J, Kang H, Mun J, Yang S, Yoon J. Mirtazapine for severe gastroparesis unresponsive to conventional prokinetic treatment. Psychosomatics. 2006;47:440–2. https://doi.org/10.1176/appi.psy.47.5.440.
7. Ramirez R, Stalcup P, Croft B, Darracq MA. Haloperidol undermining gastroparesis symptoms (HUGS) in the emergency department. Am J Emerg Med. 2017;35:1118–20. https://doi.org/10.1016/j.ajem.2017.03.015.
8. Roldan C, Chambers K, Paniagua L, Patel S, Cardenas-Turanzas M, Chathampally Y. Randomized controlled double-blind trial comparing haloperidol combined with conventional therapy to conventional therapy alone in patients with symptomatic gastroparesis. Acad Emerg Med. 2017;24:1307–14. https://doi.org/10.1111/acem.13245.
9. Phillips WJ, Tollefson B, Johnson A, Abell T, Lerant A. Relief of acute pain in chronic idiopathic gastroparesis with intravenous phentolamine. Ann Pharmacother. 2006;40:2032–6. https://doi.org/10.1345/aph.1h255.
10. Pourmand A, Mazer-Amirshahi M, Royall C, Alhawas R, Shesser R. Low dose ketamine use in the emergency department, a new direction in pain management. Am J Emerg Med. 2017;35:918–21. https://doi.org/10.1016/j.ajem.2017.03.005.
11. Ahern TL, Herring AA, Anderson ES, Madia VA, Fahimi J, Frazee BW. The first 500: initial experience with widespread use of low-dose ketamine for acute pain management in the ED. Am J Emerg Med. 2015;33:197–201. https://doi.org/10.1016/j.ajem.2014.11.010.
12. Ahern TL, Herring AA, Miller S, Frazee BW. Low-dose ketamine infusion for emergency department patients with severe pain. Pain Med. 2015;16:1402–9.

Consultant Corner: Abdominal Pain and Vomiting

40

Adam C. Ehrlich

Introduction

Adam C. Ehrlich, MD, MPH, is an Assistant Professor of Medicine in the Section of Gastroenterology (GI) at the Lewis Katz School of Medicine at Temple University. He is the Co-Medical Director of the Temple Inflammatory Bowel Disease Program and the Associate Program Director for the GI Fellowship.

Dr. Ehrlich has a number of peer-reviewed publications, serves on a variety of regional and national committees, and is a reviewer for both gastroenterology national meetings and journals. He practices at Temple University Hospital, an urban, tertiary care academic referral center that also serves as a safety-net hospital for the local community.

Answers to Key Clinical Questions

1. When do you recommend a consultation with a gastroenterologist and in what time frame?

Decisions about the need for a GI consultation should include an assessment of the underlying cause of the vomiting, need for inpatient admission, and time course of illness. Any patient that requires admission for vomiting and abdominal pain from a suspected gastroenterological source should see a gastroenterologist during the admission to help with both diagnosis and treatment. Patients that can be discharged home should most commonly be referred back to their primary care doctor. Those that have an underlying gastrointestinal diagnosis that is thought to be the cause for unscheduled acute care should be advised to follow-up with their treating gastroenterologist on a non-emergent basis.

2. What pearls can you offer emergency care providers when evaluating a patient with abdominal pain and vomiting?

My advice for emergency care providers is to take a concise and systematic history, as this will likely eliminate many of the items from the differential diagnoses. Chronicity of symptoms and other related symptoms are crucial in this puzzle.

Patients with chronic issues related to vomiting rarely need to be admitted to the hospital for workup of the underlying etiology, though they may have complications that need further inpatient treatment and/or evaluation (e.g., bleeding from a Mallory-Weiss tear).

In patients with acute symptoms, providers should identify severe or life-threatening conditions and manage them appropriately. In many circumstances, evaluation with

A. C. Ehrlich
Section of Gastroenterology, Department of Medicine, Lewis Katz School of Medicine at Temple University, Philadelphia, PA, USA
e-mail: adam.ehrlich@tuhs.temple.edu

© Springer Nature Switzerland AG 2019
A. Graham, D. J. Carlberg (eds.), *Gastrointestinal Emergencies*, https://doi.org/10.1007/978-3-319-98343-1_40

laboratory testing (CBC, CMP, lipase) +/− ultrasound will be sufficient.

Emergency care providers should have no qualms about contacting a patient's established gastroenterologist to discuss management and disposition [1].

3. What concepts do you think are key to managing a patient with abdominal pain and vomiting?

The American Gastroenterological Association's technical review on nausea and vomiting suggests a three-step approach to evaluate these symptoms. First, providers should correct any sequelae of persistent vomiting, including dehydration and electrolyte imbalances. Second, the provider should identify the underlying cause and treat as appropriate. Third, in the absence of an obvious cause, empiric medical therapy should be used [2].

4. What complications are you concerned about in this patient population?

Complications from persistent nausea and vomiting are fairly limited. Patients can have dehydration and electrolyte abnormalities. They can also develop Mallory-Weiss tears and, in very rare circumstances, esophageal rupture (Boerhaave syndrome), which is a surgical emergency [3].

Obviously, inadequate identification of the underlying disease process can result in delayed treatment and various potential complications.

5. What are the indications for imaging in the vomiting patient?

Decisions about imaging should be based on the diagnoses being considered and/or concerns about complications. Providers considering an etiology that is obstructive in nature (e.g., small bowel obstruction, gastric outlet obstruction, volvulus) should pursue cross-sectional imaging of the abdomen/pelvis to evaluate these etiologies. Suspicions about neurologic causes of vomiting (e.g., stroke, hydrocephalus, closed head injury) warrant brain imaging. Patients who present with physical exam findings suspicious for perforation should have, at a minimum, an upright abdominal X-ray and possibly a chest X-ray to exclude abdominal free air and/or Boerhaave syndrome.

6. Customizing your antiemetic: What should you consider?

Serotonin (5-HT3) antagonists like ondansetron and dopamine D2 antagonists like metoclopramide should be antiemetics of choice in the absence of absolute contraindications.

Ondansetron is well tolerated. It is available in a sublingual formulation, oral tablet, and IV infusion and is frequently cost effective in generic versions. There is a concern about QT prolongation, which seems to occur more frequently with the IV formulation and when it is given in higher doses.

Metoclopramide can also be used in oral and IV formulations and is available cheaply. The major concern is tardive dyskinesia, which generally occurs only in patients who use the medication chronically.

7. What is the best management of cyclic vomiting and cannabinoid hyperemesis syndrome?

Acute management of cyclic vomiting syndrome and cannabinoid hyperemesis syndrome should focus on managing symptoms in an effort to allow for safe discharge. Especially with prolonged symptoms, providers should assess for electrolyte abnormalities and provide both intravenous fluids and antiemetics as needed.

Long-term outpatient management may include daily prophylactic therapy for cyclic vomiting syndrome.

Cannabinoid hyperemesis syndrome patients should be counseled about the role of cannabinoids in the etiology of their disease process and should be advised to cease use.

8. What are the best antiemetics in patients with QT prolongation?

Both dopamine receptor and serotonin receptor antagonists can theoretically cause QT prolongation. As such, the only truly safe classes of medications in patients with QT prolongation are anticholinergics (e.g., scopolamine) and antihistamines (e.g., diphenhydramine and meclizine). In clinical practice, however, these medications are not particularly effective for acute nausea and vomiting.

Ondansetron has been studied extensively as to its risk of QT prolongation [4]. The FDA removed the 32 mg intravenous dose due to this risk. A meta-analysis found no reports of arrhythmia associated with a single ondansetron dose. Of the 60 unique reports of ondansetron-associated arrhythmia, the route of administration was largely intravenous, and patients frequently had concomitant use of a QT-prolonging medication or a significant medical history (especially a history of cardiac disease and/or conditions predisposing to electrolyte abnormalities). Also, the majority of patients reviewed were given ondansetron in the setting of chemotherapeutic agents or to prevent postoperative vomiting [5].

While promethazine seems to increase the QT interval, given its lack of influence on repolarization, the risk of significant arrhythmia is low [6].

In the absence of any major confounding comorbid condition like a congenital long QT syndrome, small doses of either dopamine antagonists like promethazine or serotonin antagonists like ondansetron are likely safe. With any uncertainty, checking an electrocardiogram (ECG) prior to administration and then repeating ECGs is reasonable.

9. Opiates and gastroparesis: Is there a better way?

Gastroparesis is a challenging disease with limited treatment options. While patients often present with abdominal pain, opioid pain medications likely exacerbate the problem over time, as they slow gastrointestinal motility. Society guidelines do not advocate narcotics for the treatment of these patients [7]. Non-opioid medications are recommended and may include standard non-opioid pain medications as well as tricyclic antidepressants. In the acute care setting, avoiding opioid medications is recommended. Intravenous fluids and antiemetics are recommended, as is controlling hyperglycemia when there is concomitant diabetes. Unfortunately, many patients are already taking narcotic pain medicines for gastroparesis. In these cases, while it is important to limit narcotics, care must be taken to avoid opiate withdrawal.

Suggested Resources

- Camilleri M, Parkman HP, Shafi MA, Abell TL, Gerson L. Management of gastroparesis. Am J Gastroenterol. 2013;108:18–37.
- Quigley EM, Hasler WL, Parkman HP. AGA technical review on nausea and vomiting. Gastroenterology. 2001;120:263–86.
- Scorza K, Williams A, Phillips JD, Shaw J. Evaluation of nausea and vomiting. Am Fam Physician. 2007;76:76–84.

References

1. Scorza K, Williams A, Phillips JD, Shaw J. Evaluation of nausea and vomiting. Am Fam Physician. 2007;76:76–84.
2. Quigley EM, Hasler WL, Parkman HP. AGA technical review on nausea and vomiting. Gastroenterology. 2001;120:263–86.
3. Janjua KJ. Boerhaave's syndrome. Postgrad Med J. 1997;73(859): 265–70.
4. Pourmand A, Mazer-Amirshahi M, Chistov S, Sabha Y, Vukomanovic D, Almulhim M. Emergency department approach to QTc prolongation. Am J Emerg Med. 2017; https://doi.org/10.1016/j.ajem,2017.08.044.
5. Freedman S, Uleryk E, Rumantir M, Finkelstein Y. Ondansetron and the risk of cardiac Arrythmias: a systematic review and Postmarketing analysis. Ann Emerg Med. 2014;64(1):19–25.
6. Owczuk R, Twardowski P, Dylczyk-Sommer A, Wujtewicz MA, Sawicka W, Drogoszewska B, Wujtewicz M. Influence of promethazine on cardiac repolarization: a double-blind midazolam-controlled study. Anaesthesia. 2009;64(6):609–14.
7. Camilleri M, Parkman HP, Shafi MA, Abell TL, Gerson L. Management of gastroparesis. Am J Gastroenterol. 2013;108: 18–37.

Diagnosis: What Historical Features and Laboratory Test(s) Are the Most Helpful to Make the Diagnosis? Is There Really a Normal Lipase with Active Pancreatitis? What "Red Flags" Suggest a Complicated Course?

41

Travis A. Thompson

Pearls and Pitfalls
- Pancreatitis is diagnosed with a combination of history, physical exam, pancreatic enzymes, and imaging if needed.
- Lipase levels can be normal in acute pancreatitis.
- Smoking is a cofactor with alcohol in the development of acute pancreatitis. Encouraging patients to stop smoking may decrease the likelihood of recurrent episodes.
- Evaluate patient's overall status to help predict severity rather than relying on any one lab value or clinical finding.

What Historical Features and Laboratory Test(s) Are the Most Helpful to Make the Diagnosis?

To diagnose acute pancreatitis (AP), a patient must meet two of the three following criteria:

1. *Abdominal pain characteristic of pancreatitis*
2. *Elevated lipase or amylase (>3x the upper range of normal)*
3. *Radiographic evidence of pancreatic edema on imaging*

Historical Features and Risk Factors for Acute Pancreatitis

Pain considered typical for AP is acute, epigastric, periumbilical, or left upper quadrant pain that is usually described as constant with radiation to the back, chest, or flanks. The pain is usually described as severe but can vary in intensity. The location of the pain and intensity does not correlate with the severity of pancreatitis [1]. Pain not consistent with AP is described as dull, colicky, or localized to the lower abdomen [2].

Gallstones and alcohol are the most common causes of AP [3]. Alcohol can be linked to acute pancreatitis in patients with >5 years of heavy alcohol use (generally >50 g of alcohol/day) [2, 4], while binge drinking does not lead to AP. Smoking is often overlooked as a risk factor and acts as a cofactor with alcohol consumption, increasing the risk of AP. Encouraging patients to stop smoking may decrease the likelihood of recurrent episodes [5]. Other risk factors for AP include abdominal adiposity and type II diabetes mellitus [6].

It is often difficult to determine the cause of AP, particularly in older patients [7]. If clinically equivocal, other diagnoses that can mimic AP should be considered, including myocardial infarction, peptic ulcer disease, intestinal ischemia, obstruction, or aortic aneurysm [1].

Lipase, Amylase, and Pancreatitis

Pancreatic lipase and amylase are enzymes derived from acinar cells in the pancreas. During episodes of AP, normal secretion of these enzymes is impaired which leads to extravasation and reabsorption into the systemic circulation [8]. Serum lipase and amylase levels are usually both elevated in AP, but the lipase level is generally greater than the amylase level. The level of elevation does not correlate with the severity of the acute pancreatitis episode [9].

Lipase is more specific for acute pancreatitis since amylase can also be elevated in other conditions, such as macroamylasemia, parotitis, and certain carcinomas [10]. Lipase alone is recommended as the primary lab for evaluating AP [10]. Some authors have advocated for a lipase/amylase ratio

T. A. Thompson
MedStar Washington Hospital Center, Department of Emergency Medicine, Washington, DC, USA

© Springer Nature Switzerland AG 2019
A. Graham, D. J. Carlberg (eds.), *Gastrointestinal Emergencies*, https://doi.org/10.1007/978-3-319-98343-1_41

as a method to evaluate alcoholic pancreatitis, but this method lacks sensitivity [8].

Since laboratory tests are sometimes used to screen patients with abdominal pain, lipase can be elevated in other conditions, including macrolipasemia, renal disease, appendicitis, cholecystitis, and other abdominal conditions [6]. Patients with diabetes may need a higher cutoff, 3–5 times the upper limit of normal, when compared with nondiabetic patients [11].

Imaging in Acute Pancreatitis

Imaging can be helpful in patients with an unclear diagnosis. Based on the definition of pancreatitis, it is possible to have pancreatitis with a normal lipase if there is pain typical for acute pancreatitis and signs of pancreatitis on imaging studies [10]. In cases of suspected pancreatitis but a lipase level below the threshold, computed tomography (CT) imaging with intravenous contrast is recommended [12, 13]. In cases where the diagnosis is clear, a CT is not required nor recommended [14]. CT is the only imaging modality to consistently predict extent of disease, severity, and clinical outcomes [15]. However, CT performed on admission rarely changes the clinical outcome or prognosis. In one cohort study of patients with acute pancreatitis who received a CT on admission, there was no difference in severity prognosis between CT and clinical scoring systems [15]. In patients without improvement in 48 h after presentation or with a worsening clinical picture, a CT scan is recommended to evaluate for local or systemic complications. Biliary ultrasound evaluation is recommended for all patients with first episode of acute pancreatitis since gallstone pancreatitis is the leading cause of pancreatitis and identification of a stone may change management [10].

Pancreatitis Prognostication

After diagnosing AP, it is important to assess the severity of disease. Most episodes of AP are mild, defined as a lack of organ failure or pancreatic necrosis. These patients usually have self-limited disease and require only short hospitalizations.

Severe pancreatitis has two phases; early is considered within the first week and late can last weeks to months [2, 14]. Severe pancreatitis is defined by the presence and duration of organ failure beyond 48 h [14]. Diagnosis is complicated by the fact that most patients do not have pancreatic necrosis or organ failure at presentation. Neglecting initial red flags can lead to failure to adequately rehydrate, failure to diagnose and treat associated cholangitis, and failure to treat early organ failure [2, 5].

Patient risk factors of advanced age (>55 years) and obesity (BMI > 30) increase the risk of severe AP [10]. Elevation of hematocrit [16] or BUN [17] suggests hypovolemia. Rising lab values in the setting of adequate fluid resuscitation are concerning for worsening clinical condition [9]. The presence of SIRS, pulmonary infiltrates or effusions, and altered mental status are signs of end-organ injury and advancing inflammatory process. Persistence of SIRS despite resuscitation is an important predictor of worsening condition, suggesting a more complicated course [10, 18]. While no individual labs will predict a patient trending toward organ failure, labs showing signs of dehydration or persistent inflammation are concerning.

Suggested Resource
- Tenner S, Baillie J, DeWitt J, Vege SS. American College of Gastroenterology. American College of Gastroenterology guideline: management of acute pancreatitis. Am J Gastroenterol. 2013;108(9): 1400–16.

References

1. Baillie J. Clinical pancreatology for practicing gastroenterologists and surgeons. Gastroenterology. 2005;129(4):1356.
2. Tenner S, Baillie J, DeWitt J, Vege SS. American College of Gastroenterology. American College of Gastroenterology guideline: management of acute pancreatitis. Am J Gastroenterol. 2013;108(9):1400–16.
3. Yadav D, Lowenfels AB. Trends in the epidemiology of the first attack of acute pancreatitis: a systematic review. Pancreas. 2006;33(4):323–30.
4. Coté GA, Yadav D, Slivka A, Hawes RH, Anderson MA, Burton FR, et al. Alcohol and smoking as risk factors in an epidemiology study of patients with chronic pancreatitis. Clin Gastroenterol Hepatol. 2011;9(3):266–73.
5. Apte MV, Pirola RC, Wilson JS. Mechanisms of alcoholic pancreatitis. J Gastroenterol Hepatol. 2010;25(12):1816–26.
6. Yadav D, Lowenfels AB. The epidemiology of pancreatitis and pancreatic cancer. Gastroenterology. 2013;144(6):1252–61.
7. Forsmark CE, Vege SS, Wilcox CM. Acute pancreatitis. N Engl J Med. 2016;375(20):1972–81.
8. Kwon RS, Banks PA. How should acute pancreatitis be diagnosed in clinical practice? In: Clinical pancreatology: Blackwell Publishing Ltd; Malden, Mass. 2004. p. 34–9.
9. Yadav D, Ng B, Saul M, Kennard ED. Relationship of serum pancreatic enzyme testing trends with the diagnosis of acute pancreatitis. Pancreas. 2011;40(3):383–9.
10. Banks PA, Freeman ML. The practice parameters Committee of the American College of gastroenterology. Practice guidelines in acute pancreatitis. Am J Gastroenterol. 2006;101(10):2379–400.
11. Steinberg W, De Vries H, Wadden TA, Jensen CB, Svendsen CB, Rosenstock J. Tu1502 longitudinal monitoring of lipase and amylase in adults with type 2 diabetes and obesity: evidence from two phase 3 randomized clinical trials with the once-daily GLP-1 analog liraglutide. Gastroenterology. 2012;142(5):S850–1.

12. O'Connor OJ, McWilliams S, Maher MM. Imaging of acute pancreatitis. Am J Roentgenol. 2011;197(2):W221–5.
13. Working Group IAP/APA Acute Pancreatitis Guidelines. IAP/APA evidence-based guidelines for the management of acute pancreatitis. Pancreatology. 2013;13(4 Suppl 2):e1–15.
14. Banks PA, Bollen TL, Dervenis C, Gooszen HG, Johnson CD, Sarr MG, et al. Classification of acute pancreatitis--2012: revision of the Atlanta classification and definitions by international consensus. Gut. 2013;62(1):102–11.
15. Baker M, Nelson R, Rosen M, Blake M, Cash B, Hindman N, et al. Acute pancreatitis. ACR appropriateness criteria – acute pancreatitis. 2013. Retrieved 24 Feb 2018 from https://acsearch.acr.org/docs.
16. Lankisch PG, Mahlke R, Blum T, Bruns A, Bruns D, Maisonneuve P, et al. Hemoconcentration: an early marker of severe and/or necrotizing pancreatitis? A critical appraisal. Am J Gastroenterol. 2001;96(7):2081–5.
17. Wu BU, Johannes RS, Sun X, Conwell DL, Banks PA. Early changes in blood urea nitrogen predict mortality in acute pancreatitis. Gastroenterology. 2009;137(1):129–35.
18. Mofidi R, Duff MD, Wigmore SJ, Madhavan KK, Garden OJ, Parks RW. Association between early systemic inflammatory response, severity of multiorgan dysfunction and death in acute pancreatitis. Br J Surg. 2006;93(6):738–44.

Risk Stratification and Disposition: What Is the Usual Course of Acute Pancreatitis? Which Patients Require a Higher Level of Care and Which Patients May Be Appropriate to Discharge?

Eric S. Kiechle

Pearls and Pitfalls
- Acute pancreatitis carries an overall mortality of 1%.
- About 20% of patients will have a complicated clinical course, characterized by organ failure, pancreatic necrosis, or superimposed infection, with a mortality approaching 30%.
- While many risk stratification tools are available and can suggest a complicated course, none are sufficient in isolation to predict the need for admission to an intensive care unit or higher level of care.
- Patient risk factors, labs, vital signs, and initial response to therapy can guide admission to an appropriate level of care.
- Some patients with mild pancreatitis may be safely discharged and managed as outpatients. While HAPS score can help to identify low-risk patients for progression to severe pancreatitis, clinical decision tools to guide clinicians regarding who will do well as an outpatient are lacking.

While most patients with pancreatitis will have an uncomplicated course with a brief hospitalization, about 20% will have a complicated course, with mortality in certain subgroups approaching 30% [3]. A widely adopted 2012 international consensus report on acute pancreatitis, the revised Atlanta Classification, defines three categories of AP [4]. Severity is determined by presence or absence of organ failure (e.g., cardiac, respiratory, or renal), systemic complications (e.g., exacerbation of existing cardiac, respiratory, or hepatic disease), and local complications (e.g., pseudocysts, fluid collections, pancreatic necrosis, or necrotic collections). Severe AP is defined by persistent organ failure (>48 h) [3, 4]. An alternative classification system defines "critical pancreatitis" as persistent organ failure with infected pancreatic, necrotic tissue and has a mortality of about 50% [3, 5]. The use of these classification systems is difficult in the emergency department (ED), since it is not possible to identify persistence of organ failure at the time of admission, and imaging is not routinely performed on initial evaluation. Predicting which patients may benefit from an intensive care unit (ICU) admission is of great clinical interest but has proven difficult [6].

What Is the Usual Course of Acute Pancreatitis?

The incidence of acute pancreatitis (AP) has been increasing, with around 275,000 hospitalizations in 2012 [1]. Part of this increase may stem from increasing rates of obesity and gallstone formation or from higher rates of testing and detection of milder cases [2]. Diagnosis of milder disease may also explain why the overall mortality of AP remains low, around 1% [1].

Which Patients Require a Higher Level of Care and Which Patients May Be Appropriate to Discharge?

I Think My Patient Can Be Discharged

Certain patients may be eligible for discharge and outpatient management. The Harmless Acute Pancreatitis Score (HAPS) focuses on identifying which patients will have a non-severe course – without death, need for artificial ventilation, dialysis, or presence of pancreatic necrosis. The combination of (1) absence of peritonitis (rebound tenderness or guarding), (2) normal hematocrit (< 44%), and (3) serum creatinine (≤2 mg/dL) has a 98%

E. S. Kiechle
MedStar Washington Hospital Center, Department of Emergency Medicine, Washington, DC, USA

© Springer Nature Switzerland AG 2019
A. Graham, D. J. Carlberg (eds.), *Gastrointestinal Emergencies*, https://doi.org/10.1007/978-3-319-98343-1_42

positive predictive value for a non-severe course of AP [7, 8]. The score was validated for use in stratifying level of care at admission, but experts suggest it could be used to find patients suitable for discharge [9]. We recommend that patients with AP discharged from the ED be tolerant of an oral diet, have pain controlled by oral analgesics, and have lab markers and vital signs suggestive of a mild course (e.g., normal creatinine and hematocrit, absence of local complications if imaging is obtained). Research into ED observation and discharge of such patients is ongoing [10].

My Patient Requires Admission to the Hospital, But Do They Need a Higher Level of Care?

There has been great interest in developing a tool adapted to use at admission to predict the severity of AP. Ranson's criteria was published in 1974 and defined 11 criteria that risk stratified the severity of AP, but it requires serial lab measurements at admission and at 48 h including arterial blood gas (ABG) sampling [11]. The Acute Physiology and Chronic Health Evaluation II (APACHE II) score initially developed for predicting mortality in the ICU has also been validated to predict mortality in AP but requires the collection of 12 variables including ABG sampling and complex calculations [12]. Increased availability of computed tomography (CT) led to the development of the Balthazar score, which graded severity by the extent of findings on CT [13]. However, CT findings, such as necrosis and fluid collections, are often not apparent in the first 3–5 days after admission, and few ED patients require CT imaging for AP [14].

Bedside Index for Severity in Acute Pancreatitis (BISAP) can be calculated at admission with lab results available in the ED and has been successfully validated against APACHE II [15]. Recent studies have compared many of these scoring systems and found them to be equivalent in their ability to predict persistent organ failure and mortality. However, these scores have a high rate of false positives for poor outcomes due simply to the fact that a large majority of patients have benign courses [7, 16, 17]. For this reason, the American College of Gastroenterology, the International Association of Pancreatology, and the American Pancreatic Association recommend against routine use of scoring systems (with the exception of the Systemic Inflammatory Response Syndrome (SIRS) (Table 42.1)), for predicting AP severity [14, 18]. Some commonly used risk stratification tools are listed in Table 42.2.

High-Risk Features

Certain patient risk factors and lab markers can help guide clinicians in predicting disease severity. Patient risk factors include advanced age, comorbid disease (Charlson Comorbidity Index of ≥2 (Table 42.3)), and obesity [18]. While the degree of pancreatic enzyme elevation has no prognostic utility, elevated hematocrit (>44%), BUN (>20 mg/dL), and creatinine (>1.8 mg/dL) have all been associated with severe disease [19–21]. The presence of organ failure in the ED (hypotension, hypoxia, or creatinine elevation) and an exacerbation of a patient's chronic disease

Table 42.1 Systemic Inflammatory Response Syndrome (SIRS), present if ≥2 criteria present

Temperature >38° or less <36°
Heart rate >90 beats per minute
Respiratory rate >20 or PaCO$_2$ <32 mmHg
White blood cell count >12,000/mm^3 or <4000/mm^3

Table 42.2 Common risk stratification tools and high-risk features in acute pancreatitis

Risk stratification tool	Scoring system	Evidence-based support	Advantages and limitations
Developed to identify low-risk patients with mild acute pancreatitis			
Harmless Acute Pancreatitis Score (HAPS) [1, 2]	Non-severe course predicted by presence of all three parameters: No rebound or guarding on physical exam Normal creatinine Normal hematocrit	In validation studies, HAPS score for predicting non-severe pancreatitis: Sensitivities of 24–76% (~28%) Specificities 86–97% (~97%) PPV 94–99% (~98%) NPV 10–57% (~18%)	*Advantages:* Only scoring system which could be used to identify patients suitable for discharge Ease of use with three parameters *Limitations:* Retrospectively derived through chart review Low sensitivity and NPV with potential continued overtreatment of low-risk patients with likely non-severe AP course

Table 42.2 (continued)

Risk stratification tool	Scoring system	Evidence-based support	Advantages and limitations
Developed to identify high-risk patients requiring ICU admission or possessing high risk of decompensation and death			

Ranson criteria [3–5]	One point for each of 11 parameters at admission and at 48 h
	At admission:
	  Age > 55
	  WBC >16,000/mm^3
	  Glucose >200 mg/dL
	  LDH >350 U/L
	  AST >250 U/L
	At 48 h:
	  Hct drop >10%
	  BUN rise >5 mg/dL
	  Calcium <8 mg/dL
	  pO$_2$ < 60 mmHg
	  Base deficit >4 meq/L
	  Fluid sequestration >6000 mL
		In validating study, mortality increases with increasing score, stratified into three categories:
		  Score <3 mortality 0–3%
		  Score ≥3 mortality 11–15%
		  Score ≥6 mortality 40%
			Advantages:
			  Widely recognized, one of the earliest tools in AP
			Limitations:
			  Requires extensive testing including ABG sampling at admission and at 48 h
			  Unable to use in the ED, since need delayed testing
			  Poorly predictive of severity in meta-analysis

Acute Physiology and Chronic Health Examination II (APACHE II) [6–8]	12 parameter calculator, initially designed for predicting ICU mortality
	  Rectal temperature
	  Mean arterial pressure
	  Heart rate
	  Respiratory rate
	  PaO$_2$
	  pH
	  Sodium
	  Potassium
	  Creatinine
	  Hematocrit
	  WBC count
	  Glasgow coma scale
	  Age
	  Chronic disease
		APACHE-II score of >9 at 48 h for predicting severe AP (major organ failure or pancreatic collection):
		  Sensitivity 75%
		  Specificity 92%
		  PPV 71%
		  NPV 93%
			Advantages:
			  One of the most widely used risk stratification tools in AP
			  Can be repeated daily, which could be used to determine need for change in level of care
			Limitations:
			  Requires extensive testing including ABG sampling
			  Complex to use, requires calculator

Panc 3 [9, 10]	Severe acute pancreatitis (SAP) predicted by presence of three parameters:
	  Hct > 44 mg/dL
	  BMI > 30 kg/m^2
	  Presence of pleural effusion
		Presence of criteria and LR+:
		  HCT: 14
		  BMI: 8.7
		  Pleural effusion: 9.7
		  All three criteria: 1191
			Advantages:
			  Can be used readily from the emergency department at the time of presentation
			Limitations:
			  Retrospectively derived and validated
			  Chest X-ray not routinely ordered in evaluation of AP

Glasgow-Imrie [11, 12]	Receive a point for each parameter that is positive. A score of >3 (within up to 48 h) is predictive of severe pancreatitis
	  Age > 55 year
	  WBC count >15,000
	  Calcium <8 mg/dL
	  Urea >44.8 mg/dL
	  LDH > 600 IU/L
	  Albumin <3.2 g/dL
	  Glucose >180 mg/dL
	  PaO$_2$ < 59.3 mmHg (7.9 kPa)
		Glasgow score of >3 for predicting severe AP (major organ failure, pancreatic collection, or surgical intervention needed):
		  Sensitivity 56%
		  Specificity 98%
		  PPV 94%
		  NPV 80%
			Advantages:
			  Frequently used internationally
			Limitations:
			  Calculated at 48 h after diagnosis
			  Developed prior to widespread use of imaging
			  Cumbersome to calculate and requires ABG

(continued)

Table 42.2 (continued)

Risk stratification tool	Scoring system	Evidence-based support	Advantages and limitations
Bedside Index of Severity in Acute Pancreatitis (BISAP) [8, 13, 14]	Receive a point for each parameter that is positive. BUN > 25 mg/dL Impaired mental status >/= 2 SIRS criteria Age > 60 years Presence of pleural effusion	Test characteristics of BISAP >2 for predicting mortality: Sensitivity 95% Specificity 65% PPV 36% NPV 98%	*Advantages:* Comparable to APACHE II in predicting persistent organ failure, infected pancreatic necrosis, and mortality More readily performed in the ED than other scoring systems *Limitations:* Like other scoring systems, lacks specificity for serious outcomes

Developed to predict readmission

Whitlock et al. [15]	Retrospectively derived set of criteria predictive of readmission or ED visit within 30 days of discharge: Nausea, vomiting, or diarrhea within 24 h of discharge (3 pts) Eating less than solid diet (3 pts) Pancreatic necrosis (2 pts) Received antibiotics (2 pts) Pain at discharge (1 pts)	Patient in validating cohort stratified by points: Low risk (0–1 pts) 5% readmission rate Moderate risk (2–3 pts) 18% readmission rate High risk (≥4 points) 68% readmission rate	*Advantages:* Useful to estimate readmission or ED return risk in a disease with a baseline readmission rate higher than average *Limitations:* No prospective validation yet Applies more to hospitalist than emergency clinician, though could be useful as ED observation of AP gains traction

High-risk features

Feature	Evidence-based support	Comments
Hematocrit ≥44% [16, 17]	Test parameters of Hct ≥44% at admission for organ failure: Sensitivity 60% Specificity 75% PPV 26% NPV 93%	Studies have had conflicting results regarding the predictive ability of hematocrit to predict severity in AP The evidence is most compelling for the use of a normal hematocrit to predict a non-severe course Its utility is lessened by the fact that most cases of AP are already non-severe
BUN >20 mg/dL [18, 19]	Each incremental BUN increase at admission of 5 mg/dL was associated with a mortality odds ratio of 2.9 (95% CI 1.8–4.8) A BUN at admission of >20 mg/dL was associated with a mortality odds ratio of 4.6 (95% CI 2.5–8.3)	An elevation in BUN may represent both intravascular depletion and renal failure or upper GI bleeding, all of which are associated with worse outcomes in AP
Creatinine >1.8 mg/dL [20, 21]	Test parameters of peak creatinine >1.8 mg/dL for predicting necrotizing pancreatitis Sensitivity 41% Specificity 99% PPV 93% NPV 82%	Elevated creatinine in one study was associated with pancreatic necrosis, though not all studies have found this association Studies are consistent in showing that pancreatic necrosis is very uncommon with a normal creatinine Some authors suggest that a normal creatinine obviates the need for CT imaging because of the low incidence of necrosis
SIRS [22, 23]	Test parameters of ≥2/4 SIRS criteria at admission for predicting markers of severity in AP (persistent organ failure, necrosis, need for ICU level of care or death): Sensitivities 85–100% Specificities 40–43% PPV 6–17% NPV 98–100%	Persistence of SIRS at 48 h has much more negative prognostic implications than SIRS at presentation SIRS is the only tool advocated for routine use by most professional societies such as the American College of Gastroenterology
Lactic acidosis	Lack of research evaluating predictive value of lactic acidosis and severe acute pancreatitis course	

(chronic obstructive pulmonary disease, coronary artery disease, or liver disease) are indicative of at least moderate severity AP [4]. If CT imaging is obtained, local complications defined above are associated with higher mortality [3]. Finally, presence of SIRS on admission (Table 42.1) is associated with higher mortality, especially if persistent during the hospitalization [22]. Little data exists on the predictive value of lactate in acute pancreatitis.

Cumulatively, these risk factors, lab markers, vital signs, and clinical presentation can be used to determine level of care at admission. Multiorgan dysfunction should always prompt consideration of ICU level of care.

Table 42.3 Charlson comorbidity index

Score	Condition
1	Myocardial infarction (history, ECG changes)
	Congestive heart failure
	Peripheral vascular disease (aortic aneurysm >6 cm)
	Cerebrovascular disease
	Dementia
	Chronic pulmonary disease
	Connective tissue disease
	Peptic ulcer disease
	Mild liver disease (including chronic hepatitis)
	Diabetes without end organ damage
2	Hemiplegia
	Moderate or severe renal disease
	Diabetes with end-organ damage (retinopathy, neuropathy, nephropathy, or brittle diabetes)
	Tumor without metastases (exclude if >5 years from diagnosis)
	Leukemia (acute or chronic)
	Lymphoma
3	Moderate or severe liver disease
6	Metastatic solid tumor
	AIDS (not just HIV positive)
Age	For each decade >40 years of age, a score of 1 is added to the above score

Summary

Most patients with AP will have a benign course with minimal overall mortality. While a subset of patients will have a complicated AP course with higher morbidity and mortality, existing risk stratification tools overpredict patients who may need an ICU level of care. Existing risk factors, lab markers, and vital signs can be used to make individualized decisions regarding level of care at admission. Some patients may be suitable for discharge from the ED, though this remains an area of active research.

Suggested Resources
- CORE EM, Episode 121.0 – Pancreatitis. 13 Nov 2017; https://coreem.net/podcast/episode-121-0/
- NEJM blog: acute pancreatitis. 17 Nov 2016; https://blogs.nejm.org/now/index.php/acute-pancreatitis/2016/11/17/
- New Practice Guidelines on Acute Pancreatitis Podcast, American College of Gastroenterology. 2013; https://gi.org/physician-resources/podcasts/the-american-journal-of-gastroenterology-author-podcasts/tenner-1/
- Vasudevan S, Goswami P, Sonika U, Thakur B, Sreenivas V, Saraya A. Comparison of various scoring systems and biochemical markers in predicting the outcome in acute pancreatitis. Pancreas. 2018;47:65–71.

References

1. Peery AF, Crockett SD, Barritt AS, Dellon ES, Eluri S, Gangarosa LM, et al. Burden of gastrointestinal, liver, and pancreatic diseases in the United States. Gastroenterology. 2015;149(7):1731–41.
2. Yadav D, Ng B, Saul M, Kennard ED. Relationship of serum pancreatic enzyme testing trends with the diagnosis of acute pancreatitis. Pancreas. 2011;40(3):383–9.
3. Kadiyala V, Suleiman SL, McNabb-Baltar J, Wu BU, Banks PA, Singh VK. The Atlanta classification, revised Atlanta classification, and determinant-based classification of acute pancreatitis: which is best at stratifying outcomes? Pancreas. 2016 Apr;45(4):510–5.
4. Banks PA, Bollen TL, Dervenis C, Gooszen HG, Johnson CD, Sarr MG, et al. Classification of acute pancreatitis--2012: revision of the Atlanta classification and definitions by international consensus. Gut. 2013;62(1):102–11.
5. Dellinger EP, Forsmark CE, Layer P, Levy P, Maravi-Poma E, Petrov MS, et al. Determinant-based classification of acute pancreatitis severity: an international multidisciplinary consultation. Ann Surg. 2012;256(6):875–80.
6. Chauhan S, Forsmark CE. The difficulty in predicting outcome in acute pancreatitis. Am J Gastroenterol. 2010;105(2):443.
7. Bollen TL, Singh VK, Maurer R, Repas K, Van Es HW, Banks PA, et al. A comparative evaluation of radiologic and clinical scoring systems in the early prediction of severity in acute pancreatitis. Am J Gastroenterol. 2012;107(4):612.
8. Lankisch PG, Weber–Dany B, Hebel K, Maisonneuve P, Lowenfels AB. The harmless acute pancreatitis score: a clinical algorithm for rapid initial stratification of nonsevere disease. Clin Gastroenterol Hepatol. 2009;7(6):702–5.
9. Banks PA. Acute pancreatitis: landmark studies, management decisions, and the future. Pancreas. 2016;45(5):633–40.
10. Kothari DJ, Hill M, Babineau M, Freedman SD, Shapiro N, Sheth S. Sa1351-management of mild acute pancreatitis through observation in the emergency department (ED): a novel clinical pathway. Gastroenterology. 2017;152(5):S287.
11. Ranson J. Prognostic signs and the role of operative management in acute pancreatitis. Surg Gynecol Obstet. 1974;139:69–81.
12. Al-Hadeedi S, Fan S, Leaper D. APACHE-II score for assessment and monitoring of acute pancreatitis. Lancet. 1989; 334(8665):738.
13. Balthazar EJ, Robinson DL, Megibow AJ, Ranson JH. Acute pancreatitis: value of CT in establishing prognosis. Radiology. 1990;174(2):331–6.
14. Working Group IAP/APA Acute Pancreatitis Guidelines. IAP/APA evidence-based guidelines for the management of acute pancreatitis. Pancreatology. 2013;13(4):e1–e15.
15. Wu BU, Johannes RS, Sun X, Tabak Y, Conwell DL, Banks PA. The early prediction of mortality in acute pancreatitis: a large population-based study. Gut. 2008;57(12):1698–703.
16. Papachristou GI, Muddana V, Yadav D, O'Connell M, Sanders MK, Slivka A, et al. Comparison of BISAP, Ranson's, APACHE-II, and CTSI scores in predicting organ failure, complications, and mortality in acute pancreatitis. Am J Gastroenterol. 2010;105(2):435.
17. Mounzer R, Langmead CJ, Wu BU, Evans AC, Bishehsari F, Muddana V, et al. Comparison of existing clinical scoring systems to predict persistent organ failure in patients with acute pancreatitis. Gastroenterology. 2012;142(7):1476–82.
18. Tenner S, Baillie J, DeWitt J, Vege SS. American College of Gastroenterology guideline: management of acute pancreatitis. Am J Gastroenterol. 2013;108(9):1400.
19. Brown A, Orav J, Banks PA. Hemoconcentration is an early marker for organ failure and necrotizing pancreatitis. Pancreas. 2000;20(4):367–72.

20. Muddana V, Whitcomb DC, Khalid A, Slivka A, Papachristou GI. Elevated serum creatinine as a marker of pancreatic necrosis in acute pancreatitis. Am J Gastroenterol. 2009;104(1):164.

21. Wu BU, Johannes RS, Sun X, Conwell DL, Banks PA. Early changes in blood urea nitrogen predict mortality in acute pancreatitis. Gastroenterology. 2009;137(1):129–35.

22. Mofidi R, Duff M, Wigmore S, Madhavan K, Garden O, Parks R. Association between early systemic inflammatory response, severity of multiorgan dysfunction and death in acute pancreatitis. Br J Surg. 2006;93(6):738–44.

23. Singh VK, Wu BU, Bollen TL, Repas K, Maurer R, Mortele KJ, et al. Early systemic inflammatory response syndrome is associated with severe acute pancreatitis. Clin Gastroenterol Hepatol. 2009;7(11):1247–51.

How Should I Manage My in the Pancreatitis Patients Emergency Department? Who Needs Imaging? Antibiotics? Surgery? Interventional Radiology? ERCP?

43

Travis A. Thompson

> **Pearls and Pitfalls**
> - Early, aggressive fluid resuscitation is the mainstay of treatment.
> - Rule out obstructed stones with ultrasound.
> - Withhold antibiotics unless known or suspected infection.
> - Early surgical specialist involvement is helpful, but surgical intervention will likely be delayed.

Medical Management

Intravenous Fluids

Regardless of severity, treatment for acute pancreatitis begins with aggressive fluid therapy (250–500 ml/hr) [1]. Human studies demonstrating the direct effectiveness of aggressive fluid resuscitation are lacking, but signs of hemoconcentration and a lack of resuscitation are associated with poor outcomes in multiple studies [2–4]. A randomized controlled trial of 60 patients comparing aggressive to standard fluid administration showed a significant decrease in signs of hemoconcentration and SIRS, although it did not have an effect on mortality.[5] The greatest benefit from aggressive fluid resuscitation occurs in the first 12–24 h.

Experts recommend aggressive hydration with isotonic fluids, such as normal saline or lactated Ringer's solution. In one randomized controlled trial, patients with fluid resuscitation with lactated Ringer's solution had lower rates of SIRS and greater improvement in their C-reactive protein levels (CRP), suggesting reduced systemic inflammation, compared with patients resuscitated with normal saline [6].

Fluid administration should be tailored to the patient's underlying cardiopulmonary reserve [7]. Risks of overly aggressive fluid administration include abdominal compartment syndrome and respiratory failure [7].

Pain Management

Pain management is another component of supportive care for patients with AP. Strategies for pain management are similar to other painful conditions and include opiates/opioids, nonsteroidal anti-inflammatory drugs (NSAIDs), and acetaminophen. High doses of narcotics may be required [8].

Enteral Feeding

Contrary to traditional dogma, early enteral feeding has been shown to be safe and well tolerated. In one randomized controlled trial of 72 patients with AP, early refeeding was associated with decreased length of hospital stay. Length of stay and symptoms did not change if the patient was restarted on a full diet versus a stepwise progression of feeding, i.e., advance as tolerated diet [9]. A meta-analysis of six trials comparing early versus late (after 48 h) enteral feeding showed a significant decrease in organ failure in the early refeeding group [10]. Patients do not appear to benefit from remaining nil per os (NPO) and can be given a diet, but it is unclear if the feeding should begin in the emergency department or acute care setting [7]. Total parenteral nutrition is no longer recommended as initial therapy and is associated with worse outcomes [11].

Antibiotics

Prophylactic antibiotics were previously thought to be a component of acute pancreatitis treatment [1, 12]. However, a Cochrane meta-analysis of seven randomized controlled

T. A. Thompson
MedStar Washington Hospital Center, Department of Emergency Medicine, Washington, DC, USA

trials with a total of 404 patients with CT-confirmed pancreatic necrosis showed no significant difference in mortality, infection rates, or need for operative intervention [13, 14]. This subset of patients with pancreatic necrosis was isolated to improve the likelihood of seeing an effect in the sickest patients.

Given harms associated with antibiotic use (e.g., fungal infections, diarrhea, selection of resistant organisms) and failure to improve morbidity and mortality in AP, antibiotics are not routinely recommended but reserved for cases suspicious for concomitant bacterial infections. Fever is not a reliable sign of concomitant bacterial infections given that up to 60% of patients with AP have low-grade fevers [8]. Empiric antibiotics are recommended for patients with signs of gas in peripancreatic fluid collections on CT or sepsis. Antibiotics should also be considered if there is evidence for extrapancreatic infections, such as cholangitis, catheter-acquired infections, or bacteremia. If infection is suspected, treat empirically. However, antibiotics can be discontinued if all sources are found to be negative [15].

Ertapenem, imipenem, and moxifloxacin have shown good pancreatic tissue penetration and achieve mean inhibitory concentration after just one dose [1, 14].

Imaging

Patients with AP of unknown origin will require some imaging [6]. Right upper quadrant ultrasonography (US) is routinely recommended to rule out gallstone pancreatitis, choledocholithiasis, or concurrent cholangitis [1, 16]. While not used to diagnose AP, abdominal ultrasound can visualize diffuse glandular enlargement, hypoechoic texture from interstitial edema, free fluid, or focal areas of hemorrhage/necrosis within the pancreas [8].

Conversely, computed tomography (CT) has a sensitivity and specificity of >90% for the diagnosis of AP [17]. CT is not routinely recommended unless the diagnosis of AP is uncertain or there are signs of complications such as peritonitis or shock [1, 8, 16]. CT scanning after the 48 h mark is more helpful in directing care and prognosis rather than CT at time of diagnosis [18, 19]. CT findings can be normal in patients with mild pancreatitis [8].

Magnetic Resonance Cholangiopancreatography (MRCP) is another imaging modality that evaluates the hepatobiliary tract. MRCP is recommended for patients in whom the US does not adequately visualize the common bile duct, or if the US is normal and laboratory studies suggest obstruction [12, 17, 20].

Surgical Management

Surgical intervention may be necessary for two reasons: cholecystectomy for gallstone pancreatitis and severe pancreatitis with local complications.

In gallstone pancreatitis with mild disease course, surgeons will often recommend laparoscopic cholecystectomy (LC) during their hospitalization to prevent repeat episodes of gallstone pancreatitis. Failure to perform a LC is associated with repeat episodes of acute gallstone pancreatitis (18%) based on a retrospective review of eight cohort studies and one RCT with a total of 998 patients [21]. In a retrospective review [22] of 303 patients with mild gallstone pancreatitis as well as a RCT [23] of 50 patients, there were associations with decreased hospital length of stay when LC was done within 48 h of index admission with no associated increase in morbidity or mortality. A retrospective review of 187 patients with moderate to severe gallstone pancreatitis showed worse outcomes for patients who underwent LC within 3 weeks [24]. There is potential benefit to wait 6 weeks for LC in patients with moderate to severe pancreatitis [24, 25].

Surgeons may also be part of the medical team in patients with severe pancreatitis with local complications and areas of necrosis. Current surgical recommendations suggest a delay in surgery until fluid collections have walled off and the patient is stable. A "step-up" approach to surgery, where less invasive measures are attempted first, is also recommended [26]. In patients with severe pancreatitis and decompensation, a discussion between surgery, gastroenterology, and critical care medicine is helpful to determine the best course of action.

Interventional Radiology

Interventional radiology (IR) may be involved in cases of severe pancreatitis with fluid collections suspicious for infection or as part of a "step-up" approach. This approach showed a decrease in major complications and death compared with open necrosectomy [26]. Fine needle aspiration of fluid collections under CT guidance can help distinguish between sterile and infected necrotic fluid collections. As with general surgery, delay of up to 4–6 weeks is preferable to provide time for inflammation to decrease and for fluid collections to wall off.

Endoscopic Retrograde Cholangiopancreatography (ERCP)

Most gallstones will pass into the gastrointestinal tract without intervention (1). Based on a 2012 Cochrane review, routine use of ERCP in gallstone pancreatitis does not improve outcomes. In patients with signs of cholangitis or biliary obstruction, however, there was an improvement in mortality and systemic complications [27, 28]. In patients with mild to moderate pancreatitis that cannot tolerate a cholecystectomy, ERCP with sphincterotomy showed a decrease in repeat episodes of gallstone pancreatitis [21, 29].

Summary

Early aggressive fluid therapy and pain control are the mainstays of therapy for patients that can tolerate large volume resuscitation. Antibiotics are not routinely recommended in the absence of infection, and imaging is geared at ruling out biliary obstruction, identifying local complications, or identifying alternate diagnoses. Invasive therapies, such as surgery or IR-placed drains, are usually delayed and rarely performed from the emergency department.

Suggested Resources
- NEJM blog: acute pancreatitis. 17 Nov 2016; https://blogs.nejm.org/now/index.php/acute-pancreatitis/2016/11/17/
- New Practice Guidelines on Acute Pancreatitis Podcast, American College of Gastroenterology. 2013.; https://gi.org/physician-resources/podcasts/the-american-journal-of-gastroenterology-author-podcasts/tenner-1/

References

1. Tenner S, Baillie J, DeWitt J, Vege SS, American College of Gastroenterology. American College of Gastroenterology guideline: management of acute pancreatitis. Am J Gastroenterol. 2013;108(9):1400–16.
2. Brown A, Orav J, Banks PA. Hemoconcentration is an early marker for organ failure and necrotizing pancreatitis. Pancreas. 2000;20(4):367–72.
3. Wu BU, Johannes RS, Sun X, Conwell DL, Banks PA. Early changes in blood urea nitrogen predict mortality in acute pancreatitis. Gastroenterology. 2009;137(1):129–35.
4. Muddana V, Whitcomb DC, Khalid A, Slivka A, Papachristou GI. Elevated serum creatinine as a marker of pancreatic necrosis in acute pancreatitis. Am J Gastroenterol. 2009;104(1):164–70.
5. Buxbaum JL, Quezada M, Da B, Jani N, Lane C, Mwengela D, et al. Early aggressive hydration hastens clinical improvement in mild acute pancreatitis. Am J Gastroenterol. 2017;112(5):797–803.
6. Wu BU, Hwang JQ, Gardner TH, Repas K, Delee R, Yu S, et al. Lactated ringer's solution reduces systemic inflammation compared with saline in patients with acute pancreatitis. Clin Gastroenterol Hepatol. 2011;9(8):710–7.
7. Forsmark CE, Vege SS, Wilcox CM. Acute pancreatitis. N Engl J Med. 2016;375(20):1972–81.
8. Kwon RS, Banks PA. How should acute pancreatitis be diagnosed in clinical practice? In: Clinical pancreatology: Blackwell Publishing Ltd; Malden, Mass. 2004. p. 34–9.
9. Lariño-Noia J, Lindkvist B, Iglesias-García J, Seijo-Ríos S, Iglesias-Canle J, Domínguez-Muñoz JE. Early and/or immediately full caloric diet versus standard refeeding in mild acute pancreatitis: a randomized open-label trial. Pancreatology. 2014;14(3):167–73.
10. Feng P, He C, Liao G, Chen Y. Early enteral nutrition versus delayed enteral nutrition in acute pancreatitis: a PRISMA-compliant systematic review and meta-analysis. Medicine. 2017;96(46):e8648.

11. Al-Omran M, Albalawi ZH, Tashkandi MF, Al-Ansary LA. Enteral versus parenteral nutrition for acute pancreatitis. Cochrane Database Syst Rev. 2010;(1):CD002837.
12. Sainio V, Kemppainen E, Puolakkainen P, Taavitsainen M, Kivisaari L, Valtonen V, et al. Early antibiotic treatment in acute necrotising pancreatitis. Lancet. 1995;346(8976):663–7.
13. Jiang K, Huang W, Yang X-N, Xia Q. Present and future of prophylactic antibiotics for severe acute pancreatitis. World J Gastroenterol. 2012;18(3):279–84.
14. Villatoro E, Mulla M, Larvin M. Antibiotic therapy for prophylaxis against infection of pancreatic necrosis in acute pancreatitis. Cochrane Database of Systematic Reviews 2010, Issue 5. Art. No.: CD002941.
15. Banks PA, Freeman ML. The practice parameters Committee of the American College of gastroenterology. Practice guidelines in acute pancreatitis. Am J Gastroenterol. 2006;101(10):2379–400.
16. Greenberg JA, Hsu J, Bawazeer M, Marshall J, Friedrich JO, Nathens A, et al. Clinical practice guideline: management of acute pancreatitis. Can J Surg. 2016;59(2):128–40.
17. Balthazar EJ. Acute pancreatitis: assessment of severity with clinical and CT evaluation. Radiology. 2002;223(3):603–13.
18. Bollen TL, Singh VK, Maurer R, Repas K, van Es HW, Banks PA, et al. A comparative evaluation of radiologic and clinical scoring systems in the early prediction of severity in acute pancreatitis. Am J Gastroenterol. 2012;107(4):612–9.
19. Banks PA, Bollen TL, Dervenis C, Gooszen HG, Johnson CD, Sarr MG, et al. Classification of acute pancreatitis--2012: revision of the Atlanta classification and definitions by international consensus. Gut. 2013;62(1):102–11.
20. Arvanitakis M, Delhaye M, De Maertelaere V, Bali M, Winant C, Coppens E, et al. Computed tomography and magnetic resonance imaging in the assessment of acute pancreatitis. Gastroenterology. 2004;126(3):715–23.
21. van Baal MC, Besselink MG, Bakker OJ, van Santvoort HC, Schaapherder AF, Nieuwenhuijs VB, et al. Timing of cholecystectomy after mild biliary pancreatitis: a systematic review. Ann Surg. 2012;255(5):860–6.
22. Falor AE, de Virgilio C, Stabile BE, Kaji AH, Caton A, Kokubun BA, et al. Early laparoscopic cholecystectomy for mild gallstone pancreatitis: time for a paradigm shift. Arch Surg. 2012;147(11):1031–5.
23. Aboulian A, Chan T, Yaghoubian A, Kaji AH, Putnam B, Neville A, et al. Early cholecystectomy safely decreases hospital stay in patients with mild gallstone pancreatitis: a randomized prospective study. Ann Surg. 2010;251(4):615–9.
24. Nealon WH, Bawduniak J, Walser EM. Appropriate timing of cholecystectomy in patients who present with moderate to severe gallstone-associated acute pancreatitis with peripancreatic fluid collections. Ann Surg. 2004;239(6):741–9; discussion 749–51
25. Working Group IAP/APA Acute Pancreatitis Guidelines. IAP/APA evidence-based guidelines for the management of acute pancreatitis. Pancreatology. 2013;13(4 Suppl 2):e1–15.
26. De Waele JJ. A step-up approach, or open necrosectomy for necrotizing pancreatitis. N Engl J Med. 2010;363(13):1286–7.
27. Tse F, Yuan Y. Early routine endoscopic retrograde cholangiopancreatography strategy versus early conservative management strategy in acute gallstone pancreatitis. Cochrane Database Syst Rev. 2012;(5):CD009779.
28. Fan S-T, Lai E, Mok F, Lo C-M, Zheng S-S, Wong J. Early treatment of acute biliary pancreatitis by endoscopic papillotomy. N Engl J Med. 1993;328(4):228–32.
29. Hernandez V, Pascual I, Almela P, Anon R, Herreros B, Sanchiz V, et al. Recurrence of acute gallstone pancreatitis and relationship with cholecystectomy or endoscopic sphincterotomy. Am J Gastroenterol. 2004;99(12):2417–23.

How Do I Evaluate a Patient for Chronic Pancreatitis in the Emergency Department? How Are These Patients Managed Acutely? What Therapies Exist for Long-Term Management of This Condition?

44

Nick Tsipis and Eric S. Kiechle

Pearls and Pitfalls
- Patients with chronic pancreatitis can manifest a variety of exocrine, endocrine, vascular, and other complications as a result of their long-standing inflammatory state.
- Chronic pancreatitis can result in type III diabetes mellitus (pancreaticogenic diabetes) a condition that can cause significant endocrine dysfunction and result in ketoacidosis and treatment-induced refractory hypoglycemia.
- Patients with chronic pancreatitis are at increased risk of pancreatic cancer and peptic ulcer disease.
- Pain relief is a challenging yet central focus in the management of chronic pancreatitis patients.
- Guidelines recommend stepwise escalation of analgesics, targeted surgical and medical therapies, and a multimodal, interdisciplinary approach to pain relief.

Chronic pancreatitis (CP) is a chronic inflammatory condition of the pancreas resulting in fibrosis of the pancreatic ducts and parenchyma [1]. It is characterized by a decreased quality of life [2], usually secondary to long-term, debilitating abdominal pain. The majority of patients acquire the condition from alcohol abuse (70%), with another 20% of cases described as idiopathic, and 10% caused by cystic fibrosis, autoimmune disease, hypertriglyceridemia, pancreatic resection, or other rare causes [3].

How Do I Evaluate a Patient for Chronic Pancreatitis in the Emergency Department

Multiple diagnostic modalities and algorithms are used in the initial evaluation and diagnosis of chronic pancreatitis, though this workup will rarely take place in the ED. Common imaging modalities include CT, MRI, magnetic resonance cholangiopancreatography (MRCP), endoscopic retrograde cholangiopancreatography (ERCP), and endoscopic ultrasound (EUS) [4]. Chronic pancreatitis can be confirmed and its course trended by low fecal elastase, low serum trypsin, suboptimal bicarbonate measurements following secretin administration, and other specialized pancreatic function testing through a specialist [4]. However, in the emergent setting, the most easily available and helpful tests are a comprehensive metabolic panel and lipase to evaluate for exocrine function. According to one set of international guidelines, "it is well substantiated that the state of exocrine function will deteriorate over time in the majority of patients due to disease progression" [5]. This "burnout" phenomenon means that patients may become recurrently symptomatic with lower detectable lipase levels. Trending levels from previous visits or outpatient workups may be helpful to determine trajectory of illness. Repeat imaging in the ED should be considered for atypical presentations or symptoms suggestive of an alternative diagnosis, such as pancreatic pseudocyst, viscous obstruction, biliary obstruction, cancer, or vascular involvement.

Clinical considerations:

- Vascular/hematologic – Rare but serious vascular complications have been detailed in case reports, including pseudoaneurysms of the gastroduodenal and other arteries [6, 7]. Patients with chronic pancreatitis are at a higher risk of developing peptic ulcer disease [8]. Clinical findings suspicious for acute blood loss, such as a drop in hemoglobin or positive fecal occult blood testing, should prompt gastroenterology involvement for possible esophagogastroduodenoscopy (EGD) or mesenteric angiography.

N. Tsipis (✉) · E. S. Kiechle
MedStar Washington Hospital Center, Department of Emergency Medicine, Washington, DC, USA
e-mail: nickolas.tsipis@medstar.net

© Springer Nature Switzerland AG 2019
A. Graham, D. J. Carlberg (eds.), *Gastrointestinal Emergencies*, https://doi.org/10.1007/978-3-319-98343-1_44

- Endocrine and exocrine dysfunction – Patients with CP can develop endocrine and exocrine dysfunction of the pancreas. Exocrine symptoms are characterized by malabsorption, including diarrhea, steatorrhea, weight loss, metabolic bone disease, or vitamin/mineral deficiency [9]. These conditions should be treated with pancreatic enzyme replacement containing at least 40,000–50,000 USP units of lipase, either enteric coated or paired with an H2 blocker/proton-pump inhibitor [4]. Endocrine dysfunction stems from complex cause and effect interactions between pancreatic fibrosis and both type I and type II diabetes mellitus (DM). Risk factors for CP and metabolic syndrome overlap, and these patients are more likely to develop type II DM [4, 9]. Diagnostic criteria are no different for DM associated with pancreatitis [4].
- Pancreaticogenic diabetes/type III DM – Those with CP are at risk for pancreaticogenic diabetes, also known as type III DM. This condition, also described in patients who have undergone extensive pancreatic resection, shares many clinical similarities to types I and II DM, but treatment is different. The first-line hyperglycemic treatment is metformin, and insulin should be avoided until absolutely necessary [10]. This is due to a combination of treatment-induced hypoglycemia and increased risk of malignancy with insulin treatment, specifically pancreatic carcinoma. Metformin slightly reduces neoplastic incidence [4, 10].
- Pancreatic cancer – Chronic pancreatitis is associated with a significantly increased risk of pancreatic cancer. This population has an eightfold increased risk of pancreatic cancer within 5 years of diagnosis. Part of this association may be due to a combination of increased incidence of tobacco and alcohol abuse, detection bias, and delay to diagnosis and misclassification as only chronic pancreatitis [11]. This risk profile necessitates a low threshold to evaluate patients with CP for possible malignancy.

Diagnostic Recommendations We recommend sending a complete blood count, a complete metabolic panel, and a lipase level in the evaluation of chronic pancreatitis. The value of the lipase is diminished compared to acute pancreatitis but may hold some value in trending disease course. Imaging may be required but rarely in the ED setting unless trying to rule out alternative diagnoses or evaluate for specific complications of CP.

How Are These Patients Managed Acutely? What Therapies Exist for Long-Term Management of This Condition? Pain Management Strategies?

Perhaps the most familiar symptom for patients with chronic pancreatitis is refractory abdominal pain. Pain control remains an important but challenging goal for these patients. Despite research into pain pathways and specific causative molecules, the mechanism remains poorly understood [12], and there is a lack of rigorous studies testing the efficacy of specific pain regimens. Despite the significant deleterious effects on quality of life from pain, studies of current treatment regimens, including use of narcotics, resulted in only 6% of CP patients classifying themselves as "pain-free" [5]. Many patients who arrive in the ED will have already tried multiple agents for pain relief.

Recent European evidenced-based consensus specialty guidelines advocate a multimodal, multidisciplinary approach. Medical therapy should incorporate psychological evaluation, neurologic evaluation, and stepwise escalation of analgesics. All patients should be educated on nutritional optimization as well as tobacco and alcohol cessation. Some guidelines also suggest that some patients may benefit from selective serotonin or serotonin-norepinephrine reuptake inhibitors (SSRI/SNRI), tricyclic antidepressants, or gabapentinoid therapy. One randomized double-blind, placebo-controlled study advocates for the use of pregabalin (Lyrica®), a GABA-nergic agent as adjuvant therapy for pain control, as evidenced by improved patient-reported pain scores [13]. Rarely are these patients well suited for NSAIDs or opiates. Narcotic dependence and addiction are serious concerns in these patients, as they cloud the diagnostic picture, carry serious potential for overdose, and can cause worsening gastroparesis or narcotic bowel syndrome [3, 8]. Multiple sources advocate beginning with a mild opioid agonist when narcotics are deemed necessary [1, 4, 8]. Tramadol is one such agent, as it exhibits weak mu-receptor agonism as well as SSRI/SNRI activity, with "pharmacodynamics and pharmacokinetic properties that are highly unlikely to lead to dependence" [14].

The use of pancreatic enzymes has been proposed for pain relief in addition to its aforementioned use for nutritional supplement [1, 3, 8, 15]. Various reviews of the literature have determined that any significant benefit seems to come from their effects on abdominal discomfort, like excessive gas and bloating [5]. With little downside, these supplements can decrease pancreatic secretion through the fibrotic pancreatic ducts [3, 7, 14]. A variety of pancreatic enzyme product formulations exist in differing units, but a general threshold should begin with 40,000–50,000 United States Pharmacopeia (USP) units of supplementation per meal, with half that much for snacks [4]. Common brand names for these enzymes in the United States include Creon® and Pancreaze®.

Definitive endoscopic and surgical interventions are aimed at resolving or improving symptoms resulting from pancreatic calcifications and stones or the presence of anatomic strictures. Options include extracorporeal shock wave lithotripsy (ESWL) for obstructing pancreatic stones, ERCP for stent placement, sphincterotomy of the major or minor papilla, and – finally – surgical interventions including pancreatic duct decompression, islet cell transplantation, and partial or total pancreatectomy [1, 3, 8]. Each of these interventions has varied specialist agreement on utility and patient improvement rates [1, 8].

Finally, atypical/unconventional treatments include ketamine, octreotide, clonidine, benzodiazepines, antipsychotics, or cannabinoids, but these lack definitive evidence [8]. Ultimately, many of these patients will require dedicated pain management interventions like celiac plexus blocks, splanchnic nerve ablations, or other alternative approaches to pain relief [8]. While many of the agents and modalities for pain relief clearly do not fall within the scope of practice of the emergency provider, the most helpful role of the ED may be to arrange appropriate outpatient follow-up with gastroenterology, surgery, or pain management to facilitate next steps in management.

Treatment recommendations:

- Consider short course of opioid analgesics, such as tramadol, with close outpatient follow-up.
- Refer these patients to gastroenterology, and consider pain management referral given the challenge of controlling pain in chronic pancreatitis.
- Consider initiation of pancreatic enzymes, with an enteric-coated formulation that ensures for 40,000–50,000 USP units of lipase with each meal and half that much with snacks [4].

Summary

In conclusion, patients with chronic pancreatitis warrant careful consideration of life-threatening complications of their long-standing pancreatic damage. Pain control in the ED can be challenging but should be undertaken with a multimodal and multidisciplinary approach, with appropriate integration with specialists including gastroenterology, surgery, and pain management services.

Suggested Resources
- A deep dive into consensus guidelines: Löhr JM, et al. and the HaPanEU/UEG Working Group. United European Gastroenterology evidence-based guidelines for the diagnosis and therapy of chronic pancreatitis (HaPanEU). United European Gastroenterol J. 5(2):153–199.
- Johns Hopkins Medicine Podcasts: Diagnosis and management of chronic pancreatitis by Vikesh Singh, January 25, 2018: https://podcasts.hopkins-medicine.org/ste-016/ (Just this week!).
- The National Pancreas Foundation, patient information about CP: https://pancreasfoundation.org/patient-information/chronic-pancreatitis/

References

1. Anderson MA, Akshintala V, Albers KM, Amann ST, Belfer I, Brand R, et al. Mechanism, assessment and management of pain in chronic pancreatitis: recommendations of a multidisciplinary study group. Pancreatology. 2016;16(1):83–94.
2. Olesen SS, Juel J, Nielson AK, Frokjaer JB, Wilder-Smith OH, Drewes AM. Pain severity reduces life quality in chronic pancreatitis: implications for design of future outcome trials. Pancreatology. 2014;14(6):497–502.
3. Gupta V, Toskes PP. Diagnosis and management of chronic pancreatitis. Postgrad Med J. 2005;81:491–7.
4. Forsmark CE. Management of chronic pancreatitis. Gastroenterology. 2013;144:1282–91.
5. Löhr JM, Dominquez-Munoz E, Rosendahl J, Besselink M, Mayerle J, Lerch MM, et al. United European Gastroenterology evidence-based guidelines for the diagnosis and therapy of chronic pancreatitis (HaPanEU). United European Gastroenterol J. 2017;5(2):153–99.
6. Klaub M, Heye T, Stampfl U, Grenacher L, Radeleff B. Successful arterial embolization of a giant pseudoaneurysm of the gastroduodenal artery secondary to chronic pancreatitis with literature review. J Radiol Case Rep. 2012;6(2):9–16.
7. Balachandra S, Siriwardena AK. Systemic appraisal of the management of the major vascular complications of pancreatitis. Am J Surg. 2005;190(3):489–95.
8. Drewes AM, Bouwense SAW, Campbell CM, Ceyhan GO, Delhaye M, Demir IE, et al. Guidelines for the understanding and management of pain in chronic pancreatitis. Pancreatology. 2017;17(5):720–31.
9. Yang D, Forsmark CE. Chronic pancreatitis. Curr Opin Gastroenterol. 2017;33(5):396–403.
10. Cui Y, Andersen DK. Pancreaticogenic diabetes: special considerations for management. Pancreatology. 2011;11:279–94.
11. Kirkegard J, Mortensen FV, Cronin-Fenton D. Chronic pancreatitis and pancreatic cancer risk: a systematic review and meta-analysis. Am J Gastroenterol. 2017;112(9):1366–72.
12. Pasricha PJ. Unraveling the mystery of pain in chronic pancreatitis. Nat Rev Gastroenterol Hepatol. 2012;9:140–51.
13. Olesen SS, Bouwense SA, Wilder-Smith OH, van Goor H, Drewes AM. Pregabalin reduces pain in patients with chronic pancreatitis in a randomized, controlled trial. Gastroenterology. 2011;141:536–43.
14. Dayer P, Desmueles J, Collart L. Pharmacology of tramadol. Drugs. 1997;53(Suppl 2):18–24.
15. Warshaw AL, Banks PA, Fernandez-Del CC. AGA technical review: treatment of pain in chronic pancreatitis. Gastroenterology. 1998;115(3):765–76.

Gallstone Pancreatitis: How Does Management Differ from Other Causes of Acute Pancreatitis?

45

Lindsea Abbott and Travis A. Thompson

Pearls and Pitfalls
- Gallstone pancreatitis is treated differently than alcoholic or other types of pancreatitis.
- An elevated ALT level with concomitant elevation of lipase >3x upper normal reference is highly suggestive of gallstone pancreatitis.
- The probability of a common bile duct (CBD) stone increases from 28% to 50% when the diameter cutoff of the CBD is changed from 6 mm to 10 mm.
- Imaging and surgery will be required for most patients unless unstable. Surgery is often not emergent.
- ERCP is unnecessary in most cases and comes with risk of complications.

Gallstone Pancreatitis: How Does Management Differ from Other Causes of Acute Pancreatitis?

Acute pancreatitis (AP) is generally defined as an inflammatory condition of the pancreas characterized by severe, persistent epigastric pain and elevated levels of serum pancreatic enzymes [1]. While there are many documented causes of AP, the most common cause of AP worldwide is gallstone pancreatitis (GP) [2–4]. There are two accepted theories on how gallstones induce AP. Reflux of bile into the pancreatic duct occurs due to transient or complete obstruction of the ampulla or due to edema around the ampulla after passage of the stone. Fortunately, only 3–7% of patients with gallstones will develop AP [5]. Unlike other causes of AP, GP requires a more extensive workup with labs and imaging and directed treatment course addressing the underlying cause [6]. Patients with confirmed GP have a significant risk of life-threatening complications including persistent biliary obstruction and acute cholangitis, which can lead to systemic organ failure [7, 8].

Current recommendations state that all patients with suspected common bile duct stones causing acute GP should be evaluated with liver enzyme levels and a trans-abdominal right upper quadrant ultrasound focusing on the gallbladder, searching for the presence of gallstones and the diameter of the common bile duct. [6, 9]

All patients presenting with their first attack of acute pancreatitis should be evaluated for GP [9, 10]. Furthermore, for patients with a known history of gallstones, the index of suspicion for GP should be significantly higher, and these patients may need a more extensive evaluation if initial screening tests are negative. A meta-analysis found that an alanine aminotransferase (ALT) concentration greater than 150 U/L had a positive predictive value of 95% for the diagnosis of gallstone pancreatitis when there is a concomitant elevation of serum lipase to three times the normal value [11, 12].

A dilated common bile duct (CBD) on transabdominal ultrasound is suggestive of choledocolithiasis, and classically a cutoff of 6 mm has been used to distinguish a dilated CBD (with adjustment for age); however, the probability of a CBD stone increases from 28% to 50% when the cutoff is changed from 6 mm to 10 mm [13–16]. The size of biliary stones matters. Stones with a diameter less than 5 mm are more likely to pass through the cystic duct and cause obstruction at or around the ampulla; therefore, the presence of small stones and sludge on transabdominal ultrasound are more concerning for the possibility of having common bile duct stones than the finding of a large stone within the gallbladder [17, 18]. Ultrasound is operator dependent, and limited by bowel gas and body habitus, leading to a sensitivity variation of 20–90% in various studies [19]. A 2015 Cochrane meta-analysis of 5 studies with 523 patients showed a sensitivity of 73% and specificity of 91% [20].

L. Abbott · T. A. Thompson (✉)
MedStar Washington Hospital Center, Department of Emergency Medicine, Washington, DC, USA

© Springer Nature Switzerland AG 2019
A. Graham, D. J. Carlberg (eds.), *Gastrointestinal Emergencies*, https://doi.org/10.1007/978-3-319-98343-1_45

Consultation and Disposition

For patients suspected of having acute GP, the decision to consult gastroenterology versus general surgery depends on both initial laboratory tests and ultrasound imaging, as well as level of suspicion that there is a persistent stone in the CBD. For patients with GP diagnosed by elevated liver enzymes and the presence of gallstones, dilation of the CBD, or evidence of a stone within the CBD, the current treatment guidelines recommend admitting the patient for further evaluation and management. There is no clear consensus recommendation of the most appropriate service for admission; however, there is a small observational trial of 100 patients with mild GP who were admitted to medicine versus general surgery. Those admitted to the general surgery service had a shorter length of hospital stay and shorter time to surgical intervention [21].

If there is ongoing obstruction or cholangitis, ERCP is warranted. For patients with cholangitis, ERCP should be performed as soon as possible and within 24 h. If there is obstruction only, there is no definitive time but is recommended in <72 h, which allows for brief observation period for improvement. Magnetic resonance cholangiopancreatography (MRCP) or endoscopic ultrasound (EUS) can be performed during the observation period to further eliminate those without a stone and unlikely to benefit from ERCP. For patients with suspected acute GP with liver function tests (LFTs) that have normalized and a transabdominal ultrasound that shows sludge or gallstones with a normal common bile duct diameter, literature supports performing an intraoperative cholangiogram or laparoscopic ultrasound during the cholecystectomy [22]. If a stone in the CBD is found on EUS or MRCP, current guidelines recommend ERCP for stone removal followed immediately by cholecystectomy. A Cochrane meta-analysis of 5 randomized controlled trials with 644 patients showed a significant decrease in local complications with early routine ERCP for biliary obstruction [23]. Studies have not found a benefit in overall mortality to recommend early ERCP or emergent ERCP for acute GP with biliary obstruction but no signs of systemic inflammatory response syndrome (SIRS) or acute cholangitis. MRCP does not rule out stones <5 mm so caution is warranted with negative results [24].

After acute GP, patients benefit from cholecystectomy to prevent relapse from further stones. The timing varies based on the severity of the AP. Mild pancreatitis should have a cholecystectomy during the index admissions since it has been shown to reduce recurrence without increasing morbidity or operative difficulty [25]. Patients with moderate-to-severe pancreatitis should have a cholecystectomy from 4 to 6 weeks after improvement due to higher likelihood of necrosis and secondary infection [26]. High-risk patients (elderly, multiple comorbidities) can forego cholecystectomy

but are higher risk of repeat AP, some of which is severe [10]. The risks and benefits should be discussed with the patient and surgical team.

> **Suggested Resources**
> - Core EM: https://coreem.net/core/cholangitis/
> - University of Maryland Medical Reference Guide: https://www.umm.edu/health/medical/reports/articles/gallstones-and-gallbladder-disease

References

1. Banks PA, Bollen TL, Dervenis C, Gooszen HG, Johnson CD, Sarr MG, et al. Classification of acute pancreatitis–2012: revision of the Atlanta classification and definitions by international consensus. Gut. 2013;62(1):102–11.
2. Yadav D, Lowenfels AB. Trends in the epidemiology of the first attack of acute pancreatitis: a systematic review. Pancreas. 2006;33(4):323–30.
3. Yadav D, Lowenfels AB. The epidemiology of pancreatitis and pancreatic cancer. Gastroenterology. 2013;144(6):1252–61.
4. Párniczky A, Kui B, Szentesi A, Balázs A, Szűcs Á, Mosztbacher D, et al. Prospective, multicentre, nationwide clinical data from 600 cases of acute pancreatitis. PLoS One. 2016;11(10): e0165309.
5. Moreau JA, Zinsmeister AR, Melton LJ 3rd, DiMagno EP. Gallstone pancreatitis and the effect of cholecystectomy: a population-based cohort study. Mayo Clin Proc. 1988;63(5):466–73.
6. Tenner S, Baillie J, De Witt J, Vege SS, American College of Gastroenterology. American College of Gastroenterology guideline: management of acute pancreatitis. Am J Gastroenterol. 2013;108(9):1400–15;1416.
7. Lee DWH, Chan ACW, Lam Y-H, Ng EKW, Lau JYW, Law BKB, et al. Biliary decompression by nasobiliary catheter or biliary stent in acute suppurative cholangitis: a prospective randomized trial. Gastrointest Endosc. 2002;56(3):361–5.
8. Lee BS, Hwang J-H, Lee SH, Jang SE, Jang ES, Jo HJ, et al. Risk factors of organ failure in patients with bacteremic cholangitis. Dig Dis Sci. 2013;58(4):1091–9.
9. Greenberg JA, Hsu J, Bawazeer M, Marshall J, Friedrich JO, Nathens A, et al. Clinical practice guideline: management of acute pancreatitis. Can J Surg. 2016;59(2):128–40.
10. Working Group IAP/APA Acute Pancreatitis Guidelines. IAP/APA evidence-based guidelines for the management of acute pancreatitis. Pancreatology. 2013;13(4 Suppl 2):e1–15.
11. Tenner S, Dubner H, Steinberg W. Predicting gallstone pancreatitis with laboratory parameters: a meta-analysis. Am J Gastroenterol. 1994;89(10):1863–6.
12. Baj J, Radzikowska E, Maciejewski M, Dąbrowski A, Torres K. Prediction of acute pancreatitis in the earliest stages – role of biochemical parameters and histopathological changes. Pol Przegl Chir. 2017;89(2):31–8.
13. Contractor QQ, Boujemla M, Contractor TQ, el-Essawy OM. Abnormal common bile duct sonography. The best predictor of choledocholithiasis before laparoscopic cholecystectomy. J Clin Gastroenterol. 1997;25(2):429–32.
14. Baron RL, Stanley RJ, Lee JK, Koehler RE, Melson GL, Balfe DM, et al. A prospective comparison of the evaluation of biliary

obstruction using computed tomography and ultrasonography. Radiology. 1982;145(1):91–8.

15. ASGE Standards of Practice Committee, Maple JT, Ben-Menachem T, Anderson MA, Appalaneni V, Banerjee S, et al. The role of endoscopy in the evaluation of suspected choledocholithiasis. Gastrointest Endosc. 2010;71(1):1–9.

16. Hunt DR. Common bile duct stones in non-dilated bile ducts? An ultrasound study. Australas Radiol. 1996;40(3):221–2.

17. Costi R, Sarli L, Caruso G, Iusco D, Gobbi S, Violi V, et al. Preoperative ultrasonographic assessment of the number and size of gallbladder stones. J Ultrasound Med. 2002;21(9):971–6.

18. Petrov MS, van Santvoort HC, Besselink MGH, van der Heijden GJMG, van Erpecum KJ, Gooszen HG. Early endoscopic retrograde cholangiopancreatography versus conservative management in acute biliary pancreatitis without cholangitis: a meta-analysis of randomized trials. Ann Surg. 2008;247(2):250–7.

19. Barlow AD, Haqq J, McCormack D, Metcalfe MS, Dennison AR, Garcea G. The role of magnetic resonance cholangiopancreatography in the management of acute gallstone pancreatitis. Ann R Coll Surg Engl. 2013;95(7):503–6.

20. Gurusamy KS, Giljaca V, Takwoingi Y, Higgie D, Poropat G, Štimac D, et al. Ultrasound versus liver function tests for diagnosis of common bile duct stones. Cochrane Database Syst Rev. 2015;2:CD011548.

21. Kulvatunyou N, Watt J, Friese RS, Gries L, Green DJ, Joseph B, et al. Management of acute mild gallstone pancreatitis under acute care surgery: should patients be admitted to the surgery or medicine service? Am J Surg. 2014;208(6):981–7; discussion 986–7.

22. Williams E, Beckingham I, El Sayed G, Gurusamy K, Sturgess R, Webster G, et al. Updated guideline on the management of common bile duct stones (CBDS). Gut. 2017;66(5):765–82.

23. Tse F, Yuan Y. Early routine endoscopic retrograde cholangiopancreatography strategy versus early conservative management strategy in acute gallstone pancreatitis. Cochrane Database Syst Rev. 2012.

24. Zidi SH, Prat F, Le Guen O, Rondeau Y, Rocher L, Fritsch J, et al. Use of magnetic resonance cholangiography in the diagnosis of choledocholithiasis: prospective comparison with a reference imaging method. Gut. 1999;44(1):118–22.

25. van Baal MC, Besselink MG, Bakker OJ, van Santvoort HC, Schaapherder AF, Nieuwenhuijs VB, et al. Timing of cholecystectomy after mild biliary pancreatitis: a systematic review. Ann Surg. 2012;255(5):860–6.

26. Nealon WH, Bawduniak J, Walser EM. Appropriate timing of cholecystectomy in patients who present with moderate to severe gallstone-associated acute pancreatitis with peripancreatic fluid collections. Ann Surg. 2004;239(6):741–9; discussion 749–51.

Shawn Tejiram and Laura S. Johnson

Pearls and Pitfalls

- Gallstone pancreatitis should prompt an evaluation for cholecystectomy during the index presentation.
- Computed tomography (CT) of the abdomen and pelvis may be the first imaging study obtained, but if the diagnosis of pancreatitis is confirmed, ultrasound imaging of the gallbladder and hepatobiliary tree will help identify the most common etiologies (e.g., gallstone pancreatitis).
- Resuscitation is guided by clinical markers of shock (skin perfusion, mental status, and urine output) coupled with laboratory markers of hypoperfusion (acidosis, hemoconcentration, organ failure).

Introduction

Laura S. Johnson, MD, FACS, is board certified in both general surgery and surgical critical care and is a member of the surgical team at the Burn Center at Medstar Washington Hospital Center. In addition, she is an attending surgeon in the Burns/Trauma Section of Surgery and Assistant Professor of Surgery at Georgetown University School of Medicine. Shawn Tejiram is an accomplished surgeon who is finishing his residency at Medstar Washington Hospital Center with plan to pursue a fellowship in burn/critical care surgery at University of California Davis. Dr. Johnson and Dr. Tejiram

S. Tejiram
MedStar Georgetown University Hospital - Washington Hospital Center Residency Program in General Surgery, Department of Surgery, MedStar Washington Hospital Center, Washington, DC, USA

L. S. Johnson (✉)
Georgetown University School of Medicine, Washington, DC, USA
e-mail: laura.s.johnson@medstar.net

practice in a large, urban tertiary referral hospital in Washington, DC, evaluating acute care surgical patients.

Answers to Key Clinical Questions

1. What is the surgeon's general approach to pancreatitis?

From the surgeon's perspective, the pancreas is one of the last organs in the human body to be successfully managed operatively due to its unfavorable location in the abdomen, complex anatomy, and high associated morbidity and mortality. The first documented case of surgical management of the pancreas was not until the late nineteenth century, when Dr. Karl Gussenbauer first described the treatment of a pancreatic cyst through marsupialization. Various pancreatic procedures have been described since, perhaps most famously the distal pancreatectomy by Trendelenburg and the pancreaticoduodenectomy (or Whipple procedure) by Whipple.

Initially, surgical involvement in pancreatitis trended toward management of late sequela: pancreatic necrosis, pseudocysts, or pancreatic cancer. As preoperative imaging and perioperative management have both improved, resulting in improved outcomes and survivability, surgeons have found themselves involved much earlier in the management of pancreatitis despite only operating in a small subset of patients. Today, pancreatitis requires a multidisciplinary approach to achieve optimal outcomes while minimizing potential complications.

2. When do you recommend consultation with a surgeon and in what time frame?

Consultation with specialty services should always be undertaken with specific goals for patient care in mind. Management of acute pancreatitis (AP) has become multidisciplinary, with contributions from interventional radiology, interventional gastroenterology, and surgery. Surgical consultation is useful in three specific scenarios: (1) when a surgical etiology of pancreatitis is identified, (2) when surgical complications of pancreatitis are identified, and (3) when a team approach is necessary to manage the long-term sequelae of pancreatitis. Once the specific goal is identified, early consultation is important.

In the first scenario, AP may be the result of a disease with a surgical cure, most commonly cholelithiasis. Other etiologies include traumatic injury, choledocholithiasis, choledochocysts, cholangiocarcinoma, and pancreatic cancer. *Gallstone pancreatitis should prompt an evaluation for cholecystectomy during the index presentation.*

In the second scenario, the patient may present with sequelae of pancreatitis, including peri-pancreatic fluid collections or necrosis, splenic or portal vein thrombosis, gastric outlet dysfunction, and colonic necrosis. While several of these can be managed with deliberate escalation from percutaneous to open surgical intervention, others need immediate aggressive surgical intervention.

Finally, the last scenario addresses those patients for whom the acute pancreatitis episode evolves into chronic pancreatitis. Recognition of the chronicity of the issue during an emergency department (ED) visit and the benefit to these patients of a multidisciplinary team approach should prompt referral to surgery in a health-care system where chronic pancreatitis is managed by surgeons.

3. What diagnostic testing is recommended when evaluating pancreatitis from a surgeon's perspective?

Many of the disease processes that mimic AP (perforated peptic ulcer, mesenteric ischemia, intestinal obstruction, or ruptured aortic aneurysm) also require surgical intervention, so it is helpful to obtain targeted data early to guide consultant interventions. *Computed tomography (CT) of the abdomen and pelvis may be the first imaging study obtained, but if the diagnosis of pancreatitis is confirmed, ultrasound imaging of the gallbladder and hepatobiliary tree will help identify the most common etiologies (e.g., gallstone pancreatitis).* Early engagement of surgical consultation can help direct further management including the need for additional imaging, assistance with determination of disease severity (including the risk and benefit of early surgical interventions), and enable necessary interventions in an appropriate step-up fashion.

4. What pearls of resuscitation can you offer emergency care providers when evaluating a patient with pancreatitis?

While 80% of AP is self-limited, recognizing and managing the 20% of patients who progress to moderately or severe AP can be challenging. The 2012 revised Atlanta criteria for the classification of AP have streamlined the language used by practitioners to categorize pancreatitis; while the final diagnosis takes 48 h to confirm, the initial dichotomy of "organ failure on presentation, yes/no" does allow for appropriate triage of these patients. Once patients are identified as having organ failure on admission, close attention to the trajectory of organ function, appropriate and timely escalation of care, and prompt intervention when appropriate are critical.

Fluid resuscitation should be accomplished with isotonic intravenous fluids targeting markers of adequate end-organ perfusion. Patients presenting with AP may already be "behind" several liters of fluid due to vomiting, reduced oral intake, and the SIRS response triggered by the inflammatory process. While specific goals have yet to be established, correction of systemic hypovolemia may be critical in prevention of additional pancreatic ischemia and subsequent necrosis. *With the most recent literature suggesting that both under- and over-resuscitation have negative implications for patients with AP, we recommend using clinical markers of shock (skin perfusion, mental status, and urine output) coupled with laboratory markers of hypoperfusion (acidosis, hemoconcentration, organ failure) to guide resuscitation.* Complicating the resuscitation of severe AP can be fluid overload-related respiratory failure and multifactorial cardiogenic shock; early transfer to an intensive care unit based on these concerns allows for close monitoring for adverse effects of resuscitation.

5. What concepts do you think are key to managing a patient with pancreatitis?

Early accurate triage of patients with pancreatitis is still a challenge, as scoring systems typically depend on longitudinal data that is difficult to collect in an ED setting. However, as the mortality increases from 1% to around 30% in patients who develop severe acute pancreatitis, a relatively inclusive approach to admission is currently the safest approach for patients who present without a clear-cut case of self-limited mild acute pancreatitis.

Pancreatitis leaves patients severely catabolic; traditional protocols recommended NPO status to "rest" the hepatobiliary system, but current literature suggests receipt of regular diet on admission or within 48 h of admission is associated with improved outcomes. Early enteral feeding may contribute to decreasing the incidence of infected pancreatic necrosis, as it promotes normal bowel health and minimizes bacterial overgrowth. Antibiotic use in this population has also traditionally included all patient with evidence of necrotizing pancreatitis. However, we believe this represents overuse with an unnecessary associated expense. Widespread and prolonged antibiotic use in pancreatitis may expose already-ill patients to the side effect profile introduced by antibiotic use as well as the chances of multidrug-resistant bacteremia. Current guidelines do not support the use of prophylactic antibiotics in mild or severe acute pancreatitis except in the setting of infected pancreatic necrosis. Cultures of infected collections should be obtained if possible for selection of organism-specific coverage.

Finally, while upward of 80% of acute pancreatitis will resolve without any long-term complications, for the 20% who progress toward pancreatic necrosis, the multidisciplinary approach to the management of these patients cannot be stressed enough. The step-up approach advocated by centers that routinely manage necrotizing pancreatitis suggests a patient-specific escalation of care. While mortality currently remains around 15% for this complication, morbidity can be significantly reduced.

6. What complications are you concerned about in this patient population?

Complications of AP can be grouped into both anatomic and chronicity-related subgroups. Anatomic problems can be roughly separated into three components: pancreatic complications, vascular complications, and gastrointestinal complications. Pancreatic complications include pancreatic pseudocyst formation and necrotizing pancreatitis and can result from even a single episode of AP. A "step-up" or stepwise approach using minimally invasive techniques before progressing to endoscopic, and finally surgical, management, based on patient-specific tolerance has increasingly been advocated.

Both arterial and venous complications can be seen with pancreatitis; ruptured pseudoaneurysms are the most common arterial complications, while portal and splenic vein thromboses are the most common venous complications. Early identification of arterial hemorrhage is critical, as mortality can be as high as 50%; most of these bleeds can be managed definitively by interventional radiology. Venous complications are thought to occur both from inflammation resulting in a local pro-thrombotic state and from compression by pancreatic pseudocysts. Management of venous complications is more often than not conservative, as the use of anticoagulation may precipitate bleeding into peripancreatic fluid collections and has not been shown to significantly improve venous recanalization. Splenic vein thrombosis has been associated with gastric hemorrhage after the development of gastric varices; typically these are managed endoscopically, though vascular recanalization for venous occlusion is increasingly considered in these cases.

While ileus is a frequently recognized component of pancreatitis, more concerning is the development of colonic complications. Severe AP can result in colonic ischemia, causing necrosis in the early period and stricture in a more delayed fashion, often not during the index period of pancreatitis. Colonic necrosis is typically localized to the transverse colon, anatomically the segment of colon abutting the pancreas; this clearly is an acute surgical emergency with a mortality over 50% in the literature. Clinical suspicion should be high for this complication in patients with severe acute pancreatitis; persistent sepsis and evidence of rectal bleeding should prompt timely interventions.

7. Pearls in the management of chronic pancreatitis?

While many of the anatomic problems can occur in either acute or chronic pancreatitis, chronic pancreatitis comes with added complications related to the function of pancreatic tissue. Pancreatic exocrine and endocrine function can worsen as disease progresses and can lead to "burnout" of the pancreas, resulting in both endocrinopathies such as diabetes mellitus and exocrine insufficiency manifested as fat malabsorption (abdominal bloating, cramping, weight loss, and steatorrhea).

These insufficiency syndromes will require replacement of endogenous hormones such as insulin and pancreatic enzyme replacement therapy. Repeated bouts of inflammation can also increase the risk of fibrotic stricture involving the pancreatic portion of the common bile duct. Self-expanding metal stents or plastic stents placed endoscopically have been shown to be efficacious; those with significant obstruction or not amenable to endoscopic management may need referral to a hepatobiliary specialist for consideration of a hepaticojejunostomy or pancreaticoduodenectomy. Finally, the risk of pancreatic ductal adenocarcinoma is also increased in patients with chronic pancreatitis and is exacerbated by the use of cigarette smoking, alcohol use, and diabetes mellitus.

Suggested Resources

- American College of Gastroenterology Recommendations: https://gi.org/guideline/acute-pancreatitis/
- Babu RY, Gupta R, Kang M, Bhasin DK, Rana SS, Singh R. Predictors of surgery in patients with severe acute pancreatitis managed by the step-up approach. Ann Surg. 2013;257(4):737–50.
- Greenberg JA, et al. Clinical practice guideline: management of acute pancreatitis. Can J Surg. 2016;59(2):128–40.
- Martin RF. Operative management of acute pancreatitis. Surg Clin North Am. 2013;93(3):595–610.
- Sandra van Brunschot, Janneke van Grinsven, Hjalmar C van Santvoort, Olaf J Bakker, Marc G Besselink, Marja A Boermeester, Thomas L Bollen, Koop Bosscha, Stefan A Bouwense, Marco J Bruno, Vincent C Cappendijk, Esther C Consten, Cornelis H Dejong, Casper H van Eijck, Willemien G Erkelens, Harry van Goor, Wilhelmina M U van Grevenstein, Jan-Willem Haveman, Sijbrand H Hofker, Jeroen M Jansen, Johan S Laméris, Krijn P van Lienden, Maarten A Meijssen, Chris J Mulder, Vincent B Nieuwenhuijs, Jan-Werner Poley, Rutger Quispel, Rogier J de Ridder, Tessa E Römkens, Joris J Scheepers, Nicolien J Schepers, Matthijs P Schwartz, Tom Seerden, B W Marcel Spanier, Jan Willem A Straathof, Marin Strijker, Robin Timmer, Niels G Venneman, Frank P Vleggaar, Rogier P Voermans, Ben J Witteman, Hein G Gooszen, Marcel G Dijkgraaf, Paul Fockens, Eric R Manusama, Mohammed Hadithi, Camiel Rosman, Alexander F Schaapherder, Erik J Schoon, (2018) Endoscopic or surgical step-up approach for infected necrotising pancreatitis: a multicentre randomised trial. The Lancet 391 (10115):51–58.
- Rahul Maheshwari, Ram M. Subramanian, (2016) Severe Acute Pancreatitis and Necrotizing Pancreatitis. Critical Care Clinics 32 (2):279–290.

Part VII

Bowel Obstruction

Small Bowel Obstruction: When Is X-Ray Enough?

47

Lauren M. Westafer

Pearls and Pitfalls
- Abdominal x-rays have poor sensitivity for small bowel obstruction (SBO). They are poor screening tests for SBO.
- Abdominal x-rays cannot reliably differentiate between ileus and SBO.
- Computed tomography and/or ultrasound are better tests when SBO is suspected.

Table 47.1 Performance of diagnostic modalities to diagnose Small Bowel Obstruction [8, 9]

Imaging modality	Sensitivity	Specificity
X-ray	75% (95% CI 68–80%)	66% (95%CI 55–76%)
Point-of-care ultrasound	93–97% (95% CI 89–99)	90–96% (84–99)
CT scan[a]	93–96% (80–100)	93–100% (69–100)

[a]Includes studies using current generation 64 slice CT scanners

Abdominal radiographs are often ordered in the initial workup of suspected small bowel obstruction (SBO), but their clinical utility is limited due to poor sensitivity and specificity. The historical argument for obtaining radiographs to screen for SBO is predicated on their widespread availability, low ionizing radiation, and low cost. However, the American College of Radiology (ACR) recommends that other diagnostic modalities such as computed tomography (CT) are more appropriate for patients with suspected SBO [1].

Studies assessing the performance of x-ray for diagnosing SBO yield variable results. Early studies demonstrated sensitivities as high as 86% but did not list confidence intervals [2, 3]. A meta-analysis found abdominal radiographs had a pooled sensitivity of 75% (95% CI 68–80%) in all-comers [4]. The sensitivity of abdominal x-rays may be higher in high-grade obstruction. A study reporting an overall sensitivity of 69% for SBO found that low-grade SBO was detected on only 50% of plain films, while high-grade SBO was detected in 86% of plain films [3].

The specificity of abdominal x-ray for the diagnosis of SBO is also poor, reported at 66% (95% CI 55–76%) [4]. This lack of specificity may stem partially from an inability to differentiate between ileus and mechanical obstruction [5]. Radiographs identified only 13–19% of postoperative SBOs, even when clinical context was taken into consideration [4].

In addition to difficulties reliably diagnosing the presence of SBO, abdominal x-rays often fail to identify the level and etiology of obstruction. One study found that x-ray identified the etiology of obstruction in only 7% of cases and the level of obstruction in only 66–78% of cases [6, 7]. Because x-rays rarely find the cause of obstruction and only intermittently find the level of obstruction, positive x-rays are frequently followed by more advanced imaging.

Based on available data, abdominal x-rays have insufficient sensitivity to rule out SBO and often yield inconclusive results. X-ray does not perform well enough to be used as a screening test due to the frequency of both inconclusive and false-negative results. Other diagnostic modalities such as CT and ultrasound perform far better in diagnosing SBO. Table 47.1 shows the sensitivity and specificity of x-ray, point-of-care ultrasound, and CT for diagnosing SBO.

In some institutions, patients presenting with a clinical picture of recurrent SBO with known etiology may receive only x-ray and/or ultrasound if conservative management is planned.

L. M. Westafer
Department of Emergency Medicine, Baystate Medical Center/
UMMS, Springfield, MA, USA

A. Graham, D. J. Carlberg (eds.), *Gastrointestinal Emergencies*, https://doi.org/10.1007/978-3-319-98343-1_47

Suggested Resources
- EM Lyceum GI Imaging, "Answers" (May 2014: https://emlyceum.com/2014/05/07/gi-imaging-answers/)
- FOAMcast Episode 23 (January 2015: http://foamcast.org/tag/small-bowel-obstruction/)
- Gottlieb M, Peksa GD, Pandurangadu AV, Nakitende D, Takhar S, Seethala RR. Utilization of ultrasound for the evaluation of small bowel obstruction: a systematic review and meta-analysis. Am J Emerg Med. 2018;36(2):234–42.

References

1. Ros PR, Huprich JE. ACR appropriateness criteria on suspected small-bowel obstruction. J Am Coll Radiol. 2006;3(11):838–41.
2. Fukuya T, Hawes DR, Lu CC, Chang PJ, Barloon TJ. CT diagnosis of small-bowel obstruction: efficacy in 60 patients. AJR Am J Roentgenol. 1992;158(4):765–9; discussion 771–2.
3. Maglinte DD, Reyes BL, Harmon BH. Reliability and role of plain film radiography and CT in the diagnosis of small-bowel obstruction. AJR Am J Roentgenol. 1996;167(6):1451–5.
4. Taylor MR, Lalani N. Adult small bowel obstruction. Acad Emerg Med. 2013;20(6):528–44.
5. Frager DH, Baer JW, Rothpearl A, Bossart PA. Distinction between postoperative ileus and mechanical small-bowel obstruction: value of CT compared with clinical and other radiographic findings. AJR Am J Roentgenol. 1995;164(4):891–4.
6. Suri S, Gupta S, Sudhakar PJ, Venkataramu NK, Sood B, Wig JD. Comparative evaluation of plain films, ultrasound and CT in the diagnosis of intestinal obstruction. Acta Radiol. 1999;40(4):422–8.
7. Musoke F, Kawooya MG, Kiguli-Malwadde E. Comparison between sonographic and plain radiography in the diagnosis of small bowel obstruction at Mulago Hospital, Uganda. East Afr Med J. 2003;80(10):540–5.
8. Gottlieb M, Peksa GD, Pandurangadu AV, Nakitende D, Takhar S, Seethala RR. Utilization of ultrasound for the evaluation of small bowel obstruction: a systematic review and meta-analysis. Am J Emerg Med. 2018;36(2):234–42.
9. Jang TB, Schindler D, Kaji AH. Bedside ultrasonography for the detection of small bowel obstruction in the emergency department. Emerg Med J. 2011;28(8):676–8.

What Is the Utility of Ultrasound for Small Bowel Obstruction?

48

Lauren M. Westafer

Pearls and Pitfalls
- Point-of-care ultrasound has high sensitivity and specificity for small bowel obstruction (SBO).
- SBO features on ultrasound include loops of bowel greater than 2.5 cm in diameter and abnormal peristalsis.
- Further studies are needed to ascertain ultrasound's accuracy for finding a transition point and for differentiating ileus from small bowel obstruction.

While computed tomography (CT) is the most common diagnostic modality for the diagnosis of small bowel obstruction (SBO), recent literature has shown that emergency provider performed point-of-care ultrasound (POCUS) that is accurate to both rule in and rule out SBO [1, 2].

On ultrasound (US), SBO is diagnosed by using a curvilinear probe to assess the bilateral paracolic gutters, epigastric, and suprapubic regions or by using a "mowing the lawn" technique in which the entire abdomen is assessed in sequential horizontal tracks. Small bowel obstruction is diagnosed when (1) dilated loops of bowel, which appear hypoechoic, are at least 2.5 cm in diameter and (2) a bidirectional or "to-and-fro" peristalsis is seen (Fig. 48.1) [3]. Additional findings of SBO include the "piano key" or "keyboard" sign (Fig. 48.1) and the "tanga sign" (Fig. 48.2). The piano keys represent plicae circulares, and the "tanga sign" depicts free fluid between loops of bowel [4]. Table 48.1 shows the main criteria and adjunct findings for diagnosing SBO with POCUS.

Emergency department studies assessing POCUS for SBO demonstrate a sensitivity of 93–97% (95% CI 89–99)

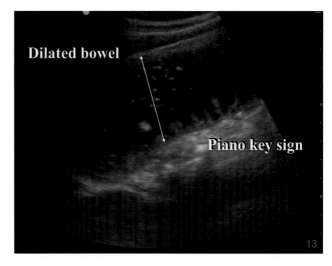

Fig. 48.1 Features of SBO on US include dilated bowel loops (>2.5 cm diameter, shown above), bidirectional peristalsis, the piano key sign (shown above), and the tanga sign

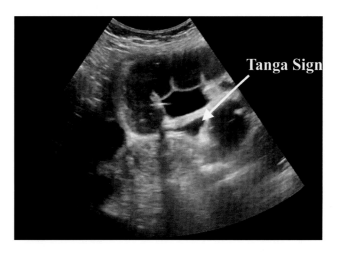

Fig. 48.2 The tanga sign on ultrasound depicts free fluid between loops of bowel and can suggest small bowel obstruction (Image courtesy of Jacob Avila, MD)

L. M. Westafer
Department of Emergency Medicine, Baystate Medical Center/ UMMS, Springfield, MA, USA

© Springer Nature Switzerland AG 2019
A. Graham, D. J. Carlberg (eds.), *Gastrointestinal Emergencies*, https://doi.org/10.1007/978-3-319-98343-1_48

Table 48.1 Ultrasound diagnosis of small bowel obstruction

Ultrasound diagnosis of SBO		
Main criteria	Dilated bowel >2.5 cm in diameter	
	Abnormal bidirectional peristalsis "to and fro"	
Adjunct findings	Piano key or keyboard sign	Fingerlike projections of the plicae circulares
	Tanga sign	Collection of intra-abdominal fluid between loops of bowel

Table 48.2 Sensitivity and specificity of diagnostic modalities for small bowel obstruction [2, 3]

Imaging modality	Sensitivity	Specificity
X-ray	75% (95% CI 68–80%)	66% (95%CI 55–76%)
Point-of-care ultrasound	93–97% (95% CI 89–99)	90–96% (84–99)
Radiology performed Ultrasound	92% (95% CI 85–96)	99% (95% CI 60–100)
CT scan[a]	93–96% (80–100)	93–100% (69–100)

[a]Includes studies using current generation 64 slice CT scanners

and a specificity of 90–96% (95% CI 84–99) [1, 2]. Further, two meta-analyses report likelihood ratios for POCUS that are far better than x-ray and that approximate CT. The positive likelihood ratio of POCUS is between 9.5 and 21.1, and the negative likelihood ratio is between 0.04 and 0.08 [1, 2]. One study found that POCUS produced fewer equivocal results than x-ray [3]. Table 48.2 compares the sensitivity and specificity of abdominal x-ray, US, and CT for SBO.

The primary limitation of US for SBO diagnosis is difficulty identifying the level and etiology of the obstruction. Studies assessing the ability of US for this purpose have focused on trained radiology technicians rather than POCUS [5–8]. In these studies, US underperforms CT, with approximately 70–80.5% of USs identifying the level of obstruction and only 23–62% identifying the cause of obstruction. Lastly, no studies assess the acute care provider's ability to differentiate between ileus and SBO using US.

POCUS for SBO requires training beyond the American College of Emergency Physicians' core applications of US. However, this training can be completed in a 10-min session with 5–10 USs performed [3].

Compared with other diagnostic modalities such as x-ray and CT, POCUS requires provider presence at the bedside, although the US can be performed concurrent with the history in certain circumstances.

Based on available studies, US is an adequate means of diagnosing SBO and performs better as a screening test than abdominal x-ray. Additional imaging may be necessary to localize a transition point and identify the cause of the obstruction; however, the ability to rapidly rule out SBO is advantageous when this diagnosis is high in the differential. POCUS may be integrated into the workflow by using this test for bedside screening during the history and physical assessment with follow-up imaging ordered as needed. In such cases where the etiology is already known, such as recurrent SBO, further imaging beyond POCUS may be unnecessary.

Suggested Resources
- FOAMcast. Episode 23: SBO and Mesenteric Ischemia. January 2015: http://foamcast. org/2015/01/26/episode-23-sbo-and-mesenteric-ischemia/
- Taylor MR, Lalani N. Adult small bowel obstruction. Acad Emerg Med. 2013;20(6):528–44.

References

1. Taylor MR, Lalani N. Adult small bowel obstruction. Acad Emerg Med. 2013;20(6):528–44.
2. Gottlieb M, Peksa GD, Pandurangadu AV. Utilization of ultrasound for the evaluation of small bowel obstruction: a systematic review and meta-analysis. Am J Emerg Med. Forthcoming 2017.
3. Jang TB, Schindler D, Kaji AH. Bedside ultrasonography for the detection of small bowel obstruction in the emergency department. Emerg Med J. 2011;28(8):676–8.
4. Mizio R. Small bowel obstruction CT features with plain film and US correlations. Milan: Springer; 2007. Print.
5. Suri S, Gupta S, Sudhakar PJ, Venkataramu NK, Sood B, Wig JD. Comparative evaluation of plain films, ultrasound and CT in the diagnosis of intestinal obstruction. Acta Radiol. 1999; 40(4):422–8.
6. Musoke F, Kawooya MG, Kiguli-Malwadde E. Comparison between sonographic and plain radiography in the diagnosis of small bowel obstruction at Mulago Hospital, Uganda. East Afr Med J. 2003;80(10):540–5.
7. Frager DH, Baer JW, Rothpearl A, Bossart PA. Distinction between postoperative ileus and mechanical small-bowel obstruction: value of CT compared with clinical and other radiographic findings. AJR Am J Roentgenol. 1995;164(4):891–4.
8. Schmutz GR, Benko A, Fournier L, Peron JM, Morel E, Chiche L. Small bowel obstruction: role and contribution of sonography. Eur Radiol. 1997;7(7):1054–8.

So I am Getting a CT for Small Bowel Obstruction, Do I Need Oral Contrast? IV Contrast?

49

Cameron Gettel and Catherine Cummings

Pearls and Pitfalls
- Recent guidelines suggest against using oral contrast in patients requiring computed tomography (CT) for suspected small bowel obstruction (SBO).
- Intravenous contrast does not increase the sensitivity of CT but does allow for assessment of bowel ischemia.
- Nearly 70% of emergency medicine providers continue to administer oral contrast when obtaining CT for suspected SBO.

I am Getting a CT for Small Bowel Obstruction, Do I Need Oral Contrast?

Prior studies and clinical practice guidelines have suggested the use of intravenous (IV) contrast, oral contrast (e.g., gastrografin, barium), or both for the diagnosis of small bowel obstruction (SBO) by abdominal computed tomography (CT).

Oral contrast typically requires an observation period following its administration to allow opacification of the small bowel and passage of contrast into the colon to exclude complete or high-grade obstruction [1]. In addition to this required delay, contrast ingestion itself may take a significant amount of time, especially in patients with SBO. A recent study showed a median time of greater than 100 min for oral contrast ingestion, even with prophylactic antiemetics. Oral contrast resulted in delayed diagnosis and increased emergency department length of stay [2]. A frequent argument against oral contrast is that the diagnosis of SBO with CT can be made by the presence of secreted fluids and ingested air, which are already present in the bowel lumen and provide sufficient contrast to detect bowel dilation [3].

The American College of Radiology (ACR) Appropriateness Criteria guidelines suggest against administering oral contrast in patients suspected of small bowel obstruction because it "will not reach the site of obstruction, wastes time, adds expense, can induce further patient discomfort, will not add to diagnostic accuracy, and can lead to complications, particularly vomiting and aspiration" [4].

Despite the ACR's recommendation, a recent study showed that 69% of emergency medicine providers continue to administer oral contrast when obtaining CT for SBO [5].

IV Contrast?

Recent literature has shown that the average sensitivity of an entirely non-contrast CT for SBO is 88.1% [6]. Adding IV contrast does not significantly alter CT's sensitivity for SBO, but it does improve assessment for bowel ischemia, an important sequela of SBO that generally requires urgent operative intervention.

After IV contrast administration, small bowel with an intact blood supply appears with a thin and complete bright wall on CT. The absence of enhancement is highly specific for bowel wall ischemia. Sometimes administration of oral contrast can make differentiating between healthy and ischemic bowel difficult because it hinders the ability to determine whether there is appropriate bowel wall enhancement after IV contrast [7]. For this reason, many argue that oral contrast should be avoided if suspecting an SBO [7]. The IV contrast-enhanced CT shown in Fig. 49.1 depicts an SBO.

In conclusion, evidence-based literature suggests that CT for suspected SBO should be performed with IV contrast whenever possible. Oral contrast does not provide benefit and may cause harm.

C. Gettel (✉) · C. Cummings
Department of Emergency Medicine, Alpert Medical School of Brown University, Providence, RI, USA
e-mail: cameron_gettel@brown.edu

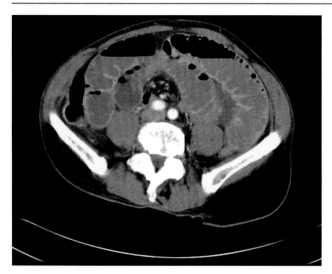

Fig. 49.1 CT with IV contrast and without oral contrast showing a SBO with pneumatosis intestinalis and some bowel wall thickening. IV contrast improves evaluation of the bowel wall. Oral contrast may hinder evaluation of the bowel wall. (Photo courtesy of Robert Tubbs, MD)

Suggested Resource
• Broder J. CT of small bowel obstruction. Emergency physicians monthly. October 2015: http://epmonthly. com/article/ct-of-small-bowel-obstruction/

References

1. Paulson EK, Thompson WM. Review of small-bowel obstruction: the diagnosis and when to worry. Radiology. 2015;275(2):332–42.
2. Garra G, Singer AJ, Bamber D, Chohan J, Troxell R, Thode HC Jr. Pretreatment of patients requiring oral contrast abdominal computed tomography with antiemetics: a randomized controlled trial of efficacy. Ann Emerg Med. 2009;53:528–33.
3. Furukawa A, Yamasaki M, Takahashi M, Nitta N, Tanaka T, Yokoyama K, Murata K, Sakamoto T. CT diagnosis of small bowel obstruction: scanning technique, interpretation and role in the diagnosis. Semin Ultrasound CT MR. 2003;24(5):336–52.
4. National Guideline Clearinghouse (NGC). Guideline summary: ACR Appropriateness Criteria® suspected small-bowel obstruction. In: National Guideline Clearinghouse (NGC). Rockville (MD): Agency for Healthcare Research and Quality (AHRQ); 2013. [cited 2017 Jul 17]. Available: https://www.guideline.gov
5. Broder JS, Hamedani AG, Liu SW, Emerman CL. Emergency department contrast practices for abdominal/pelvic computed tomography-a national survey and comparison with the American College of Radiology Appropriateness Criteria. J Emerg Med. 2013;44:423–33.
6. Atri M, McGregor C, McInnes M, Power N, Rahnavardi K, Law C, Kiss A. Multidetector helical CT in the evaluation of acute small bowel obstruction: comparison of non-enhanced (no oral, rectal or IV contrast) and IV enhanced CT. Eur J Radiol. 2009;71:135–40.
7. Sheedy SP, Earnest F, Fletcher JG, Fidler JL, Hoskin TL. CT of small-bowel ischemia associated with obstruction in emergency department patients: diagnostic performance evaluation. Radiology. 2006;241:729–36.

Does Everyone with a Small Bowel Obstruction Need a Nasogastric Tube? What Is the Safest Way to Place It?

Ashley Gray and Jessica L. Smith

Pearls and Pitfalls
- Nontoxic patients with small bowel obstruction (SBO) should undergo a trial of conservative management before operative intervention.
- Patients with SBO and significant symptoms should undergo intestinal decompression with nasogastric (NG) intubation.
- SBO patients who remain asymptomatic may benefit from a trial without NG intubation.
- The need for NG intubation in the non-vomiting patient remains a clinical judgment by practitioners involved in the patient's care.
- NG tubes should be removed at first evidence of return of bowel function.

Does Everyone with an SBO Need a Nasogastric Tube?

Small bowel obstruction is a common diagnosis in the acute care setting. While estimates vary, up to 15% of emergency department visits for abdominal pain are attributable to obstruction [1]. Patients with high-risk features such as peritonitis, metabolic acidosis, fever, and tachycardia should undergo emergent surgical intervention regardless of degree of obstruction in order to prevent strangulation, intestinal ischemia, and perforation [2]. For those with low-risk profiles, it is standard to initially trial nonoperative therapy [3]. While the duration of observation prior to surgical intervention is still debated, 24–48 h of conservative management is generally recommended. Beyond 3 days there is an increased morbidity in those requiring surgical intervention [4].

A. Gray (✉) · J. L. Smith
Department of Emergency Medicine, Alpert Medical School of Brown University, Providence, RI, USA

For patients undergoing conservative management, the first-line approach is intestinal decompression via nasogastric (NG) intubation, intravenous hydration, and electrolyte repletion.

The benefit of NG intubation has been well established for patients who are significantly symptomatic. Intestinal decompression may provide relief of nausea, vomiting, and sensation of bloating [5]. It can also reduce air swallowing [5]. Intermittent wall suction can evacuate gastric contents and lead to better optimization of fluid repletion [5].

However, in a recent study of patients without active emesis, NG decompression was associated with increased rates of pneumonia and respiratory failure [6]. Furthermore, NG tubes are not entirely benign. They have been shown to cause gastric bleeding and irritation due to suctioning, and they can impair the lower esophageal sphincter, leading to reflux and esophagitis [7]. In those with SBO but without vomiting, the decision for or against NG intubation should be made based on the clinical judgment of the providers caring for the patient.

What Is the Safest Way to Place It?

If an NG tube is inserted, a large bore double lumen 14 or 16 French Salem sump tube is generally preferred. Insertion depth should be approximated by measuring from the ear to the nose to the xiphoid [7]. The alert patient should be sitting up with head flexed slightly forward. The tube should be directed toward the back of the naris and then advanced. Patients should then be instructed to swallow and may benefit from drinking water to help guide placement. Prophylactic use of anesthetizing spray or mucosal lidocaine may help dampen the gag reflex. Antiemetics may also improve patient comfort [8]. Accidental tracheal placement of an NG tube is possible, even in endotracheally intubated patients [9].

© Springer Nature Switzerland AG 2019
A. Graham, D. J. Carlberg (eds.), *Gastrointestinal Emergencies*, https://doi.org/10.1007/978-3-319-98343-1_50

Confirmation of NG tube placement is crucial, as complications with malpositioned tubes include pneumothorax and bronchial administration of medications [7, 10]. Auscultation of instilled air alone is unreliable for placement verification. Absence of end tube capnography helps confirm tube location, as does suctioning acidic contents (pH < 5) [8, 10]. X-ray may be used to confirm appropriate location and depth.

Once the NG tube is placed, securing it with tape is effective and offers the fewest complications. Suturing the tube in place or using a bridle is not recommended [7]. Attaching the tube too tightly may lead erosion and alar necrosis.

Once the NG tube is placed, serial abdominal exams should be performed, as should aspiration of gastric contents at least every 4 h. NG tubes should be removed as soon as patients demonstrate return of bowel function [7].

Suggested Resources
- Fonseca AL, Schuster KM, Maung AA, Kaplan LJ, Davis KA. Routine nasogastric decompression in small bowel obstruction: is it really necessary? Am Surg. 2013;79(4):422–8.
- Nickson C. Nasogastric and orogastric tubes. Life in the fast lane medical blog [internet]. 2017 [cited 31 August 2017]. Available from: https://lifeinthefastlane.com/ccc/nasogastric-tube-insertion/

References

1. Jackson P, Raiji M. Evaluation and management of intestinal obstruction. Am Fam Physician. 2011;83(2):159–65.
2. Maung A, Johnson D, Piper G, Barbosa R, Rowell S, Bokhari F, et al. Evaluation and management of small-bowel obstruction. J Trauma Acute Care Surg. 2012;73:S362–9.
3. Diaz JJ Jr, Bokhari F, Mowery NT, Acosta JA, Block EF, Bromberg WJ, Collier BR, Cullinane DC, Dwyer KM, Griffen MM, Mayberry JC, Jerome R. Guidelines for management of small bowel obstruction. J Trauma. 2008;64(6):1651–64.
4. Keenan J, Turley R, McCoy C, Migaly J, Shapiro M, Scarborough J. Trials of nonoperative management exceeding 3 days are associated with increased morbidity in patients undergoing surgery for uncomplicated adhesive small bowel obstruction. J Trauma Acute Care Surg. 2014;76(6):1367–72.
5. Overview of management of mechanical small bowel obstruction in adults [internet]. 2017 [cited 31 August 2017]. Available from: https://www.uptodate.com/contents/overview-of-management-of-mechanical-small-bowel-obstruction-in-adults?source=search_result&search=sbo&selectedTitle=1~150
6. Fonseca A, Schuster K, Maung A, Kaplan L, Davis K. Routine nasogastric decompression in small bowel obstruction: is it really necessary? Am Surg. 2013;79:422–8.
7. Nasogastric and nasoenteric tubes [internet]. 2017 [cited 31 August 2017]. Available from: https://www.uptodate.com/contents/nasogastric-and-nasoenteric-tubes?source=search_result&search=ngt&selectedTitle=1~150
8. Nickson C. Nasogastric and orogastric tubes [internet]. 2017 [cited 31 August 2017]. Available from: https://lifeinthefastlane.com/ccc/nasogastric-tube-insertion/
9. Wang P, Tseng G, Yang H, Chou K, Chen C. Inadvertent tracheobronchial placement of feeding tube in a mechanically ventilated patient. J Chin Med Assoc. 2008;71(7):365–7.
10. Pillai J, Vegas A, Brister S. Thoracic complications of nasogastric tube: review of safe practice. Interact Cardiovasc Thorac Surg. 2005;4(5):429–33.

Atypical Obstructions: What Do Emergency Providers Need to Know About Incarcerated and Strangulated Hernia, Closed Loop Obstruction, Volvulus, and Internal Hernia? What Is the Prognostic Value of a Lactate?

Jessie Werner and Jane Preotle

Pearls and Pitfalls

- In incarcerated hernia, time from symptom onset to surgery is important in patient outcomes, particularly in patients with symptoms >8 h, comorbid conditions, high ASA scores, presence of strangulation, and advanced age.
- Computed tomography is the preferred imaging modality for diagnosing and characterizing bowel obstructions.
- Closed loop obstructions have higher rates of ischemia and perforation than uncomplicated small bowel obstructions.
- Sigmoid volvulus and cecal volvulus are the two most common types of volvulus. Sigmoid volvulus occurs more often in the elderly, and cecal volvulus occurs more often in younger patients (20–60 years old).
- Abdominal surgeries, especially liver transplants and Roux-en-Y gastric bypasses, predispose to internal hernias in adults. Internal hernias can also occur in patients without any prior abdominal surgery.
- Elevated lactate can suggest intestinal ischemia, but it is neither sensitive nor specific.

J. Werner (✉) · J. Preotle
Department of Emergency Medicine, Alpert Medical School of Brown University, Providence, RI, USA
e-mail: jpreotle@lifespan.org

What Do Emergency Providers Need to Know About Incarcerated and Strangulated Hernia, Closed Loop Obstruction, Volvulus, and Internal Hernia?

Incarcerated and Strangulated Hernia

An abdominal wall hernia arises from a weakness in the anterior abdominal wall that allows bulging of intraabdominal tissue. These hernias are classified as groin (e.g., inguinal and femoral) and ventral (e.g., epigastric, umbilical, Spigelian (lateral to rectus muscle), lumbar, incisional, and parastomal) [1]. The estimated lifetime risk of an abdominal wall hernia is 5% [2]. Of the estimated 2.3 million abdominal hernia repairs performed between 2001 and 2010, 576,000 were performed emergently, with the highest rate of emergent surgery in patients greater than 65 years old [3].

An incarcerated hernia develops when hernia's contents are irreducible. Incarcerated hernias classically present with an abdominal bulge associated with varying degrees of abdominal pain. These incarcerated hernias may become strangulated, meaning that the blood supply to the incarcerated omentum and/or bowel becomes compromised. Strangulated hernias generally present with intractable pain and tenderness.

In many cases, ultrasound will be able to detect abdominal wall hernias in adults. Added benefits with ultrasound include the lack of ionizing radiation and the capability to utilize Valsalva maneuvers to dynamically assess for hernias [2]. CT identifies hernias and may also reveal sequelae including bowel obstruction and advanced bowel ischemia.

Time from symptom onset to surgery is important in patient outcomes, particularly in patients with symptoms >8 h, comorbid conditions, high ASA scores, presence of strangulation or necrosis, and advanced age [1, 4].

Signs of SIRS with an incarcerated hernia should raise the suspicion for strangulation with bowel compromise, but these are neither sensitive nor specific enough to be used in isolation to differentiate an incarcerated hernia from a strangulated one [1, 5, 6]. Other laboratory markers that have been shown to be helpful in determining whether an incarcerated hernia is strangulated include creatine phosphokinase, white blood cell count, and D-dimer [1, 7–9]. Lactate <2 mm/L has been associated with intestinal viability [10]. The final section of this chapter discusses the utility of lactate in greater detail.

It is often safe to discharge patients with surgical referral, generally after reduction of an incarcerated hernia. However, one retrospective study of 111 patients found that 28 patients (25%) returned to the emergency department with a hernia-related complaint. Some patients returned multiple times. Nine of these patients (32%) required emergency surgery. While 76 patients (68%) were lost to follow-up, limiting the generalizability of this study, it highlights the fact that patients with symptomatic hernias often return for unscheduled care, with some requiring emergent surgery. Thus, a discussion with surgical colleagues to secure close follow-up, consultation, or admission, especially for high-risk patients and those with continued pain, may be beneficial [11].

Closed Loop Obstruction

A small bowel obstruction (SBO) is classified as "closed loop" when a section of bowel is obstructed at two adjacent points. If the resulting incarcerated bowel loop rotates on its axis, it becomes a volvulus [12]. Closed loop obstructions, unlike uncomplicated SBOs, are often complete – there is no passage of contents beyond the point of obstruction. This results in a significantly higher rate of complications, morbidity, and mortality. Closed loop obstruction can be challenging to diagnose on both exam and imaging. Because of its higher rate of ischemia and perforation compared to uncomplicated SBO, closed loop obstruction is a surgical emergency [13]. On computed tomography (CT) closed loop obstructions often present as distended, fluid-filled loops of bowel that may appear in a C or U shape with a "whirl sign," which occurs when the bowel rotates around its mesentery, resembling a whirlpool [14]. Figure 51.1 shows two examples of a whirl sign on CT.

Volvulus

Volvulus accounts for about 5% of adult obstructions in the United States and is most often located in the sigmoid colon or cecum. Patients typically present with colicky abdominal pain and a distended abdomen [15].

Sigmoid volvulus typically occurs in elderly and nursing home patients and is classically associated with the "kidney-bean sign" or "coffee-bean sign," which appears as a distended loop arising from the pelvis and encompassing the entire abdomen (Fig. 51.2) [16]. Sigmoid volvulus may be treated with decompression via colonoscopy or rectal tube beyond the point of volvulus, but this often results in recurrence, so sigmoid resection and primary anastomosis are often the preferred treatment [15].

Cecal volvulus typically occurs in younger patients (20–60 years), and X-ray findings are generally most apparent in the left upper quadrant (Fig. 51.3). Cecal volvulus typically

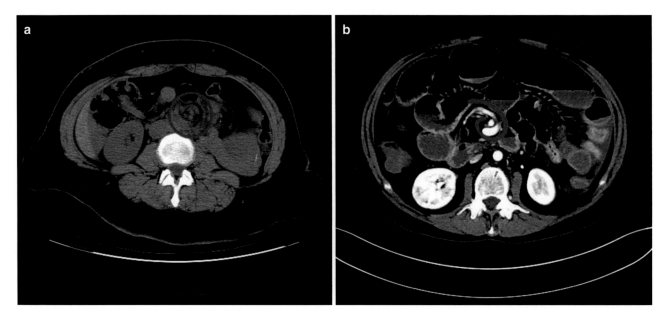

Fig. 51.1 Panel (**a**): Whirl sign on non-contrast-enhanced CT. Panel (**b**): Whirl sign on CT with IV contrast. Note the IV contrast curling with the twisted mesentery. (Image courtesy of Robert Tubbs, MD)

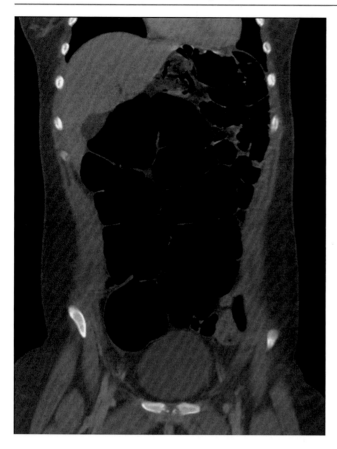

Fig. 51.2 The "coffee-bean" or "kidney-bean" sign is often seen on imaging in sigmoid volvulus. It can be seen on X-ray or reconstructed CT (above). (Image courtesy of Robert Tubbs, MD)

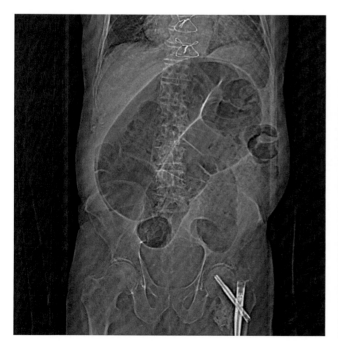

Fig. 51.3 Cecal volvulus, arising from the right lower quadrant and extending into the left upper quadrant. (Image courtesy of Robert Tubbs, MD)

requires partial colon resection or surgical reduction with anchoring of the cecum to the abdominal wall [15, 17].

Internal Hernia

An internal hernia occurs when a section of intestine or another abdominal organ protrudes through an opening in the peritoneum or mesentery [18]. Internal hernias are a rare cause of intestinal obstruction in adults (0.5–5.8%), but if strangulated and untreated, they have a mortality exceeding 50% [19].

Internal hernias may result from congenital anomalies, iatrogenic (postsurgical) changes, trauma, or infection. In adults, the majority of internal hernias are acquired and result from previous abdominal surgeries, including Whipple procedures, liver transplants, and gastric bypasses. The highest-risk surgeries are laparoscopic bowel altering procedures that cause mesenteric defects, which are generally not closed intraoperatively. An internal hernia develops when a loop of bowel passes into the residual mesenteric defect, placing it at high risk of both obstruction and strangulation. Obstructed internal hernia after Roux-en-Y gastric bypass is increasingly encountered as the laparoscopic approach has become more common [20]. Congenital internal abdominal hernias also occur.

Internal hernias may be challenging to diagnose because of their nonspecific symptoms. Patients may have intermittent obstruction without radiographic abnormalities. CT is the most useful imaging study for identifying internal hernia with obstruction (Fig. 51.4), but CT may not distinguish

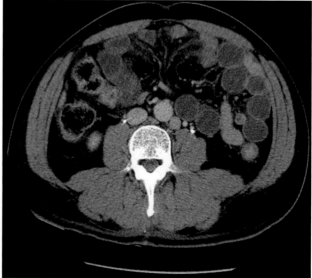

Fig. 51.4 Internal hernia with closed loop obstruction. Note the central mesentery erupting from the internal hernia with obstructed bowel loops on the right and left. (Image courtesy of Robert Tubbs, MD)

between a simple obstruction caused by adhesions and an internal hernia with closed loop obstruction and impending strangulation. Early emergent surgical consultation is recommended for the SBO patient with severe symptoms and a previous high-risk surgery, as this may indicate an obstructed internal hernia not apparent on CT. Diagnostic delays may result in ischemia, necrosis, and the need for bowel resection; therefore, early surgical intervention is critical [19, 21]. It is important for the acute care provider to keep internal hernia in the differential when evaluating patients with abdominal pain, nausea, and/or vomiting, even when patients have no prior history of surgery or trauma.

Lactic Acid in Bowel Obstruction: What Is the Prognostic Value of a Lactate?

Elevated lactate is a sign of tissue hypoxia and has been used as a marker for mesenteric ischemia. In closed loop obstruction, internal hernia, and volvulus, the supply of oxygen to tissue may be limited secondary to strangulation, which may result in elevated lactate [22]. However, lactate is nonspecific and may not rise until advanced injury has already occurred. This makes lactate less useful for diagnosis in the acute setting. Furthermore, although L-lactate is the routinely measured stereoisomer of lactate, recent studies suggest that D-lactate may actually be more specific. Despite the better specificity of D-lactate, there is no single serum marker that is sensitive or specific enough to diagnose early intestinal injury from bowel obstruction. Various studies are ongoing to identify improved serum markers for intestinal ischemia [23].

Suggested Resources
- Mancuso N, Sweeney M. The sick bowel obstruction patient. EM Docs. 2017. http://www.emdocs.net/sick-bowel-obstruction-patient/
- Weingrow D, McCague A, Shah R, Lalezarzadeh F. Delayed presentation of a sigmoid volvulus in a young woman. West J Emerg Med. 2012;13:100–2.

References

1. Birindelli A, Sartelli M, Di Saverio S, et al. 2017 update of the WSES guidelines for emergency repair of complicated abdominal wall hernias. World J Emerg Surg. 2017;12:37.
2. Murphy K, O'Connor O, Maher M. Adult abdominal hernias. AJR Am J Roentgenol. 2014;202(6):w506–22.
3. Beadles C, Meagher A, Charles A. Trends in emergent hernia repair in the United States. JAMA Surg. 2015;150(3):194–200.
4. Derici H, Unalp HR, Bozdag AD, Nazli O, Tansug T, Kamer E. Factors affecting morbidity and mortality in incarcerated abdominal wall hernias. Hernia. 2007;11(4):341–6. https://doi.org/10.1007/s10029-007-0226-3.
5. Tsumura H, Ichikawa T, Hiyama E, Murakami Y, Sueda T. Systemic inflammatory response syndrome (SIRS) as a predictor of strangulated small bowel obstruction. Hepato-Gastroenterology. 2004;51(59):1393–6.
6. Sarr MG, Bulkley GB, Zuidema GD. Preoperative recognition of intestinal strangulation obstruction. Prospective evaluation of diagnostic capability. Am J Surg. 1983;145(1):176–82. https://doi.org/10.1016/0002-9610(83)90186-1.
7. Icoz G, Makay O, Sozbilen M, et al. Is D-dimer a predictor of strangulated intestinal hernia? World J Surg. 2006;30(12):2165–9. https://doi.org/10.1007/s00268-006-0138-x.
8. Kahramanca S, Kaya O, Ozgehan G, et al. Are fibrinogen and complete blood count parameters predictive in incarcerated abdominal hernia repair? Int Surg. 2014;99(6):723–8.
9. Graeber G, O'Neil J, Wolf R, Wukich D, Caffery P, Harman J. Elevated levels of peritoneal serum creatine phosphokinase with strangulated small bowel obstruction. Arch Surg. 1983;118:837–40.
10. Tanaka K, Hanyu N, Iida T, et al. Lactate levels in the detection of preoperative bowel strangulation. Am Surg. 2012;78(1):86–8.
11. Spence L, Pillado E, Kim D, Plurad D. Follow-up trends after emergency department discharge for acutely symptomatic hernias. Am J Surg. 2017;214(6):1018–21. https://doi.org/10.1016/j.amjsurg.2017.08.028.
12. Chick JFB, Mandell JC, Mullen KM, Khurana B. Classic signs of closed loop bowel obstruction. Intern Emerg Med. 2013;8:263.
13. Kulaylat MN, Doerr RJ. Small bowel obstruction. Surgical treatment: evidence-based and problem-oriented. Zuckschwerdt: Munich; 2001.
14. Paulson E, Thompson W. Review of small-bowel obstruction: the diagnosis and when to worry. Radiology. 2015;275(2):332–42.
15. Gingold D, Murrell Z. Management of colonic volvulus. Clin Colon Rectal Surg. 2012;25(4):236–44.
16. Scharl M, Biedermann L. A symptomatic coffee bean: acute sigmoid volvulus. Case Rep Gastroenterol. 2017;11(2):348–51.
17. Gündeş E, Akgul N, Mazican M, Aday U, Cetin DA, Ciyiltepe H. Acute abdomen in a mentally retarded patient: cecal volvulus. Prz Gastroenterol. 2017;12(2):159–61.
18. Kar S, Mohapatra C, Rath PK. A rare type of primary internal hernia causing small intestinal obstruction. Case Rep Surg. 2016;2016:3540794.
19. Martin L, Merkle E, Thompson W. Review of internal hernias: radiographic and clinical findings. Am J Roentgenol. 2006;186(3):703–17.
20. Al-Mansour MR, Mundy R, Canoy JM, Dulaimy K, Kuhn JN, Romanelli J. Internal hernia after laparoscopic antecolic Roux-en-Y gastric bypass. Obes Surg. 2015;25(11):2106–11.
21. Mancuso N, Sweeney M. The sick bowel obstruction patient [Internet]. 2017 [cited 2017 Sept 24]. Available from: http://www.emdocs.net/sick-bowel-obstruction-patient/
22. Lange H, Jäckel R. Usefulness of plasma lactate concentration in the diagnosis of acute abdominal disease. Eur J Surg. 1994;160(6–7):381–4.
23. Demir IE, Ceyhan GO, Friess H. Beyond lactate: is there a role for serum lactate measurement in diagnosing acute mesenteric ischemia? Dig Surg. 2012;29(3):226–35.

Large Bowel Obstruction, Ogilvie Syndrome, and Stercoral Colitis: When Is Dilatation Pathologic? How Are These Conditions Managed?

Scott H. Pasichow and Angela F. Jarman

Pearls and Pitfalls
- 6 cm of dilation in the large intestine or 9 cm in the cecum is considered pathologic.
- Common mechanical causes of large bowel obstruction (LBO) include neoplasm, sigmoid volvulus, and diverticular complications such as stricture or abscess.
- LBO can be associated with electrolyte abnormalities including hypomagnesemia, hypokalemia, and hypercalcemia. It is also associated with hypothyroidism.
- Iatrogenic pharmacologic causes include opiates, anticholinergics, antihistamines, antipsychotics, and tricyclic antidepressants.
- Neostigmine is reserved for colonic pseudo-obstruction with either more than 12 cm of dilation or failure of conservative management.
- Failure of pharmacologic therapies for colonic pseudo-obstruction may require colonoscopy or surgery for decompression.

Large Bowel Obstruction, Ogilvie Syndrome, and Stercoral Colitis: When Is Dilatation Pathologic?

Large bowel obstruction (LBO) is a condition characterized by abdominal distention and failure to pass flatus due to a blockage in the large intestine. Abdominal pain, nausea, vomiting, and constipation are commonly described, though the absence of any of these symptoms does not rule out the diagnosis. In one case series, 41% of patients with large bowel obstruction had diarrhea [1]. More than half LBOs are related to cancer, but infection, hernia, strictures, and volvulus are other common causes [2]. When no structural abnormality can be found, LBO is termed Ogilvie syndrome or colonic pseudo-obstruction. This condition has multiple etiologies: electrolyte abnormalities, endocrine disorders, neurologic disorders, inflammatory bowel disease such as ulcerative colitis, medications that slow gut motility such as opioids, and anticholinergic medications [3, 4]. As these obstructions progress, increased pressure on the bowel wall may cause edema and inflammation. This condition is known as stercoral colitis, defined as 3 mm or more of bowel wall edema. Stercoral colitis rarely causes ischemia, and perforation occurs ~0.5% of the time [5]. The routine use of antibiotics is not indicated in these conditions; however, when complications develop, antibiotic use and surgical consultation for source control may be warranted.

Dilation of ≥ 6 cm in the large bowel or ≥ 9 cm in the cecum defines LBO [6]. When colonic dilation reaches ≥ 12 cm, risk of colonic perforation significantly increases. Computed tomography is the most useful imaging study, as it may identify the transition point, potential causes, and evidence of perforation. Intravenous contrast aides in identifying bowel wall involvement and/or inflammation [7].

How Are These Conditions Managed?

The treatment of LBO is determined by the etiology. Mechanical causes such as neoplasm or mass generally require surgical intervention. However, cases of pseudo- or functional obstruction often respond well to conservative management, consisting of bowel rest, nasogastric and/or rectal tube decompression, removal of potential causative agents, disimpaction, and tap water enemas [1]. As these conditions generally do not resolve quickly, patients are usually kept in the hospital in either observation or full admission status.

S. H. Pasichow (✉) · A. F. Jarman
Department of Emergency Medicine, Alpert School of Medicine of
Brown University, Providence, RI, USA
e-mail: Scott.Pasichow@lifespan.org; Angela.Jarman@
lifespan.org

© Springer Nature Switzerland AG 2019
A. Graham, D. J. Carlberg (eds.), *Gastrointestinal Emergencies*, https://doi.org/10.1007/978-3-319-98343-1_52

If conservative treatment of Ogilvie syndrome does not resolve the obstruction within 48 h or if there is severe dilation (greater than 12 cm), neostigmine is indicated. Neostigmine is an acetylcholinesterase inhibitor, which increases acetylcholine levels in the gut and thus stimulates gastrointestinal motility. Two milligrams are administered IV over 5 min, and the patient must be maintained on cardiac monitoring during and for 30 min after delivery [8]. Since neostigmine can cause bradycardia, atropine should be available; however, dosing glycopyrrolate with the neostigmine may reduce this side effect [9]. It is important to avoid neostigmine for structural obstructions, as it may cause perforation. When used appropriately, neostigmine is up to 90% effective. After successful treatment, adding propylene glycol helps prevent recurrence [10, 11]. Colonoscopy with placement of a decompression tube or surgery is sometimes needed if conservative management is not successful or if there is recurrence [12].

Perforation of the colon associated with LBO, Ogilvie syndrome, or stercoral colitis requires surgical management. Even with treatment, mortality rates have been reported as high as 53%, with long segments of dilated bowel (>40 cm) associated with higher mortality. Early diagnosis is paramount [7].

Suggested Resources

- Chong JCF. Megacolon. 2017 [cited 2017 Aug 31]. Available from: http://www.emnote.org/emnotes/megacolon
- Maloney N, Vargas HD. Acute intestinal pseudo-obstruction (Ogilvie's syndrome). Clin Colon Rectal Surg. 2005;18(2):96–101.
- Nickson C. Illeus [internet]. 2017 [cited 2017 Aug 31]. Available from https://lifeinthefastlane.com/ccc/ileus/
- Thurson M, Jones J. Large bowel obstruction [internet]. 2017 [cited 2017 Aug 31]. Available from: https://radiopaedia.org/articles/large-bowel-obstruction

References

1. Vanek VW, Al-Salti M. Acute pseudo-obstruction of the colon (Ogilvie's syndrome). An analysis of 400 cases. Dis Colon Rectum. 1986;29(3):203–10.
2. Ballantyne GH. Review of sigmoid volvulus. Clinical patterns and pathogenesis. Dis Colon Rectum. 1982;25(8):823–30.
3. Shera IA, Vyas A, Bhat MS, Yousuf Q. Unusual case of Hashimoto's encephalopathy and pseudo-obstruction in a patient with undiagnosed hypothyroidism: a case report. J Med Case Rep. 2014;8:296.
4. Weinstock LB, Chang AC. Methylnaltrexone for treatment of acute colonic pseudo-obstruction. J Clin Gastroenterol. 2011;45(10):883.
5. Ünal E, Onur MR, Balcı S, Görmez A, Akpinar E, Boge M. Stercoral colitis: diagnostic value of CT findings. Diagn Interv Radiol. 2017 Jan;23(1):5–9.
6. Jaffe T, Thompson WM. Large-bowel obstruction in the adult: classic radiographic and CT findings, etiology, and mimics. Radiology. 2015;275(3):651–63.
7. Khurana B, Ledbetter S, McTavish J, Wiesner W, Rose PR. Bowel obstruction revealed by multidetector CT. Am J Roentgenol. 2002;178:1139–44.
8. Saunders MD, Kimmey MB. Systematic review: acute colonic pseudo-obstruction. Aliment Pharmacol Ther. 2005;22(10):917.
9. Korsten MA, Rosman AS, Ng A, Cavusoglu E, Spungen AM, Radulovic M, Wecht J, Bauman WA. Infusion of neostigmine-glycopyrrolate for bowel evacuation in persons with spinal cord injury. Am J Gastroenterol. 2005;100(7):1560.
10. Ponec RJ, Saunders MD, Kimmey MB. Neostigmine for the treatment of acute colonic pseudo-obstruction. N Engl J Med. 1999;341(3):137.
11. Sgouros SN, Vlachogiannakos J, Vassiliadis K, Bergele C, Stefanidis G, Nastos H, Avgerinos A, Mantides A. Effect of polyethylene glycol electrolyte balanced solution on patients with acute colonic pseudo obstruction after resolution of colonic dilation: a prospective, randomised, placebo controlled trial. Gut. 2006;55(5):638.
12. Acute CM. Colonic pseudo-obstruction (Ogilvie's syndrome) [internet]. 2017 [updated 2017 July 5; cited 2017 Aug 31]. Available from: https://www.uptodate.com/contents/acute-colonic-pseudo-obstruction-ogilvies-syndrome

Who Gets Constipation? What Are the Causes? What Is an Evidence-Based Approach Management?

53

Jaclyn Caffrey and Gita Pensa

Pearls and Pitfalls
- Constipation is common among adults and can occur secondary to other more severe medical disorders.
- Work-up for constipation includes history and physical examination, including rectal examination.
- For constipation, first-line treatments include diet changes, bulk-forming laxatives, and non-bulk-forming laxatives.
- For severe constipation, treatment often includes suppositories, enemas, and manual disimpaction.
- Manual disimpaction is indicated for fecal impaction.
- Enemas should be avoided in patients who are non-compliant, have rectal tumors, are undergoing chemotherapy, are immunocompromised, or have active coronary artery disease.
- Complications of enemas include colonic perforation.

Who Gets Constipation?

Constipation has an estimated prevalence of 2–28% in the adult population [1–3]. That percentage increases in nursing home residents and the elderly. Some sources report constipation in up to 74% of long-term care facility residents [4]. Risk factors for constipation include female sex, older age, low income or socioeconomic status, prolonged immobility, low-fiber diet, and low-calorie intake [5]. Untreated severe constipation and fecal impaction can lead to urinary retention, stercoral ulcers, and colonic perforation. Management of constipation in the acute care setting may prevent significant morbidity and mortality [8].

J. Caffrey · G. Pensa (✉)
Department of Emergency Medicine, Alpert Medical School of Brown University, Providence, RI, USA
e-mail: Jaclyn.Caffrey@lifespan.org

What Are the Causes?

Primary constipation is divided into three classes: normal transit constipation, slow transit constipation, and defecatory disorders. While these classifications are important in the outpatient setting, they have less relevance in the acute care setting. Secondary causes of constipation are listed in Table 53.1 which include hypothyroidism, diabetes mellitus, Hirschsprung disease, spinal cord injury, Parkinson's disease, and pregnancy, and medications associated with constipation are listed in Table 53.2 [1, 5, 6].

Workup for constipation should include a thorough history and physical exam assessing for secondary causes of constipation. Anal and rectal exam should evaluate for fissure, hemorrhoid, fecal impaction, rectal mass, and proctitis. Imaging with computed tomography is indicated when

Table 53.1 Secondary causes of constipation [1, 5, 6]

Anal fissures
Autonomic neuropathy
Cerebrovascular disease
Cognitive impairment
Congenital malformations
Colon cancer
Depression
Diabetes mellitus
Hypercalcemia
Hypokalemia
Hypomagnesemia
Hypothyroidism
Immobility
Irritable bowel syndrome
Medications
Multiple sclerosis
Parkinson's disease
Pregnancy
Scleroderma
Spinal cord injury
Stricture
Rectal prolapse

© Springer Nature Switzerland AG 2019
A. Graham, D. J. Carlberg (eds.), *Gastrointestinal Emergencies*, https://doi.org/10.1007/978-3-319-98343-1_53

Table 53.2 Medications associated with constipation [1, 5, 6]

Antacids, especially containing calcium
Anticholinergic agents
Anticonvulsants
Antidiarrheal agents
Antihistamines
Antiparkinsonian agents
Antipsychotics
Antirheumatic drugs
Beta-blockers
Calcium channel blockers
Calcium supplements
Diuretics
Iron supplements
NSAIDs
Opioids
Sympathomimetics
Tricyclic antidepressants

Table 53.3 Oral laxatives [1, 6]

Bulk-forming laxatives
Psyllium
Methylcellulose
Polycarbophil
Wheat dextrin
Osmotic laxatives
Lactulose
Glycerin
Magnesium oxide, magnesium citrate, magnesium sulfate
Polyethylene glycol
Sorbitol
Stimulant laxatives
Bisacodyl
Senna
Sodium picosulfate
Surfactants
Docusate sodium
Docusate calcium

clinicians suspect intestinal obstruction or other significant pathology [4].

Constipation may be a symptom of malignancy, and patients presenting with hematochezia, weight loss of ten pounds or more, family history of colon cancer, iron-deficiency anemia, positive fecal occult blood testing, or advanced age should be referred for additional outpatient workup.

What Is an Evidence-Based Approach Management?

First-line treatments of chronic constipation are dietary changes, bulk-forming laxatives, and non-bulk-forming laxatives. Dietary changes primarily consist of increasing fiber and water intake. Oral laxatives typically take as long as 24 h to work and do not treat fecal impaction; thus their ability to adequately treat severe symptomatic constipation in the acute care setting is limited [1, 4, 6]. Oral medications for constipation are listed in Table 53.3.

Recommendations for management of severe constipation include rectal suppositories, enemas, and manual disimpaction. Commonly used rectal suppositories include glycerin and bisacodyl [1]. Enemas directly stimulate colonic smooth muscle. Many types of enemas are used by acute care providers, including phosphate enemas, soapsuds enemas, saline enemas, milk and molasses enemas, gastrografin enemas, mineral oil enemas, and the so-called "bubble gum" and "SMOG" combination enemas.

Few studies have evaluated the efficacy of suppositories and enemas; however, several publications describe the safety and complication rates of these treatments. Niv et al. assessed perforation and mortality rates after cleansing enemas for acute constipation and showed hypophosphatemia

and phosphate nephropathy associated with phosphate enemas. They recommended against use of a phosphate enemas in all patients [2]. Vilke et al. evaluated the safety and efficacy of milk and molasses enemas in the emergency department. They found an 87.5% success rate for this enema when used alone and an 82.4% success rate when used after another treatment. They were ultimately unable to prove safety [7].

Enemas should be reserved for appropriate patient populations. They should not be used in patients who are comatose or non-compliant. Patients with rectal tumors or rectal prolapse should not receive enemas, and enemas should be avoided in patients on chemotherapy, immuno-compromised patients, and patients with active coronary artery disease [2].

Complications of enemas include bowel perforation, hyperphosphatemia, phosphate nephropathy, and brady-cardia. Hyperphosphatemia and phosphate nephropathy only occur with phosphate-containing enemas, and elderly patients, those with renal disease, and those on angiotensin-converting enzyme inhibitors are at highest risk [2]. Because there is limited research on enemas, accurate complication rates and side effects are not fully understood.

Manual disimpaction, otherwise known as manual fragmentation, is indicated for fecal impaction. Often disimpaction alone is not sufficient to relieve severe constipation. Disimpaction should be followed by an enema or oral laxatives. One study recommended an oil retention enema 30 min prior to manual disimpaction to soften stool. That study also recommended pre-treatment of the rectum with topical pain relief products typically used in the treatment of hemorrhoidal pain [4]. Providers should consider giving an anxiolytic or analgesic prior to disimpaction, but they should avoid opioids because opioids may worsen constipation.

When constipation treatment is not successful in the acute care setting, patients may require fluoroscopic enema, fragmentation via flexible or rigid sigmoidoscopy, or, in severe cases, surgical relief [6, 8]. Patients with severe constipation refractory to treatment modalities need gastroenterology follow-up [3].

Suggested Resources
- Fisher W. Disimpaction action. [cited 2017 Sept 24]. Available from: https://www.youtube.com/watch?v=bU8kdrX-0pI
- Garfinkle M. A constipation cocktail. [cited 2017 Sept 24]. Available from: http://www.foamem.com/2012/12/23/a-constipation-cocktail/
- Orman R. Constipation manifesto. [cited 2017 Sept 24]. Available from: http://blog.ercast.org/the-constipation-manifesto/

References

1. Krogh K, Chaironi G, Whitehead W. Management of chronic constipation in adults. United European Gastroenterol J. 2017;5(4):465–72.
2. Niv G, Tamar G, Dickman R, Wasserberg N, Yaron N. Perforation and mortality after cleansing enema for acute constipation are not rare but preventable. Int J Gen Med. 2013;6:323–8.
3. Bharucha A, Dorn S, Lembo A, Pressman A. American Gastroenterological Association medical position statement on constipation. Gastroenterology. 2013;144(1):211–7.
4. Somes J, Donatelli N. Constipation and the geriatric patient: treatment in the emergency department. J Emerg Nurs. 2013;39:372–5.
5. Jamshed N, Zone-En L, Olden K. Diagnostic approach to chronic constipation in adults. Am Fam Physician. 2011;84(3):299–306.
6. Wald A. Management of chronic constipation in adults [internet]. 2017 [updated 2017 Feb 1; cited 2017 Sept 24 2017]. Available from: http://www.uptodate.com/contents/management-of-chronic-constipation-in-adults
7. Vilke G, Demers G, Patel N, Castillo E. Safety and efficacy of milk and molasses enemas in the emergency department. J Emerg Med. 2015;48(6):667–70.
8. Corban C, Sommers T, Segupta N, Jones M, Cheng V, Friedlander E, Bollom A, Lembo A. Fecal impaction in the emergency department: an analysis of frequency and associated charges in 2011. J Clin Gastroenterol. 2016;50:572–7.

Consultant Corner: Bowel Obstruction

54

Eric Benoit

Pearls and Pitfalls
- Bowel obstruction is a surgical disease and surgical consultation should occur early in management.
- The goals in treating bowel obstruction are to relieve intraluminal pressure by nasogastric decompression, resuscitate the patient, and intervene before ischemia, necrosis, and perforation occur.
- The complications of bowel obstruction are ischemia, perforation, sepsis, and death.
- Signs of bowel strangulation, ischemia, and perforation are all similar and include peritonitis, fever, tachycardia, leukocytosis, acidosis, and/or hemodynamic instability.
- Bariatric surgery patients, elderly and diabetic patients, and patients with obstruction due to malignancy require a higher degree of suspicion for complications and special considerations in management.

Introduction

Eric Benoit, MD, is a surgeon specializing in trauma, acute care surgery, and surgical critical care. He graduated from The Ohio State University School of Medicine and completed his surgical residency at Brigham and Women's Hospital and Tufts Medical Center. Dr. Benoit completed a surgical critical care fellowship at Rhode Island Hospital where he remains on staff and is an assistant professor of surgery in the Division of Trauma and Surgical Critical Care at the Alpert Medical School of Brown University. He practices at a busy urban academic level I trauma center with high volume and acuity. Dr. Benoit has a professional inter-

est in using the tools of personalized medicine to identify trauma and surgical patients at risk for complications. He particularly enjoys teaching residents about altered physiology, damage control surgery, and the importance of situational awareness in treating critically ill patients.

Answers to Key Clinical Questions

1. When do you recommend consultation with a surgeon and in what time frame?

Bowel obstruction is a surgical disease. The primary goals in treating bowel obstructions are relieving intraluminal pressure, resuscitating the patient, and intervening before ischemia, necrosis, and perforation occur. The need for operation must be addressed at every step in the evaluation; therefore, a surgeon should be consulted early when an obstruction is suspected or diagnosed.

2. What pearls can you offer emergency care providers when evaluating a patient with bowel obstruction?

The major determination providers must make in the patient with bowel obstruction is whether or not the bowel is strangulated. Strangulated bowel mandates urgent surgery to prevent or manage the complications of perforation. Patients requiring emergency surgery have higher rates of bowel resection and morbidity. Patients without evidence of strangulation or perforation, however, may undergo a trial of non-operative management. Recognizing when this approach has failed is often a complex decision that requires a surgeon to assess the risks and benefits of surgery.

Admission to a surgical service is associated with decreased time to the operating room, decreased hospital length of stay, lower 30-day mortality, and lower readmission rates when compared with medical admissions [1, 2]; therefore, it is preferable to admit to a surgical service rather than to a medical service with surgical consult.

E. Benoit
Division of Trauma & Surgical Critical Care, Alpert Medical School of Brown University, Providence, RI, USA
e-mail: Eric_Benoit@brown.edu

© Springer Nature Switzerland AG 2019
A. Graham, D. J. Carlberg (eds.), *Gastrointestinal Emergencies*, https://doi.org/10.1007/978-3-319-98343-1_54

3. What patient populations are at high risk? What factors should help guide evaluation and management of these patients?

Special consideration should be taken with bariatric surgery patients, elderly and diabetic patients, and patients with bowel obstructions due to malignancy.

Bariatric surgery patients are at risk for obstruction due to internal hernia, which may not be appreciated on physical exam or routine imaging. Tachycardia may be the only significant clinical finding. Because of their altered anatomy, these patients are often unable to be adequately decompressed with a nasogastric (NG) tube. These patients should be approached with a high degree of suspicion and a low threshold to proceed to surgery.

Elderly and diabetic patients both have altered visceral sensitivity and a blunted inflammatory response to injury. Therefore they may present later in the course of disease or with a fairly benign clinical picture despite bowel strangulation. A high index of suspicion is required to identify obstruction and intervene before complications occur.

Malignant bowel obstruction is often a preterminal event [3]. Surgery may be directed at palliation but carries a high complication rate. Management of malignant obstruction frequently involves goals of care conversation.

4. How should emergency care providers approach the diagnosis and management of patients with suspected or proven bowel obstruction?

Providers should inquire whether the patient has history of prior surgeries and perform an examination for scars and hernias, as over 50% of small bowel obstructions (SBOs) in the United States are due to postoperative adhesions [4]. Obstruction without prior surgery raises a concern for malignancy, and a thorough history should seek to elucidate potential signs and symptoms of malignant disease.

Each patient should be assessed for evidence of bowel strangulation, ischemia, and/or perforation as these patients require emergency surgery. Signs include peritonitis, fever, tachycardia, leukocytosis, acidosis, and/or hemodynamic instability.

In conjunction with history and physical exam, the diagnosis of bowel obstruction should be made with laboratory and radiologic testing. An elevated lactate may be present with bowel ischemia, although the absence of an elevated lactate does not exclude it and may be falsely reassuring.

In patients with a history of bowel obstruction, plain radiographs may be sufficient for diagnosis, and an upright chest x-ray may identify free air under the diaphragm in cases of perforation. However, computed tomography (CT) is the imaging modality of choice because it has a greater sensitivity and provides more information about bowel perfusion, transition point, and etiology. CT should be performed with IV contrast (if not contraindicated) to evaluate bowel wall perfusion. Lack of appropriate bowel wall enhancement indicates ischemia and may change the management plan. CT findings concerning for threatened bowel include decreased bowel wall enhancement, mesenteric edema, and the absence of the small bowel feces sign. CT readily identifies the level and location of obstruction and has a 90% sensitivity and specificity for identifying bowel ischemia [5].

Bowel obstruction is a dynamic process that may progress; therefore, patients should have frequent reevaluations including serial abdominal examinations in the acute care setting prior to admission.

A gastrografin challenge given on the day after admission may be used to predict failure of non-operative management. Passage of contrast into the colon within 24 h suggests resolution of obstruction, whereas failure of the contrast to reach the cecum predicts failure of non-operative management, and these patients should proceed to surgery.

5. What complications are you concerned about in patients with bowel obstructions?

Bowel strangulation, ischemia, and perforation are the complications of bowel obstruction which may result in sepsis and death.

6. Does everyone with a small bowel obstruction need a nasogastric tube?

In the setting of an SBO being managed non-operatively, an NG tube should be placed to decompress the bowel proximally and reduce intraluminal pressure. Failure to place an NG tube exposes patients to the risks of vomiting, aspiration, and progression of obstruction to bowel strangulation.

7. Atypical obstructions: What do emergency providers need to know about large bowel obstruction, closed-loop obstruction, volvulus, and internal hernia?

Different types of obstructions mandate different surgical management considerations. In the setting of SBOs, while 75% of patients resolve with proximal decompression via NG tube and non-operative management, the challenge lies in promptly identifying patients who progress to needing surgery prior to the development of complications such as perforation [6]. Closed-loop and large bowel obstructions have a higher risk of ischemia due to buildup of pressure that cannot be decompressed proximally with an NG tube. Therefore these conditions are surgical emergencies. The cecum is the most likely site of perforation regardless of the site of the large bowel obstruction. A cecal diameter >12 cm mandates intervention to avoid perforation. While distal colonic obstruction or volvulus may be decompressed colonoscopically, these patients may ultimately require surgery due to a high recurrence rate.

Suggested Resources

- Aquina CT, Becerra AZ, Probst CP, Xu Z, Hensley BJ, Iannuzzi JC, Noyes K, Monson JR, Fleming FJ. Patients with adhesive small bowel obstruction should be primarily managed by a surgical team. Ann Surg. 2016;264(3):437–47.
- Millet I, Taourel P, Ruyer A, Molinari N. Value of CT findings to predict surgical ischemia in small bowel obstruction: A systematic review and meta-analysis. Eur Radiol. 2015;25(6):1823–35.
- Winner M, Mooney SJ, Hershman DL, Feingold DL, Allendorf JD, Wright JD, Neugut AI. Management and outcomes of bowel obstruction in patients with stage IV colon cancer: a population-based cohort study. Dis Colon Rectum. 2013;56(7):834–43.

2. Bilderback PA, Massman JD 3rd, Smith RK, La Selva D, Helton WS. Small bowel obstruction is a surgical disease: patients with adhesive small bowel obstruction requiring operation have more cost-effective care when admitted to a surgical service. J Am Coll Surg. 2015;221(1):7–13.
3. Winner M, Mooney SJ, Hershman DL, Feingold DL, Allendorf JD, Wright JD, Neugut AI. Management and outcomes of bowel obstruction in patients with stage IV colon cancer: a population-based cohort study. Dis Colon Rectum. 2013;56(7):834–43.
4. ten Broek RP, Issa Y, van Santbrink EJ, Bouvy ND, Kruitwagen RF, Jeekel J, Bakkum EA, Rovers MM, van Goor H. Burden of adhesions in abdominal and pelvic surgery: systematic review and meta-analysis. BMJ. 2013;347:f5588.
5. Millet I, Taourel P, Ruyer A, Molinari N. Value of CT findings to predict surgical ischemia in small bowel obstruction: a systematic review and meta-analysis. Eur Radiol. 2015;25(6):1823–35.
6. Foster NM, McGory ML, Zingmond DS, Ko CY. Small bowel obstruction: a population-based appraisal. J Am Coll Surg. 2006;203(2):170–6.

References

1. Aquina CT, Becerra AZ, Probst CP, Xu Z, Hensley BJ, Iannuzzi JC, Noyes K, Monson JR, Fleming FJ. Patients with adhesive small bowel obstruction should be primarily managed by a surgical team. Ann Surg. 2016;264(3):437–47.

What Is the Utility of the Murphy's Sign and Does It Change with Pain Medication?

55

Yiju Teresa Liu

Key Concepts
- While Murphy's sign is a helpful tool in the diagnosis of acute cholecystitis (AC), it lacks the sensitivity and specificity to rule in or rule out AC.
- The sonographic Murphy's sign is more accurate than the Murphy's sign found on physical exam.
- Neither Murphy's sign is affected by the administration of analgesia.

What Is the Utility of the Murphy's Sign?

Acute cholecystitis (AC) is a morbid cause of abdominal pain seen in the emergency care setting. Clinical gestalt based on classic clinical and laboratory findings can be predictive of AC with a positive likelihood ratio (LR+) of 25–30 [1]. However, many patients do not present classically, requiring clinicians to risk stratify patients and determine the need for further diagnostic imaging.

Murphy's Sign on Physical Examination

The Murphy's sign has been described as the most helpful physical exam finding for AC and occurs when a patient feels pain as the right upper quadrant is palpated under the costal margin during inspiration, resulting in an arrest of inspiration [2]. This maneuver is supposed to compress the gallbladder and, thus, pain would suggest acute inflammation consistent with AC.

The Murphy's sign has been shown to have a high positive predictive value for AC in some studies [3, 4] but has been questioned due to its lack of consistent application and

reproducibility [1]. There have also been concerns of bias in trials of its accuracy [1]. Existing literature places its LR+ between 1.88 and 15.64 in the general population [1, 4, 5] and ~ 2.3 in the elderly [6]. Its negative likelihood ratio (LR–) is between 0.06 and 0.5 in the general population [1, 4, 5] and ~ 0.7 in the elderly [6]. However, in most of these studies, the confidence intervals cross 1, raising the concern that a Murphy's sign may not actually be predictive for AC. Thus, the Tokyo guidelines for diagnosing and determining the severity of AC state that while a positive Murphy's sign can help diagnose AC, its absence does not rule out the disease [7].

Sonographic Murphy's Sign

The sonographic Murphy's sign is an analogous diagnostic maneuver and occurs when the point of maximal pain is caused by compression of the gallbladder under sonographic visualization [3]. The sonographic Murphy's sign combined with the presence of gallstones on ultrasound is very predictive of AC [3, 8]. The sonographic Murphy's sign has LR+ that ranges between 1.32 and 9.84 and LR– that ranges between 0.19 and 0.4, [3, 9, 10] which, at first glance, appears comparable to a Murphy's sign on physical exam, but a sonographic Murphy's sign has improved confidence intervals, suggesting that it is a more reliable finding.

Does the Murphy's Sign Change with Pain Medication?

Administration of analgesia for abdominal pain has become common practice, but some fear that opioids could lead to misdiagnosis or mask findings of peritonitis on physical exam [11, 12]. This has been studied extensively and disproven [11, 12]. Likewise, while the reliability of the sonographic Murphy's sign after analgesia delivery has been questioned [8], this is not supported by the literature. One

Y. T. Liu
Harbor-UCLA Medical Center, David Geffen School of Medicine at UCLA, Torrance, CA, USA
e-mail: tliu@emedharbor.edu

retrospective study of 119 patients failed to show any change in the sonographic Murphy's sign after treatment with opioid analgesia [13], while another small prospective study of patients with right upper quadrant pain also concluded that analgesic administration did not affect its accuracy [14]

Suggested Resources
- Acute Cholecystitis. CORE EM. April 2016. https://coreem.net/core/acute-cholecystitis/
- Gall Bladder Disease. RCEM Learning. October 2017. https://www.rcemlearning.co.uk/references/gall-bladder-disease/
- Strasberg SM. Acute calculous cholecystitis. N Engl J Med. 2008;358(26):2804–11.

References

1. Trowbridge RL, Rutkowski NK, Shojania KG. Does this patient have acute cholecystitis? JAMA. 2003;289(1):80–6.
2. Avegno J, Carlisle M. Evaluating the patient with right upper quadrant abdominal pain. Emerg Med Clin. 2016;34(2):211–28.
3. Ralls PW, Colletti PM, Lapin SA, Chandrasoma PA, Boswell WD Jr, Ngo C, Radin DR, Halls JM. Real-time sonography in suspected acute cholecystitis. Prospective evaluation of primary and secondary signs. Radiology. 1985;155(3):767–71.
4. Singer AJ, McCracken G, Henry MC, Thode HC, Cabahug CJ. Correlation among clinical, laboratory, and hepatobiliary scanning findings in patients with suspected acute cholecystitis. Ann Emerg Med. 1996;28(3):267–72.
5. Jain A, Mehta N, Secko M, Schechter J, Papanagnou D, Pandya S, Sinert R. History, physical examination, laboratory testing, and emergency department ultrasonography for the diagnosis of acute cholecystitis. Acad Emerg Med. 2017;24(3):281–97.
6. Adedeji OA, McAdam WA. Murphy's sign, acute cholecystitis and elderly people. J R Coll Surg Edinb. 1996;41(2):88–9.
7. Yokoe M, Takada T, Strasberg SM, Solomkin JS, Mayumi T, Gomi H, Pitt HA, Garden OJ, Kiriyama S, Hata J, Gabata T. TG13 diagnostic criteria and severity grading of acute cholecystitis (with videos). J Hepatobiliary Pancreat Sci. 2013;20(1):35–46.
8. Bennett GL. Evaluating patients with right upper quadrant pain. Radiol Clin N Am. 2015;53(6):1093–130.
9. Bree RL. Further observations on the usefulness of the sonographic Murphy sign in the evaluation of suspected acute cholecystitis. J Clin Ultrasound. 1995;23(3):169–72.
10. Ralls PW, Halls J, Lapin SA, Quinn MF, Morris UL, Boswell W. Prospective evaluation of the sonographic Murphy sign in suspected acute cholecystitis. J Clin Ultrasound. 1982;10(3):113–5.
11. Attard AR, Corlett MJ, Kidner NJ, Leslie AP, Fraser IA. Safety of early pain relief for acute abdominal pain. BMJ. 1992;305(6853):554–6.
12. Thomas SH, Silen W, Cheema F, Reisner A, Aman S, Goldstein JN, Kumar AM, Stair TO. Effects of morphine analgesia on diagnostic accuracy in emergency department patients with abdominal pain: a prospective, randomized trial. J Am Coll Surg. 2003;196(1):18–31.
13. Nelson BP, Senecal EL, Hong C, Ptak T, Thomas SH. Opioid analgesia and assessment of the sonographic Murphy sign. J Emerg Med. 2005;28(4):409–13.
14. Noble VE, Liteplo AS, Nelson BP, Thomas SH. The impact of analgesia on the diagnostic accuracy of the sonographic Murphy's sign. Eur J Emerg Med. 2010;17(2):80–3.

Is a Negative CT Good Enough to Rule Out Acute Cholecystitis?

56

Yiju Teresa Liu

Pearls and Pitfalls
- Ultrasound is the first-line diagnostic study for acute biliary disorders.
- Computed tomography (CT) plays a supplemental role and is especially useful in cases when ultrasound and cholescintigraphy are nondiagnostic.
- CT has an overall diagnostic sensitivity of 70–100% for acute cholecystitis.
- CT can detect complications associated with acute biliary disorders.

Ultrasound is the first-line imaging study for patients with suspected biliary disease.

Computed tomography (CT) often finds biliary disease in patients evaluated for both (1) undifferentiated abdominal complaints and (2) suspected non-biliary abdominal pain (e.g., ureterolithiasis). CT may aid in the diagnosis of cholecystitis when ultrasound and cholescintigraphy are nondiagnostic. Additionally, CT may demonstrate complications related to biliary disease such as gallstone pancreatitis, gallstone ileus, emphysematous cholecystitis, and pneumobilia.

Few studies have directly compared ultrasound and CT for acute cholecystitis. The largest study to date retrospectively evaluated 101 patients with pathology-confirmed acute cholecystitis who had both CT and US. It found that CT had a higher sensitivity than ultrasound for acute cholecystitis (92% vs. 79%, $p = 0.015$), but ultrasound outperformed CT for diagnosing cholelithiasis (sensitivity 87% vs. 60%, $p < 0.01$) [1].

A multicenter trial evaluating 52 patients with cholecystitis found that CT and ultrasound had identical sensitivities for the diagnosis [2]. Most other studies report similar sensitivities between CT and ultrasound for acute cholecystitis (70–100% vs. 82–91%) [3–6].

The two modalities, however, may not be truly comparable. CT is generally more sensitive than ultrasound for detecting complications associated with acute cholecystitis, such as pericholecystic abscesses, pericholecystic gas, gallbladder wall thickening, and extra-biliary stones [7]. Cholelithiasis, the predominant cause of cholecystitis, is better diagnosed with ultrasound [1]. CT should be considered in patients at risk for acalculous cholecystitis.

CT may miss cases of acute cholecystitis subsequently found on cholescintigraphy.

Since a negative CT does not fully rule out acute cholecystitis, further testing should be obtained following a negative CT in patients with continued suspicion based on history, physical exam, and laboratory findings. Additional testing may include ultrasound and/or cholescintigraphy as indicated by the clinical situation.

Suggested Resources
- Acute Cholecystitis. Radiopaedia. https://radiopaedia.org/articles/acute-cholecystitis
- Trowbridge RL, Rutkowski NK, Shojania KG. Does this patient have acute cholecystitis? JAMA. 2003;289(1):80–6.

Y. T. Liu
Harbor-UCLA Medical Center, David Geffen School of Medicine at UCLA, Torrance, CA, USA
e-mail: tliu@emedharbor.edu

References

1. Fagenholz PJ, Fuentes E, Kaafarani H, Cropano C, King D, deMoya M, Butler K, Velmahos G, Chang Y, Yeh DD. Computed tomography is more sensitive than ultrasound for the diagnosis of acute cholecystitis. Surg Infect. 2015;16:509–12.
2. van Randen A, Lame'ris W, van Es HW, et al. A comparison of the accuracy of ultrasound and computed tomography in

common diagnoses causing acute abdominal pain. Eur Radiol. 2011;21:1535–45.

3. De Vargas MM, Lanciotti S, De Cicco ML, et al. Ultrasonographic and spiral CT evaluation of simple and complicated acute cholecystitis: diagnostic protocol assessment based on personal experience and review of the literature. Radiol Med. 2006;111:167–80.

4. Kiewiet JJ, Leeuwenburgh MM, Bipat S, Bossuyt PM, Stoker J, Boermeester MA. A systematic review and meta-analysis of diagnostic performance of imaging in acute cholecystitis. Radiology. 2012;264:708–20.

5. Shea JA, Berlin JA, Escarce JJ, et al. Revised estimates of diagnostic test sensitivity and specificity in suspected biliary tract disease. Arch Intern Med. 1994;154:2573–81.

6. Jain A, Mehta N, Secko M, Schechter J, Papanagnou D, Pandya S, Sinert R. History, physical examination, laboratory testing, and emergency department ultrasonography for the diagnosis of acute cholecystitis. Acad Emerg Med. 2017;24:281–97.

7. Chawla A, Bosco JI, Lim TC, Srinivasan S, Teh HS, Shenoy JN. Imaging of acute cholecystitis and cholecystitis-associated complications in the emergency setting. Singap Med J. 2015;56(8):438.

57

When Is Acute Intervention (Interventional Radiology/Surgery) Necessary for Acute Cholecystitis? Can Acute Cholecystitis Be Managed at Home with Oral Antibiotics?

Veronica Solorio and Andrea Wu

Key Concepts

- Treatment for acute cholecystitis remains primarily surgical, with early laparoscopic cholecystectomy having the best outcomes.
- In elderly or immunocompromised patients who are poor surgical candidates, parenteral antibiotics with or without percutaneous cholecystostomy may be an alternative treatment option.
- There is little to no role for outpatient oral antibiotics in acute cholecystitis.

Cholecystitis occurs when the gallbladder is unable to empty appropriately, allowing for buildup of bile and development of inflammation. The inflamed gallbladder becomes a nidus for infection and can become pressurized.

Cholecystitis is typically diagnosed by a composite of findings that includes the following:

1. Local signs of inflammation – focal tenderness over the gallbladder
2. Systemic signs of inflammation – fever, leukocytosis, abnormal liver function tests, and/or an elevated C-reactive protein
3. Radiographic findings of inflammation – gallbladder wall thickening, pericholecystic fluid, pneumobilia, and/or a sonographic Murphy's sign

V. Solorio (✉)
Department of Emergency Medicine, Harbor-UCLA Medical Center, Torrance, CA, USA
e-mail: Vsolorio@dhs.lacounty.gov

A. Wu
Department of Emergency Medicine, David Geffen School of Medicine at UCLA, Harbor-UCLA Medical Center, Torrance, CA, USA
e-mail: awu@emedharbor.edu

When Is Acute Intervention (Surgery/Interventional Radiology) Necessary for Acute Cholecystitis?

Traditionally, the treatment for acute cholecystitis has been surgical. Early laparoscopic cholecystectomy (ELC) has the best outcomes [1, 2]. A recent meta-analysis comparing ELC to delayed laparoscopic cholecystectomy (DLC) found that ELC (surgery within 7 days of admission) was associated with a lower risk of wound infections, lower hospital costs, shorter hospital stays, and greater patient satisfaction [3]. Further studies showed that complications including common bile duct injury, bowel perforation, and need to convert from laparoscopic to open cholecystectomy are lower in patients who undergo surgery within 2 days of admission [4, 5]. There is a slightly higher risk of adverse outcomes when operative management occurs on the day of admission, highlighting the importance of resuscitation and optimizing the patient's volume status and comorbidities [4].

An important component of the resuscitation is initiation of antimicrobial therapy. Per IDSA guidelines, patients with suspected community-acquired cholecystitis can be treated with cefazolin, cefuroxime, or ceftriaxone. In patients with more severe infections (severe physiologic disturbances, immunosuppression, advanced age, and/or ascending cholangitis), antibiotic therapy should be escalated and include metronidazole plus either a carbapenem, cefepime, or piperacillin-tazobactam [6].

The importance of definitive management via cholecystectomy has been highlighted in various studies. Among those who did not undergo cholecystectomy during their index admission, 19% had a gallstone-related emergency department visit or hospital admission within 3 months, and 30% had a gallstone-related emergency department visit or hospital admission within 1 year [7]. Nearly one-third of these returns involved biliary obstruction or pancreatitis [7].

© Springer Nature Switzerland AG 2019
A. Graham, D. J. Carlberg (eds.), *Gastrointestinal Emergencies*, https://doi.org/10.1007/978-3-319-98343-1_57

Special Populations

Although definitive treatment is preferred, special consideration must be given to those older than 65, the immunecompromised, and those with certain comorbid conditions.

Research comparing cholecystectomy to non-operative management of acute cholecystitis in those 65 years or older found that postoperative complications were significant, even among those who were considered the best surgical candidates [8]. Among the elderly, those who underwent conservative management with either parenteral antibiotics alone or with parenteral antibiotics and biliary decompression via percutaneous cholecystostomy had fewer complications, including death, without an increase in recurrent acute cholecystitis [8]. However, other studies suggested that readmissions for gallbladder-related disease, the rate of conversion from laparoscopic to open cholecystectomy, and overall cost increased among elderly patients who did not undergo cholecystectomy during their index presentations [9]. Thus, the decision whether or not to operate on this group continues to be challenging. Cholecystitis in the elderly is discussed in Chap. 63 of this textbook.

Emerging endoscopic techniques may provide safer alternatives for patients unable to undergo traditional surgery. Natural orifice transluminal endoscopic surgery and endoscopic transpapillary drainage may offer alternatives for those who are poor surgical candidates due to comorbid conditions such as ascites and coagulopathy. While these methods are not yet widely available [1], they are likely to become more common as the populations of both the elderly and those with comorbid conditions increase.

Can Acute Cholecystitis Be Managed at Home with Oral Antibiotics?

While a minimally invasive approach might be indicated for some patients, oral antibiotics alone have never been shown to provide adequate treatment for acute cholecystitis.

Conclusion

For younger acute cholecystitis patients without significant comorbidities, surgical management with early laparoscopic cholecystectomy has the best outcomes after appropriate resuscitation. In elderly patients and/or poor surgical candidates, surgical intervention may carry too much risk, and alternative treatment may include parenteral antibiotics +/− either percutaneous cholecystostomy or an emerging endoscopic procedure.

> **Suggested Resources**
> - EM@3 AM – Acute Cholecystitis. emDocs. March 2017. http://www.emdocs.net/em3am-acute-cholecystitis/
> - Episode 117.0 – Acute Cholecystitis. Core EM. October 2017. https://coreem.net/podcast/episode-117-0/
> - Ultrasound for the Win Case – 46F with Abdominal Pain. Academic life in emergency medicine. April 2015. https://www.aliem.com/2015/04/ultrasound-for-the-win-46f-abdominal-pain/

References

1. Baron TH, Grimm IS, Swanstrom LL. (2015). Interventional approaches to gallbladder disease. N Engl J Med. 2015;373:357–65.
2. Zafar SN, Obirieze A, Adesibikan B, Cornwell EE, Fullum TM, Tran DD. Optimal time for early laparoscopic cholecystectomy for acute cholecystitis. JAMA Surg. 2015;150:129–36.
3. Wu XD, Tian X, Liu MM, Wu L, Zhao S, Zhao L. Meta-analysis comparing early versus delayed laparoscopic cholecystectomy for acute cholecystitis. Br J Surg. 2015;102:1302–13.
4. Österberg J, Sandblom G, Lundell L, Hedberg M, Enochsson L. The sooner, the better? The importance of optimal timing of cholecystectomy in acute cholecystitis: data from the national Swedish registry for gallstone surgery, GallRiks. J Gastrointest Surg. 2017;21:33–40.
5. Banz V, Gsponer T, Candinas D, Guller U. Population-based analysis of 4113 patients with acute cholecystitis: defining the optimal time-point for laparoscopic cholecystectomy. Ann Surg. 2011;254:964–70.
6. Solomkin K, Mazuski JE, Bradley JS, Rodvold KA, Goldstein EJC, Baron EJ, O'Neill PJ, Chow AW, Dellinger EP, Eachempati SR, Gorbach S, Hilfiker M, May AK, Nathens AB, Sawyer RG, Bartlett JG. Diagnosis and management of complicated intra-abdominal infection in adults and children: guidelines by the surgical infection society and the Infectious Diseases Society of America. Clin Infect Dis. 2010;50:133–64. https://doi.org/10.1086/649554.
7. de Mestral C, Rotstein OD, Laupacis A, Hoch JS, Zagorski B, Nathens AB. A population-based analysis of the clinical course of 10,304 patients with acute cholecystitis, discharged without cholecystectomy. J Trauma Acute Care Surg. 2013;74:26–31.
8. McGillicuddy EA, Schuster KM, Barre K, Suarez L, Hall MR, Kaml GJ, Davis KA, Longo WE. Non-operative management of acute cholecystitis in the elderly. Br J Surg. 2012;99:1254–61.
9. Riall TS, Zhang D, Townsend CM, Kuo YF, Goodwin JS. Failure to perform cholecystectomy for acute cholecystitis in elderly patients is associated with increased morbidity, mortality, and cost. J Am Coll Surg. 2010;210:668–77.

Is There a Role for HIDA Scan in the Emergency Setting?

58

Manpreet Singh

Key Concepts
- The hydroxy iminodiacetic acid (HIDA) scan has significantly higher sensitivity and specificity than ultrasound for acute cholecystitis. It also has better positive and negative predictive values.
- HIDA should be considered in patients with equivocal ultrasound findings or when ultrasound findings do not fit the clinical presentation.

Cholescintigraphy or hepatobiliary scintigraphy is a nuclear study in which the patient receives hydroxy iminodiacetic acid (HIDA), a radioactive compound that is taken up by the liver and excreted into the biliary tract [1, 2]. Thus, it is commonly referred to as a HIDA scan.

Normally, in the first phase of the study, the gallbladder becomes visible approximately 1 h after injection. However, in the setting of cholecystitis or cystic duct obstruction, visualization is either delayed or completely absent.

Abnormal gallbladder filling and visualization on the HIDA scan have a sensitivity of >95% and a specificity of >90% for cholecystitis [1–3], making it more accurate than ultrasound [4–7]. HIDA scan also has better positive and negative predictive values. Therefore, while ultrasound is the initial imaging modality of choice, some believe the HIDA scan should be considered instead due to its better test characteristics for cholecystitis [4].

In the second phase of the HIDA scan, the patient is given cholecystokinin, which contracts the gallbladder, causing it to empty within several hours, expel the HIDA, and be no longer visualized. However, in the setting of biliary dysfunction or sphincter of Oddi spasm, the gallbladder continues to be visualized because the emptying is either delayed or absent, and the HIDA is retained in the gallbladder.

While biliary dysfunction and sphincter of Oddi spasm can cause chronic, intermittent pain, they rarely require emergent intervention. These patients generally do not require admission, and these conditions are not associated with significant mortality. Thus, in the acute care setting, the most important part of the HIDA scan is the first phase involving gallbladder filling.

There are several disadvantages to the HIDA scan which continue to limit its utilization as a primary imaging modality in the acute setting [8, 9]:

1. Hepatitis and prolonged fasting can cause delayed gallbladder emptying.
2. It is more expensive than ultrasound.
3. It requires more technician time (typically 3–4 h).
4. It exposes the patient to ionizing radiation.
5. It may be unavailable at night or on weekends.
6. It is less accurate for diagnosing symptomatic cholelithiasis without cholecystitis.
7. It does not assess for alternative diagnoses that can mimic cholecystitis, such as hepatic abscess, cholangiocarcinoma, pancreatitis, and obstructive uropathy.

Given its limitations and disadvantages, HIDA scan should be reserved for when ultrasound is equivocal or ultrasound findings do not fit the clinical presentation. For example, a patient with chronic ascites due to alcohol abuse may have elevated transaminases, gallbladder wall thickening, and pericholecystic fluid at baseline, and these findings on ultrasound may not be related to acute cholecystitis. Likewise, these findings could also be present on computed tomography at a patient's baseline, limiting its utility for acute cholecystitis. Thus, HIDA scan would be helpful in determining if there were delayed or absent gallbladder filling to suggest true cholecystitis.

M. Singh
Department of Emergency Medicine, David Geffen School of Medicine at UCLA, Harbor-UCLA Medical Center,
Torrance, CA, USA
e-mail: masingh@dhs.lacounty.gov

© Springer Nature Switzerland AG 2019
A. Graham, D. J. Carlberg (eds.), *Gastrointestinal Emergencies*, https://doi.org/10.1007/978-3-319-98343-1_58

Suggested Resources

- Cholescintigraphy. Radiopaedia. https://radiopaedia. org/articles/cholescintigraphy
- Normal HIDA scan for gallbladder dysfunction. Radiopaedia. https://radiopaedia.org/cases/normal-hida-scan-for-gallbladder-dysfunction

References

1. Missiroli C, Mansouri M, Singh A. Emergencies of the biliary tract. In: Singh A, editor. Emergency radiology. Cham: Springer; 2018.
2. Elwood DR. Cholecystitis. Surg Clin North Am. 2008;88(6):1241–52. https://doi.org/10.1016/j.suc.2008.07.008.
3. Graff LG, Robinson D. Abdominal pain and emergency department evaluation. Emerg Med Clin North Am. 2001;19:123–36.
4. Alobaidi M, Gupta R, Jafri SZ, Fink-Bennet DM. Current trends in imaging evaluation of acute cholecystitis. Emerg Radiol. 2004;10:256–8.
5. Trowbridge RL, Rutkowski NK, Shojania KG. Does this patient have acute cholecystitis? JAMA. 2003;289:80–6.
6. Behnia F, Gross JA, Ragucci M, Monti S, Mancini M, Elman S, Vesselle H, Mannelli L. Nuclear medicine and the emergency department patient: an illustrative case-based approach. Radiol Med. 2015;120:158–70.
7. Jain A, Mehta N, Secko M, Schechter J, Papanagnou D, Pandya S, Sinert R. History, physical examination, laboratory testing, and emergency department ultrasonography for the diagnosis of acute cholecystitis. Acad Emerg Med. 2017;24:281–97. https://doi.org/10.1111/acem.13132.
8. Kaoutzanis C, Davies E, Leichtle SW, Welch KB, Winter S, Lampman RM, Franz MG, Arneson W. Is hepato-imino diacetic acid scan a better imaging modality than abdominal ultrasound for diagnosing acute cholecystitis? Am J Surg. 2015;210:473–82. https://doi.org/10.1016/j.amjsurg.2015.03.005.
9. Mujoomdar M, Russell E, Dionne F, Moulton K, Murray C, McGill S, Lambe K. Optimizing health system use of medical isotopes and other imaging modalities. CADTH optimal use reports. Canadian Agency for Drugs and Technologies in Health: Ottawa; 2012.

59

What Is Acalculous Cholecystitis? What Are Its Implications? How Is It Managed?

Manpreet Singh

Pearls and Pitfalls

- Acalculous cholecystitis (ACC) is usually associated with severe underlying, comorbid medical or surgical disease.
- ACC is associated with increased morbidity and mortality compared to calculous cholecystitis and is more likely to perforate or develop necrotizing complications.
- Though cholecystectomy is the treatment of choice for ACC, patients who are unstable or poor surgical candidates are often treated initially with percutaneous intervention and antibiotics.

What Is Acalculous Cholecystitis?

Acalculous cholecystitis (ACC) occurs when the gallbladder develops inflammation without evidence of gallstones or cystic duct obstruction. The inflammation becomes a nidus for infection.

ACC frequently occurs in patients with severe underlying chronic comorbid medical or surgical conditions such as malnutrition, TPN use, sepsis, significant burns, multitrauma, and HIV [1, 2]. It is believed that these many different, unrelated underlying comorbidities cause increased bile viscosity, resulting in stagnant bile, which accumulates and becomes increasingly pressurized [3–6]. The gallbladder wall subsequently becomes edematous, inflamed, and ischemic, predisposing to gallbladder infection [3–6].

Acute or acute on chronic illness can also play a significant role in the development of ACC. Fever and dehydration can lead to increased bile viscosity. Decreased oral intake can lead to decreased cholecystokinin production and, thus, decreased cholecystokinin-induced biliary contraction [3–6]. When these febrile and dehydrated patients with poor oral intake develop increased bile viscosity and bile stasis, the accumulated bile distends the gall bladder and places stress on the gall bladder wall, causing reactive inflammation and increasing the risk of subsequent gallbladder infection [3–6].

Likewise, poor circulation and/or organ perfusion can contribute to gallbladder edema, which weakens the gall bladder wall, leading to distension and accumulation of bile, resulting in inflammation and risk of gallbladder infection [3–6].

What Are Its Implications?

ACC accounts for 5–10% of all cases of acute cholecystitis, and it is more common among the elderly, even when comorbid conditions are taken into account. ACC is associated with increased morbidity and mortality compared to calculous cholecystitis (cholecystitis due to gallstones) [1, 2]. Mortality is more than ten times greater in ACC. Gangrenous and necrotizing complications are six times more common and gallbladder perforation more likely [1, 2].

How Is It Managed?

Rapid identification and treatment are essential in ACC. Complete blood count (CBC) and liver function tests (LFTs) are often used to screen for ACC but are frequently abnormal due to the underlying, comorbid conditions that make ACC more likely. This makes it difficult to diagnose ACC in the very patients most at risk for it. Therefore, ACC should be considered in all elderly, hospitalized, or immune-compromised patients with fever and abdominal pain, especially if the pain is localized to the right upper quadrant.

M. Singh
Department of Emergency Medicine, David Geffen School of Medicine at UCLA, Harbor-UCLA Medical Center, Torrance, CA, USA
e-mail: masingh@dhs.lacounty.gov

© Springer Nature Switzerland AG 2019
A. Graham, D. J. Carlberg (eds.), *Gastrointestinal Emergencies*, https://doi.org/10.1007/978-3-319-98343-1_59

Evaluation is based on ultrasound (US), cholescintigraphy (HIDA), and/or computed tomography (CT) based on the clinical situation. When ACC is suspected, US is usually the initial diagnostic imaging of choice. Its sensitivity ranges from 30% to 98%, and its specificity ranges from 89% to 100%. When the diagnosis is uncertain after US or when patients have vague, nonspecific symptoms, a CT may be performed to evaluate for ACC and other potential causes of fever and abdominal pain. When both US and CT are unrevealing and suspicion for ACC persists, a HIDA scan be obtained. Sensitivity of HIDA ranges from 67% to 100%, and specificity ranges from 58% to 88%.

Regardless of the imaging modality chosen, it is key to understand that imaging alone is not specific enough to make the diagnosis. Imaging should be interpreted in the context of the clinical presentation, and alternate diagnoses should be excluded.

Once diagnosed, treatment should include:

1. Immediate antibiotic coverage, as ascending infection, abdominal sepsis, and shock can develop rapidly
2. Generous fluid resuscitation, as hypovolemia and dehydration are important predisposing factors
3. Consultation with a hepatobiliary surgeon, gastroenterologist, and/or interventional radiologist
4. Management of comorbid factors and concurrent acute disease processes [7–10]

Cholecystectomy is the preferred definitive treatment, but the patients who develop ACC are often unstable or poor surgical candidates due to the comorbidities that made them susceptible to developing ACC in the first place [10]. Nonsurgical interventions may be necessary and should be considered early. Endoscopic gallbladder stent placement or endoscopic ultrasonography-guided transmural gallbladder drainage with a lumen-apposing metal stent may be performed by a gastroenterologist [11, 12]. Percutaneous cholecystostomy and drain placement may be performed by an interventional radiologist [7–9]. Though nonsurgical approaches are not better than cholecystectomy, they provide a survival benefit compared to antibiotics alone and are important considerations in poor surgical candidates [10].

Suggested Resources
- Acalculous Cholecystitis. Life in the Fastlane. Feb 2017. https://lifeinthefastlane.com/ccc/acalculous-cholecystitis
- Acute Acalculous Cholecystitis. Radiopaedia. https://radiopaedia.org/articles/acute-acalculous-cholecystitis

References

1. Barie PS, Eachempati SR. In: Dultz LA, Todd SR, Eachempati SR, editors. Acute cholecystitis. Cham: Springer International Publishing; 2015.
2. Treinen C, Lomelin D, Krause C, Goede M, Oleynikov D. Acute acalculous cholecystitis in the critically ill: risk factors and surgical strategies. Langenbeck's Arch Surg. 2015;400:421–7. https://doi.org/10.1007/s00423-014-1267-6.
3. Tana M, Tana C, Cocco G, Iannetti G, Romano M, Schiavone C. Acute acalculous cholecystitis and cardiovascular disease: a land of confusion. J Ultrasound. 2015;18(4):317–20.
4. Theodorou P, Maurer CA, Spanholtz TA, et al. Acalculous cholecystitis in severely burned patients: incidence and predisposing factors. Burns. 2009;35(3):405–11.
5. Hamp T, Fridrich P, Mauritz W, Hamid L, Pelinka LE. Cholecystitis after trauma. J Trauma. 2009;66(2):400–6.
6. Gu MG, Kim TN, Song J, Nam YJ, Lee JY, Park JS. Risk factors and therapeutic outcomes of acute acalculous cholecystitis. Digestion. 2014;90(2):75–80.
7. Joseph T, Unver K, Hwang GL, et al. Percutaneous cholecystostomy for acute cholecystitis: ten-year experience. J Vasc Interv Radiol. 2012;23(1):83–8.e1.
8. Chung YH, Choi ER, Kim KM, et al. Can percutaneous cholecystostomy be a definitive management for acute acalculous cholecystitis? J Clin Gastroenterol. 2012;46(3):216–9.
9. Noh SY, Gwon DI, Ko GY, Yoon HK, Sung KB. Role of percutaneous cholecystostomy for acute acalculous cholecystitis: clinical outcomes of 271 patients. Eur Radiol. 2018;28(4):1449–55.
10. Soria Aledo V, Galindo Iniguez L, Flores Funes D, Carrasco Prats M, Aguayo Albasini JL. Is cholecystectomy the treatment of choice for acute acalculous cholecystitis? A systematic review of the literature. Rev Esp Enferm Dig. 2017;109(10):708–18.
11. Irani S, Baron TH, Grimm IS, Khashab MA. EUS-guided gallbladder drainage with a lumen-apposing metal stent (with video). Gastrointest Endosc. 2015;82(6):1110–5.
12. Anderson JE, Inui T, Talamini MA, Chang DC. Cholecystostomy offers no survival benefit in patients with acute acalculous cholecystitis and severe sepsis and shock. J Surg Res. 2014;190(2):517–21.

What Is the Optimal Management for Biliary Colic and Who Requires Admission?

60

Anthony Scarcella

Key Concepts
- The initial management of biliary colic in the emergency setting includes IV fluids, analgesics, and antiemetics as needed.
- Evaluation should include laboratory studies and diagnostic imaging.
- Patients with uncomplicated biliary colic who have no signs of complications and whose pain has resolved can be discharged with outpatient follow-up.
- Patients with uncontrolled pain should be admitted.
- Patients with complications such as cholecystitis, choledocholithiasis, cholangitis, or gallstone pancreatitis require hospital admission and often require specialty consultation.

The evaluation and initial management of upper abdominal pain due to suspected biliary colic is similar to the evaluation and initial management of other biliary pathologies. Severity of the symptoms, gallstone location, and complications dictate management [1].

Patients presenting with acute symptoms due to possible biliary colic often receive intravenous fluids, analgesics, and antiemetics. Intravenous (IV) fluids are given to maintain adequate hydration and provide volume resuscitation in those with suspected hypovolemia. Analgesics and antiemetics are given as needed for symptom relief. In general, patients are not given oral intake (except for oral contrast if indicated) until morbid causes of pain have been reasonably excluded.

The typical laboratory work-up for biliary colic and other biliary diseases includes a complete blood count, comprehensive metabolic panel, and lipase. If bilirubin is elevated, a conjugated bilirubin helps differentiate among potential causes. An EKG, cardiac enzymes, and cardiac monitoring may be indicated in the elderly and those with cardiac risk factors [2, 3]. These tests either assess for complications of gallstone disease or assess for alternate diagnoses, rather than diagnosing biliary colic itself.

Conversely, biliary ultrasound can visualize gallstones, as well as concomitant signs of inflammation and some complications. It is often the first imaging test used [1–4]. In certain settings, computed tomography (CT) may be obtained instead of ultrasound [1, 2, 4]; however, one study showed that CT demonstrated gallstones in only 87 out of 110 patients (79%) who had gallstones identified via other modalities (ultrasound and/or direct visualization intraoperatively) [5]. An in-depth approach to liver and biliary imaging is discussed in Chap. 70 of this textbook.

Patients presenting with biliary colic with resolved symptoms, no obvious complications, and normal labs can be discharged with analgesics, antiemetics, outpatient surgical follow-up, and advice to avoid triggers (e.g., dietary fat) [3]. NSAIDs are generally the first-line therapy, as they may be equally effective as narcotics in relieving biliary pain with fewer adverse effects [6, 7]. Narcotic pain medications may be added as necessary.

Admission for uncomplicated biliary colic is indicated when pain is not controlled. Admission is frequently indicated when a gallstone is impacted in the neck of the gallbladder. Impacted stones place patients at risk for recurrent attacks, and if patients with impacted stones are discharged (pain free and without complications), urgent surgical follow-up should be ensured and strict return precautions should be provided.

Medical management of gallstones has declined in recent years, but it may be a useful alternative in patients who are poor surgical candidates or who are unwilling to undergo operative intervention. Medical management includes oral bile acid therapy and extracorporeal shockwave lithotripsy. These treatments, however, are not generally initiated in the emergency setting [8].

A. Scarcella
Department of Emergency Medicine, Eisenhower Medical Center, Rancho Mirage, CA, USA
e-mail: ascarcella@eisenhowerhealth.org

Suggested Resources

- Acute Cholecystitis and Biliary Colic. Medscape. Jan 2017. https://emedicine.medscape.com/article/1950020-overview
- Podcast: Biliary Colic and Cholecystitis. Surgery 101. Jan 2018. http://surgery101.org/podcast/biliary-colic-and-cholecystitis/

References

1. Abraham S, Rivero H, Erlikh I, et al. Surgical and nonsurgical management of gallstones. Am Fam Physician. 2014;89:795–802.
2. Alam HB, Demehri FR, Repaskey WT, et al. Evaluation and management of gallstone-\related diseases in non-pregnant adults. Ann Arbor, MI: Faculty Group Practice, University of Michigan Health System; 2014. Available from the National Guideline Clearinghouse at www.guideline.gov/content.aspx?id=48262
3. Demehri F, Alam H. Evidence-based management of common gallstone-related emergencies. J Intensive Care Med. 2016;31:3–13.
4. Tomizawa M, Shinozaki F, Hasegawa R, et al. Abdominal ultrasonography for patients with abdominal pain as a fist-line diagnostic imaging modality. Exp Ther Med. 2017;13:1932–6.
5. Barakos JA, Ralls PW, Lapin SA, et al. Cholelithiasis: evaluation with CT. Radiology. 1987;162(2):415–8.
6. Henderson SO, Swardron S, Newton E. Comparison of intravenous ketorolac and meperidine in the treatment of biliary colic. J Emerg Med. 2002;23:237–41.
7. Johnston MJ, Fitzgerald JE, Bhangu A, et al. Outpatient management of biliary colic: a prospective observational study of prescribing habits and analgesia effectiveness. Int J Surg. 2014;12:169–76.
8. Tazuma S, Unno M, Igarashi Y, et al. Evidence-based clinical practice guidelines for cholelithiasis 2016. J Gastroenterol. 2017;52(3):276–300.

What Is Gallstone Ileus and What Are Its Implications?

61

Bryan Sloane and Andrea Wu

Key Concepts
- Gallstone ileus is a rare etiology for bowel obstruction that disproportionately affects elderly women.
- Patients often present with a subacute onset of vague symptoms, making diagnosis difficult.
- Gallstone ileus is caused by a large gallstone, typically >2.5 cm, which passes through a biliary-enteric fistula and impacts in the bowel.
- Diagnosis is best made by CT and treatment is surgical.
- Mortality is ~30%.

Gallstone ileus, a mechanical bowel obstruction due to an intraluminal ectopic gallstone, is a rare cause of bowel obstruction that is highly morbid and often difficult to diagnose [1]. Recent literature shows that less than 1% of all mechanical bowel obstructions in the United States result from gallstone impaction, although prior research had suggested a frequency as high as 5% [1]. Older women are most typically affected, with a female to male ratio of 6:1. Patients are typically over 60 years old, with most patients in their 70s [1, 2]. Mortality had been reported as high as 60% but more recently has been estimated at 30% [1]. This decrease in mortality may be due to earlier detection and intervention, [1] although patients often present with subacute nonspecific symptoms that make diagnosis difficult. The mean time from symptom onset to diagnosis is 4 days.

The etiology of gallstone ileus is complex. Chronic inflammation of the gallbladder leads to local irritation of the abdominal viscera. This gallbladder and intestinal inflammation, combined with pressure necrosis from a large gallstone pressing against the gallbladder wall, eventually leads to formation of a fistula between the gallbladder and the intestine. If the gallstone passes through this fistula into the gastrointestinal tract and becomes impacted, it causes a gallstone ileus [3].

Most often, the fistula occurs between the gallbladder and the duodenum given their close proximity. However, the fistula can form between the gallbladder and any other portion of the GI tract, including the stomach and colon, with the former leading to Bouveret's syndrome, which is a gastric outlet obstruction from an impacted gallstone [3].

The most common sites of obstruction are in the terminal ileum and at the ileocecal valve, which are the narrowest segments of intestine. Impactions also occur at sites of pre-existing stricture.

The majority of cases are caused by gallstones greater than 2.5 cm, with large gallstones (>5 cm) especially likely to become impacted and not spontaneously pass [3].

The most reliable means for diagnosing a gallstone ileus is computerized tomography (CT), which outperforms both plain films and ultrasound and has a 93% sensitivity [3, 4]. The classic radiographic findings of pneumobilia, ectopic stone, and obstructed bowel form Rigler's triad, which is found in 15% of abdominal plain films of gallstone ileus and 78% of CTs [2, 4]. Abdominal ultrasonography may show the impacted stone and demonstrate the location of the fistula, but it provides less information than CT. Ultrasound is not the imaging of choice for gallstone ileus [4].

Figure 61.1 shows a gallstone ileus visualized by CT

Timely surgical consultation for stone removal is necessary for patients with suspected or confirmed gallstone ileus. While small gallstones may pass spontaneously, stones larger than 2.5 cm are less likely to pass and more likely to result in obstruction, requiring removal. Surgical intervention may consist of simple enterolithotomy or an

B. Sloane (✉)
Department of Emergency Medicine, Harbor-UCLA Medical Center, Torrance, CA, USA

A. Wu
Department of Emergency Medicine, David Geffen School of Medicine at UCLA, Harbor-UCLA Medical Center, Torrance, CA, USA
e-mail: awu@emedharbor.edu

© Springer Nature Switzerland AG 2019
A. Graham, D. J. Carlberg (eds.), *Gastrointestinal Emergencies*, https://doi.org/10.1007/978-3-319-98343-1_61

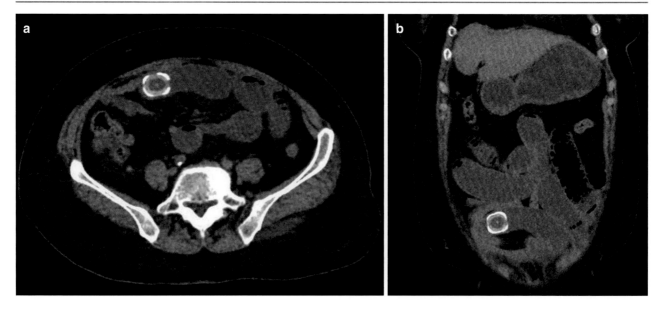

Fig. 61.1 Axial (**a**) and coronal (**b**) CT images of a gallstone ileus caused by a large gallstone impacted in the distal small bowel

enterolithotomy and fistula repair [3–5]. Less invasive procedures such as endoscopic retrieval of ectopic gallstones have been performed successfully and may become the treatment of choice in stable, nontoxic patients [3].

Suggested Resources

- Gallstone ileus – causes, symptoms, diagnosis, treatment & pathology. YouTube. Oct 2016. https://www.youtube.com/watch?v=96Cj6SWAOjM
- Gallstone ileus. Emergency Physicians Monthly. May 2012. http://epmonthly.com/article/gallstone-ileus/
- Gallstone ileus. Radiopaedia. https://radiopaedia.org/articles/gallstone-ileus

References

1. Halabi WJ, Kang CY, Ketana N, et al. Surgery for gallstone ileus. Ann Surg. 2014;259(2):329–35. https://doi.org/10.1097/SLA.0b013e31827eefed.
2. Lassandro F, Gagliardi N, Scuderi M, Pinto A, Gatta G, Mazzeo R. Gallstone ileus analysis of radiological findings in 27 patients. Eur J Radiol. 2004;50(1):23–9. https://doi.org/10.1016/j.ejrad.2003.11.011.
3. Nuño-Guzmán CM, Marín-Contreras ME, Figueroa-Sánchez M, Corona JL. Gallstone ileus, clinical presentation, diagnostic and treatment approach. World J Gastrointest Surg. 2016;8(1):65–76. https://doi.org/10.4240/wjgs.v8.i1.65.
4. Ayantunde AA, Agrawal A. Gallstone ileus: diagnosis and management. World J Surg. 2007;31(6):1292–7. https://doi.org/10.1007/s00268-007-9011-9.
5. Ravikumar R, Williams JG. The operative management of gallstone ileus. Ann R Coll Surg Engl. 2010;92(4):279–81. https://doi.org/10.1308/003588410X12664192076377.

What Is Emphysematous Cholecystitis Diagnosis and Management?

62

Manpreet Singh

Emphysematous cholecystitis is a surgical emergency that occurs in 1 in 100 cases of acute cholecystitis [1]. It is the most morbid of cholecystitis entities with a mortality approaching 25% due to gangrene of the gallbladder wall, subsequent perforation, and a resulting release of toxins, inflammatory cells, and bacteria into the intraperitoneal cavity [1].

Typically, emphysematous cholecystitis is missed on the initial presentation because it most often presents in immune-compromised patients with decreased visceral sensation, such as elderly, obese men with uncontrolled diabetes. Thus, the classic presentation is insidious with vague complaints that mislead physicians until rapid progression leads to clinical deterioration and sudden cardiovascular collapse [2].

In emphysematous cholecystitis, gangrene develops in the gallbladder wall, which increases the risk and rate of perforation. Subsequently, perforation results in a release of toxins, inflammatory mediators, and bacteria into the peritoneal cavity.

Emphysematous cholecystitis may be caused by several overlapping, comorbid co-contributing factors [3]:

- Vascular insufficiency from cystic artery occlusion or stenosis, hepatic artery embolization, or endoarteritis obliterans can cause edema of the gallbladder wall due to micro-ischemia. This creates an anaerobic environment that promotes growth of anaerobic bacteria such as *Escherichia coli* and clostridia while also allowing for translocation of bacteria. The edematous gallbladder wall can also become a nidus for other co-infecting bacteria.
- Stagnant bile, caused by poor nutrition or chronic debility, becomes alkalinized, which promotes bacterial growth.
- Obstructing or impacted cholelithiasis can cause local gallbladder wall edema, which can lead to gallbladder wall ischemia, potentially leading to subsequent additional vascular compromise. However, this typically only occurs in those with chronic vasculopathy and is not a common complication of cholelithiasis in those who are otherwise young and healthy.
- Immunecompromise, especially diabetes and old age, increases the risk of emphysematous cholecystitis, but this may not be an independent risk factor once vascular co-morbidities are accounted for.
- Gas-forming bacteria such as clostridia, *Klebsiella*, *Bacteroides fragilis*, and *E. coli* are the most common bacteria associated with emphysematous cholecystitis. These bacteria may infect the gallbladder primarily, causing gas formation and gangrene, subsequently increasing the risk of perforation. These bacteria may also seed an ischemic gallbladder and subsequently cause gangrene and perforation.

Most cases of emphysematous cholecystitis occur in elderly males with underlying diabetes and obesity [4]. Patients tend to be deconditioned and may not mount a febrile response, making diagnosis more challenging. A third of patients with emphysematous cholecystitis may be afebrile

M. Singh
Department of Emergency Medicine, David Geffen School of Medicine at UCLA, Harbor-UCLA Medical Center, Torrance, CA, USA
e-mail: masingh@dhs.lacounty.gov

without localized tenderness, presenting instead with vague, generalized abdominal pain. Thus, the key to diagnosis is a high index of suspicion followed by confirmation of gallbladder emphysema.

Ultrasound is frequently diagnostic, with gas starting in the lumen, progressing into the wall, and then spreading through pericholecystic tissue [5]. Air caused by gas-forming bacteria disperses or scatters sonographic waves so sonographers rely on the dispersion of signal in the gallbladder fossa to make the diagnosis. However, this "nonvisualization of the gall bladder" can also be due to adjacent bowel gas, and, thus, false negatives are not uncommon [5]. Although ultrasound has a high specificity for emphysematous cholecystitis, the rate of false negatives gives it a low sensitivity. Therefore, negative ultrasound exams should be followed by further imaging in patients at risk for emphysematous cholecystitis [5, 6].

Computed tomography is a useful diagnostic test for emphysematous cholecystitis because it easily identifies air in the gallbladder and gallbladder wall, differentiates adjacent bowel gas from intra-biliary gas, and often identifies precipitating causes such as vascular occlusion. [7, 8] Furthermore, computed tomography can better identify complications of emphysematous cholecystitis such as perforation, local abscess formation, and concomitant pyelonephritis or hepatitis.

Treatment for emphysematous cholecystitis is similar to treatment for acalculous cholecystitis, discussed in Chap. 59 of this textbook. Cholecystectomy is the definitive treatment [6], but may not be preferred in poor surgical candidates. In these cases, percutaneous and endoscopic alternatives should be considered [9].

Suggested Resources
- Bennett GL, Balthazar EJ. Ultrasound and CT evaluation of emergent gallbladder pathology. Radiol Clin N Am. 2003;41(6):1203–16.
- Chuang C, Hsieh H, Wu H, et al. Management of emphysematous cholecystitis. Chir Gastroenterol. 2007;23:75–8.

References

1. Mentzer RM Jr, Golden GT, Chandler JG, et al. A comparative appraisal of emphysematous cholecystitis. Am J Surg. 1975;129(1):10–5.
2. Gill KS, Chapman AH, Weston MJ. The changing face of emphysematous cholecystitis. Br J Radiol. 1997;70(838):986–91.
3. Garcia-Sancho Tellez L, Rodriguez-Montes JA, Fernandez de Lis S, Garcia-Sancho Martin L. Acute emphysematous cholecystitis. Report of twenty cases. Hepatogastroenterology. 1999;46(28):2144–8.
4. Lorenz RW, Steffen HM. Emphysematous cholecystitis: diagnostic problems and differential diagnosis of gallbladder gas accumulations. Hepatogastroenterology. 1990;37(Suppl 2):103–6.
5. Bloom RA, Libson E, Lebensart PD, et al. The ultrasound spectrum of emphysematous cholecystitis. J Clin Ultrasound. 1989;17(4):251–6.
6. Chuang C, Hsieh H, Wu H, et al. Management of emphysematous cholecystitis. Chir Gastroenterol. 2007;23:75–8.
7. Andreu J, Perez C, Caceres J, Llauger J, Palmer J. Computed tomography as the method of choice in the diagnosis of emphysematous cholecystitis. Gastrointest Radiol. 1987;12(4):315–8. [Medline]
8. Bennett GL, Balthazar EJ. Ultrasound and CT evaluation of emergent gallbladder pathology. Radiol Clin North Am. 2003;41(6):1203–16.
9. Slot WB, Ooms HW, Van der Werf SD, et al. Percutaneous gallbladder drainage in emphysematous cholecystitis. Neth J Med. 1995;46(2):86–9.

Acute Cholecystitis in the Elderly Patient: How Is It Different?

63

Andrea J. Hladik and Matthias Barden

Pearls and Pitfalls
- The diagnosis of acute cholecystitis, while common in elderly patients, is often missed on initial presentation, and treatment may be delayed.
- A high index of suspicion and a broad differential diagnosis should be employed when evaluating elderly patients with vague complaints.
- Computed tomography may be the better initial test in evaluating these patients.
- Once the diagnosis is made, treatment is dependent on the patient's overall condition and comorbidities. Initial cholecystostomy with drain placement may be advantageous over immediate surgical intervention in some patients.

The "classic" presentation of acute cholecystitis includes right upper quadrant abdominal pain with nausea, vomiting, and fever. Elderly patients commonly present atypically with vague and nonspecific symptoms; therefore, providers should approach this population with a high index of suspicion [1]. Elderly patients with abdominal pain experience greater morbidity than their younger counterparts, with a higher rate of admission (up to one-half) and a greater need for surgical intervention (one-third of those admitted) [2, 3].

The incidence of cholecystitis increases with age due to an increased prevalence of gallstones, increased lithogenicity of bile, and reduced gallbladder motility. Complications, such as acalculous cholecystitis, emphysematous cholecystitis, and gallbladder perforation, are more likely in elderly patients, and mortality rates are higher [2]. The greater morbidity and mortality among the elderly are due in part to an increased prevalence of comorbid diseases [4].

A. J. Hladik (✉) · M. Barden
Department of Emergency Medicine, Eisenhower Medical Center,
Rancho Mirage, CA, USA
e-mail: ahladikpotz@emc.org

Elderly patients with acute cholecystitis are harder to diagnose because.

1. Differences in pain perception can lead to delays in seeking medical care.
2. Physiologic changes of aging and the use of a polypharmacy may lead to fewer vital sign abnormalities.
3. Vomiting, leukocytosis, and a positive Murphy's sign occur less frequently [5].

Due to the limitations of the physical exam and laboratory testing in the elderly, providers should take a more aggressive approach with imaging. The American College of Radiology recommends ultrasound (US) as the most appropriate diagnostic modality in patients with right upper quadrant pain [1], but computed tomography (CT) is indicated in the evaluation of nonspecific abdominal pain and, therefore, may be the more appropriate initial imaging modality in elderly patients. While US is more sensitive and specific for determining the presence of gallstones, CT is more sensitive for detecting gallbladder wall thickening, pericholecystic fluid, pneumobilia, and gall bladder perforation [6, 7]. It can also demonstrate ductal dilation [7] and often helps identify alternate diagnoses.

The geriatric population has the same morbidity and mortality as the general population for symptomatic cholelithiasis without concurrent infection when treated with elective, outpatient cholecystectomy [8]. However, elderly patients with acute cholecystitis have an increased morbidity and mortality when undergoing cholecystectomy compared to the general population [8]. Thus, elderly patients found to have gallstones may benefit more from undergoing expedited/semi-elective surgery before complications such as acute cholecystitis develop [8].

Elderly patients with acute cholecystitis should have intravenous antibiotics initiated upon diagnosis and receive early surgical consultation. While the definitive treatment for acute cholecystitis is cholecystectomy (typically laparoscopic), it is associated with increased morbidity and mortality in the elderly, the severely ill, and those with significant comorbidities [4, 5, 9]. Thus, some favor a less invasive initial approach with intravenous antibiotics +/− either percutaneous cholecystostomy or endoscopic intervention [10–12]. After antimicrobial treatment and gallbladder decompression, poor surgical candidates can be optimized for delayed or interval cholecystectomy. Optimal timing and management strategies remain controversial [13].

Suggested Resources
- Abdominal pain in the elderly. EM:RAP C3 Project. Sept 2012. https://www.emrap.org/episode/september2012/c3project1
- Cholangitis: deadly cause of right upper quadrant abdominal pain. emDocs. Feb 2016. http://www.emdocs.net/cholangitis-deadly-cause-of-right-upper-quadrant-abdominal-pain/
- Geriatric gastroenterology: series #19 – Billiary disease in the elderly. Practical gastroenterology. Sept 2008. http://www.practicalgastro.com/pdf/September08/ShahArticle.pdf

References

1. Ozeki M, Takeda Y, Morita H, et al. Acute cholecystitis mimicking or accompanying cardiovascular disease among Japanese patients hospitalized in a hospital Cardiology Department. BMC Res Notes. 2015;8:805.
2. Leuthauser A, McVane B. Abdominal pain in the geriatric patient. Emerg Med Clin N Am. 2016;34:363–75.
3. Magidson PD, Martinez JP. Abdominal pain in the geriatric patient. Emerg Med Clin N Am. 2016;34:559–74.
4. Zhang ZM, Liu Z, Liu LM, et al. Therapeutic experience of 289 elderly patients with biliary diseases. World J Gastroenterol. 2017;23:2424–34.
5. Spangler R, Van Pham T, Khoujah D, et al. Abdominal emergencies in the geriatric patient. Int J Emerg Med. 2014;7:43.
6. Fagenholz PJ. Computed tomography is more sensitive than ultrasound for the diagnosis of acute cholecystitis. Surg Infect. 2015;16:509–12.
7. Pinto A, Reginelli A, Cagini L, et al. Accuracy of ultrasonography in the diagnosis of acute calculous cholecystitis: review of the literature. Crit Ultrasound J. 2013;5:S11.
8. Hsieh YC, Chen CK, Su CW, et al. Outcome after percutaneous cholecystostomy for acute cholecystitis: a single-center experience. J Gastrointest Surg. 2012;16:1860–8.
9. Lee SI, Na BG, Yoo YS, et al. Clinical outcome for laparoscopic cholecystectomy in extremely elderly patients. Ann Surg Treat Res. 2015;88:145–51.
10. Venara A, Carretier V, Lebigot J, Lermite E. Technique and indications of percutaneous cholecystostomy in the management of cholecystitis in 2014. J Visc Surg. 2014;151:435–9.
11. Lee S, Park DH, Hwang CY, et al. EUS-guided transmural cholecystostomy as rescue management for acute cholecystitis in elderly or high-risk patients: a prospective feasibility study. Gastrointest Endosc. 2007;66:1008–12.
12. Cherng N, Witkowski ET, Sneider EB, et al. Use of cholecystostomy tubes in the management of patients with primary diagnosis of acute cholecystitis. J Am Coll Surg. 2012;214:196–201.
13. Wang CH, Wu CY, Yang JCT, et al. Long-term outcomes of patients with acute cholecystitis after successful percutaneous cholecystostomy treatment and the risk factors for recurrence: a decade experience at a single center. PLoS One. 2016;11:e0148017.

Consultant Corner: Gallbladder Disease

64

Robert Riviello and Timothy Jang

Pearls and Pitfalls

- Symptomatic cholelithiasis, cholecystitis, choledocholithiasis, and cholangitis overlap in presentation but are managed differently, requiring accurate diagnosis.
- Etiologies such as hepatitis, cirrhosis, Fitz-Hugh-Curtis syndrome, decompensated heart failure, chronic AIDS, and cholangiocarcinoma can cause symptoms, laboratory abnormalities, and radiographic findings similar to biliary disease. Emergent surgery in these patients is generally not indicated and risks significant complications.
- Lactated Ringer's solution should be considered in place of normal saline for patients with an anion gap, low bicarbonate, or low pH.
- Comorbid conditions must often be managed before surgery can be safely pursued.

Introduction

Robert Riviello, MD, MPH, is an Assistant Professor of Surgery and an Assistant Professor of Global Health and Social Medicine at the Harvard University School of Medicine. He practices at Brigham and Women's Hospital in Boston, MA, where he is an acute care and burn surgeon. Dr. Riviello is board certified in general surgery and in surgical critical care. Brigham and Women's Hospital is a large, urban tertiary referral hospital.

R. Riviello
Harvard University School of Medicine, Brigham and Women's Hospital, Boston, MA, USA
e-mail: rriviello@bwh.harvard.edu

T. Jang (✉)
Harbor-UCLA Medical Center, David Geffen School of Medicine at UCLA, Torrance, CA, USA
e-mail: tbj@g.ucla.edu

Answers to Key Clinical Questions

1. What concepts do you think are key to managing a patient with acute biliary disease?

Patients with acute biliary disease (which includes diseases of the gallbladder and biliary tree) who require surgery may rapidly develop sepsis and decompensate. Local inflammation or obstruction of the biliary tree can become a nidus for infection that can form local abscesses, spread to the liver and surrounding structures, and cause ascending infection with systemic consequences of sepsis and shock.

Patients with acute biliary disease often present with upper abdominal pain, nausea, and vomiting. However, the exact cause of their symptoms can vary. Symptomatic cholelithiasis, though painful for the patient, does not require emergent intervention. Cholelithiasis, however, is the most common cause of cholecystitis and cholangitis, which often present similarly but have significantly greater morbidity and mortality. Likewise, cholelithiasis can cause pancreatitis and small bowel obstruction (commonly called gallstone ileus), important extra-biliary complications that require additional care to avoid further morbidity.

Thus, the first step in optimizing these patients is accurate diagnosis. Since these causes of acute pain overlap in presentation, appropriate laboratory evaluation and radiographic imaging are essential.

2. What pearls can you offer emergency care providers when evaluating a patient with acute biliary disease?

Unfortunately, other etiologies such as hepatitis, cirrhosis, Fitz-Hugh-Curtis syndrome, decompensated heart failure, chronic AIDS, and cholangiocarcinoma can cause symptoms, laboratory abnormalities, and radiographic findings similar to biliary disease. Emergent surgery in these patients with biliary disease mimics is generally not indicated and risks significant complications. Thus, clinicians must consider laboratory and radiographic abnormalities in light of these possible diagnostic alternatives.

© Springer Nature Switzerland AG 2019
A. Graham, D. J. Carlberg (eds.), *Gastrointestinal Emergencies*, https://doi.org/10.1007/978-3-319-98343-1_64

3. How should I approach volume resuscitation in the systemically ill patient with acute biliary disease?

Since patients with acute biliary disease typically present after several days of worsening symptoms, they are often hypovolemic due to oral intolerance and possibly vomiting. Thus, volume resuscitation should be considered in all such patients, including those with congestive heart failure and end-stage renal disease. Appropriate fluid administration helps clear a metabolic acidosis and is essential for maintaining appropriate tissue perfusion.

Most patients should be given a 20 mL/kg bolus of an isotonic crystalloid solution unless they also have overt signs of fluid overload due to their comorbid conditions. Following this initial bolus, they should be reassessed and given additional fluids until they are clinically euvolemic and able to maintain an adequate urine output.

The choice of resuscitative fluids should be made judiciously. Normal saline (NS) has a pH of 5.0 and osmolarity of 308 mOsm/L, so patients receiving large volumes of NS develop a metabolic acidosis, which has been associated with increased morbidity in critically ill patients. Lactated Ringer's (LR) solution, on the other hand, has a pH of 6.5 and is hypo-osmolar (272 mOsm/L) and is considered a "balanced fluid" because it has the same level of bicarbonate as plasma [1]. Thus, LR should be considered in place of NS for patients with an anion gap, low bicarbonate, or low pH. LR administration has been associated with improved outcomes in some patients. In a pig model, LR was associated with improved acid clearance and hemodynamics [1]. Conversely, the use of NS rather than a balanced fluid like LR is associated with worsened acidosis, increased acute kidney injury, the need for renal replacement therapy, worsened mortality, increased postoperative complications, and the need for hemodialysis [2–5].

4. How do I optimize a patient's antibiotic regimen in acute biliary disease?

Antibiotics should be administered in all patients with suspected infection and all who may require urgent interventional or surgical procedures. Ascending infection causing sepsis can be rapidly fatal, and timely antibiotic administration is essential for minimizing morbidity. The most common bacteria of the biliary tree are the gram-negative anaerobes *Escherichia coli* and *Klebsiella pneumoniae* [6, 7]. Thus, common treatment regimens include metronidazole with a second- or third-generation cephalosporin or a fluoroquinolone. However, *Bacteroides fragilis* is also a common coinfecting bacteria, and ESBL-producing organisms are becoming increasingly common, necessitating broad-spectrum antibiotic coverage that may include piperacillin/tazobactam, tigecycline, or meropenem [6, 7].

5. When is an initial interventional radiology or endoscopic approach superior to an initial surgical approach for acute biliary disease?

Although surgical care is often required for definitive management, immediate surgery is not the treatment of choice in every case. Cholangitis, for example, is often better treated with endoscopic or percutaneous drainage for sepsis source control, followed by delayed cholecystectomy. Likewise, many patients with gallstone pancreatitis will improve with endoscopic treatment and can undergo delayed cholecystectomy.

6. What comorbidities place patients at high risk for surgical management of acute biliary disease, and how can the emergency provider help optimize these?

Surgical outcomes improve when patient comorbidities are optimally managed. Gastrointestinal surgery is associated with a moderate cardiac risk [8], which can be worse in the critically ill and is often higher in at-risk populations such as the elderly and deconditioned. Unfortunately, patients with complicated diseases such as acalculous cholecystitis, emphysematous cholecystitis, and gallstone pancreatitis are more likely to have cardiac comorbidities. This requires emergency providers to both consider treatment alternatives (e.g., percutaneous drainage) and consider which medications to continue or avoid. For example, diuretics are generally contraindicated due to the risk of intraoperative hypovolemia, but continuing beta-blockers has been associated with fewer dysrhythmias.

Other common and important comorbidities to address include diabetes, renal insufficiency, and pulmonary disease.

Hyperglycemia should be managed as severe hyperglycemia can diminish immune function and worsen metabolic derangements, increasing the risk of morbid complications.

Renal insufficiency should be addressed as uremia, acidosis, and poor renal clearance can impact the postoperative course.

Pulmonary disease should especially be addressed as impaired oxygen delivery is associated with worse outcomes [9].

While this management is often deferred to the primary admitting team, patients who remain in the emergency care setting while awaiting final disposition and/or an inpatient bed will need to have these conditions addressed to prevent delays in care.

Suggested Resources

- Bochwerg B, Alhazzani W, Sindi A, et al. Fluid resuscitation in sepsis: a systematic review and network meta-analysis. Ann Intern Med. 2014;161:347–55.
- Sartelli M, VIale P, Koike K, Pea F, Tumietto F, vanGoor H, et al. WSES consensus conference: guidelines for first-line management of intra-abdominal infections. World J Emerg Surg. 2011;6:2.
- Yunos NM, Bellomo R, Hegarty C. Association between a chloride-liberal vs. chloride-restrictive intravenous fluid administration strategy and kidney injury in critically ill adults. JAMA. 2012;255:821–9.

References

1. Martini WZ, Cortez DS, Dubick MA. Comparisons of normal saline and lactated ringer's resuscitation on hemodynamics, metabolic response, and coagulation in pigs after severe hemorrhagic shock. Scand J Trauma Resusc Emerg Med. 2013;21:86.

2. Lobo DN, Awad S. Should chloride-rich crystalloids remain the mainstay of fluid resuscitation to prevent "pre-renal" acute kidney injury? Kidney Int. 2014;86:1096–105.
3. Yunos NM, Bellomo R, Hegarty C. Association between a chloride-liberal vs. chloride-restrictive intravenous fluid administration strategy and kidney injury in critically ill adults. JAMA. 2012;255:821–9.
4. Shaw AD, Bagshaw SM, Goldstein SL, et al. Major complications, mortality, and resource utilization after open abdominal surgery: 0.9% saline compared to plasma-lyte. Ann Surg. 2012;255:821–9.
5. Bochwerg B, Alhazzani W, Sindi A, et al. Fluid resuscitation in sepsis: a systematic review and network meta-analysis. Ann Intern Med. 2014;161:347–55.
6. Fuks D, Cossee C, Regimbeau JM. Antimicrobial therapy in acute calculous cholecystitis. J Visc Surg. 2013;150:3–8.
7. Sartelli M, VIale P, Koike K, Pea F, Tumietto F, vanGoor H, et al. WSES consensus conference: guidelines for first-line management of intra-abdominal infections. World J Emerg Surg. 2011;6:2.
8. Grade M, Quintel M, Ghadimi BM. Standard perioperative management in gastrointestinal surgery. Langenbeck's Arch Surg. 2011;396:591–606.
9. Daveis SJ, Wilson RJT. Preoperative optimization of the high-risk surgical patient. Br J Anaesth. 2004;93:121–8.

How Do I Resuscitate the Crashing Cirrhotic Patient?

65

Krystle Shafer

Pearls and Pitfalls

- Occult gastrointestinal bleeding is frequently a source of shock in cirrhotic patients.
- Coagulopathy should not preclude emergent, life-saving procedures.
- Fungal bacteremia, most commonly from fungal peritonitis, is an important cause of sepsis in cirrhotic patients.
- Diagnostic paracentesis has great utility in septic patients with ascites.
- While these patients are frequently total body fluid overloaded, they are often intravascularly volume deplete and fluid responsive in the acute shock phase.

Pathophysiology

The normal liver contains reticuloendothelial cells, which are crucial for clearing bacteria. When the liver becomes cirrhotic and reticuloendothelial cells decrease, an immune dysfunction syndrome develops with a decreased ability to clear cytokines, bacteria, and endotoxins from the circulation [1]. Thus, cirrhotics are at high risk of developing infection. In fact, infections occur in ~33% of hospitalized patients with cirrhosis and in 45% of hospitalized cirrhotic patients with gastrointestinal hemorrhage [2].

Additionally, hepatic structural changes from cirrhosis result in increased resistance to portal blood flow, which causes portal hypertension [3]. As the portal pressure rises, the venous blood that normally drains into the portal circulation becomes redirected and stagnant, resulting in venous distension. Thus, 50% of patients with cirrhosis will develop varices, which will hemorrhage at a rate of 5–15% annually.

Additionally, endothelial dysfunction resulting from portal hypertension creates arteriolar vasodilation with pooling of blood in the splanchnic system, leading to under-filling in the rest of the body's arterial circulation. Cardiac output increases to compensate for the low arterial blood pressure and reduced splanchnic vascular resistance [4]. The resulting neurohumoral response leads the kidneys to avidly retain sodium and water, which plays a role in the development of ascites [4]. Severe peripheral (non-splanchnic) vasoconstriction develops as the body attempts to maintain arterial blood pressure, leading to less effective filtration by the kidneys. Eventually the renal injury known as hepatorenal syndrome develops.

Slowed intestinal motility and resulting bacterial overgrowth allows for bacterial translocation into ascitic fluid and subsequent spontaneous bacterial peritonitis [1].

All of these physiologic changes should be considered when formulating the differential diagnosis for the acutely ill cirrhotic patient. These patients have a high risk for septic shock, variceal hemorrhage, and renal failure.

Resuscitation

For the undifferentiated liver patient in shock, fluid resuscitation is vital, even with significant peripheral edema and ascites. Although patients may have total body fluid overload, they are generally intravascularly dry in acute shock. This especially holds true in septic and hemorrhagic shock. Providers should take both fluid responsiveness and the patient's baseline blood pressure into account when determining how much volume to provide and when to add vasopressors. There is no role for N-acetylcysteine in resuscitating the crashing cirrhotic patient.

Determining the cause of shock is vital.

Hemorrhagic shock should lead to a quick transition from IV fluids to blood products, with a special focus on reversing coagulopathy. Vitamin K administration has utility in patients

K. Shafer
Department of Emergency Medicine, Critical Care Intensivist, OHICU and MSICU, WellSpan York Hospital, York, PA, USA
e-mail: kshafer@wellspan.org

© Springer Nature Switzerland AG 2019
A. Graham, D. J. Carlberg (eds.), *Gastrointestinal Emergencies*, https://doi.org/10.1007/978-3-319-98343-1_65

with elevated baseline INR. Octreotide or somatostatin bolus and infusion may help reduce portal venous pressure for variceal hemorrhage patients. Combining octreotide or somatostatin with vasopressin has meta-analysis data demonstrating decreased mortality, improved bleeding control, and decreased hospital length of stay in cirrhotic patients with variceal hemorrhage [5]. Prophylactic antibiotics should be given while awaiting endoscopic intervention.

For septic shock, recent studies have demonstrated that cirrhotics should generally receive the same care as noncirrhotics. Antibiotics, fluid administration, vasopressor use, mechanical ventilation, and renal replacement therapies are all the same [6]. However, fungal infections occur with a much higher prevalence in cirrhotics (6.8%) compared to the general population [6]. Fungal cultures should thus be ordered routinely when a diagnostic paracentesis is performed and antifungal treatment should be added empirically to the septic cirrhotic patient who is unresponsive to standard antimicrobial therapy [7]. Cirrhotic patients are more likely to have sepsis-induced adrenal insufficiency [8], and they may be resistant to the vasopressor effects of norepinephrine and vasopressin [4].

Selecting resuscitation fluids for liver patients in septic shock requires careful consideration. Normal saline may pose a risk because its sodium concentration is 154 mEq/L, and many cirrhotic patients are hyponatremic at baseline. Rapidly rising sodium levels (greater than 8 mEq/L within 24 h) risks causing osmotic demyelination syndrome. With lactated ringers, sodium lactate can theoretically accumulate in the patient with severe, acute liver failure, but this has never been demonstrated as unsafe in the medical literature. Balanced crystalloids such as lactated ringers and plasmalyte are increasingly recommended in cirrhotic patients with sepsis due to concerns that unbalanced crystalloids are associated with increased acute kidney injury, increased bleeding risk, and increased mortality [9].

Providers may also choose albumin for the resuscitation of cirrhotic patients. Studies performed in both medical and surgical ICU patients both with and without cirrhosis demonstrated no difference in mortality comparing colloid use versus crystalloid use [10]. Considering the cost difference between the two options, most providers within the United States often choose crystalloids for resuscitation. However, patients with cirrhosis have low albumin levels and arguably third space crystalloids faster than non-cirrhotic patients. Colloids have been demonstrated to have longer intravascular half-lives in comparison to crystalloids [11], and the oncotic pressure difference produced by colloids helps pull third-space fluids from the interstitial space into the intravascular space. This effect is transient, as colloids eventually leave the intravascular space. While using albumin for septic shock in cirrhosis has not been directly studied, using albumin prevents paracentesis-induced

circulatory dysfunction, prevents renal failure in patients with spontaneous bacterial peritonitis, and treats hepatorenal syndrome [4]. Colloid use is thus worth considering as adjunctive therapy for resuscitation in cirrhotic patients.

Finally, many patients with shock require procedural intervention. The baseline thrombocytopenia and elevated INR in cirrhotic patients often results in concerns for bleeding complications. However, this increased bleeding risk has been repeatedly debunked in the medical literature, with no strong evidence to support correcting this coagulopathy before performing a procedure [12]. As a result, it is unclear what INR or platelet count threshold (if any) should spark transfusion prior to a procedure [12]. In emergencies, lifesaving procedures should be performed regardless of platelet count or INR. In the elective setting, the choice for reversal agents depends on the type of procedure, provider comfort, and institutional guidelines.

Suggested Resources
- Al-Khafaji A, Huang DT. Critical care management of patients with end-stage liver disease. Crit Care Med. 2011;39:1157–66.
- Coagulopathy management in the bleeding cirrhotic: seven pearls and one crazy idea. EMCrit. Dec 2015. https://emcrit.org/pulmcrit/coagulopathy-bleeding-cirrhotic-inr/.
- Spontaneous bacterial peritonitis-pearls & pitfalls. emDocs. July 2016. http://www.emdocs.net/spontaneous-bacterial-peritonitis-pearls-pitfalls/.

References

1. Bonnel A, Bunchorntavakul C, Reddy KR. Immune dysfunction and infections in patients with cirrhosis. Clin Gastroenterol Heptaol. 2011;9:727–38.
2. Tandon P, Guadalupe G. Bacterial infections, sepsis, and multiorgan failure in cirrhosis. Semin Liver Dis. 2008;28(1):26–42.
3. García-Pagán JC, Gracia-Sancho J, Bosch J. Functional aspects on the pathophysiology of portal hypertension in cirrhosis. J Hepatol. 2012;57(2):458–61.
4. Polli F, Gattinoni L. Balancing volume resuscitation and ascites management in cirrhosis. Curr Opin Anaesthesol. 2010;23:151–8.
5. Wells M, Chande N, Adams P, et al. Meta-analysis: vasoactive medications for the management of acute variceal bleeds. Aliment Pharmacol Ther. 2012;35(11):1267–78.
6. Galbois A, Aegerter P, Martel-Samb P, et al. Improved prognosis of septic shock in patients with cirrhosis: a multicenter study. Crit Care Med. 2014;42(7):1666–74.
7. Bucsics T, Schwabl P, Mandorfer M, Peck-Radosavljevic M. Prognosis of cirrhotic patients with fungiascites and spontaneous fungal peritonitis. J Hepatol. 2016;64(6):1452–4.
8. Gustot T, Durand F, Lebrec D, Vincent JL, Moreau R. Severe sepsis in cirrhosis. Hepatology. 2009;50(6):2022–33.

9. Correa T, Calvalcanti A, Cesar M. Balanced crystalloids for septic shock resuscitation. Rev Bras Ter Intensiva. 2016;28(4):463–71.

10. Annane D, Siami D, Jaber S, et al. Effects of fluid resuscitation with colloids versus crystalloids on mortality in critically ill patients presenting with hypovolemic shock: the CRISTAL randomized trial. JAMA. 2013;310(17):1809–17.

11. Vercueil A, Grocott M, Mythen M. Physiology, pharmacology, and rationale for colloid administration for the maintenance of effective hemodynamic stability in critically ill patients. Transfus Med Rev. 2005;19:93–109.

12. Van de Weeerdt E, Beimond B, Baake B, Vermin B, Binnekade J, et al. Central venous catheter placement in coagulopathic patients: risk factors and incidence of bleeding complications. Tranfusion. 2017;57(10):2512–25.

How Do I Diagnose and Manage Acute Cholangitis?

66

Jessica Riley, KinWah Chew, and Timothy Jang

> **Pearls and Pitfalls**
> - The diagnosis of acute cholangitis is made by the presence of systemic inflammation plus laboratory findings of cholestasis and/or imaging showing biliary dilation or bile duct obstruction.
> - Antibiotics for acute cholangitis should target common gastrointestinal flora and expand to cover resistant organisms in certain clinical settings.
> - The absence of Charcot's triad or Reynold's pentad should not rule out acute cholangitis.

Acute cholangitis is an infectious process characterized by biliary obstruction leading to cholestasis and increased pressure in the biliary tree, which subsequently allows bacterial ascension and transmission into the venous and lymphatic system. This produces a systemic inflammatory response [1]. Biliary obstruction is caused by biliary stones more than 60% of the time. Other causes include malignancy, obstruction of a preexisting stent, and stent dislodgement [2].

Diagnosis

The 2013 Tokyo Guidelines (TG13) are internationally accepted criteria for diagnosing acute cholangitis and grading its severity [3]. The TG13 are based on three key factors:

J. Riley (✉) · K. Chew
WellSpan York Hospital, Department of Emergency Medicine, York, PA, USA
e-mail: jriley@wellspan.org; kchew@wellspan.org

T. Jang
Harbor-UCLA Medical Center, David Geffen School of Medicine at UCLA, Torrance, CA, USA
e-mail: tbj@g.ucla.edu

1. Signs of systemic inflammation: fever, leukocytosis, and/or elevated C-reactive protein
2. Evidence of cholestasis: jaundice, hyperbilirubinemia, transaminitis, and/or other elevated liver function tests (gamma-glutamyl transferase and alkaline phosphatase)
3. Biliary obstruction: gallstone pancreatitis, biliary dilation, and/or other evidence of obstruction (biliary stent migration on plain radiograph, stricture seen on cholangiopancreatography) [4].

Acute cholangitis should be suspected when there is systemic inflammation and evidence of either cholestasis or biliary obstruction. Acute cholangitis is confirmed when there is systemic inflammation and evidence of both cholestasis and obstruction [4].

A multicenter TG13 validation study conducted in Japan showed a sensitivity of 91.8% and a specificity of 77.7% for acute cholangitis, though the gold standard comparison was not clearly identified [4].

Imaging helps determine the source of biliary obstruction and may identify sequelae of acute cholangitis. Computed tomography (CT) may demonstrate biliary stones, pneumobilia, or mass. It may also find bile duct dilation, wall thickening, obstruction, or stenosis. Noncalcified biliary stones are radiolucent and may require ultrasound or magnetic resonance imaging (MRI) for visualization [4]. Specific identification of inflammation in the biliary tree itself requires specialized dynamic CT or magnetic resonance cholangiopancreatography (MRCP).

In addition to establishing acute cholangitis diagnostic criteria, the TG13 grade disease severity, and this subsequently guides treatment (Table 66.1). Grade 3, the most severe form of acute cholangitis, is associated with significant end-organ dysfunction. Grade 2 identifies individuals at high risk for decompensation and/or disease progression. Grade 1 is mild cholangitis [4].

Hyperbilirubinemia (total bilirubin ≥ 5 mg/dL), coagulopathy (INR ≥ 1.5), and the presence of abscess are associated with a high mortality rate, while an elevated alanine

Table 66.1 Grading of cholangitis severity and associated management [5]

Grade	Findings	Management
Grade 1 – mild	None of the below findings	Antibiotics Supportive care +/− biliary drainage
Grade 2 – moderate	WBC > 12,000/μL WBC < 4000/μL Temperature > 39 °C Age > 75 years Bilirubin > 5 mg/dL Hypoalbuminemia	Antibiotics Supportive care Early biliary drainage
Grade 3 – severe	Vasopressor requirement Altered mental status PaO₂/FiO₂ < 300 Oliguria or creatinine > 2.0 INR > 1.5 Platelet count < 100,000	Antibiotics Supportive care Urgent biliary drainage

WBC white blood cell count, *PaO₂* arterial partial pressure of oxygen, *FiO₂* fraction of inspired oxygen, *INR* international normalized ratio

aminotransferase and leukocytosis predict benefit from early biliary decompression and drainage [4, 6]. Other factors associated with increased morbidity and mortality include:

1. Age ≥75 years old
2. Fever ≥39 °C
3. Hypoalbuminemia
4. Acute renal dysfunction
5. Cardiopulmonary compromise
6. Altered level of consciousness [4]

Charcot's triad (fever, jaundice, and right upper quadrant pain) and Reynold's pentad (Charcot's triad plus altered mental status and hypotension) may aid in the diagnosis of acute cholangitis. However, multiple studies have shown that neither has high sensitivity. A recent review found a sensitivity of 36.3% and a specificity of 93.2% for Charcot's triad, suggesting that, while the presence of Charcot's triad may support a diagnosis of acute cholangitis, its absence does not rule out the disease. Reynold's pentad had an even lower sensitivity for acute cholangitis at 4.82% [7]. The TG13 advise against the use of Charcot's triad when evaluating for acute cholangitis. They note that, in addition to a high false-negative rate, Charcot's triad will identify nearly 12% of acute cholecystitis patients (who do not have concomitant cholangitis) [4].

Management

Cholangitis is frequently complicated by sepsis, and appropriate resuscitation should begin early.

Treatment of acute cholangitis targets the two main components of the disease process: (1) bacterial infection of the biliary tree necessitates systemic antibiotics, and (2) biliary obstruction generally requires decompression. Antibiotics for acute cholangitis help control systemic inflammation and sepsis. They may not sterilize bile [8].

The TG13 provide management guidance for acute cholangitis based on severity (Table 66.1) [5]. Antibiotic selection should target the most commonly identified organisms: gastrointestinal flora. In a recent study, *E. coli* was the most commonly identified organism, followed by several *Klebsiella* species [2]. *Bacteroides fragilis* and other anaerobes have also been implicated [9, 10]. Thus, common treatment regimens include ceftriaxone with metronidazole, ciprofloxacin with metronidazole, and ampicillin/sulbactam [10]. In the critically ill, those with signs of sepsis, and those with high-risk features such as potential hospital-acquired infection, piperacillin/tazobactam is preferred over ceftriaxone and ciprofloxacin [10]. In the setting of risk factors for extended-spectrum beta-lactamase-producing bacteria, some authors recommend tigecycline [10], but meropenem may also be used.

The optimal duration of antibiotic therapy for acute cholangitis is unclear. Current recommendations suggest 4–7 days of antimicrobial treatment after source control is obtained. The TG13 guidelines recommend at least 14 days of treatment when bacteremia is present; however, recent literature suggests that a shorter course of treatment may be equally effective [11].

There are many acceptable approaches to draining the biliary system in acute cholangitis, including endoscopic, percutaneous, and surgical techniques. For cholangitis due to a biliary stone, elective laparoscopic cholecystectomy is recommended [12].

Endoscopic retrograde cholangiopancreatography (ERCP) and image-guided percutaneous drain placement are much more common than surgical techniques and are typically considered first-line treatment [13]. No head-to-head studies have compared ERCP with percutaneous drainage; however, complication rates of hemorrhage and peritonitis are higher with percutaneous treatment. Therefore, if available, ERCP is preferred [13].

The optimal timing of biliary drainage is not fully established. Mild disease can often be treated initially with antibiotics alone, with the obstructive pathology addressed later [5]. While patients with moderate to severe cholangitis require early biliary decompression, the TG13 do not set specific time windows for drainage [5]. One study defined early ERCP to be less than 24 h from admission and found an associated significant reduction in 30-day mortality [14]. Another study found that delays in ERCP, defined as 48 h or more, were associated with a significant increase in length of hospital stay [15]. Further delay to 72 h from admission was associated with increased vasopressor requirement and a possible trend toward increased mortality [15]. Based on this data, biliary drainage within 24 h of hospitalization for moderate to severe cholangitis appears to be a reasonable goal.

ERCP complications include post-ERCP cholangitis (1%), significant bleeding (0.1–0.5%), perforation of the duodenum, bile duct or pancreatic duct (1%), biliary stricture (<8%), and post-ERCP pancreatitis. The incidence of post-ERCP pancreatitis can range from 1% to 15% depending on patient and procedural characteristics [16].

Suggested Resources
- Acute cholangitis. Life in the fast lane. Aug 2014. https://lifeinthefastlane.com/ccc/acute-cholangitis/.
- Afdhal N, Chopra S, Grover S. Acute cholangitis. UpToDate. Mar 2016. https://www.uptodate.com/contents/acute-cholangitis.

References

1. Kiriyama S, Takada T, Hwang T, Akazawa K, Miura F, Gomi H, et al. Clinical application and verification of the TG13 diagnostic and severity grading criteria for acute cholangitis: an international multicenter observational study. J Hepatobiliary Pancreat Sci. 2017;24:329–37.
2. Gomi H, Takada T, Hwang T, Akazawa K, Mori R, Endo I, et al. Updated comprehensive epidemiology, microbiology, and outcomes among patients with acute cholangitis. J Hepatobiliary Pancreat Sci. 2017;24:310–8.
3. Wada K, Takada T, Kawarada Y, Nimura Y, Miura F, Yoshida M, et al. Diagnostic criteria and severity assessment of acute cholangitis: Tokyo guidelines. J Hepato-Biliary-Pancreat Surg. 2007;14:52–8.
4. Kiriyama S, Takada T, Strasberg SM, Solomkin JS, Mayumi T, Pitt HA, et al. TG13 guidelines for diagnosis and severity grading of acute cholangitis. J Hepatobiliary Pancreat Sci. 2013;20:24–34.
5. Miura F, Takada T, Strasberg SM, Solomkin JS, Pitt HA, Gouma DJ. TG13 flowchart for the management of acute cholangitis and cholecystitis. J Hepatobiliary Pancreat Sci. 2013;20:47–54.
6. Salek J, Livote E, Sideridis K, Bank S. Analysis of risk factors predictive of early mortality and urgent ERCP in acute cholangitis. J Clin Gastroenterol. 2009;43:171–5.
7. Rumsey S, Winders J, MacCormick AD. Diagnostic accuracy of Charcot's triad. ANZ J Surg. 2017;87:232–8.
8. Lan Cheong Wah D, Christophi C, Muralidharan V. Acute cholangitis: current concepts. ANZ J Surg. 2017;87:554–9.
9. Fuks D, Cossee C, Regimbeau JM. Antimicrobial therapy in acute calculous cholecystitis. J Visc Surg. 2013;150:3–8.
10. Sartelli M, VIale P, Koike K, Pea F, Tumietto F, vanGoor H, et al. WSES consensus conference: Guidelines for first-line management of intra-acbdominal infections. World J Emerg Surg. 2011;6:2.
11. Uno S, Hase R, Kobayashi M, Shiratori T, Nakaji S, Hirata N, et al. Short-course antimicrobial treatment for acute cholangitis with gram-negative bacillary bacteremia. Int J Infect Dis. 2017;55:81–5.
12. Li V, Yum J, Yeung Y. Optimal timing of elective laparoscopic cholecystectomy after acute cholangitis and subsequent clearance of choledocholithiasis. Am J Surg. 2010;200:483–8.
13. Mosler P. Diagnosis and management of acute cholangitis. Curr Gastroenterol Rep. 2011;13:166–72.
14. Tan M, Schaffalitzky de Muckadell O, Laursen S. Association between early ERCP and mortality in patients with acute cholangitis. Gastrointest Endosc. 2018;87(1):185–92.
15. Hou L, Laine L, Motamedi N, Sahakian A, Lane C, Buxbaum J. Optimal timing of endoscopic retrograde cholangiopancreatography in acute cholangitis. J Clin Gastroenterol. 2017;51:534–8.
16. Szary NM, Al-Kawas FH. Complications of endoscopic retrograde cholangiopancreatography: how to avoid and manage them. Gastroenterol Hepatol (NY). 2013;9:496–504.

How Do I Diagnose and Manage Acute Hepatic Encephalopathy?

Brent A. Becker

Hepatic encephalopathy (HE) represents a clinical state of cerebral dysfunction that occurs in the setting of liver disease and/or portosystemic shunting. It comprises a spectrum of cognitive and behavioral abnormalities ranging from subtle subclinical changes to profound coma [1–3]. The pathophysiology is complex, but in the simplest terms, HE arises from excess ammonia, glutamine, and other neurotoxins in the circulation due to impaired liver metabolic function [4–6]. Subsequent inflammation, oxidative stress, and osmolar gradients lead to neuronal dysfunction and potential brain edema [5–7].

HE classification is based on underlying causes: *A*cute/ fulminant hepatic failure (type A), portosystemic shunting/ *B*ypass (type B), and *C*hronic/cirrhotic liver disease (type C) [1, 7, 8]. Type A confers a greater risk of cerebral edema and increased intracranial pressure (ICP) [8].

B. A. Becker
WellSpan York Hospital, Department of Emergency Medicine,
York, PA, USA
e-mail: bbecker2@wellspan.org

Patients with HE are likely to seek acute medical care. Approximately 20–40% of cirrhotic patients will develop HE at some point and severe HE portends a 1-year mortality greater than 50% [9, 10]. It is essential that emergency providers facilely diagnose and manage HE.

How Do I Diagnose Acute Hepatic Encephalopathy?

The clinical presentation of HE is highly variable and dependent on disease severity. *Covert HE*, also termed minimal HE, is defined as mild neuropsychiatric abnormalities that are clinically undetectable outside of specialized neuropsychological assessment. *Overt HE* refers to patients with perceivable changes to their personality, cognitive abilities, and neurologic function [5–7, 9, 11]. Expert consensus associates *overt HE* with disorientation or asterixis [8, 12].

The West Haven Criteria, shown in Table 67.1, provides a grading system for HE that illustrates the continuum of clinical signs and symptoms [5, 6, 8]. Psychomotor slowing is an early finding, followed by cognitive impairment, sleep-wake cycle disruption, and personality changes [7, 8, 13]. Patients become increasingly disoriented and progress to somnolence, stupor, and coma [7, 8].

Unfortunately, precise staging of HE severity is hampered by the unpredictable order in which features develop in individual patients [5, 8].

Asterixis ("liver flap" or "flapping tremor") is a classic finding in mild-to-moderate HE, although it is not pathognomonic. It is characterized by low amplitude, alternating flexion and extension of the wrists (arrhythmic negative myoclonus) when the patient attempts to hold them in extension. Subtle asterixis can be difficult to perceive visually and may be more easily felt by the examiner [7, 8].

Pupils usually dilate and become less reactive in grades III and IV [5, 13]. Hyperreflexia or hyporeflexia may be present, with the latter being more common as patients become more comatose [8]. Other neurologic findings, such

Table 67.1 Grading of acute hepatic encephalopathy

WHC grade	ISHEN consensus	Clinical features
Minimal	Covert HE	No overt clinical abnormalities
Grade I		Mild unawareness Euphoria or anxiety Shortened attention span Impairment of addition or subtraction Altered sleep rhythm
Grade II	Overt HE	Lethargy or apathy Disorientation for time Obvious personality change Inappropriate behavior Dyspraxia Asterixis
Grade III		Somnolence to stupor Responsive to stimuli Confusion Gross disorientation Bizarre behavior
Grade IV		Coma

Modified from Ref. [8]

HE hepatic encephalopathy, *ISHEN* International Society for Hepatic Encephalopathy and Nitrogen Metabolism, *WHC* West Haven Criteria

Table 67.2 Precipitating factors for acute hepatic encephalopathy

Infection/inflammation	Constipation
Gastrointestinal bleeding	Surgery
Dehydration/overdiuresis	TIPS
Electrolyte disorders	Alcohol/benzodiazepines
Noncompliance with secondary prophylaxis	Other psychoactive drugs
	Withdrawal syndromes

TIPS transjugular intrahepatic portosystemic shunt

as upgoing Babinski reflex or gaze deviation, can be seen in more severe HE; however, these are generally transient and typically resolve as hyperammonemia corrects, even in cases of decerebrate and decorticate posturing [5, 7, 11, 13].

HE rarely causes overt seizures. When they do occur, seizures most frequently present in cases of acute liver failure (type A) with more significant cerebral edema. Generalized seizures in HE usually suggest a separate pathologic process; however, subclinical seizures may occur in up to 15% of severe HE cases and often go underrecognized [7, 8, 13].

The overall likelihood of HE relates to the degree of underlying liver insufficiency and portosystemic shunting, but myriad conditions can significantly increase this risk (Table 67.2) [8]. Infection, gastrointestinal (GI) bleeding, electrolyte disorders, dehydration, and constipation are among the most common precipitants of acute HE; however, the cause for decompensation in some patients remains unidentified [7–9, 11]. Patients with transjugular intrahepatic portosystemic shunt (TIPS) placement are at particularly high risk for HE, with a 10–50% median 1-year incidence following the procedure [14].

Altered mental status in the patient with liver insufficiency confers a vast differential diagnosis, shown in

Table 67.3 Differential diagnosis for acute hepatic encephalopathy (non-exhaustive)

Category	Diagnosis
Drugs/toxins	Alcohol/benzodiazepine intoxication or withdrawal Metronidazole encephalopathy Opioids/other psychoactive drugs Neuroleptics Wernicke's encephalopathy/other micronutrient deficiency
Endocrine	Hypoglycemia Thyroid dysfunction
Infection	Encephalitis Meningitis Sepsis from any source
Metabolic	Hyperosmolar states Ketoacidosis Electrolyte disorders (hyponatremia, hypercalcemia)
Neurologic	Central pontine myelinolysis Cerebral hypoperfusion Dementia Intracranial bleeding Neoplasm Nonconvulsive seizures/postictal state Normal pressure hydrocephalus Stroke Wilson's disease
Psychiatric	Depression Psychosis
Respiratory	Hypoxemia Obstructive sleep apnea

Table 67.3. Acute HE remains largely a diagnosis of exclusion and rigorous evaluation is often required to evaluate for alternate etiologies [8, 9, 15].

Elevated serum ammonia is classically associated with acute HE, but higher levels do not necessarily correlate with greater clinical severity or worse prognosis in chronic liver disease patients. In these patients, acute HE is possible even with normal serum ammonia levels [5, 11, 16]. Conversely, a serum ammonia concentration above 150–200 µmol/L in acute liver failure is associated with an increased risk of cerebral edema and elevated ICP [5, 11].

Additional laboratory testing is vital in assessing for alternate causes of cognitive and neurologic dysfunction, such as hypoglycemia, electrolyte derangements, acute renal insufficiency, thyroid dysfunction, and toxic exposures [11, 13].

Infectious workup should be directed by clinical symptoms and might include blood cultures, chest radiography, lumbar puncture, paracentesis, *Clostridium difficile* screening, and urinalysis [11, 13].

Neuroimaging is frequently warranted in patients with suspected acute HE to assess for cerebral edema and other intracranial pathology. While imaging might be deferred in patients with a history of HE and a typical presentation, neuroimaging is generally indicated in patients with a first-time episode of HE, focal neurologic findings, trauma, severe/worsening symptoms, or failure to improve with adequate HE treatment [7, 8]. Computed tomography (CT) is typically the first-line modality given its speed, availability, and capability to detect acute bleeding; however, CT is relatively insensitive for the subtle changes seen in early cerebral edema. Magnetic resonance imaging (MRI) or invasive ICP monitoring should be considered if clinical suspicion is high [11, 13].

Electroencephalography (EEG) is typically abnormal in acute HE, but findings are nonspecific and generally not useful in establishing the diagnosis [7, 8, 13]. Currently, the role of EEG in HE is mainly limited to evaluating for suspected subclinical seizures [5, 7].

How Do I Manage Acute Hepatic Encephalopathy?

The initial treatment of acute HE parallels that of any patient with altered mental status, including assessment and management of the airway, breathing, and circulation. Patients with evidence of cerebral edema should receive standard management strategies for increased ICP [5, 11, 15]. It is critical to identify and correct precipitating factors, as patients often improve significantly with reversal of the underlying condition alone [7–9].

Lactulose, a nonabsorbable disaccharide, is considered first-line empiric treatment for acute HE. Recommended initial oral dosing is 20 mL every hour until a bowel movement is achieved, followed by a reduction to standard dosing of 20–30 mL every 8–12 h, titrated to 2–3 soft or loose bowel movements daily [5, 7, 8, 15, 17]. A naso-/orogastric tube can be used in obtunded patients, although rectal lactulose (300 mL in 700 mL of saline) is often recommended in severe HE (grade III/IV). Providers should observe for complications of therapy, including aspiration, dehydration, and electrolyte disturbances [8, 11, 18].

Rifaximin, a nonabsorbed semisynthetic antibiotic, provides a beneficial adjunct to lactulose therapy. Standard oral dosing is 550 mg twice daily. Dual treatment with lactulose and rifaximin appears more effective than lactulose alone, although there is no evidence for rifaximin monotherapy [5, 7, 8, 11, 17, 19]. Neomycin and metronidazole are alternative choices, but rifaximin is currently the preferred antibiotic due to greater tolerability and safety [6–8, 11, 19].

Many adjunctive therapies for HE are the subjects of ongoing study, including oral branched-chain amino acids (BCAA), intravenous L-ornithine-L-aspartate (LOLA), probiotics, polyethylene glycol, flumazenil, zinc, and others. None are widely used due to limited, preliminary, or scant evidence [6, 8, 9, 17, 19].

Invasive options for severe disease that fails to respond to medical treatment include continuous venovenous hemofiltration, albumin dialysis with a molecular adsorbent recirculating system (MARS), and percutaneous embolization of large portosystemic shunts; however, the roles of these therapies lack consensus [7, 9, 11, 15, 17, 19].

Liver transplantation remains the only definitive treatment for refractory HE [7, 11].

Disposition of patients with acute HE depends on the severity of symptoms and the social support system available. While a majority of patients will require hospitalization, those with minor symptoms, an identified and correctable precipitating condition, and reliable follow up can be considered for discharge [20]. All patients with HE should remain on lactulose prophylaxis and be referred to gastroenterology or hepatology if specialty care has not already been established. Referral to palliative care should be considered in patients with advanced liver disease, recurrent episodes of HE, and/or life expectancy of less than 1 year [7, 8]. Patients with prior episodes of acute HE will likely benefit from adding rifaximin to their regimen [5, 7–9, 17].

Suggested Resources
- American Association for the Study of Liver and European Association for the Study of the Liver Diseases. Hepatic encephalopathy in chronic liver disease: 2014 practice guideline by the European Association for the Study of the Liver and the American Association for the Study of Liver Diseases. J Hepatol. 2014;61:642–59.
- Wijdicks EF. Hepatic encephalopathy. N Engl J Med. 2016;375:1660–70.
- Swaminathan A (2015) Episode 24.0: hepatic encephalopathy. CORE EM. Available at https://coreem.net/podcast/episode-24-0-hepatic-encephalopathy/. Accessed Feb 21 2018.

References

1. Ferenci P, Lockwood A, Mullen K, Tarter R, Weissenborn K, Blei AT. Hepatic encephalopathy--definition, nomenclature, diagnosis, and quantification: final report of the working party at the 11th world congresses of gastroenterology, Vienna, 1998. Hepatology. 2002;35:716–21.
2. Cordoba J. New assessment of hepatic encephalopathy. J Hepatol. 2011;54:1030–40.
3. Weissenborn K, Ennen JC, Schomerus H, Ruckert N, Hecker H. Neuropsychological characterization of hepatic encephalopathy. J Hepatol. 2001;34:768–73.
4. Oja SS, Saransaari P, Korpi ER. Neurotoxicity of Ammonia. Neurochem Res. 2017;42:713–20.
5. Wijdicks EF. Hepatic encephalopathy. N Engl J Med. 2016;375:1660–70.

6. Hadjihambi A, Arias N, Sheikh M, Jalan R. Hepatic encephalopathy: a critical current review. Hepatol Int. 2018;12:135–47.
7. Ellul MA, Gholkar SA, Cross TJ. Hepatic encephalopathy due to liver cirrhosis. BMJ. 2015;351:h4187.
8. American Association for the Study of Liver and European Association for the Study of the Liver Diseases. Hepatic encephalopathy in chronic liver disease: 2014 practice guideline by the European Association for the Study of the Liver and the American Association for the Study of Liver Diseases. J Hepatol. 2014;61:642–59.
9. Shawcross DL, Dunk AA, Jalan R, Kircheis G, de Knegt RJ, Laleman W, et al. How to diagnose and manage hepatic encephalopathy: a consensus statement on roles and responsibilities beyond the liver specialist. Eur J Gastroenterol Hepatol. 2016;28:146–52.
10. Jepsen P, Ott P, Andersen PK, Sorensen HT, Vilstrup H. Clinical course of alcoholic liver cirrhosis: a Danish population-based cohort study. Hepatology. 2010;51:1675–82.
11. Kandiah PA, Kumar G. Hepatic encephalopathy-the old and the new. Crit Care Clin. 2016;32:311–29.
12. Bajaj JS, Cordoba J, Mullen KD, Amodio P, Shawcross DL, Butterworth RF, et al. Review article: the design of clinical trials in hepatic encephalopathy--an International Society for Hepatic Encephalopathy and Nitrogen Metabolism (ISHEN) consensus statement. Aliment Pharmacol Ther. 2011;33:739–47.
13. Datar S, Wijdicks EF. Neurologic manifestations of acute liver failure. Handb Clin Neurol. 2014;120:645–59.
14. Bai M, Qi X, Yang Z, Yin Z, Nie Y, Yuan S, et al. Predictors of hepatic encephalopathy after transjugular intrahepatic portosystemic shunt in cirrhotic patients: a systematic review. J Gastroenterol Hepatol. 2011;26:943–51.
15. Nadim MK, Durand F, Kellum JA, Levitsky J, O'Leary JG, Karvellas CJ, et al. Management of the critically ill patient with cirrhosis: a multidisciplinary perspective. J Hepatol. 2016;64:717–35.
16. Arora S, Martin CL, Herbert M. Myth: interpretation of a single ammonia level in patients with chronic liver disease can confirm or rule out hepatic encephalopathy. CJEM. 2006;8:433–5.
17. Fukui H, Saito H, Ueno Y, Uto H, Obara K, Sakaida I, et al. Evidence-based clinical practice guidelines for liver cirrhosis 2015. J Gastroenterol. 2016;51:629–50.
18. Patidar KR, Bajaj JS. Covert and overt hepatic encephalopathy: diagnosis and management. Clin Gastroenterol Hepatol. 2015;13:2048–61.
19. Suraweera D, Sundaram V, Saab S. Evaluation and management of hepatic encephalopathy: current status and future directions. Gut Liver. 2016;10:509–19.
20. Marx JA, Hockberger RS, Walls RM, Adams J, Rosen P. Rosen's emergency medicine: concepts and clinical practice. 7th ed. Philadelphia: Mosby/Elsevier; 2010.

What Do I Need to Know About Primary Sclerosing Cholangitis and Primary Biliary Cirrhosis?

68

Bob Stuntz

Pearls and Pitfalls
- Primary sclerosing cholangitis is a rare idiopathic fibrotic condition with a male predominance that leads to intra- and extrahepatic biliary strictures. It is strongly associated with inflammatory bowel disease.
- Primary biliary cirrhosis is a rare autoimmune condition with a strong female predominance leading to destruction of the cells lining intrahepatic bile ducts.
- Both conditions can lead to cirrhosis. Additionally, primary sclerosing cholangitis has a strong association with cholangiocarcinoma and colorectal cancer.
- Treatment of cholestatic pruritus leads to improved quality of life and should be approached in a stepwise fashion.

Table 68.1 Differentiation between primary sclerosing cholangitis (PSC) and primary biliary cirrhosis (PBC) [1–4]

	PSC	PBC
Age and gender	30s–40s, predominantly male	Middle age, predominantly female
Site of pathogenesis	Intra- and extrahepatic biliary system	Intrahepatic biliary system
Cause of pathogenesis	Fibrosis and stricture formation	Autoimmune destruction of cells lining intrahepatic bile ducts
Diagnostic buzzwords	Beaded appearance on ERCP/MRCP	Antimitochondrial antibodies (AMA)
Associated conditions	Inflammatory bowel disease	Other autoimmune conditions
Complications	Cirrhosis, cholangiocarcinoma, and colorectal cancer	Cirrhosis

ERCP endoscopic retrograde cholangiopancreatography, *MRCP* magnetic resonance cholangiopancreatography

Primary sclerosing cholangitis (PSC) and primary biliary cirrhosis (now more commonly referred to as primary biliary cholangitis (PBC)) are both rare progressive disorders that ultimately lead to cirrhosis [1, 2]. Table 68.1 summarizes features of the two conditions.

Primary Sclerosing Cholangitis

PSC is an idiopathic fibrotic condition with a variable history: some patients suffer from an aggressive progression, while others may have long symptom-free periods [3]. It is defined by both intra- and extrahepatic bile duct fibrosis, which leads to beading and stricture formation and causes the characteristic beaded appearance of bile ducts on endoscopic or magnetic resonance cholangiopancreatography. These strictures lead to recurrent biliary obstruction and cholangitis. Hallmarks of PSC include its episodic nature and the fact that episodes cannot be attributed to any other cause. PSC may lead to end-stage liver disease [3, 4].

PSC is a rare condition, with a prevalence of between 0.4 and 2 per 100,000 patients in the United States. There is a strong association between PSC and inflammatory bowel disease (IBD), as PSC occurs in up to 8% of IBD patients. PSC is typically seen in males between 30 and 40 years of age [3, 4]. Up to 25% will have a concomitant unrelated autoimmune disorder [4].

Primary Biliary Cirrhosis

PBC is an autoimmune disease in which antimitochondrial antibodies attack the cells lining the intrahepatic bile ducts, leading to cholestasis. PBC may occur concomitantly

B. Stuntz
Department of Emergency Medicine, WellSpan York Hospital, York, PA, USA
e-mail: rstuntz@wellspan.org

© Springer Nature Switzerland AG 2019
A. Graham, D. J. Carlberg (eds.), *Gastrointestinal Emergencies*, https://doi.org/10.1007/978-3-319-98343-1_68

with other autoimmune disorders [1]. While prevalence varies widely, it is highest in the United States with 402 cases per million inhabitants. It is ten times more common in women [1].

Diagnosis

Both PSC and PBC are unlikely to be diagnosed in the acute care setting, as both require multimodal diagnostic approaches, including studies likely unavailable to emergency providers. Other causes of cholestasis, including inflammatory, toxic, infectious, and obstructive, should be excluded with imaging and laboratory evaluation. Patients may present with symptoms of cholestasis, including pruritus, jaundice, and cholangitis. Laboratory evaluation of liver enzymes will likely show an obstructive pattern.

The acute care provider should evaluate for a history of recurrent episodes of cholestasis or a history of previous episodes without definite causes, especially in patients with known IBD or other autoimmune disorders. This may help create diagnostic momentum when patients are admitted for further workup and treatment.

Management

Both conditions lack definitive chronic treatment, and both may lead to cirrhosis and require liver transplant [1, 4]. Patients with new cirrhosis, acute cholangitis, or other acute complications should be treated in the standard fashion.

Pruritus secondary to cholestasis can be seen in either condition, but it is more common in PBC [1]. These patients will complain of pruritus that is not associated with any dermatologic changes. Scratching does not tend to relieve symptoms [5]. Treatment of pruritus in patients with PBC is important to quality of life and should progress in a stepwise fashion. Initial treatment with bile acid resins, most commonly cholestyramine, is recommended. Rifampicin can be added in those who do not respond to cholestyramine. Naltrexone can be considered if these treatments fail, as endogenous opioids likely play some role in the pathogenesis of pruritus. Sertraline may help in non-responders. Liver transplant is the ultimate treatment for patients who have failed the above therapies [5].

Because PSC confers a high risk of cholangiocarcinoma and colorectal cancer, these conditions should be considered in patients with PSC and symptoms suggestive of malignancy [4].

In patients with end-stage PSC or PBC, clinicians should evaluate for and treat complications or sequelae of cirrhosis, including hepatic encephalopathy, spontaneous bacterial peritonitis, and gastrointestinal bleeding.

Suggested Resources
- Karlsen T, Folserias T, Thorburn D, Vesterhus M. Primary sclerosing cholangitis – a comprehensive review. J Hepatol. 2017;67:1298–323.
- Lleo A, Marzorati S, Anaya J, Gershwin M. Primary biliary cholangitis: a comprehensive overview. Hepatol Int. 2017;11:485–99.

References

1. Lleo A, Marzorati S, Anaya J, Gershwin M. Primary biliary cholangitis: a comprehensive overview. Hepatol Int. 2017;11:485–99.
2. Williamson K, Chapman R. Primary sclerosing cholangitis: a clinical update. Br Med Bull. 2015;114:53–64.
3. Lindor K, Kowdley K, Harrison M. ACG clinical guideline: primary sclerosing cholangitis. Am J Gastroenterol. 2015;110:646–59.
4. Karlsen T, Folserias T, Thorburn D, Vesterhus M. Primary Sclerosing cholangitis – a comprehensive review. J Hepatol. 2017;67:1298–323.
5. Hegade V, Bolier R, Elferink R, Beurs U, Kendrick S, Jones D. A systematic approach to the management of cholestatic pruritus in primary biliary cirrhosis. Frontline Gastroenterol. 2016;7:158–66.

When Does Transaminitis Become Acute Hepatic Failure? What Is the Management of Transaminitis and Acute Hepatic Failure?

Michelle A. Hieger

Pearls and Pitfalls
- Acute liver failure is a common pathway for many conditions and insults, leading to massive hepatic necrosis and/or loss of normal hepatic function.
- Transaminases can be elevated secondary to many intra- and extrahepatic causes.
- The level of transaminitis should not be the sole determinant in management and disposition.
- Patients with acute liver failure should be considered for early transfer to a liver transplant center, ideally prior to elevation in intracranial pressure or the development of severe coagulopathy.

When Does Transaminitis Become Acute Hepatic Failure?

Transaminases (aspartate aminotransferase (AST) and alanine aminotransferase (ALT)) are frequently obtained in the acute care setting [1–3]. Non-toxicological causes of elevated transaminases include infection, ischemia, metabolic derangement, malignancy, autoimmune disease, and primary graft failure after transplant [1].

Acute Hepatic Failure

Non-toxicological causes of acute liver failure are listed in Table 69.1 [1]. Toxicological causes of acute liver failure are listed in Table 69.2 [1]. Viral hepatitis is the most common cause of acute liver failure worldwide, while acetaminophen is the most common cause of acute liver failure in the United States [3]. Acute liver failure is a common pathway for many conditions and insults, leading to massive hepatic necrosis and/or loss of normal hepatic function.

Acute liver failure can be classified into subgroups by acuity of encephalopathy. Hyperacute liver failure is encephalopathy within 1 week of jaundice onset. Acute liver failure is encephalopathy within 8–28 days of jaundice onset. Subacute liver failure is encephalopathy within 5–12 weeks of jaundice onset [4, 5].

Complications

Each subgroup has its own set of complications. Hyperacute and acute liver failure have an increased incidence of cerebral edema, but hyperacute liver failure patients are more likely to survive with supportive care, and acute liver failure patients are more likely to die without liver transplant. Subacute liver failure patients have increased mortality, less cerebral edema, and increased likelihood of portal hypertension, leading to ascites and renal failure [5].

Other complications from acute liver failure include [5]:

- Bleeding (including exsanguination)
- Cardiovascular derangements
- Pulmonary and ventilatory derangements
- Central nervous system dysfunction (temperature dysregulation causing hypothermia, disruption of the blood-brain barrier, and increased intracranial pressure leading to encephalopathy)
- Metabolic derangements
- Infection

The higher the number of complications, the more likely the patient will not survive [1].

Overall, outcomes have improved due to earlier identification of causes, earlier initiation of treatment, improved intensive care, and improved transplant science. Formerly, mortality was 55–95%, and now mortality is 30–40% [4, 6].

M. A. Hieger
Section of Toxicology, Department of Emergency Medicine, WellSpan Health, York Hospital, York, PA, USA
e-mail: mhieger@wellspan.org

Table 69.1 Non-toxicological causes of acute liver failure[a]

Infection	Ischemia	Metabolic derangements	Malignancy	Autoimmune problems	Primary graft failure after transplant
Viral hepatitis (hepatitis A&E most common)	Disruption of portal vein or hepatic artery	Acute fatty liver of pregnancy	Any malignancy causing obstruction or liver damage	Autoimmune hepatitis	Liver transplant failure
Herpes simplex, EBV, varicella zoster, CMV, parvovirus (usually immunocompromised if acute liver failure occurs from these)	Prolonged hypotension (overdose, cardiac arrest, intraoperative, AMI, PE)	HELLP syndrome			
Rare: *Coxiella burnetii*, *Plasmodium falciparum*, amebic abscesses, disseminated TB, *Bacillus cereus*	Veno-occlusive disease (chemotherapy or bone marrow transplant related)	Reye's syndrome			
	Budd-Chiari syndrome	Wilson's disease			
	Exertional heat stroke				

EBV Epstein-Barr virus, *CMV* cytomegalovirus, *TB* tuberculosis, *AMI* acute myocardial infarction, *PE* pulmonary embolism, *HELLP* hemolysis, elevated liver enzymes, low platelets

[a]Not an all-inclusive list

Table 69.2 Toxicological causes of acute liver failure[a]

Pharmaceuticals	Drugs of abuse	Chemicals	Biologic agents
Acetaminophen	Cocaine	CCl₄	Sea anemone sting
Rare/idiosyncratic/unpredictable (valproic acid, troglitazone, amiodarone)	MDMA	Chloroform	Mushrooms (cyclopeptides)
Hypersensitivity reactions (phenytoin, para-aminosalicylate, chlorpromazine, sulfonamides)	PCP	Halothane	
Halogenated anesthetics (enflurane, methoxyflurane, isoflurane, halothane): toxic hepatitis, rare FHF	TCE (inhaled)	Cleaning solvents with fluorinated or halogenated hydrocarbons	
NSAIDs: sulindac, diclofenac	Toluene (inhaled)		
Macrolides (erythromycin, clarithromycin): cholestasis, rare hepatic necrosis	Ethanol		
Other medications: aspirin, amoxicillin-clavulanate, azathioprine, infliximab, carbamazepine, captopril, tetracycline, zidovudine, dantrolene, herbal meds (kava), dapsone, diltiazem, statins, methimazole, MAOIs, methotrexate, nitrofurantoin, TCAs, phenothiazines, gold, propylthiouracil, isoniazid, rifampin, ketoconazole, methyldopa			

FHF fulminant hepatic failure, *NSAIDs* nonsteroidal anti-inflammatory drugs, *MAOIs* monoamine oxidase inhibitors, *TCAs* tricyclic antidepressants, *MDMA* 3,4-methylenedioxymethamphetamine, *PCP* phencyclidine, *TCE* trichloroethylene

[a]Not an all-inclusive list

Laboratory Abnormalities

Liver failure generally results in laboratory abnormalities beyond transaminitis. Blood work in acute liver failure may show [1, 7]:

- Synthetic dysfunction, which is usually the first sign of impending liver failure – decreased albumin and clotting factor levels, increased coagulation profiles
- Defects in gluconeogenesis – decreased serum glucose
- Worsening toxicant metabolism – increased ammonia
- Decreased hepatic excretory function – increased bilirubin
- Decreased renal function – elevated creatinine from prerenal azotemia, acute tubular necrosis, and/or hepatorenal syndrome

Table 69.3 reviews the utility of labs, imaging, and other ancillary tests in the evaluation of potential acute hepatic failure [1, 3, 8].

Non-hepatic Transaminitis

In the appropriate clinical setting, elevations in AST and ALT should prompt the clinician to consider rhabdomyolysis

Table 69.3 Initial diagnostic testing in fulminant hepatic failure

Parameter	Rationale
Electrolytes and minerals	Imbalances are common. Abnormalities can cause arrhythmias and worsen encephalopathy. Hypophosphatemia is common in acetaminophen overdose
BUN/creatinine	Renal failure is frequent and affects management and prognosis. Etiology (e.g., toxic effect of ingested substances) may alter therapy (e.g., hemodialysis)
Glucose	Hypoglycemia is common and can produce permanent neurologic sequelae
CBC with platelets	Assess for sepsis (leukocytosis), GI bleeding (anemia), and risk of hemorrhage (thrombocytopenia)
Liver profile	Assess for degree of damage and follow course of illness. Elevated transaminases are generally due to hepatocyte damage. Increase in alkaline phosphatase is usually due to cholestasis or biliary obstruction. Increased bilirubin with indirect/direct can guide differential
Ammonia	Increased in hepatic metabolic failure. Poor prognosis if significantly increased in fulminant hepatic failure
Coagulation profile	Serve as prognostic indicators (protime, factor V level) and assess risk of hemorrhage
Arterial blood gases	Prognostic significance (lactic acidosis). Derangements are common
Blood group	Preparation for transplantation. Type and crossmatch in anticipation of bleeding
Toxicology, virology, autoimmune panel, ceruloplasmin, medication history	Etiology affects management (e.g., NAC for acetaminophen, charcoal for *Amanita*) and prognosis
Blood and urine cultures	Surveillance for sepsis; aggressive treatment warranted if positive
ECG	May affect management. Preparation for transplantation
Chest radiograph	Sepsis surveillance. Evaluate for ARDS and pulmonary edema
Abdominal ultrasound	Evaluate for vascular thrombosis and infection. Preparation for transplantation
Intracranial pressure	Assess ICP if stage III–IV encephalopathy present. Cerebral edema is the most common cause of death

ARDS adult respiratory distress syndrome, *BUN* blood urea nitrogen, *CBC* complete blood count, *ECG* electrocardiogram, *ALF* acute liver failure, *GI* gastrointestinal, *ICP* intracranial pressure, *NAC* N-acetylcysteine, *PT* prothrombin time

Table 69.4 Stages of clinical hepatic encephalopathy

Stage	Level of consciousness	Neuromuscular changes	Behavioral/intellectual changes
I	Reversal of sleep pattern Mild confusion	Mild asterixis Impaired handwriting	Euphoria/depression Short-term memory lapses
II	Slow responses Increasing drowsiness	Asterixis/ataxia Slurred speech	Inappropriate behavior Loss of time/amnesia
III	Disorientation Somnolence	Rigidity/spasticity Loss of continence	Stuporous/incoherent Marked confusion/paranoia
IV A/B	Comatose A: Responds to pain B: No response to pain	Decorticate/decerebrate posturing Hyperreflexic	Comatose

and order a creatinine kinase level. Rhabdomyolysis-induced transaminitis occurs secondary to AST (and some ALT) release from muscle breakdown. In the past, ALT was considered liver-specific, but ALT elevations may occur in patients with myopathy but no liver disease [9]. Hypoperfusion from other medical issues can lead to transaminitis as well.

Prognostication

The King's College Criteria is used to determine potential for liver transplant in both acetaminophen toxicity and other causes of acute liver failure.

The King's College Criteria for acetaminophen toxicity suggests transplant if [4, 10]:

- pH <7.3 (irrespective of other factors)
- Grade III–IV encephalopathy (Table 69.4) *and* protime >100 s *and* serum creatinine >3.4 mg/dL

The King's College Criteria for non-acetaminophen toxicity suggests transplant if [4, 10]:

- PT >35 s
- INR >7.7
- Any three of the following:
  - Age <10 or >40 years old
  - Unfavorable etiology (non-A and non-B hepatitis, idiosyncratic drug reaction, halothane hepatitis, Wilson's disease)

- Serum bilirubin >17 mg/dL
- Time from jaundice to encephalopathy >7 days
- INR >4

The Acute Physiology and Chronic Health Evaluation III Score (APACHE III Score) may also identify those in need of liver transplant [11].

What Is the Management of Transaminitis and Acute Hepatic Failure?

Transaminitis

Initial management of acute transaminitis includes fluid resuscitation, pain management, and nausea management. Generally, the cause of transaminitis will determine treatment and disposition. Transaminase values alone do not determine disposition. Admission is recommended for higher-risk (elderly and pregnant) patients or when there is no response or poor response to supportive care. It is also recommended for bilirubin ≥20 mg/dL, PT >50% above normal, hypoglycemia, spontaneous bacterial peritonitis, new or worsening hepatic encephalopathy, hepatorenal syndrome, or coagulopathy with bleeding. Additionally, the patient should be admitted if the he or she cannot ambulate safely or if there is an unsafe home condition. Any patient with acetaminophen toxicity (using the Rumack-Matthew nomogram) should be admitted, even if the transaminases and coagulation factors are normal [8].

Acute Hepatic Failure

Patients with acute liver failure should be considered for early transfer to a liver transplant center, ideally prior to intracranial pressure elevation or development of severe coagulopathy [1]. Prophylactic treatment of coagulopathy is unnecessary. Fresh frozen plasma or factor VII should be given if there is active bleeding or before invasive procedures [12]. Patients with grade IV encephalopathy generally require intubation. Providers should elevate the head of bed to 10–20 ° and consider avoiding positive end-expiratory pressure if possible (grade III recommendation) [13]. With cerebral edema, intracranial pressure monitoring and decompression may be necessary.

Antidotes and Specific Treatments

Specific antidotes exist for acetaminophen toxicity (n-acetylcysteine) and for *Amanita* mushroom poisoning (silibinin and intravenous penicillin G). Shock liver will improve with the restoration of perfusion. Herpes causing transaminitis can be treated with acyclovir. Acute Budd-

Chiari syndrome (thrombosis of the hepatic veins) can be treated with transjugular intrahepatic portosystemic shunt (TIPS), surgical decompression, or thrombolysis. Autoimmune hepatitis can be treated with steroids. Idiosyncratic drug-induced transaminitis can be treated with withdrawal of the drug. Rechallenge of the drug should not be performed unless there is no alternate therapy [1].

Suggested Resources

- Interpretation of liver function tests. (2013). http://www.oscestop.com/LFT_interpretation.pdf.
- Bernal W, Wendon J. Acute liver failure. N Engl J Med. 2013;369:2525–34.
- Farkas S, Hackl C, Schlitt HJ. Overview of the indications and contraindications for liver transplantation. Cold Spring Harb Perspect Med. 2014;4

References

1. Dalhoff K. Toxicant-induced hepatic failure. In: Brent J, et al., editors. Critical care toxicology. Cham: Springer International Publishing; 2016. p. 385–408.
2. Moore P, Burkhart K. Adverse drug reactions in the ICU. In: Brent J, et al., editors. Critical care toxicology. Cham: Springer International Publishing; 2016. p. 693–741.
3. Aghababian RV. Essentials of emergency medicine. Hepatitis. Sudbury: Jones & Bartlett Learning; 2010.
4. O'Grady JG, et al. Early indicators of prognosis in fulminant hepatic failure. Gastroenterology. 1989;97(2):439–45.
5. O'Grady JG, Schalm SW, Williams R. Acute liver failure: redefining the syndromes. Lancet. 1993;342(8866):273–5.
6. Murali AR, Narayanan Menon KV (2017) Acute liver failure [cited 4 Mar 2018]; Available from: http://www.clevelandclinicmeded.com/medicalpubs/diseasemanagement/hepatology/acute-liver-failure/.
7. O'Grady JG, Williams R. Management of acute liver failure. Schweiz Med Wochenschr. 1986;116(17):541–4.
8. Susan R, O'Mara KG. Hepatic disorders. In: Tintinalli JE, et al., editors. Tintinalli's emergency medicine: a comprehensive study guide. New York: McGraw-Hill Education. p. 525–33.
9. Delaney KA. Hepatic principles. In: Hoffman RS, editor. Goldfrank's toxicologic emergencies. New York: McGraw-Hill Education. p. 302–11.
10. McPhail MJ, Wendon JA, Bernal W. Meta-analysis of performance of Kings's college hospital criteria in prediction of outcome in non-paracetamol-induced acute liver failure. J Hepatol. 2010;53(3):492–9.
11. Fikatas P, et al. APACHE III score is superior to King's college hospital criteria, MELD score and APACHE II score to predict outcomes after liver transplantation for acute liver failure. Transplant Proc. 2013;45(6):2295–301.
12. Shami VM, et al. Recombinant activated factor VII for coagulopathy in fulminant hepatic failure compared with conventional therapy. Liver Transpl. 2003;9(2):138–43.
13. Muñoz SJ. Difficult management problems in fulminant hepatic failure. In: Seminars in liver disease. New York: Thieme Medical Publishers; 1993.

How Should I Image the Patient with Suspected Liver or Biliary Disease?

70

Thompson Kehrl, Mark Collin, and Timothy Jang

Pearls and Pitfalls
- Right upper quadrant (RUQ) pain is often best initially imaged with ultrasound (US), and US has very good accuracy for cholelithiasis.
- If US is negative or nondiagnostic, computed tomography has utility in assessing for potential etiologies.
- As with any test, US risks false-positive and false-negative results.

Patients with right upper quadrant (RUQ) pain frequently present for emergency care. Although gallbladder pathology and biliary pathology generally reside at the top of the differential diagnosis in many of these patients, other important diagnoses must be considered, and clinicians frequently turn to imaging to supplement laboratory workup. The American College of Radiology lists ultrasound (US) as the initial test of choice for all of the clinical scenarios presented in its Appropriateness Criteria for the evaluation of patients with RUQ pain [1].

US is the preferred first-line imaging because:

1. It is relatively inexpensive when compared to computed tomography (CT), cholescintigraphy, and magnetic resonance imaging (MRI).
2. It does not deliver ionizing radiation.
3. It does not require contrast administration.
4. It can be completed at the bedside by emergency physicians with comparable accuracy to radiology-performed US [2].

Gallbladder and Biliary Pathology

When evaluating specifically for gallbladder and biliary pathology, with minimal concern for other etiologies of RUQ pain, US is especially useful. Physical exam and laboratory testing lack the sensitivity and specificity to accurately diagnose biliary disease [3]. US is better at visualizing gallstones than CT and cholescintigraphy. In addition to detecting gallstones, US can detect ductal dilation, gallbladder polyps, biliary carcinoma, and pneumobilia.

Choledocholithiasis and Cholecystitis

US is the optimal test in the acute evaluation for gallbladder pathology. It helps evaluate for gallstones, gallbladder sludge, gallbladder distension and wall thickening, pericholecystic fluid, and a sonographic Murphy's sign. US interpretation may be challenging in certain cases, and supplementation with CT and/or cholescintigraphy may be useful.

An abnormal US may not correlate with acute clinical disease for patients with certain comorbid conditions. For example, gallbladder wall thickening, which is suggestive of acute cholecystitis, can also be seen in chronic cholecystitis, AIDS, cirrhosis, ascites, pancreatitis, chronic right-sided heart failure, and hepatitis [4]. Likewise, pericholecystic

T. Kehrl (✉) · M. Collin
Section of Emergency Ultrasound, York Hospital Emergency Ultrasound Fellowship, York Hospital Emergency Medicine Residency, York Hospital Department of Emergency Medicine, York, PA, USA
e-mail: tkehrl@wellspan.org; mcollin6@wellspan.org

T. Jang
Harbor-UCLA Medical Center, David Geffen School of Medicine at UCLA, Torrance, CA, USA
e-mail: tbj@g.ucla.edu

© Springer Nature Switzerland AG 2019
A. Graham, D. J. Carlberg (eds.), *Gastrointestinal Emergencies*, https://doi.org/10.1007/978-3-319-98343-1_70

fluid, another sign of acute cholecystitis, can also be seen in hepatitis, pancreatitis, ascites, AIDS, Fitzgerald-Hugh-Curtis syndrome, adjacent colitis, and hepatic abscess [4]. Many of these patients are also likely to have baseline laboratory abnormalities, making it difficult to diagnose acute cholecystitis based on laboratory findings and US results.

Choledocholithiasis

Evaluation for choledocholithiasis can be challenging in the acute care setting. RUQ US is insensitive for common bile duct (CBD) stones, with sensitivities ranging from 22 to 75%, mainly due to limitations from overlying bowel gas [5, 6]. Specificity is higher at 91% [7]. Figure 70.1 shows a CBD stone on US. Measurement of the CBD is typically performed during RUQ US, and dilation of the CBD (>6 mm) is potentially suggestive of choledocholithiasis. The CBD also dilates with age and after cholecystectomy [8].

Most retained CBD stones after cholecystectomy tend to present within a few years after surgery [9]. CT is generally the preferred imaging modality to evaluate RUQ pain after cholecystectomy [10].

Magnetic resonance cholangiopancreatography (MRCP) is highly sensitive for choledocholithiasis but is generally not immediately available in the acute setting.

Cholangitis

Cholangitis usually results from biliary stasis and obstruction of the biliary tree, frequently by biliary calculi [11]. Diagnosis and evaluation of suspected cholangitis is chal-lenging and frequently requires imaging. US, CT, and MRCP all play a role, but US and CT have the most utility in the acute setting.

Liver Pathology

There are a number of important non-biliary liver-related diseases to consider in the acute evaluation of RUQ pain.

Budd-Chiari syndrome (thrombosis of the hepatic veins) is best assessed by RUQ US with Doppler of the hepatic venous circulation.

Portal vein thrombosis is caused by a number of different diseases and occurs in up to 15% of patients with cirrhosis. RUQ US with Doppler of the portal venous system assesses for portal vein thrombosis [12].

Hepatitis may be caused by many disease processes, and imaging is generally performed to evaluate for potential causes of hepatitis or complications thereof.

Pyogenic liver abscess, shown in Fig. 70.2, is the most common type of visceral abscess and can be evaluated with either US or CT [13].

Imaging Modalities

Ultrasound

US is the preferred first-line imaging modality for RUQ pain; however, other imaging modalities may have utility in evaluating RUQ pain as well.

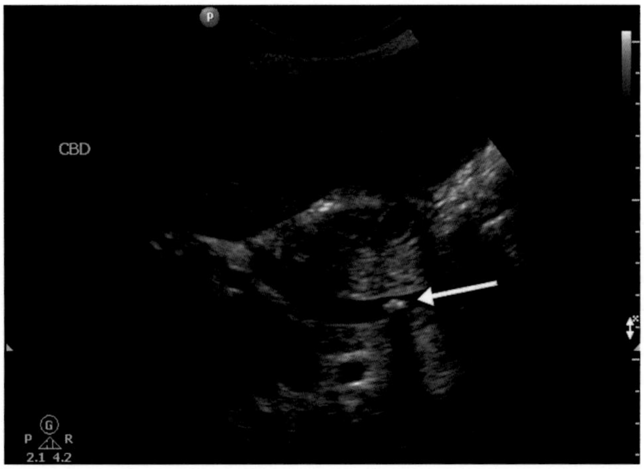

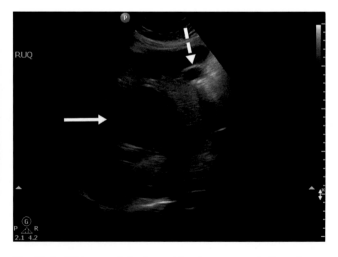

Fig. 70.1 US image of the common bile duct with a strongly echogenic stone noted in the lumen of the duct (arrow) with dense shadowing noted posterior to the stone

Fig. 70.2 US image of the liver with a large pyogenic liver abscess (arrow). Note the complex internal echoes. The gallbladder is noted in near-field (dashed arrow)

Computed Tomography

CT can be performed in patients difficult to ultrasound due to habitus and is better for diagnosing gallbladder and biliary complications such as pneumobilia, gallstone pancreatitis, gallstone ileus, emphysematous cholecystitis, gallbladder abscess, cholecystoenteric fistula, and gallbladder perforation. It also evaluates for other etiologies of abdominal pain that can mimic biliary disease, including right-sided diverticulitis, transverse colitis, gastric perforation, ureterolithiasis, and abdominal aortic aneurysm.

Some consider CT the primary imaging modality in all elderly patients with suspected biliary disease and those with increased risk for biliary complications [14].

Unfortunately, many patients with comorbid diseases (e.g., chronic pancreatitis, hepatitis, congestive heart failure, and AIDS) have chronic CT findings that mimic cholecystitis, including gallbladder wall thickening and pericholecystic fluid.

Furthermore, CT has several disadvantages compared to US, including:

1. Lower sensitivity for cholelithiasis [15]
2. Increased cost
3. Exposure to ionizing radiation
4. Potential need for intravenous contrast to improve accuracy

Cholescintigraphy

When US and/or CT findings are equivocal or the patient's etiology of symptoms remains unclear due to underlying comorbid conditions (e.g., ascites or hepatitis), many clinicians consider cholescintigraphy, also known as a HIDA (hepatobiliary iminodiacetic acid) scan, as their next step. Non-visualization of the gallbladder during the first phase of this test has a sensitivity of 96% and specificity of 90% for acute cholecystitis [16]. Abnormal emptying of the gallbladder in the second phase is associated with chronic acalculous cholecystitis as well as sphincter of Oddi dysfunction and predicts those most likely to benefit from cholecystectomy [17, 18]. More importantly, those with normal filling but abnormal emptying rarely require emergent surgery. However, HIDA requires ionizing radiation, takes up to four hours to perform, and does not evaluate for as many alternative diagnoses as CT and MRI. HIDA is discussed further in Chap. 58 of this book.

Magnetic Resonance Imaging

MRI is comparable to US for diagnosing acute cholecystitis, [16] can be done in patients difficult to ultrasound due to habitus, and has better diagnostic accuracy for detecting CBD stones when MRCP is performed [19]. MRI can also be utilized in patients with equivocal ultrasounds when attempting to minimize radiation (e.g., children and pregnant women). However, MRI and MRCP are not commonly done in the acute setting due to increased cost, lack of availability, and increased study time.

Suggested Resources
- Biliary colic mimics: what you don't want to miss. emDocs. June 2017. http://www.emdocs.net/biliary-colic-mimics-dont-want-miss/.
- Missiroli C, Singh A. Emergencies of the biliary tract. In: Singh A, editor. Emergency radiology: imaging of acute pathologies. New York: Springer Science; 2013. p. 11–25.
- Cirrhosis. Radiopedia. https://radiopaedia.org/articles/cirrhosis.

References

1. Yarmish GM, Smith MP, Rosen MP, et al. ACR appropriateness criteria right upper quadrant pain. J Am Coll Radiol. 2014;11:316–22.
2. Ross M, Brown M, McLaughlin K, Atkinson P, Thompson J, Powelson S, Clark S, Lang E. Emergency physician-performed ultrasound to diagnose cholelithiasis: a systemic review. Acad Emerg Med. 2011;18:227–35.
3. Jain A, Mehta N, Secko M, Schechter J, Papanagnou D, Pandya S, Sinert R. History, physical examination, laboratory testing, and emergency department. Ultrasonography for the diagnosis of acute cholecystitis. Acad Emerg Med. 2017;24(3):281–97.
4. Bisset RA, Khan AN. Differential diagnosis in abdominal ultrasound, vol. 202. Long: WB Saunders. p. 159–80.
5. Scott MA, Farrands PA, Guyer PB, et al. Ultrasound of the common bile duct in patients undergoing cholecystectomy. J Clin Ultrasound. 1991;19:73–6.
6. Dong B, Chen M. Improved sonographic visualization of choledocholithiasis. J Clin Ultrasound. 1987;15:185–90.
7. Gurusamy KD, Giljaca V, Takwoingi Y, et al. Ultrasound versus liver function tests for diagnosis of common bile duct stones. Cochrane Database Syst Rev. 2015;2:1–57.
8. Lal N, Mehra S, Lal V. Ultrasonographic measurement of normal common bile duct diameter and its correlation with age, sex and anthropometry. J Clin Diagn Res. 2014;8:AC01–4.
9. Lee DH, Ahn YJ, Lee HW, et al. Prevalence and characteristics of clinically significant retained common bile duct stones after

laparoscopic cholecystectomy for symptomatic cholelithiasis. Ann Surg Treat Res. 2016;91:239–46.

10. Thurley PD, Dhingsa R. Laparoscopic cholecystectomy: post-operative imaging. Am J Roentgenol. 2008;191:794–801.

11. Kimura Y, Takada T, Kawarada Y, et al. Definitions, pathophysiology, and epidemiology of acute cholangitis and cholecystitis: Tokyo guidelines. J Hepato-Biliary-Pancreat Surg. 2007;14:15–26.

12. Amitrano L, Guardascione MA, Brancaccio V, et al. Risk factors and clinical presentation of portal vein thrombosis in patients with liver cirrhosis. J Hepatol. 2004;40:736–41.

13. Altemeier WA, Culbertson WR, Fullen WD, et al. Intra-abdominal abscesses. Am J Surg. 1973;125:70–9.

14. Bloom AA, Remy P. Emphysematous cholecystitis. Medscape 2015 https://emedicine.medscape.com/article/173885. Accessed 20 Dec 2017.

15. Paulson EK. Acute cholecystitis: CT findings. Semin Ultrasound CT MR. 2000;21:56–63.

16. Kiewiet JJ, Leeuwenburgh MM, Bipat S, Bossuyt PM, Stoker J, Boermeester MA. A systematic review and meta-analysis of diagnostic performance of imaging in acute cholecystitis. Radiology. 2012;264:708–20.

17. Sorenson MK, Fancher S, Lang NP, Eidt JF, Broadwater JR. Abnormal gallbladder nuclear ejection fraction predicts success of cholecystectomy in patients with biliary dyskinesia. Am J Surg. 1993;166:672–4.

18. Mahid SS, Jafri NS, Brangers BC, Minor KS, Hornung CA, Galandiuk S. Meta-analysis of cholecystectomy in symptomatic patients with positive hepatobiliary iminodiacetic acid scan results without gallstones. Arch Surg. 2009;144:180–7.

19. Aube C, Delorme B, Yzet T, et al. MR cholangiopancreatography versus endoscopic sonography in suspected common bile duct lithiasis: a prospective, comparative study. Am J Roentgenol. 2005;184:55–62.

What About Point-of-Care Ultrasound for Right Upper Quadrant Pain? What Do I Need to Know About Image Interpretation?

Mark Collin and Thompson Kehrl

Pearls and Pitfalls
- Point-of-care ultrasound (PoCUS) allows the provider with the best understanding of the clinical picture to interpret the imaging study.
- Other benefits include cost savings and throughput improvements.
- Training is not onerous, and, once providers are trained, PoCUS compares favorably to other diagnostic imaging studies for identifying biliary pathology.
- The clinical context, including physical exam and laboratory values, must always be kept in mind. PoCUS may help guide the provider to a diagnosis, but a false negative PoCUS is also possible.

What About Point-of-Care Ultrasound for Right Upper Quadrant Pain?

Point-of-care ultrasound (PoCUS) (as opposed to radiology-performed ultrasound (US)) is part of the emergency care provider's toolset for evaluating right upper quadrant (RUQ) abdominal pain.

Benefits of PoCUS for biliary pathology have been enumerated in the literature, including [1–4]:

1. Significantly reduced length of stay, particularly during radiology off-hours
2. Reduced cost
3. Increased confidence in the medical competence of the provider performing PoCUS by patients
4. Accuracy comparable to both radiology-performed studies and pathology reports when PoCUS is performed by trained emergency physicians

Ultrasound is both scanner and reader-dependent, adding a layer of complexity to the study that is often overlooked. The traditional imaging model uses the technologist as the image obtainer and the radiologist as the image interpreter. PoCUS combines these two roles. Additionally, PoCUS places imaging in the hands of the clinician with direct patient care experience. Unlike a radiologist, the provider performing PoCUS has evaluated the patient and is therefore in a position to interpret the study in the context of the clinical presentation.

Barriers to POCUS

Real and perceived barriers may hinder use of RUQ PoCUS.

The training barrier is relatively low. Teaching clinicians to perform RUQ PoCUS is fairly straightforward, and one can become competent after performing and interpreting as few as 25 scans [5].

Another barrier is the expense of ultrasound equipment purchase and upkeep [6], but this may be defrayed over time by billing for PoCUS and by improved patient throughput times.

Avoiding RUQ PoCUS because of concerns about missing clinically significant extra-biliary pathology may be an overly cautious approach due to the low prevalence and frequently benign nature of these findings [7].

M. Collin (✉) · T. Kehrl
Section of Emergency Ultrasound, York Hospital Emergency Ultrasound Fellowship, York Hospital Emergency Medicine Residency, York Hospital Department of Emergency Medicine, York, PA, USA
e-mail: mcollin6@wellspan.org; tkehrl@wellspan.org

© Springer Nature Switzerland AG 2019
A. Graham, D. J. Carlberg (eds.), *Gastrointestinal Emergencies*, https://doi.org/10.1007/978-3-319-98343-1_71

What Do I Need to Know About Image Interpretation?

Acute care providers planning to perform PoCUS should take into account potential pitfalls in diagnosing gallbladder disease with US.

Evaluating and managing a patient with a disparate exam, laboratory findings, and sonographic findings can pose significant challenges. Importantly, no single sonographic sign is pathognomonic for acute cholecystitis; however, as the number of secondary signs increases, the likelihood of cholecystitis increases [8].

Stones lodged in the neck of the gallbladder are shown in Fig. 71.1. These stones, which are the most likely to cause symptoms, are easily missed and lead to significant morbidity.

Gallbladder wall thickening can be seen in many conditions, making it sensitive but not specific for cholecystitis [9].

The gallbladder can be difficult to identify when contracted around or filled with a large stone burden because the stones may obscure the bile-filled lumen. On US this appears as a gallbladder wall with a hyperechoic structure immediately behind, followed by shadowing. This sonographic sign, shown in Fig. 71.2, is called the "WES" (wall, echo, shadow) sign and can easily be mistaken for bowel.

Fluid-filled bowel, shown in Fig. 71.3, can easily be misinterpreted as the gallbladder.

Emphysematous cholecystitis is shown in Fig. 71.4. Air in the gallbladder wall can be confused with bowel gas.

Gallbladder polyps can mimic stones, but will typically not shadow and will not be mobile or gravitationally dependent.

When a RUQ US shows no signs of gallstones, wall edema, pericholecystic fluid, or transducer elicited tenderness, an alternative diagnosis should be sought. Alternatively, in patients with significant symptoms, lab abnormalities, and comorbidities, acute care providers need to consider the possibility of a false negative US.

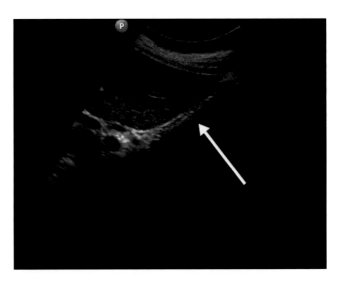

Fig. 71.2 Ultrasound of the gallbladder in long axis with a wall-echo-shadow sign (arrow). Note that there is no anechoic fluid in the gallbladder lumen, which is completely filled with stones. Also note the dense posterior shadowing

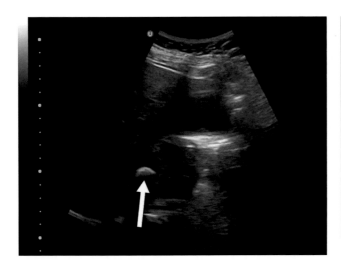

Fig. 71.1 Ultrasound of the gallbladder in long axis with a large stone lodged in the neck (arrow). Failing to image the neck of the gallbladder can lead to false negative scans

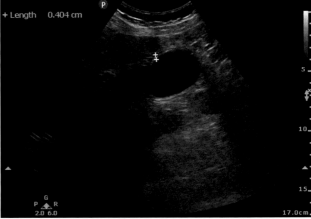

Fig. 71.3 Ultrasound of the duodenum, which was thought to be the gallbladder. Fluid-filled small bowel, particularly the duodenum, can be easily mistaken for the gallbladder. The sonographer went as far as measuring the wall thickness of the duodenum

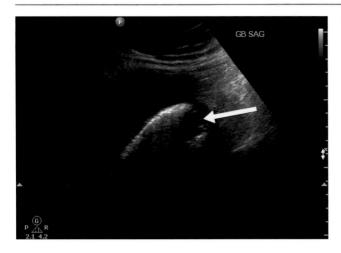

Fig. 71.4 Ultrasound of the gallbladder in long axis (arrow) with a significant amount of air in the anterior wall. Findings are consistent with emphysematous cholecystitis

Suggested Resources

- Bedside biliary ultrasound. ACEP Now. Nov 2010. http://www.acepnow.com/article/bedside-biliary-ultrasound/4/?singlepage=1.
- Summers SM, Scruggs W, Menchine MD, et al. A prospective evaluation of emergency department bedside ultrasonography for the detection of acute cholecystitis. Ann Emerg Med. 2010;56:114–22.

References

1. Blaivas M, Harwood RA, Lambert MJ. Decreasing length of stay with emergency ultrasound examination of the gallbladder. Acad Emerg Med. 1999;6:1020–3.
2. Durston W, Carl ML, Guerra W, et al. Comparison of quality and cost effectiveness in the evaluation of symptomatic cholelithiasis with different approaches to ultrasound availability in the ED. Am J Emerg Med. 2001;19:260–9.
3. Claret PG, Bobbia X, Le Roux S, et al. Point-of-care ultrasonography at the ED maximizes patient confidence in emergency physicians. Am J Emerg Med. 2016;34:657–9.
4. Summers SM, Scruggs W, Menchine MD, et al. A prospective evaluation of emergency department bedside ultrasonography for the detection of acute cholecystitis. Ann Emerg Med. 2010;56:114–22.
5. Gaspari RJ, Dickman E, Blehar D. Learning curve of bedside ultrasound of the gallbladder. J Emerg Med. 2009;37:51–6.
6. Sanders JL, Noble VE, Raja AS, et al. Access to and use of point-of-care ultrasound in the emergency department. West J Emerg Med. 2015;16:747–52.
7. Becker BA, Fields WA, Pfisterer L, et al. Extrabiliary pathology identified by right upper quadrant abdominal ultrasound in emergency department patients. J Emerg Med. 2016;50:92–8.
8. Ralls P, Colletti P, Lapin S, et al. Real-time sonography in suspected acute cholecystitis. Prospective evaluation of primary and secondary signs. Radiology. 1985;155:767–71.
9. Elyaderani MK. Accuracy of cholecystosonography with pathologic correlation. W V Med J. 1984;80:111–5.

Who Needs a Paracentesis? How Do I Optimize Safety? How Do I Interpret the Results?

Thomas Yeich

Pearls and Pitfalls
- Paracentesis in the acute care setting is primarily performed to evaluate for peritonitis.
- Ascites is sterilized within 6 h after receipt of the first dose of antibiotic. Ideally, paracentesis should be performed prior to antibiotic therapy.
- Current guidelines do not support prophylactic platelet transfusion or correcting INRs below 2.5 prior to emergent paracentesis.
- Ultrasound helps localize fluid and helps prevent complications.

Who Needs Paracentesis?

Half of patients diagnosed with cirrhosis will develop ascites over 10 years. Of those, 10–30% will develop spontaneous bacterial peritonitis (SBP), which carries a 20–40% mortality [1–3]. 12–20% of hospitalized patients with ascites have SBP, and ascitic fluid is sterilized within 6 h after receipt of the first antibiotic dose [4, 5]. Ideally, paracentesis should be performed prior to antibiotic therapy (Class I Level B). Timely and accurate diagnosis of and therapy for SBP improve survival [4]. Risk factors for SBP include prior history of SBP, low-protein ascites, and acute GI bleeding [5, 6]. It is important to differentiate SBP from *secondary* bacterial peritonitis. The former is typically mono-microbial, whereas the latter, typically due to bowel perforation, is polymicrobial and often represents a surgical emergency.

Paracentesis is classified as either "diagnostic" or "therapeutic/large volume."

Diagnostic paracentesis is performed to identify the etiology of ascites and/or to evaluate for infection. It should be performed for new onset ascites, as well as for ascites with either (1) abdominal pain, (2) clinical deterioration (e.g., GI bleed, encephalopathy, sepsis, acute renal failure), or (3) hospitalization [5].

Physician judgment regarding the presence or absence of SBP has been shown as inaccurate, and therefore providers should have a low threshold to perform diagnostic paracentesis [4, 6]. One retrospective analysis identified an increased risk of SBP in patients with deeper ascitic fluid pockets and/or abdominal pain. It also showed a "near negligible" risk of SBP when ascitic fluid pockets measure less than 5 cm on ultrasound [7].

Indications for large-volume paracentesis relate to patient comfort. Emergent therapeutic paracentesis is primarily done to alleviate dyspnea or severe pain. Depending on the conditions at the time of diagnostic paracentesis, some practitioners might offer large-volume drainage simultaneously to save the patient a second procedure; however, large-volume drainage is often time-consuming and may strain resources.

How Do I Optimize Safety?

While there are several relative contraindications to paracentesis, the primary absolute contraindications are (1) presence of a surgical abdomen and (2) presence of disseminated intravascular coagulation (DIC) [8].

The literature comparing safety of paracentesis in the emergency department (ED) versus elsewhere in the hospital is sparse. However, one small single-center observational study enrolled 399 patients undergoing thoracentesis, paracentesis, and lumbar puncture to assess time to procedure completion, cost, length of stay (LOS), and complications. The study revealed an approximately 4 h (40%) reduction in time to procedure completion and a 38% ($500) cost reduction if the procedure was completed at

T. Yeich
Department of Emergency Medicine, WellSpan York Hospital, York, PA, USA
e-mail: tyeich@wellspan.org

© Springer Nature Switzerland AG 2019
A. Graham, D. J. Carlberg (eds.), *Gastrointestinal Emergencies*, https://doi.org/10.1007/978-3-319-98343-1_72

bedside in the ED as compared to in diagnostic radiology. There was no difference in hospital LOS. Complication rates were not statistically significant between the ED and other locations; however the study was underpowered to fully assess for this [9].

Complications of paracentesis are similar to those of any invasive procedure and include bleeding, infection, and injury to adjacent organs (including bowel perforation). Additionally, large-volume paracentesis, defined as the removal of greater than 5 L of ascites, increases the risk of paracentesis-induced circulatory dysfunction (PICD), which can lead to hepatorenal syndrome, encephalopathy, recurrent ascites, and death. For every liter of ascites removed above 5 L, these patients should receive 6–8 g of 25% albumin (Class IIa Level A). Albumin infusion for lower-volume paracenteses may not be indicated (Class I Level C) [4, 10, 11]. Other colloid preparations are not considered superior to albumin in preventing PICD [12]. In an effort to reduce patient exposure to blood products, there is promising preliminary research indicating a post-procedure course of terlipressin (1 mg every 4 h for 48 h) as a viable alternative to albumin [13–16].

Since cirrhotic patients often have decreased clotting factors, the concern for bleeding as a complication of paracentesis has been well addressed in the literature. Bleeding complications include abdominal wall hematoma (52% of bleeding complications), hemoperitoneum (41%), and pseudoaneurysm (7%). Operator inexperience, lack of knowledge of abdominal wall vasculature, and failure to use ultrasound guidance correlate with an increased risk of hemorrhagic complications [7, 17]. Therapeutic paracentesis also carries a slightly increased risk of bleeding complications compared to diagnostic paracentesis [17]. The incidence of bleeding after paracentesis is 0–0.97%; thus, it is not necessary to check coagulation studies or provide procoagulant agents (e.g., fresh frozen plasma) on a routine basis (Class III, Level C) [4, 17]. Elevated plasma creatinine/low GFR (<60) is an identified risk factor for of bleeding, and renal disease patients should be observed post-procedure. Additionally, patients with acute disseminated intravascular coagulation (DIC) should not undergo paracentesis [17]. If available, euglobulin clot lysis time can be obtained on patients in DIC, and, if shortened (<120 min), this can be corrected with aminocaproic acid prior to performing paracentesis [4]. Caution should be exercised in patients with renal disease, history of severe thrombocytopenia (platelets <20k), and history of INR greater than 2; however the current guidelines do not support prophylactic platelet transfusion or correcting INRs below 2.5 [4, 8, 16].

In order to avoid adjacent organ injury, care should be taken in approaching those with organomegaly, bowel and urinary obstruction, or significant abdominal wall surgeries that could predispose to adhesions. Care must also be taken in pregnant patients. Steps to mitigate adjacent organ injury

such as nasogastric tube aspiration, bladder catheterization, and avoidance of surgical scars at the point of needle insertion should be considered in high-risk patients. Additionally, the use of ultrasound guidance reduces the incidence of such complications [8, 17–19].

Infectious complications can be reduced via sterile technique and avoidance of needle placement through potentially infected structures (e.g., abdominal wall cellulitis).

As with all emergent procedures, informed consent should be obtained, sterile technique should be employed, and adequate local anesthesia should be provided. Ultrasound guidance, either to mark the insertion site in advance or to actively visualize needle insertion, while not mandatory, reduces the risk of complications.

Needle insertion sites are generally in the lower abdomen, either [20]:

1. The right or left lower abdomen, lateral to the rectus musculature (and associated inferior epigastric arteries) and 2–4 cm cephalad and medial to the anterior iliac crest
2. Midline through the relatively avascular linea alba, 2 cm caudal to the umbilicus

The latter approach may reduce the risk of hemorrhagic complications [20]. Engorged veins on the abdominal wall should be avoided. Figure 72.1 shows potential locations for

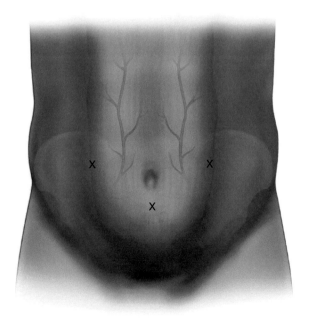

Fig. 72.1 Needle insertion sites for paracentesis are generally in the lower abdomen, either (1) the right or left lower abdomen, lateral to the rectus musculature (and associated inferior epigastric arteries) and 2–4 cm cephalad and medial to the anterior iliac crest, or (2) midline through the relatively avascular linea alba, 2 cm caudal to the umbilicus. Ultrasound guidance is helpful in choosing the exact site of needle insertion

needle insertion. In obese patients the left lateral approach may be preferred due to a potentially deeper pocket of ascites and thinner abdominal wall [21]. Use of longer (3.5 in.) and Caldwell-type catheters increases the rate of first attempt success [19].

Two methods of needle insertion attempt to reduce the risk of post-procedure ascites leak. The z-track method begins with the operator pulling the skin 2 cm caudal and then inserting the needle into the peritoneum at a 90° angle to the skin surface. This allows the skin to form a seal over the puncture wound when the needle is withdrawn. The angular or coaxial technique entails inserting the needle at a 45° angle to the skin, thereby offsetting the skin and peritoneal puncture points [18, 22]. Post-procedural ascites leak was 13% in either method; however pain scores were statistically lower in patients who underwent the angular approach [23]. Negative pressure should be applied to the syringe during needle insertion.

Providers should ensure they have an adequately sized syringe to collect the desired amount of ascites and a needle or IV catheter of sufficient length to penetrate the peritoneum. As cultures are generally required for emergent diagnostic paracentesis, appropriate culture bottles should be at the bedside and inoculated immediately upon acquisition with 10 mL of ascites. This has been demonstrated to improve diagnostic yield, with sensitivities approaching 80% [4, 19].

Using a premanufactured paracentesis kit, accompanied by an appropriate number of vacuum bottles to collect fluid, helps facilitate therapeutic paracentesis. These kits usually have large-bore catheters with multiple fenestrations and safety features such as blunt retractable obturators. They allow for greater first-time success and have lower complication rates [18]. If vacuum bottles are not readily available, many kits have gravity collection bags included. A makeshift vacuum system can also be configured using wall suction and several large-volume wall suction collection canisters connected in serial formation. The canister "train" is then attached to the catheter hub by placing the end of the suction hose into an appropriately sized syringe with plunger removed [24]. In the absence of a specialized paracentesis kit, one author proposed using a 20-gauge spinal needle with the protective sheath cut to approximate abdominal wall thickness to act as a safety stop. The needle can be connected via sterile IV tubing to drain by gravity into a Foley catheter bag [25].

How Do I Interpret the Results?

For patients with established etiologies of their ascites, the main goal of diagnostic paracentesis is evaluation for infectious peritonitis. Therefore, providers should send fluid for cell count, differential, gram stain, and culture. Additional testing can be performed as the clinical situation dictates.

The generally accepted cutoff for peritonitis is a polymorphonuclear cell count (PMN) >250 cells per microliter (µL). In the case of a traumatic tap, the PMN count can be reduced by 1 for every 250 erythrocytes present in the fluid. Several authors have studied a cutoff of 500 PMN/µL, which provides a better positive likelihood ratio (LR) and a similar negative LR [19]. Absolute white blood cell count (WBC) >500/µL demonstrates LRs similar to PMN >250/µL [19]. Ascitic fluid pH <7.35 was found to have statistically significant positive and negative LRs in one small study; however the current guidelines do not advocate for testing ascitic pH [4, 19].

When suspicion exists for secondary bacterial peritonitis, ascites should be tested for glucose, lactate dehydrogenase (LDH), and total protein.

An elevated amylase level suggests pancreatitis or hollow viscus perforation [18].

Table 72.1 depicts LRs for different WBC and PMN cutoffs for SBP, as well as ascitic laboratory findings concerning for secondary bacterial peritonitis.

Occasionally emergency providers will encounter patients with ascites from an unknown origin. If the clinical situation necessitates determining the cause of ascites, providers should first evaluate the fluid's serum-ascites albumin gradient (SAAG), which is the absolute difference between the albumin level in the patient's serum and ascites (SAAG = serum albumin minus ascites albumin). If SAAG ≥ 1.1 g/dL, portal hypertension most likely caused the ascites. SAAG is more accurate than the traditional transudate/exudate categorization of ascites [4].

The differential diagnosis for portal hypertension includes cirrhosis, alcoholic liver disease, cardiac ascites, portal vein thrombosis, Budd-Chiari syndrome, and metastatic liver disease.

The differential diagnosis for non-portal hypertension ascites includes infectious peritonitis, carcinomatosis, nephrotic syndrome, serositis, and pancreatic, biliary, and chylous ascites.

Table 72.1 Laboratory values for ascitic fluid in the evaluation of bacterial peritonitis

Suggestive of bacterial peritonitis			Suggestive of secondary bacterial peritonitis (in addition to cell counts at left)
PMN > 250 cells/µL;	+LR 6.4	−LR 0.20	• Total protein >1 g/dL
PMN > 500 cells/µL;	+LR 10.6	−LR 0.16	• LDH > upper level of normal serum level
WBC > 500 cells/µL;	+LR 5.9	−LR 0.21	• Glucose <50 mg/dL • Alkaline phosphatase
WBC > 1000 cells/µL;	+LR 9.1	−LR 0.25	>240 U/L • Polymicrobial

LR likelihood ratio, *LDH* lactate dehydrogenase, *PMN* polymorphonuclear cell, *WBC* white blood cell count

Additional testing for non-portal hypertension ascites may include evaluation for SBP, tuberculosis testing, amylase, bilirubin, and triglycerides. A separate 50 mL fluid sample for cytology should also be considered when there is concern for malignancy.

Approximately 5% of patients with ascites present with multiple etiologies simultaneously [4, 18].

Suggested Resources

- Wilkerson RG, Sinert R. The use of paracentesis in the assessment of the patient with ascites. Ann Emerg Med. 2009;54:465–8.
- Ultrasound-guided paracentesis. ACEP Now. Nov 2012. http://www.acepnow.com/article/ultrasoundg uidedparacentesis/?singlepage=1&theme=pr int-friendly.
- Management of adult patients with ascites due to cirrhosis: update 2012. Bruce Runyon. American Association for the Study of Liver Diseases. https:// www.aasld.org/sites/default/files/guideline_docu- ments/adultascitesenhanced.pdf.
- Paracentesis. N Engl J Med Video Clin Med. Nov 2006. http://www.nejm.org/doi/full/10.1056/ NEJMvcm062234.

References

1. Gines P, Quintero E, Arroyo V, et al. Compensated cirrhosis: natural history and prognostic factors. Hepatology. 1987;7:122–8.
2. Rimola A, Garcia-Tsao G, Navasa M, et al. Diagnosis, treatment and prophylaxis of spontaneous bacterial peritonitis: a consensus document. International Ascites Club. *J Hepatol*. 2000;32:142–53.
3. Thuluvath PJ, Thompson R. Spontaneous bacterial peritonitis: in-hospital mortality, predictors of survival, and health care costs from 1988 to 1998. Am J Gastroenterol. 2001;96:1232–6.
4. Runyon BA. AASLD practice guideline: management of adult patients with ascites due to cirrhosis: update 2012. Hepatology. 2013:1–96.
5. Sanyal A. Filling and draining the water balloon in symposia 1a: portal hypertension: pressure and leak. Am Coll Gastroenterol. 2010:15–17. http://universe-syllabi.gi.org/acg2010_08_nar.pdf
6. Chinnock B, et al. Physician clinical impression does not rule out spontaneous bacterial peritonitis in patients undergoing emergency department paracentesis. Ann Emerg Med. 2008;52:268–73.
7. Sideris A, et al. Imaging and clinical predictors of spontaneous bacterial peritonitis diagnosed by ultrasound-guided paracentesis. Proc (Bayl Univ Med Cent). 2017;30(3):262–4.
8. Scheer D, et al. Ultrasound-guided paracentesis [Internet] (1 Nov 2012 by ACEP Now). Available from: http://www.acepnow.com/article/ultrasoundguidedparacentesis/?singlepage=1&theme=pr int-friendly.
9. Kay C, et al. Examining invasive bedside procedure performance at an academic medical center. South Med J. 2016;109(7):402–7.
10. Bernardi M, et al. Does the evidence support a survival benefit of albumin infusion in patients with cirrhosis undergoing large-volume paracentesis? Expert Rev Gastroenterol Hepatol. 2017;11(3):191–2.
11. Bernardi M, et al. Albumin infusion in patients undergoing large-volume paracentesis: a meta-analysis of randomized trials. H. 2012;55:1172–81.
12. Widjaja FF, et al. Colloids versus albumin in large volume paracentesis to prevent circulatory dysfunction: evidence-based case report. Acta Med Indones Indones J Intern Med. 2016;48(2):148–55.
13. Shah R, et.al. Ascites treatment & management. [Internet] Medscape, 24 Aug 2016; Available from: http://emedicine.med-scape.com/article/170907-treatment.
14. Lata J, et al. The efficacy of terlipressin in comparison with albumin in the prevention of circulatory changes after the paracentesis of tense ascites--a randomized multicentric study. Hepato-Gastroenterology. 2007;54(79):1930–3.
15. Singh V, et al. Terlipressin versus albumin in paracentesis-induced circulatory dysfunction in cirrhosis: a randomized study. J Gastroenterol Hepatol. 2006;21(1 pt 2):303–7.
16. Moreau R, et al. Comparison of the effect of terlipressin and albumin on arterial blood volume in patients with cirrhosis and tense ascites treated by paracentesis: a randomised pilot study. Gut. 2002;50(1):90–4.
17. Wolfe KS, Kress JP. Risk of procedural hemorrhage. Chest. 2016;150(1):237–46.
18. Thomsen TW, et al. Paracentesis. N Engl J Med. 2006;355:e21.
19. Wilkerson RG, Sinert R. The use of paracentesis in the assessment of the patient with ascites. Ann Emerg Med. 2009;54:465–8.
20. Marx JA. Peritoneal procedures. In: Roberts JR, Hedges J, editors. Clinical procedures in emergency medicine. 4th ed. Philadelphia: Saunders; 2004. p. 851–6.
21. Runyon BA. Management of adult patients with ascites due to cirrhosis. Hepatology. 2004;39:841–56.
22. Thomsen TW, et al. Paracentesis. Videos in clinical medicine[Internet]. N Engl J Med. 2006;355:e21. Available from: http://www.nejm.org/doi/full/10.1056/NEJMvcm062234
23. Shriver AR, et al. A randomized controlled trial of procedural techniques for large volume paracentesis. Ann Hepatol. 2017;16(2):279–84.
24. Jeong J, et al. How to use continuous wall suction for paracentesis. [Internet] ACEP Now, 9 July 2014. Available from: http://www.acepnow.com/article/use-continuous-wall-suction-paracentesis/?si nglepage=1&theme=print-friendly.
25. Fisher W. Road map for a makeshift tap. [Internet] ACEP Now, 1 Nov 2012. Available from: http://www.acepnow.com/article/road-map-makeshift-tap/?singlepage=1&theme=print-friendly.

What Medications Commonly Given in the Acute Care Setting Are Safe in Liver Failure and Cirrhosis? In What Doses?

73

Amber Ruest

Pearls and Pitfalls
- The majority of common medications given in the acute care setting can be safely used in patients with cirrhosis, including those that are potentially hepatotoxic, but lower dose or reduced frequency is recommended.
- Acetaminophen should be considered the first-line treatment for acute pain and can be used safely at low doses ($\leq$2–3 g daily) for short durations.
- Medications that can precipitate gastrointestinal bleeding, renal failure, spontaneous bacterial peritonitis, and encephalopathy should be avoided.
- Cirrhotic patients may take prophylactic medications, and adverse effects of these medications should be considered.

Only a small number of drugs have been reported (with adequate evidence) to increase the risk of hepatotoxicity in chronic liver disease [1]. These include antituberculosis drugs (e.g., isoniazid, pyrazinamide, rifampicin), nevirapine (a drug used in highly active antiretroviral therapy), methimazole, methotrexate, nefazodone, propoxyphene, valproate, and vitamin A [1]. However, significant pharmacokinetic changes occur in patients with cirrhosis, requiring medication dose adjustments to ensure safe administration [2]. Several comprehensive reviews have evaluated the effects of antidepressants, anxiolytics, opioids, and other classes used to treat pain. These should be used with caution in cirrhotic patients as they can precipitate hepatic encephalopathy [1].

Regarding opioids specifically [3–6]:

- Morphine dosing and frequency should be reduced by half.
- Fentanyl does not require adjustment for single dosing.
- Codeine should be avoided.
- Oxycodone dosing should be reduced.
- Tramadol should be avoided in decompensated cirrhotics and in those at risk for seizures.
- Hydromorphone has limited data.

Acetaminophen is probably the most feared drug by patients and physicians; however, most data suggests that it is safe to administer to cirrhotic patients when used in low doses (<2–3 g/day) and in limited duration [1].

Ibuprofen and other nonsteroidal anti-inflammatory drugs (NSAIDs) might lead to or worsen gastrointestinal hemorrhage in patients with underlying gastropathy and coagulopathy. Therefore, acetaminophen is preferred over NSAIDs [7]. Additionally, NSAIDs are not recommended in cirrhosis due to the risk of renal failure [3].

Proton pump inhibitors have been linked to a greater risk of spontaneous bacterial peritonitis in cirrhotics and should be used with caution or avoided entirely [1].

Cirrhotic patients may take certain medications as prophylaxis, and clinicians should consider potential adverse effects and complications of these drugs when evaluating cirrhotic patients.

Nonselective beta-blockers reduce portal pressures and are used in the primary and secondary prophylaxis of variceal hemorrhage [8, 9]. However, various studies caution against the use of beta-blockers in situations such as decompensated cirrhosis with refractory ascites, hypotension, hepatorenal syndrome, spontaneous bacterial peritonitis, and severe alcoholic hepatitis [10, 11].

Patients with cirrhosis who have a history of hypertension gradually become normotensive and eventually hypotensive as cirrhosis progresses; therefore antihypertensive agents should be discontinued in patients with ascites or hypotension

A. Ruest
Department of Emergency Medicine, Wellspan York Hospital, York, PA, USA
e-mail: aruest@wellspan.org

© Springer Nature Switzerland AG 2019
A. Graham, D. J. Carlberg (eds.), *Gastrointestinal Emergencies*, https://doi.org/10.1007/978-3-319-98343-1_73

[10, 11]. In patients with stable hypotension, midodrine may improve splanchnic and systemic hemodynamic variables, renal function, and sodium excretion [12]. The combination of octreotide and midodrine is used for the treatment of type 1 hepatorenal syndrome [13].

Antibiotic prophylaxis may reduce the risk of bacterial infection, including spontaneous bacterial peritonitis; it may also increase survival rates in certain scenarios. Selective intestinal decontamination with trimethoprim-sulfamethoxazole or ciprofloxacin increases short-term survival and reduces the risk of bacterial infection in patients with a history of SBP and among hospitalized patients with ascitic fluid protein <1.5 g/dL [14]. Otherwise, routine antibiotic prophylaxis should be avoided to minimize the risk of antibiotic-resistant infection [15].

Diuretics have been the mainstay of noninvasive management of ascites [16]. Spironolactone is preferred for the initial treatment of ascites due to cirrhosis [16]. The most frequent side effects of spironolactone are due to its antiandrogenic activity: decreased libido, impotence, and gynecomastia in men and menstrual irregularity in women [16]. Hyperkalemia is a significant complication that frequently limits the use of spironolactone in the treatment of ascites [17]. Because of its low efficacy when used alone in cirrhosis, furosemide is generally used adjunctively with spironolactone. High doses of furosemide are associated with severe electrolyte disturbances and metabolic alkalosis; thus, high doses should be used cautiously [16].

Lactulose is effective for primary prevention of overt hepatic encephalopathy in patients with cirrhosis [18]. The side effects of lactulose (including excessively sweet taste and gastrointestinal side effects such as bloating, flatulence, and severe and unpredictable diarrhea possibly leading to dehydration) often lead to noncompliance [18]. Rifaximin has a protective effect against episodes of hepatic encephalopathy and reduces the risk of hospitalization related to hepatic encephalopathy [19]. Some fear that rifaximin will predispose to *Clostridium difficile* infection and bacterial resistance induction, especially if used long term [20].

Suggested Resources
- Ge PS, Runyon BA. A review article: treatment of patients with Cirrhosis. N Engl J Med. 2016;375:767–77.
- Lewis JH, Stine JG. Review article: Prescribing medications in patients with cirrhosis-a practical guide. Aliment Pharmacol Ther. 2013;37:1132.

References

1. Lewis JH, Stine JG. Review article: prescribing medications in patients with cirrhosis-a practical guide. Aliment Pharmacol Ther. 2013;37:1132.
2. Verbeeck RK. Pharmacokinetics and dosage adjustments in patient with hepatic dysfunction. Eur J Clin Pharmacol. 2008;64:1147–61.
3. Bosilkovska M, Walder B, Besson M, et al. Analgesics in patients with hepatic impairment: pharmacology and clinical implications. Drugs. 2012;72:1645–69.
4. Tegeder I, Lotsch J, Geisslinger G. Pharmacokinetics of opioids in liver disease. Clin Pharmacokinet. 1999;37:17–40.
5. Smith HS. Opioid metabolism. Mayo Clin Proc. 2009;84:613–24.
6. Murphy EJ. Acute pain management pharmacology for the patient with concurrent renal or hepatic disease. Anesth Intensive Care. 2005;33:311–22.
7. Lee YC, Chang CH, Lin JW, et al. Non-steroidal anti-inflammatory drugs use and risk of upper gastrointestinal adverse events in cirrhotic patients. Liver Int. 2012;32:859–66.
8. Lebrec D, Poynard T, HIllon P, Benhamou J-P. Propranolol for prevention of recurrent gastrointestinal bleeding in patents with cirrhosis-a controlled study. N Engl J Med. 1981;305:1371–4.
9. Pascal J-P, Cales P, Multicenter Study Group. Propranolol in the prevention of first upper gastrointestinal tract hemorrhage in patients with cirrhosis of the liver and esophageal varices. N Engl J Med. 1987;317:856–61.
10. Krag A, Wiest R, Albillos A, Gluud LL. The window hypothesis: haemodynamic and non-haemodynamic effects of beta-blockers improve survival of patients with cirrhosis during a window in the disease. Gut. 2012;61:967–9.
11. Ge PS, Runyon BA. The changing role of beta-blocker therapy in patients with cirrhosis. J Hepatol. 2014;60:643–53.
12. Ge PS, Runyon BA. A review article: treatment of patients with cirrhosis. N Engl J Med. 2016;375:767–77.
13. Angeli P, Volpin R, Gerunda G, et al. Reversal of type 1 hepatorenal syndrome with the administration of midodrine and octreotide. Hepatology. 1999;29:1690–7.
14. Saab S, Hernandez JC, Chi AC, Tong MJ. Oral antibiotic prophylaxis reduces spontaneous bacterial peritonitis occurrence and improves short-term survival in cirrhosis: a meta-analysis. Am J Gastroenterol. 2009;104:993–1001.
15. O'Leary JG, Reddy KR, Wong F, et al. Long-term use of antibiotics and proton pump inhibitors predict development of infections in patients with cirrhosis. Clin Gastroenterol Hepatol. 2015;13(4):753–9. e1.
16. Moore KP, Aithal GP. Guidelines on the management of ascites in cirrhosis. Gut. 2006;55(Suppl 6):vi1–vi12.
17. Sungaila I, Bartle WR, Walker SE, et al. Spironolactone pharmacokinetics and pharmacodynamics in patients with cirrhotic ascites. Gastroenterology. 1992;102:1680–5.
18. Sharma P, Sharma BC, Agrawal A, Sarin SK. Primary prophylaxis of overt hepatic encephalopathy in patients with cirrhosis: an open labeled randomized controlled trial of lactulose versus no lactulose. J Gastroenterol Hepatol. 2012;27(8):1329–35.
19. Bass NM, Mullen KD, Sanyal A, et al. Rifaximin treatment in hepatic encephalopathy. N Engl J Med. 2010;362:1071–81.
20. Zullo A, Hassan C, Ridola L, Lorenzetti R, Campo SM, Riggio O. Rifaximin therapy and hepatic encephalopathy: Pros and cons. World J Gastrointest Pharmacol Ther. 2012;3(4):62–7.

Consultant Corner: Hepatology

74

Rajesh Panchwagh

Pearls and Pitfalls

- Many liver disease patients, especially those with variceal bleeding and cholangitis, have an extremely high mortality. Early and aggressive management may help reduce mortality.
- Providers should focus on their institution's resources, such as the availability of ERCP, as sicker patients may need to be transferred to larger facilities.
- The encephalopathic patient with a high INR, renal failure, and/or a Model for End-Stage Liver Disease (MELD) score greater than 20 should be considered for immediate transfer to a liver transplant center.
- Patients with advanced hepatic encephalopathy require ICU admission and frequently require endotracheal intubation.
- Transaminase levels five to ten times above the upper limit of normal frequently require observation or admission, as these levels raise concern for toxin-induced injury, shock liver, obstructive process, or infiltrative process.
- Acetaminophen at a dose of 2 grams or less daily is safe.

Introduction

Rajesh Panchwagh, D.O., is an attending physician at WellSpan Gastroenterology (GI) and is also the Associate Medical Director of WellSpan Population Health Services. He trained in internal medicine from 1996 to 1999 at Penn State Hershey Medical Center and subsequently completed a fellowship in GI/Hepatology/Nutrition at the University of Pittsburgh from 1999 to 2002. He has practiced as a gastroenterologist in York, PA, since 2002. His practice focuses on hepatology. He commonly performs therapeutic advanced endoscopy and endoscopic retrograde cholangiopancreatography (ERCP).

Answers to Key Clinical Questions

1. When do you recommend consultation with a specialist, and in what time frame?

The encephalopathic patient with a high INR, renal failure, and/or a Model for End-Stage Liver Disease (MELD) score greater than 20 should be considered for immediate transfer to a liver transplant center for advanced specialist consultation.

The crashing cirrhotic patient requires early gastroenterology/hepatology consultation, ideally after airway, breathing, and circulation have been controlled.

Patients with ascending cholangitis require GI consultation as well. The sicker a patient is, the earlier consultation should occur. While ERCP will generally be required, the patient must be stabilized first. Facilities without ERCP capability should urgently transfer patients to institutions able to perform the procedure.

Hepatic encephalopathy generally requires GI or hepatology consultation.

With primary sclerosing cholangitis (PSC), acute ascending cholangitis and sepsis may occur, so GI consultation for ERCP and biliary drainage may be needed if there is obstructive jaundice and/or cholangitis. For stable admitted PSC or primary biliary cholangitis (also known as primary biliary cirrhosis) patients, GI consultation within 12 h of admission is reasonable. PSC and primary biliary cholangitis (PBC) patients not showing signs of infection, encephalopathy, cholangitis, or gastrointestinal bleeding may be spared admission depending on the clinical situation.

R. Panchwagh
WellSpan Gastroenterology, WellSpan Population Health Services, WellSpan York Hospital, York, PA, USA
e-mail: rpanchwagh@wellspan.org

© Springer Nature Switzerland AG 2019
A. Graham, D. J. Carlberg (eds.), *Gastrointestinal Emergencies*, https://doi.org/10.1007/978-3-319-98343-1_74

2. What pearls can you offer emergency care providers when evaluating a patient with liver disease?

Providers should focus on their institution's resources, such as the availability of ERCP, as sicker patients may need to be transferred to larger facilities.

3. What concepts do you think are key to managing a patient with liver disease?

Unfortunately, many of these patients, especially those with variceal bleeds and cholangitis, have an extremely high mortality. Early and aggressive management may help reduce morbidity and mortality.

4. How do I resuscitate the crashing cirrhotic patient?

One key is to identify whether the patient is unstable due to encephalopathy, GI bleeding, or sepsis related to spontaneous bacterial peritonitis (SBP). These are the most likely situations. Other less common situations include acute toxin-induced injury and fulminant liver failure (which may also be toxin-induced).

Acute resuscitation includes the usual algorithm of airway management, fluid resuscitation, and blood products as needed, along with the following special considerations: nasogastric tube for lactulose administration and lactulose enemas in encephalopathic patients, octreotide and a proton pump inhibitor for gastrointestinal bleeding, and N-acetylcysteine (NAC) when toxin-induced injury is suspected. If SBP with sepsis and/or gastrointestinal bleeding is suspected, then broad-spectrum antibiotics should be given.

5. How do I diagnose and manage acute cholangitis?

Providers should be especially concerned for ascending cholangitis when WBC > 16,000/μL, fever >38.3 °C, and bilirubin >4 mg/dL. Tachycardia and/or hypotension should increase this suspicion even further.

These patients require fluid resuscitation, airway management, and immediate broad-spectrum antibiotics.

While ERCP with stent is generally necessary, patients should be stabilized first. In some instances, pressors may be required to maintain blood pressure and urine output. These critically ill patients should receive early GI consultation.

6. How do I diagnose and manage acute hepatic encephalopathy?

If a patient is encephalopathic, providers should stage the level of encephalopathy. Zero represents minimal encephalopathy, and 4 represents coma. If stage 3 or 4, the patient will likely need to be admitted to the ICU with intubation for airway protection. If he or she is stage 1 or 2, then lactulose given orally, rectally, or by nasogastric tube is standard.

The other important factor is assessing why the patient is encephalopathic, as encephalopathy may be caused by medications, infection, gastrointestinal bleeding, toxic ingestion, worsening liver failure, infiltrative processes, etc. If infection is suspected, immediate cultures should be drawn, and paracentesis should be considered.

7. What do I need to know about primary sclerosing cholangitis and primary biliary cirrhosis?

Both PSC and PBC can present with jaundice, pruritus, elevated alkaline phosphatase, and elevated bilirubin. Later in both disease processes, signs of cirrhosis (encephalopathy, SBP, or gastrointestinal bleeding) may develop.

8. When does transaminitis become acute hepatic failure? What is the management of transaminitis and acute hepatic failure?

Transaminase levels five to ten times the upper limit of normal should raise concern for toxic injury, shock liver, obstructive process, or infiltrative process. These patients generally require either observation or admission. Drug-induced liver injury should be strongly considered, especially acetaminophen toxicity. The need for admission or a GI consultation boils down to the root cause of elevated transaminases and patient stability.

9. How should I image the patient with suspected liver or biliary disease?

Ultrasound (US) is best if providers are worried about biliary obstruction or gallbladder pathology. Computed tomography may be utilized in most other instances. Magnetic resonance cholangiopancreatography (MRCP) can be ordered when concerned about a biliary stricture and/or PSC.

10. Who needs a paracentesis? How do I optimize safety? How do I interpret the results?

A diagnostic paracentesis should be done any time SBP is suspected. A large-volume paracentesis should be done for a tense abdomen with respiratory compromise, including significant orthopnea. An US-guided approach is safest, if available. Sterile technique is required.

11. What medications commonly given in the acute care setting are safe in liver failure and cirrhosis? In what doses?

When medicating cirrhotic patients, providers should consider providing short acting medications. Opioids should be avoided whenever possible. Acetaminophen at a dose of 2 grams or less daily is safe. Nonsteroidal anti-inflammatory drugs (NSAIDS) should be avoided, as renal injury and GI bleeding can occur. Most antibiotics are safe.

Part X

Appendicitis

What Patients Will Have an "Atypical" Presentation for Appendicitis? What Are Those Presentations?

75

Stephen D. Lee

Pearls and Pitfalls

- Appendicitis presents with classic symptoms only about half the time.
- Variable lie of the appendix can result in atypical symptoms, including diarrhea and urinary symptoms, as adjacent structures may become inflamed.
- Patients with atypical or altered anatomy, including pregnant patients, may present with atypical location of pain, including in the right upper quadrant.
- Appendicitis in pregnancy may lack the classic pain presentation due to downregulation of pain receptors and increased distance to the parietal peritoneum.
- Pediatric appendicitis frequently presents without many classic symptoms, and the youngest patients may present with nonspecific signs, from irritability to hip pain and limping.
- Elderly patients with appendicitis present with classical symptoms only 26% of the time, generally present later in the disease process, and—along with pregnant patients and diabetics—have higher rates of perforation.

Classic Appendicitis

The "classic" presentation of appendicitis begins with vague periumbilical abdominal pain that migrates to the right lower quadrant, often associated with nausea and/or vomiting, anorexia, and low-grade fever [1]. However, this classic combination of symptoms occurs in only 50% of patients [1];

thus, a significant number of patients with appendicitis will present atypically, creating a diagnostic challenge for clinicians.

Anatomic Variations

Patients with anatomic variations will logically present more frequently with atypical features, as the location of the appendix will affect both pain localization and associated symptoms. These associated symptoms vary depending on which adjacent structures become inflamed.

Those with retrocecal appendicitis may present with pain in the right flank or costovertebral angle. They may also have psoas irritation or pain referred to the right testicle or adnexa [1, 2]. A subcecal/pelvic appendicitis may abut the ureter or bladder, resulting in potential pyuria on urinalysis and urinary frequency or dysuria as a primary complaint [2, 3]. Alternately, irritation of the nearby rectum may result in diarrhea [1]. Figure 75.1 demonstrates potential locations of the appendix and adjacent structures.

Both congenital and acquired anatomic abnormalities may cause atypical pain. Appendicitis patients with situs inversus generally complain of pain in the left abdomen. Patients with solid organ transplant may have the appendix displaced by the donor organ; however, appendicitis in transplant patients is rare [5].

Pregnancy

Owing somewhat to altered anatomy, pregnant patients with appendicitis may present atypically, as the gravid uterus increasingly displaces the appendix superiorly [6].

S. D. Lee
Department of Emergency Medicine, University of Maryland School of Medicine, Baltimore, MD, USA
e-mail: stephenlee@som.umaryland.edu

Fig. 75.1 Appendix location can influence signs and symptoms in acute appendicitis. Retrocecal appendicitis may cause right flank pain, costovertebral pain, psoas irritation, or pain referred to the scrotum/adnexa. Peri-ileal appendicitis may be relatively asymptomatic but can cause vomiting and diarrhea. Subcecal/pelvic appendicitis may irritate the bladder or ureter, causing dysuria and abnormal urinalysis. It may also irritate the rectum, causing diarrhea [1, 2, 4]

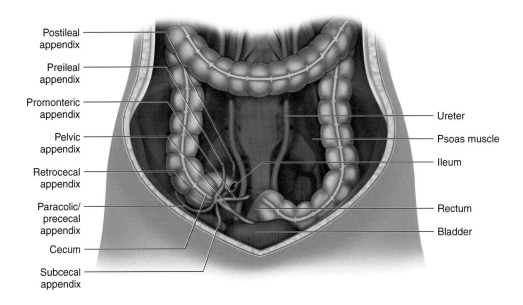

Particularly by the third trimester, appendiceal pain may localize to the right upper quadrant (Fig. 75.2) [7]. Discomfort has also been described in the right flank and right lumbar region [8]. Additionally, appendicitis in pregnancy may present later and with more severe systemic illness, as appendiceal rupture is more common in pregnancy, particularly in the third trimester [7]. This may be due to delayed diagnosis and treatment, given that many findings associated with appendicitis (nausea, vomiting, abdominal pain, tachycardia, and leukocytosis) are not uncommon in gravid patients [6–9]. Paradoxically, abdominal pain may be absent in pregnant appendicitis patients, as stretching of the abdominal wall may downregulate the pain receptor response to peritoneal irritation and may increase the distance between the inflamed appendix and the parietal peritoneum [7, 9].

Children

Children with appendicitis may present atypically as well, with initial misdiagnosis rates in children ≤12 years old ranging from 28% to 57% [10]. One study found that many classic symptoms were absent in these pediatric patients, including fever (absent in 83%), rebound tenderness (52%), pain migration (50%), anorexia (40%), maximal pain in the right lower quadrant (32%), and nausea/vomiting (29%) [11]. In a meta-analysis of pediatric emergency department patients, the most common individual findings in appendicitis were cough/hop pain (positive likelihood ratio [LR+] = 7.6), pain migration (LR+ = 4.8), and Rovsing's sign (LR+ = 3.5) [12]. Children may also provide a limited

or incomplete history, either due to apprehension or a limited ability to articulate symptoms, particularly at younger ages [11, 13]. With neonates and infants, appendicitis may present with nonspecific features, including irritability, lethargy, abdominal distension, grunting, cough, hip pain, and limp [10].

Elderly and Diabetics

Elderly patients also may present atypically, with one study reporting only 26% of patients over 60 years old presenting with classic symptoms [14]. Older patients tend to present later in their disease course and have a higher incidence of perforation. Up to 70% have perforation at 48 h after symptom onset, vs. ~20% of all comers [14, 15].

Similar to the elderly, diabetic patients present more frequently with perforation (39%); thus diabetics may arrive with more systemic or peritoneal signs. However, diabetics present with classic symptoms at a rate similar to the general population [16].

Summary

Many of the presenting symptoms of appendicitis, typical or otherwise, depend on the anatomic location of the appendix. While anatomy is variable in the general population, further alterations due to pregnancy or transplant result in additional atypical presentations of appendicitis. Patients at the extremes of age can be diagnostically challenging, with limitations in the attainable history as a contributing factor.

Fig. 75.2 As pregnancy progresses, the appendix is displaced superiorly. In late pregnancy it is often located in the right upper quadrant

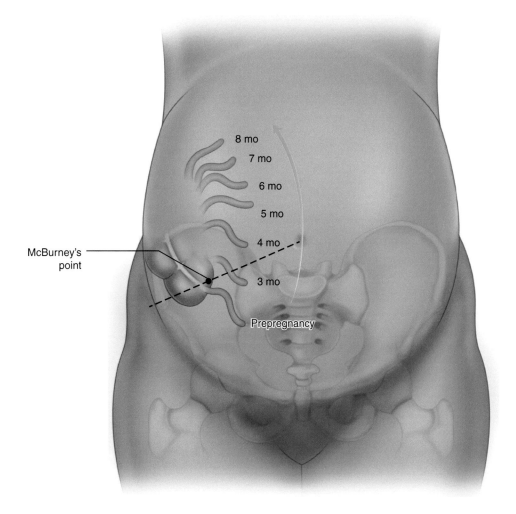

Maintaining a high index of suspicion, especially in at-risk patient populations, is important in the evaluation for potential appendicitis.

Suggested Resources
- Chase C, Koyfman A, Long B. Appendicitis Mimics: ED Focused Management. 2017 Jun 14. Available from: http://www.emdocs.net/appendicitis-mimics-ed-focused-management/.
- Silen W, Cope Z. Cope's early diagnosis of the acute abdomen. New York: Oxford University Press; 2010.
- Wagner J, McKinney W, Carpenter J. Does this patient have appendicitis? JAMA. 1996;276(19):1589–94.

References

1. Humes D, Simpson J. Acute appendicitis. BMJ. 2006;333(7567):530–4.
2. Petroianu A. Invited review: diagnosis of acute appendicitis. Int J Surg. 2012;10(3):115–9.
3. Puskar D, Bedalov G, Fridrih S, et al. Urinalysis, ultrasound analysis, and renal dynamic scintigraphy in acute appendicitis. Urology. 1995;45:108–12.
4. Humes DJ, Simpson J. Clinical presentation of acute appendicitis: clinical signs—laboratory findings—clinical scores, Alvarado score and derivate scores. In: Keyzer C, Gevenois P, editors. Imaging of acute appendicitis in adults and children. Medical radiology. Berlin/Heidelberg: Springer; 2012.
5. Wei C, Chang C, Lee C, Chen J, Yin W. Acute appendicitis in organ transplantation patients: a report of two cases and a literature review. Ann Transplant. 2014;19:248–52.
6. Flexer S, Tabib N, Peter M. Review: suspected appendicitis in pregnancy. Surgeon. 2014;12(2):82–6.
7. Franca Neto AH, Amorim MM, Nóbrega BM. Acute appendicitis in pregnancy: literature review. Rev Assoc Med Bras (1992). 2015;61(2):170–7.
8. Bouyou J, Gaujoux S, Marcellin L, Leconte M, Goffinet F, Chapron C, Dousset B. Review: abdominal emergencies during pregnancy. J Visc Surg. 2015;152(6 Suppl):S105–15.
9. Sinclair J, Marzalik P. Suspected appendicitis in the pregnant patient. J Obstet Gynecol Neonatal Nurs. 2009;38(6):723–9.
10. Rothrock S, Pagane J. Acute appendicitis in children: emergency department diagnosis and management. Ann Emerg Med. 2000;36(1):39–51.
11. Becker T, Kharbanda A, Bachur R. Atypical clinical features of pediatric appendicitis. Acad Emerg Med. 2007;14(2):124–9.
12. Benabbas R, Hanna M, Shah J, Sinert R. Diagnostic accuracy of history, physical examination, laboratory tests, and point-of-care

ultrasound for pediatric acute appendicitis in the emergency department: a systematic review and meta-analysis. Acad Emerg Med.
2017;24(5):523–51.

13. Glass C, Rangel S. Overview and diagnosis of acute appendicitis in
children. Semin Pediatr Surg. 2016;25(4):198–203.

14. Storm-Dickerson T, Horattas M. What have we learned over
the past 20 years about appendicitis in the elderly? Am J Surg.
2003;185(3):198–201.

15. Segev L, Keidar A, Schrier I, Rayman S, Wasserberg N, Sadot
E. Acute appendicitis in the elderly in the twenty-first century. J
Gastrointest Surg. 2015;19(4):730–5.

16. Bach L, Donovan A, Loggins W, Thompson S, Richmond
B. Appendicitis in diabetics: predictors of complications and their
incidence. Am Surg. 2016;82(8):753–8.

Radiation: When Can Patients Be Spared CT? Alvarado Score? Ultrasound?

76

Katharine Meyer and David Carlberg

Pearls and Pitfalls
- CT with intravenous contrast is the most sensitive and specific test for appendicitis.
- A CT of the abdomen and pelvis is approximately 10–30 mSv of radiation. By comparison, a chest X-ray is 0.02 mSv.
- Using the Alvarado score as an appendicitis "ruleout" risks missed appendicitis, and if the score is used, it should be done cautiously while taking into account the entire clinical picture.
- The accuracy of ultrasound has been reported as high as 93%, but the test is user dependent.
- Combining the Alvarado score and ultrasound for an appendicitis "ruleout" has shown promise in a small study and should be further researched.

Acute appendicitis is the most common cause of surgical abdominal pain in the emergency department [1]. The gold standard for diagnosing appendicitis is histological review after surgery; however this is not feasible for emergency physicians. Since the advent of modern imaging technology, physicians continue striving to minimize the negative appendectomy rate (NAR) from the historically accepted 20–30%. Computerized tomography (CT) has decreased the NAR to 3–10% [1].

Radiation

While CT is the most sensitive and specific test for diagnosing appendicitis and, as a result, provides the lowest NAR [2], it exposes patients to ionizing radiation and frequently to intravenous contrast dye. According to the American College of Radiology (ACR), a CT of the abdomen and pelvis delivers ~10–30 mSv of radiation, which likely causes a small increase in a patient's lifetime cancer risk [3]. By contrast, a chest X-ray delivers only ~0.02 mSv. Because of its risks, CT may not be the ideal stand-alone approach for appendicitis evaluation. Many studies have evaluated other modalities, including clinical prediction rules (CPR) and ultrasound (US).

Alvarado Score?

The Alvarado score is a CPR that features a 10-point scoring system, which combines signs, symptoms, and diagnostic testing to risk stratify patients by likelihood of having appendicitis (Table 76.1) [4]. Based on Alvarado's work, a score of 1–4 was associated with a 3.5% likelihood of appendicitis; a score of 5–6 was associated with a 15.4% likelihood of appendicitis; and a score of 7–10 was associated with an 81.1% likelihood of appendicitis [4].

Table 76.1 Alvarado score [4]

Pain migration	1
Anorexia	1
Nausea/vomiting	1
Right lower quadrant tenderness	2
Rebound pain	1
Fever	1
Leukocytosis	2
Left shift	1
Total score	10

Reproduced from Alvarado [4] with automatic permission from Elsevier through the STM signatory guidelines

K. Meyer · D. Carlberg (✉)
Department of Emergency Medicine, MedStar Georgetown University Hospital & Washington Hospital Center, Washington, DC, USA

© Springer Nature Switzerland AG 2019
A. Graham, D. J. Carlberg (eds.), *Gastrointestinal Emergencies*, https://doi.org/10.1007/978-3-319-98343-1_76

A 2011 meta-analysis of 42 studies determined that the sensitivity of an Alvarado score ≤ 4 for ruling out appendicitis was 96–99% [5]. No optimal score was found to "rule in" appendicitis [5]. The study also showed that the score performs best in men, overpredicts the risk of appendicitis in women of childbearing age, and does not perform well enough to use in children [5].

Other sources, including the American College of Emergency Physicians clinical policy on patients with suspected appendicitis, argue that the Alvarado score has too many false negatives to be used in isolation for excluding appendicitis [6–8].

Similar to the Alvarado score, other appendicitis scoring systems such as the Pediatric Appendicitis Score and the Appendicitis Inflammatory Response Score carry a relatively high risk of false negatives [9, 10].

Clinicians choosing to use a CPR as part of their reason for avoiding CT should ensure they take the entire clinical picture into account. Discharged patients should be counseled appropriately and given strict return precautions.

Ultrasound?

US is an imaging modality that is increasingly used to diagnose appendicitis, potentially reducing CT utilization. On US, the diagnosis is made when the appendix has a thickened wall, is >6 mm in diameter, and is shown to be a non-compressible, non-peristalsing structure (Fig. 76.1) [11]. Even if the appendix is not visualized, secondary signs such

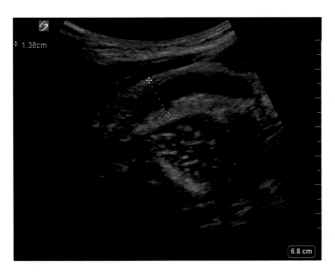

Fig. 76.1 Appendicitis seen on long-axis US view. Note the structure is blind-ending with wall thickening and dilation to 1.38 cm. This structure was non-compressible

as inflammation of surrounding tissues and fluid in the abdomen may suggest the diagnosis [11]. According to the ACR, US is an appropriate first-line test for many patients with suspected acute appendicitis [12]. An US showing acute appendicitis in the right clinical setting generally warrants surgical evaluation and treatment.

One significant challenge with US is that full visualization of the appendix is largely operator dependent. The rate of non-visualization can be as high as 75.6% [6]; however, one study showed an accuracy of 93% for appendicitis when US was performed by an experienced operator [12]. Its operator-dependent nature may contribute to US's wide range of both sensitivity (55–96%) and specificity (72–98%) [11]. Non-visualization is more likely to occur with excess intra-abdominal fat, significant bowel gas, and an atypical position of the appendix [12]. The ability to detect appendicitis using US also varies based on the skill and experience of the radiologist reading the study [2].

The appendix in pediatric patients is more frequently identified than it is in adults. This is likely due to the smaller body habitus of children and makes US a suggested first-line imaging modality for this population when available [6].

Even when the appendix is visualized by US and reported as normal, there is still a risk of a false negative result. One study described 105 US that reported a normal appendix, and 18 of these were false negatives [13]. Therefore, even with a negative ultrasound, an appendicitis workup should continue if there is significant clinical suspicion based on history and serial abdominal examinations.

When Can Patients Be Spared CT?

Combining Alvarado score and US as part of appendicitis "ruleout" has shown promise in a small Turkish study [11], but data to suggest implementing this into clinical practice is still lacking.

The push to find sensitive and specific CT-sparing modalities for the evaluation of potential appendicitis has shown promise. Studies on the Alvarado score have been mixed, and US is both operator and radiologist dependent. Continued research may show that, in the hands of an experienced operator and radiologist, ultrasound alone may be sufficiently sensitive to "rule out" appendicitis. It may also show that combining the Alvarado score and US may be of benefit. Currently, however, if clinical suspicion persists despite a negative Alvarado score and/or ultrasound, evaluation for potential appendicitis should continue.

Suggested Resources

- U.S. Food & Drug Administration - What are the Radiation Risks from CT? - https://www.fda.gov/radiationemittingproducts/radiationemittingproductsandprocedures/medicalimaging/medicalx-rays/ucm115329.htm.
- Howell JM, Eddy OL, Lukens TW, Thiessen ME, Weingart SD, Decker WW. American College of Emergency Physicians. Clinical policy: Critical issues in the evaluation and management of emergency department patients with suspected appendicitis. Ann Emerg Med. 2010;55(1):71–116.

References

1. Debnath CJ, George CR, Ravikumar BR. Imaging in acute appendicitis: what, when and why? Med J Armed Forces India. 2016;73(1):74–9.
2. Ozkan S, Duman A, Durukan P, Yildirim A, Ozbakan O. The accuracy rate of Alvarado score, ultrasonography and computerized tomography in the diagnosis of acute appendicitis in our center. Niger J Clin Pract. 2013;17(4):413–8.
3. Smith M, Katz D, Lalani T, Carucci L, Cash B, Kim D, et al. ACR appropriateness criteria right lower quadrant pain – suspected appendicitis. Am Coll Radiol Ultrasound Q. 2015;31(2):85–91.
4. Alvarado A. A practical score for the early diagnosis of acute appendicitis. Ann Emerg Med. 1986;15(5):557–64.
5. Ohle R, Oreilly F, Obrien KK, Fahey T, Dimitrov BD. The Alvarado score for predicting acute appendicitis: a systematic review. BMC Med. 2011;9(139):1–13.
6. Carlberg DJ, Lee SD, Dubin JS. Lower abdominal pain. Emerg Med Clin North Am. 2016;34(2):229–49.
7. Howell JM, Eddy OL, Lukens TW, Thiessen ME, Weingart SD, Decker WW, American College of Emergency Physicians. Clinical policy: critical issues in the evaluation and management of emergency department patients with suspected appendicitis. Ann Emerg Med. 2010;55(1):71–116.
8. Shogilev D, Duus N, Odom S, Shapiro N. Diagnosing appendicitis: evidence-based review of diagnostic approach in 2014. West J Emerg Med. 2014;15(7):859–71.
9. Mandeville K, Pottker T, Bulloch B, et al. Using appendicitis scores in the pediatric ED. Am J Emerg Med. 2011;29:972–7.
10. Kollár D, McCartan DP, Bourke M, et al. Predicting acute appendicitis? A comparison of the alvarado score, the appendicitis inflammatory response score and clinical assessment. World J Surg. 2015;39:104–9.
11. Unluer E, Urnal R, Eser U, Bilgin S, Hacryanh M, Oyar O, et al. Application of scoring systems with point-of-care ultrasonography for bedside diagnosis of appendicitis. World J Emerg Med. 2016;7(2):125–9.
12. Bachar I, Perry Z, Dukhno L, Mizrahi S, Kirshtein B. Diagnostic value of laparoscopy, abdominal computed tomography, and ultrasonography in acute appendicitis. J Laparoendosc Adv Surg Tech. 2013;23(12):1–8.
13. Leeuwenburgh MM, Stockmann HB, Bouma WH, et al. A simple clinical decision rule to rule out appendicitis in patients with nondiagnostic ultrasound results. Acad Emerg Med. 2014;21:488–96.

MRI for Appendicitis: Gold Standard or Emerging Technology with Limited Role?

Maria Dynin and David Carlberg

Pearls and Pitfalls
- MRI is a safe and effective imaging modality to diagnose acute appendicitis.
- MRI does not emit ionizing radiation.
- Unlike ultrasound, MRI allows visualization of alternate diagnoses.
- CT and MRI have similar sensitivity and specificity for appendicitis.
- MRI takes longer to perform and may be costlier than CT.

Appendicitis is commonly seen in the acute care setting, and physicians should be prepared to make a timely and accurate diagnosis whenever possible. The increased availability of advanced imaging has led to a significant decline in the negative appendectomy rate over the last two decades [1]. Computed tomography (CT) is the preferred imaging modality for diagnosing appendicitis in most adults, yet CT delivers ionizing radiation and therefore likely increases cancer risk [2]. For this reason, demand has increased for imaging tools that avoid radiation while preserving sensitivity and specificity for appendicitis. Ultrasound spares radiation but has limitations in the adult population due to its high rate of indeterminate results, especially in patients with larger body habitus [3]. Magnetic resonance imaging (MRI), which has become more available in the acute care setting, has been suggested as a radiation-sparing alternative to CT for the diagnosis of acute appendicitis.

Because it provides visualization of both intra- and extra-abdominal structures, MRI has the potential to show both acute appendicitis and potential alternate diagnoses. It is frequently performed without gadolinium when evaluating for acute appendicitis, meaning it can be performed in both pregnancy and renal disease. Intravenous gadolinium may be added if non-contrast MRI is nondiagnostic [4].

A meta-analysis of MRI for appendicitis reported a sensitivity of 96% (95% CI 95 to 97%) and a specificity of 96% (95% CI 95 to 97%) [5]. In comparison, a meta-analysis evaluating CT for appendicitis reported a sensitivity of 95% (95% CI 95 to 97%) and a specificity of 96% (95% CI 93 to 97%) [6]. Hence, CT and MRI have both very high and very similar diagnostic accuracy for acute appendicitis.

One unfortunate drawback with MRI is that its accuracy may be reader dependent. One study reported an MRI sensitivity of 89% when read by general radiologists and 97% when read by MRI experts [7]. Another drawback is the risk of a nondiagnostic exam. One study that evaluated the T1 spin echo sequences of 71 randomly selected MRIs looking for a normal appendix showed that the appendix was not visualized 22% of the time [4]. Yet, Kearl et al. found that even when the appendicitis was not visualized, MRI had 100% diagnostic accuracy for ruling out acute appendicitis when no secondary signs were seen [8]. Additionally, with increasing availability of MRI, radiologists are likely to become more comfortable reading them for appendicitis, and the visualization, sensitivity, and specificity will likely improve in future studies [9].

Three factors that significantly limit the use of MRI for appendicitis in the acute care arena are cost, availability, and test duration [10]. One study found the technical cost of an examination with US, CT, and MRI at a tertiary care center was $50, $112, and $267, respectively [11]. MRI may not be feasible in patients with metallic foreign bodies or certain implanted medical devices. Furthermore, a full abdominal MRI requires ~1 h to complete, which can be difficult for patients who are acutely ill and in pain or who have claustrophobia. However, protocols have been developed that

M. Dynin (✉)
Department of Emergency Medicine, MedStar Washington Hospital Center & MedStar Georgetown University Hospital, Washington, DC, USA

D. Carlberg
Department of Emergency Medicine, MedStar Georgetown University Hospital & Washington Hospital Center, Washington, DC, USA
e-mail: david.carlberg@gunet.georgetown.edu

© Springer Nature Switzerland AG 2019
A. Graham, D. J. Carlberg (eds.), *Gastrointestinal Emergencies*, https://doi.org/10.1007/978-3-319-98343-1_77

decrease study duration. Many institutions focus MRI images in the right lower quadrant when evaluating for appendicitis, and the duration of these focused MRIs has decreased to ~10–20 min [12].

While MRI is often used for evaluating potential appendicitis in children and pregnant women, it has not become the standard in nonpregnant adults. Its broader use is currently limited by cost, availability, and study time. If these improve, MRI may eventually supplant CT in the appendicitis workup because of its similar accuracy combined with its lack of ionizing radiation. Currently, MRI is a reasonable alternative to CT in the acute care setting if it is available, especially when read by an abdominal MRI-trained radiologist.

Suggested Resources
- Kearl YL, Claudius I, Behar S, Cooper J, et al. Accuracy of Magnetic Resonance Imaging and Ultrasound for Appendicitis in Diagnostic and Nondiagnostic Studies. Acad Emerg Med. 2016 Feb;23(2):179–85.
- Kulaylat AN, Moore MM, Engbrecht BW, et al. An implemented MRI program to eliminate radiation from the evaluation of pediatric appendicitis. J Pediatr Surg. 2015;50(8):1359–63.

References

1. Lu Y, Friedlander S, Lee SL. Negative appendectomy: clinical and economic implications. Am Surg. 2016;82(10):1018–22.
2. Smith MP, Katz DS, Lalani T, Carucci LR, Cash BD, Kim DH, Piorkowski RJ, Small WC, Spottswood SE, Tulchinsky M, Yaghmai V, Yee J, Rosen MP. ACR appropriateness criteria®right lower quadrant pain--suspected appendicitis. Ultrasound Q. 2015;31(2):85–91.
3. Mallin M, Craven P, Ockerse P, Steenblik J, Forbes B, Boehm K, Youngquist S. Diagnosis of appendicitis by bedside ultrasound in the ED. Am J Emerg Med. 2015;33(3):430–2.
4. Nikolaidis P, Hammond N, Marko J, et al. Incidence of visualization of the normal appendix on different MRI sequences. Emerg Radiol. 2006;12:223.
5. Duke E, Kalb B, Arif-Tiwari H, Daye ZJ, Gilbertson-Dahdal D, Keim SM, Martin DR. A systematic review and meta-analysis of diagnostic performance of MRI for evaluation of acute appendicitis. AJR Am J Roentgenol. 2016;206(3):508–17.
6. Dahabreh IJ, Adam GP, Halladay CW, Steele DW, Daiello LA. Diagnosis of right lower quadrant pain and suspected acute appendicitis [internet]. AHRQ Comparative Effectiveness Reviews. 2015;Report No: 15(16)-EHC025-EF.
7. Leeuwenburgh MMN, Wiarda BM, Jensch S, van Es HW, Stockmann HBAC, Gratama JWC, Cobben LPJ, Bossuyt PMM, Boermeester MA, Stoker J. Accuracy and interobserver agreement between MR-non-expert radiologists and MR-experts in reading MRI for suspected appendicitis. Eur J Radiol. 2015;83(1):103–10.
8. Kearl YL, Claudius I, Behar S, Cooper J, et al. Accuracy of magnetic resonance imaging and ultrasound for appendicitis in diagnostic and nondiagnostic studies. Acad Emerg Med. 2016;23(2):179–85.
9. Leeuwenburgh MMN, Wiarda BM, Bipat S, Yung Nio C, Bollen TL, Joost Kardux J, Jensch S, Bossuyt PMM, Boermeester MA, Stoker J. Acute appendicitis on abdominal MR images: training readers to improve diagnostic accuracy. Radiology. 2012;264(2):455–63.
10. Leeuwenburgh MM, Laméris W, van Randen A, Bossuyt PM, Boermeester MA, Stoker J. Optimizing imaging in suspected appendicitis (OPTIMAP-study): a multicenter diagnostic accuracy study of MRI in patients with suspected acute appendicitis. Study protocol. BMC Emerg Med. 2010;10:19. https://doi.org/10.1186/1471-227X-10-19.
11. Saini S, Seltzer SE, Bramson RT, et al. Technical cost of radiologic examinations: analysis across imaging modalities. Radiology. 2000;216(1):269–72.
12. Kulaylat AN, Moore MM, Engbrecht BW, et al. An implemented MRI program to eliminate radiation from the evaluation of pediatric appendicitis. J Pediatr Surg. 2015;50(8):1359–63.

What About Appendicitis and Pregnancy? Is There a Systematic Approach to Save Time, Reduce Radiation, and Make Everyone Happy?

Philippa N. Soskin

Pearls and Pitfalls
- The risk of fetal mortality increases significantly with ruptured appendicitis. A negative appendectomy also has risk to the fetus.
- Ultrasound has high specificity but also has high rates of non-visualization, particularly as pregnancy progresses.
- Ultrasound and MRI are recommended initial diagnostic tests.
- Radiation exposure from a standard CT abdomen/pelvis is ~14 mSv. In utero exposure to radiation at this level has not been shown to increase the risk of prenatal death, malformation, or impaired mental development.
- The small risk of childhood malignancy doubles with in utero radiation exposure; however, this risk is far less than the risk of fetal mortality with ruptured appendicitis.

What About Appendicitis and Pregnancy?

Appendicitis is the most common non-obstetric surgical emergency in pregnancy. Clinical diagnosis can be challenging given alternative etiologies of abdominal pain, potential displacement of the appendix as pregnancy progresses, and variable data on the clinical utility of signs including fever and leukocytosis [1–5].

Data on fetal mortality in pregnancy varies greatly, but studies show a risk of 1.5–9% in uncomplicated appendicitis, with risk rising to as much as 36% in cases of ruptured appendicitis [6–12]. A negative appendectomy is also associated with an increased risk of fetal loss [13].

Is There a Systematic Approach to Save Time, Reduce Radiation, and Make Everyone Happy?

Given the challenges of clinical diagnosis and increased risk of fetal mortality with both appendicitis and negative appendectomy, timely and accurate preoperative diagnosis is essential. The importance of making an accurate diagnosis must be balanced with the theoretical harm to the fetus from in utero radiation exposure. Guidelines from both the obstetrics and radiology literature recommend ultrasound (US) and magnetic resonance imaging (MRI) as preferred initial diagnostic imaging modalities [14–17]. Figure 78.1 depicts a suggested algorithm for evaluation of appendicitis in pregnancy.

Ultrasound

US has become the first-line diagnostic modality for evaluation of right lower quadrant pain in pregnancy given its safety profile, low cost, and accessibility. Studies show sensitivities as low as 18% and as high as 100% with specificities generally higher, from 80% to 100% [18–20]. There can be a high rate of non-visualization of the appendix using US, particularly as pregnancy progresses, and therefore an inconclusive study or a non-visualized appendix requires further diagnostics [21–23]. Additionally, false negative studies occur even when the appendix is visualized and read as normal; therefore if clinical suspicion remains, continued workup for appendicitis should continue despite negative ultrasound [24].

Magnetic Resonance Imaging

MRI poses minimal risk to the fetus and is an effective diagnostic imaging technique with lower rates of non-visualization compared to US and generally high sensitivity

P. N. Soskin
MedStar Georgetown University Hospital and Washington Hospital Center, Washington, DC, USA

© Springer Nature Switzerland AG 2019
A. Graham, D. J. Carlberg (eds.), *Gastrointestinal Emergencies*, https://doi.org/10.1007/978-3-319-98343-1_78

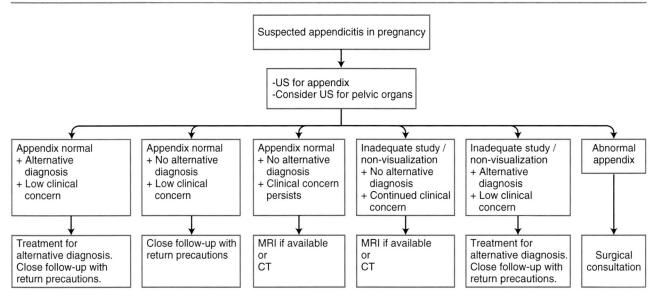

Fig. 78.1 Potential algorithm for evaluation of suspected appendicitis in pregnancy

(60–100%) and specificity (93–100%) [18, 19, 25, 26]. While MRI is diagnostically superior to US, obtaining MRI as an initial test may be unrealistic given its lack of accessibility and high cost. MRI for appendicitis during pregnancy does not require gadolinium, and since gadolinium is not recommended in pregnancy, it should only be used if expected to greatly improve maternal and fetal outcomes [15].

Computed Tomography

CT is considered the gold standard imaging modality for diagnosing appendicitis in the general population. However, given the risk of teratogenesis and carcinogenesis from in utero radiation exposure, CT is recommended when alternative modalities are unavailable or inconclusive [14, 15]. The baseline risk of developing childhood malignancy is 0.2–0.3%. Exposure to 10 mSv increases this risk by ~ 0.3%–0.7% [14, 27]. While this doubles the relative risk, the overall risk is much lower than the risk of ruptured appendicitis, which carries a fetal mortality of up to 36% [6–12].

In utero exposure to radiation from diagnostic imaging has not been found to increase the risk of prenatal death, malformation, or impairment of central nervous system development. No adverse effects have been seen with exposure to 50–100 mSv during 0–2 weeks' gestation and 18–27 weeks' gestation; effects at 3–18 weeks are uncertain and probably too small to be clinically detectable. Exposure to greater than 100 mSv may increase the possibility of spontaneous abortion, malformation, and diminishing IQ [27]. This exposure is significantly higher

than the radiation from most diagnostic imaging tests. The radiation dose from a single CT abdomen/pelvis is ~14 mSv.

Suggested Resources
- EM:RAP. RLQ pain in the pregnant patient. Episode 123. (December 2011: https://www.emrap.org/episode/december2011/rlqpaininthe?emrap=ekp5qfv2go7mnqhh2ktts67vn7).
- ERCAST. RLQ pain in pregnancy. (November 11, 2011: http://blog.ercast.org/rlq-pain-in-pregnancy/).

References

1. Cardall T, Glasser J, Guss D. Clinical value of the total white blood cell count and temperature in the evaluation of patients with suspected appendicitis. Acad Emerg Med. 2004;11(10):1021–7.
2. Erkek A, Anik Ilhan G, Yildizhan B, Aktan A. Location of the appendix at the third trimester of pregnancy: a new approach to old dilemma. J Obstet Gynaecol. 2015;35(7):688–90.
3. House J, Bourne C, Seymour H, Brewer K. Location of the appendix in the gravid patient. J Emerg Med. 2014;46(5):741–4.
4. Mourad J, Elliott J, Erickson L, Lisboa L. Appendicitis in pregnancy: new information that contradicts long-held clinical beliefs. Am J Obstet Gynecol. 2000;182(5):1027–9.
5. Theilen L, Mellnick V, Shanks A, Tuuli M, Odibo A, Macones G, Cahill A. Acute appendicitis in pregnancy: predictive clinical factors and pregnancy outcomes. Am J Perinatol. 2017;34(6):523–8.
6. Al-Fozan H, Tulandi T. Safety and risks of laparoscopy in pregnancy. Curr Opin Obstet Gynecol. 2002;14(4):375–9.
7. Al-Mulhim A. Acute appendicitis in pregnancy. A review of 52 cases. Int Surg. 1996;81(3):295–7.

 8. Mazze R, Källén B. Appendectomy during pregnancy: a Swedish registry study of 778 cases. Obstet Gynecol. 1991;77(6):835–40.
 9. Hée P, Viktrup L. The diagnosis of appendicitis during pregnancy and maternal and fetal outcome after appendectomy. Int J Gynecol Obstet. 1999;65(2):129–35.
10. Ueberrueck T, Koch A, Meyer L, Hinkel M, Gastinger I. Ninety-four appendectomies for suspected acute appendicitis during pregnancy. World J Surg. 2004;28(5):508–11.
11. Yilmaz H, Akgun Y, Bac B, Celik Y. Acute appendicitis in pregnancy — risk factors associated with principal outcomes: a case control study. Int J Surg. 2007;5(3):192–7.
12. Zhang Y, Zhao Y, Qiao J, Ye R, Wei Y. O1050 the diagnosis of appendicitis during pregnancy and perinatal outcome in late pregnancy. Int J Gynecol Obstet. 2009;107:S392.
13. McGory M, Zingmond D, Tillou A, Hiatt J, Ko C, Cryer H. Negative appendectomy in pregnant women is associated with a substantial risk of fetal loss. J Am Coll Surg. 2007;205(4):534–40.
14. ACR-SPR practice parameter for imaging pregnant or potentially pregnant adolescents and women with ionizing radiation. Revised 2013 (Resolution 48). [cited 2017 Sep 23] Available from: http://www.acr.org/~/media/9e2ed55531fc4b4fa53ef3b6d3b25df8.pdf.
15. Guidelines for diagnostic imaging during pregnancy and lactation. Committee opinion no. 723. American College of Obstetricians and Gynecologists. Obstet Gynecol. 2017;130:e210–6.
16. Patel S, Reede D, Katz D, Subramaniam R, Amorosa J. Imaging the pregnant patient for nonobstetric conditions: algorithms and radiation dose considerations. Radiographics. 2007;27(6):1705–22.
17. Smith M, Katz D, Lalani T, Carucci L, Cash B, Kim D, et al. ACR appropriateness criteria® right lower quadrant pain—suspected appendicitis. Ultrasound Q. 2015;31(2):85–91.
18. Israel G, Malguria N, McCarthy S, Copel J, Weinreb J. MRI vs. ultrasound for suspected appendicitis during pregnancy. J Magn Reson Imaging. 2008;28(2):428–33.
19. Konrad J, Grand D, Lourenco A. MRI: first-line imaging modality for pregnant patients with suspected appendicitis. Abdom Imaging. 2015;40(8):3359–64.
20. Lim H, Bae S, Seo G. Diagnosis of acute appendicitis in pregnant women: value of sonography. Am J Roentgenol. 1992;159(3):539–42.
21. Lehnert B, Gross J, Linnau K, Moshiri M. Utility of ultrasound for evaluating the appendix during the second and third trimester of pregnancy. Emerg Radiol. 2012;19(4):293–9.
22. Tamir IL, Bongard FS, Klein SR. Acute appendicitis in the pregnant patient. Am J Surg. 1990;160(6):575–6.
23. Theilen L, Mellnick V, Longman R, Tuuli M, Odibo A, Macones G, et al. Utility of magnetic resonance imaging for suspected appendicitis in pregnant women. Am J Obstet Gynecol. 2015;212(3):345.e1–345.e6
24. Leeuwenburgh MM, Stockmann HB, Bouma WH, et al. A simple clinical decision rule to rule out appendicitis in patients with nondiagnostic ultrasound results. Acad Emerg Med. 2014;21:488–96.
25. Kereshi B, Lee K, Siewert B, Mortele K. Clinical utility of magnetic resonance imaging in the evaluation of pregnant females with suspected acute appendicitis. Abdom Radiol. 2017;43:1446. https://doi.org/10.1007/s00261-017-1300-7.
26. Patel D, Fingard J, Winters S, Low G. Clinical use of MRI for the evaluation of acute appendicitis during pregnancy. Abdom Radiol. 2017;42(7):1857–63.
27. International commission on radiological protection. Biological effects after prenatal irradiation (embryo and fetus). Bethesda: ICRP Publication; 2003. vol 90. p. 1–200.

What About Kids and Appendicitis? Small Adults or Different Approach?

79

Meredith C. Thompson and David Carlberg

Pearls and Pitfalls
- The appendix assumes adult shape and becomes susceptible to appendicitis at ages 1–2.
- The classic description of periumbilical pain migrating to the right lower quadrant with fever comes from studies in adults and occurs in less than half of children.
- Perforation risk in children rises linearly and substantially with time.
- Transfer to a pediatric center should be considered before imaging when evaluating for appendicitis in children.

Although appendicitis is often considered in the assessment of children presenting with abdominal pain, its diagnosis remains challenging and often requires intricate evaluation and refined clinical decision-making in this population of varying ages and stages of development.

Typically, appendicitis occurs due to obstruction of the appendiceal lumen, classically with a fecalith or lymphoid hyperplasia. Appendicitis is rare during infancy due to this group's liquid diet, infrequent illness, and funnel-shaped appendix; however, between ages 1 and 2, the appendix assumes an adult shape and becomes susceptible [1]. Lymphoid follicular size increases gradually and peaks in adolescence, corresponding to the period of highest appendicitis incidence [1].

Diagnostic Challenges

The classic history of periumbilical pain migrating to the right lower quadrant (RLQ) with vomiting and fever comes from studies in adults and occurs in less than half of children [2].

Atypical features are common. One study of children diagnosed with appendicitis found that atypical features included absence of fever (83%), tenderness not maximal in the RLQ (32%), and presence of diarrhea (16%). 44% had multiple atypical features [2]. Another study warned that exclusion of appendicitis should be undertaken with caution in children with abdominal pain and concurrent respiratory infection. 23% of children with appendicitis missed on the initial visit had concurrent upper respiratory symptoms. The same study showed that up to 30% of children with missed appendicitis had an abnormal urinalysis, as an inflamed appendix may cause ureteral irritation, leading to pyuria and/or dysuria [3].

Misdiagnosis and delayed diagnosis of pediatric appendicitis, which occurs with a frequency of 28–57%, are associated with increased risk of perforation, morbidity, and mortality [1, 3]. In children the risk of perforation increases linearly from 7.7% at 24 hours to 44% at 36 hours, compared to adults where the risk of rupture is only 5% over the first 36 hours [4]. 80% of those under age 4 present with perforation [1]. Not surprisingly, appendicitis follows only meningitis in common pediatric malpractice claims involving emergency departments [5].

Laboratory Tests and Decision Rules

Many studies have attempted to elicit clinical and laboratory features to aid in diagnosis of pediatric appendicitis. A large meta-analysis found that if present, fever was the single most useful sign suggesting appendicitis [1]. While several studies have demonstrated that a normal white blood cell count and

M. C. Thompson (✉)
Department of Emergency Medicine, University of Virginia Health System, Charlottesville, VA, USA
e-mail: mac2rx@hscmail.mcc.virginia.edu

D. Carlberg
Department of Emergency Medicine, MedStar Georgetown University Hospital & Washington Hospital Center, Washington, DC, USA

© Springer Nature Switzerland AG 2019
A. Graham, D. J. Carlberg (eds.), *Gastrointestinal Emergencies*, https://doi.org/10.1007/978-3-319-98343-1_79

negative inflammatory markers each reduce the likelihood of appendicitis, these findings are weak individual discriminators and should not be used in isolation to diagnose or exclude appendicitis [1, 2]. Clinical decision rules (e.g. Alvarado Score, Pediatric Appendicitis Score) have been developed; however subsequent studies have questioned their usefulness due to inadequate predictive value, variable interrater reliability, and similar performance to clinical judgment [6–8].

Computed Tomography

Given the high risk of misdiagnosis and sometimes limited utility of the history and clinical exam, physicians must frequently turn to imaging to diagnose or exclude appendicitis. Although computed tomography (CT) has high sensitivity and specificity for appendicitis in children, it is a suboptimal initial imaging modality as it exposes children to ionizing radiation. One fatal cancer may develop per 1000 CTs performed in young children [9, 10].

Ultrasound

Ultrasound (US) has become the preferred initial imaging modality in children, largely due to its lack of ionizing radiation [9, 11, 12]. Unfortunately, US does have some limitations in excluding appendicitis. The greatest challenge is that US is highly operator dependent, with one study reporting non-visualization of the appendix in 75.6% of children [13]. Pediatric sonographers are better at identifying the appendix than adult sonographers [13]. The reported sensitivity of US for appendicitis in children is variable, ranging between 81.7% and 99.5% with complete visualization [12, 14, 15]. As there is potential for false negative US, if significant clinical suspicion for appendicitis remains, clinicians should consider observation or additional imaging. In a well-appearing child with a benign exam, a negative US is sufficient to exclude appendicitis, and discharge with strict return precautions and close follow-up is appropriate. A positive US with an appropriate clinical picture should prompt surgical consultation and treatment for acute appendicitis.

Magnetic Resonance Imaging

Although the current American College of Radiology recommendation is that a nondiagnostic ultrasound be followed by CT, there is evidence that magnetic resonance imaging (MRI) may be the better secondary imaging modality. It provides similar sensitivity and specificity to CT without radiation exposure [11, 16].

Transfer and Definitive Management

Due to the complex clinical decision-making that may occur with an equivocal ultrasound, some authors have advocated for early transfer of any child with suspected appendicitis to a pediatric center prior to imaging [17].

Admission for serial examinations by a pediatric surgeon remains a safe and acceptable disposition decision.

Appendectomy is the mainstay of treatment for pediatric appendicitis. Although there is emerging evidence for the use of antibiotics alone to treat uncomplicated appendicitis in children, lack of prospective studies and randomized controlled trials limits the generalizability of these results [18, 19].

Suggested Resources
- Bundy DG, Byerley JS, Liles EA, Perrin EM, Katznelson J, Rice HE. Does this child have appendicitis? JAMA. 2007;298(4):438–51.
- Pediatric EM. Morsels. Appendicitis clinical decision rules. (October 2014: http://pedemmorsels. com/appendicitis-clinical-decision-rules/).

References

1. Bundy DG, Byerley JS, Liles EA, Perring EM, Katznelson J, Rice HE. Does this child have appendicitis? JAMA. 2007;298(4):438–51.
2. Becker T, Kharbanda A, Bachur R. Atypical clinical features of pediatric appendicitis. Acad Emerg Med. 2007;14(2):124–9.
3. Rothrock SG, Skeoch G, Rush JJ, Johnson NE. Clinical features of misdiagnosed appendicitis in children. Ann Emerg Med. 1991;20(1):45–50.
4. Narsule CK, Kahle EJ, Kim DS, Anderson AC, Luks FI. Effect of delay in presentation on rate of perforation in children with appendicitis. Am J Emerg Med. 2011;29(8):890–3.
5. Selbst SM, Friedman MJ, Singh SB. Epidemiology and etiology of malpractice lawsuits involving children in US emergency departments and urgent care centers. Pediatr Emerg Care. 2005;21(3):165–9.
6. Mandeville K, Pottker T, Bulloch B, Liu J. Using appendicitis scores in the pediatric ED. Am J Emerg Med. 2011;29(9):972–7.
7. Ebell MH, Shinholser J. What are the most clinically useful cutoffs for the alvarado and pediatric appendicitis scores? A systematic review. Ann Emerg Med. 2014;64(4):365–72.
8. Kharbanda AB. Appendicitis: do clinical scores matter? Ann Emerg Med. 2014;64(4):373–5.
9. Doria AS, Moineddin R, Kellenberger CJ, Epelman M, Beyene J, Schuh S, Babyn PS, Dick PT. US or CT for diagnosis of appendicitis in children and adults? A Meta-Analysis. Radiology. 2006;241(1):83–94.
10. Rice HE, Frush DP, Farmer D, Waldhausen JH, APSA Education Committee. Review of radiation risks from computed tomography: essentials for the pediatric surgeon. J Pediatr Surg. 2007;42(4):603–7.
11. Smith MP, Katz DS, Lalani T, Carucci LR, Cash PD, Kim DH, Piorkowski RJ, Small WC, Spottswood SE, Tulchinski M,

Yaghmai V, Yee J, Rosen MP. ACR appropriateness criteria® right lower quadrant pain--suspected appendicitis. Ultrasound Q. 2015;31(2):85–91.

12. Pacham P, Ying J, Linam LE, Brody AS, Babcock DS. Sonography in the evaluation of acute appendicitis: are negative sonographic findings good enough? J Ultrasound Med. 2010;29(12):1749–55.

13. Trout AT, Sanchez R, Ladino-Torres MF, et al. A critical evaluation of US for the diagnosis of pediatric acute appendicitis in a real-life setting: how can we improve the diagnostic value of sonography? Pediatr Radiol. 2012;42:813–23.

14. D'Souza N, D'Souza C, Grant D, et al. The value of ultrasonography in the diagnosis of appendicitis. Int J Surg. 2015;13:165–9.

15. Ross MJ, Liu H, Netherton SJ, Eccles R, et al. Outcomes of children with suspected appendicitis and incompletely visualized appendix on ultrasound. Acad Emerg Med. 2014;21:538–42.

16. Kim JR, Suh CH, Yoon HM, Jung AY, Lee JS, Kim JH, Lee JY, Cho YA. Performance of MRI for suspected appendicitis in pediatric patients and negative appendectomy rate: a systematic review and meta-analysis. J Magn Reson Imaging. 2018;47(3):767–78.

17. Badru F, Piening N, To A, Xu P, Fitzpatrick C, Chatoorgoon K, Villalona G, Greespon J. Imaging for acute appendicitis at non-pediatric centers exposes children to excess radiation. J Surg Res 2017;216:201–06.

18. Bachur RG, Lipsett SC, Monuteaux MC. Outcomes of nonoperative management of uncomplicated appendicitis. Pediatrics. 2017;140(1):e20170048.

19. Georgiou R, Eaton S, Stanton MP, et al. Efficacy and safety of nonoperative treatment for acute appendicitis: a meta-analysis. Pediatrics. 2017;139(3):e20163003.

Is There a Role for Medical Management in Acute Appendicitis?

80

Jonathan Watson and David Carlberg

Pearls and Pitfalls
- Treatment of acute appendicitis with antibiotics has been shown to improve quality of life, lower healthcare costs, and allow for earlier return to normal activities.
- Patients treated with antibiotics have a higher risk of recurrent appendicitis.
- No single superior antibiotic regimen has been established (drug, route of delivery, duration).
- Further research is required to identify which patients will have the greatest benefit and highest likelihood for treatment success.

Acute appendicitis is the most frequent cause of acute abdomen in emergency departments in North America and Europe, with a lifetime risk ranging from 6.7% to 8.6% [1]. Appendectomy has been the gold standard for treatment for acute appendicitis, but there are concerns about adverse outcomes including negative appendectomy (appendix free of disease when removed), development of adhesions, and surgical wound infection. New evidence shows that not all cases of uncomplicated appendicitis progress to perforation, and spontaneous resolution may be common. This challenges the classic teaching that appendectomy is indicated to prevent inevitable perforation and/or abscess [2]. Because of this, there is growing interest in the use of antibiotic therapy as a noninvasive treatment alternative for acute appendicitis. Although there have been successful reports of an "antibiotics-first" strategy for complicated appendicitis (evidence of perforation, abscess, or phlegmon) [3], it is cur-

rently more generally accepted that surgery and/or interventional radiology approaches are the appropriate treatment for complicated appendicitis [4]. Therefore this chapter will focus on uncomplicated appendicitis.

A randomized controlled trial (RCT) in *JAMA* in 2015 studied 530 patients with uncomplicated appendicitis confirmed by abdominal CT and determined the treatment failure rate and complication rate for patients receiving antibiotic therapy. Of the 257 patients who received antibiotic therapy (IV ertapenem × 3 days, followed by 7 days of oral levofloxacin and metronidazole), 73% did not require further treatment, but 27% required appendectomy within the 1-year follow-up period. No patients in this group developed intra-abdominal abscess or other major acute complication. Those randomized to the surgical group had more abdominal pain, more incisional pain, more frequent surgical site infections, and took more sick leave. The acute complication rate in the surgical group was 20.5%, while the acute complication rate in the nonsurgical group was 2.8% [5].

The Non-Operative Treatment for Acute Appendicitis study demonstrated initial resolution of appendicitis within a 1-week follow-up period for 88.1% of the 159 enrolled patients with suspected appendicitis. These patients were discharged and treated with amoxicillin/clavulanate for 7 days as an outpatient. After 2 years, the overall recurrence rate of acute appendicitis was 13.8%. In the 22 patients that developed recurrent appendicitis, a repeat course of antibiotics successfully treated 14 of the 22 (63.6%) [6].

An RCT published in *Annals of Emergency Medicine* in 2017 randomized 15 patients with CT-proven appendicitis to an antibiotic treatment group (IV ertapenem × 2 doses, followed by 8 days of oral antibiotics). Two patients had recurrence in the 30-day follow-up period. One was treated with appendectomy, and the other had resolution of symptoms with further antibiotics. The non-operative management group had more pain-free days, faster return to normal activities, and less missed work. This is the only randomized trial in which patients were treated on an exclusively outpatient basis, with the initial doses of IV antibiotics delivered in the

J. Watson (✉) · D. Carlberg
Department of Emergency Medicine, MedStar Georgetown University Hospital & Washington Hospital Center, Washington, DC, USA
e-mail: jonathan.m.watson@medstar.net; david.carlberg@medstar.net

© Springer Nature Switzerland AG 2019
A. Graham, D. J. Carlberg (eds.), *Gastrointestinal Emergencies*, https://doi.org/10.1007/978-3-319-98343-1_80

emergency department followed by discharge [7]. Criticisms of this study include its single-center design, small sample size, and short follow-up period [8]. Previous studies have shown higher failure rates with an antibiotics-only approach during a 2-year follow-up period [6].

A study in the pediatric population has shown similar results. Families were given the choice between non-operative management and urgent appendectomy. Non-operative management was successful in 89.2% at 30 days and 75.7% at 1 year. Children managed non-operatively had fewer disability days and lower appendicitis-related healthcare costs [9].

Growing evidence suggests that there is a conditional role for an antibiotics-only approach to managing acute appendicitis. The decision to treat appendicitis with antibiotics should be individualized to the specific patient based on his or her wishes, medical history, and current clinical condition. Patients who wish to avoid surgery for personal preference, have other comorbid conditions, are able to easily return if treatment fails (if discharged), have appropriate close follow-up (if discharged), and accept the treatment failure risk are candidates for initial treatment with antibiotics [10, 11].

The challenge moving forward will be to identify which patients and antibiotic regimens/doses will have the greatest likelihood of producing a long-lasting cure. Additional studies are needed that focus on the antibiotics-only approach in the elderly, immunocompromised, and other poor surgical candidates.

Suggested Resources
- EM:RAP Paper Chase 3: Antibiotics for appendicitis. (December 2014: https://www.emrap.org/episode/december2014/paperchase3)
- R.E.B.E.L. EM Episode 35: Nonoperative treatment of appendicitis (April 2017: http://rebelem.com/episode-35-non-operative-treatment-of-appendicitis-nota/)

References

1. Addis D, Shaffer N, Fowler B, Tauxe R. The epidemiology of appendicitis and appendectomy in the United States. Am J Epidemiol. 1990;132(5):910–25.
2. Andersson R. The natural history and traditional management of appendicitis revisited: spontaneous resolution and predominance of prehospital perforations imply that a correct diagnosis is more important than an early diagnosis. World J Surg. 2006;31(1):86–92.
3. Aranda-Narváez J, González-Sánchez A, Marín-Camero N, Montiel-Casado C, López-Ruiz P, Sánchez-Pérez B, et al. Conservative approach versus urgent appendectomy in surgical management of acute appendicitis with abscess or phlegmon. Rev Esp Enfer Dig. 2010;102(11):648–52.
4. Simillis C, Symeonides P, Shorthouse A, Tekkis P. A meta-analysis comparing conservative treatment versus acute appendectomy for complicated appendicitis (abscess or phlegmon). Surgery. 2010;147(6):818–29.
5. Salminen P, Paajanen H, Rautio T, Nordström P, Aarnio M, Rantanen T, et al. Antibiotic therapy vs appendectomy for treatment of uncomplicated acute appendicitis. JAMA. 2015;313(23):2340.
6. Di Saverio S, Sibilio A, Giorgini E, Biscardi A, Villani S, Coccolini F, et al. The NOTA study (non operative treatment for acute appendicitis). Ann Surg. 2014;260(1):109–17.
7. Talan D, Saltzman D, Mower W, Krishnadasan A, Jude C, Amii R, et al. Antibiotics-first versus surgery for appendicitis: a US pilot randomized controlled trial allowing outpatient antibiotic management. Ann Emerg Med. 2017;70(1):1–11.
8. Kharbanda A, Schmeling D. Are antibiotics a feasible therapeutic option for appendicitis? Ann Emerg Med. 2017;70(1):15–7.
9. Minneci P, Mahida J, Lodwick D, Sulkowski J, Nacion K, Cooper J, et al. Effectiveness of patient choice in nonoperative vs surgical management of pediatric uncomplicated acute appendicitis. JAMA Surg. 2016;151(5):408–15.
10. Flum D. Acute appendicitis — appendectomy or the "antibiotics first" strategy. N Engl J Med. 2015;372(20):1937–43.
11. Di Saverio S, Birindelli A, Kelly M, Catena F, Weber D, Sartelli M, et al. WSES Jerusalem guidelines for diagnosis and treatment of acute appendicitis. World J Emerg Surg. 2016;11(1):34.

Is Surgery for Appendicitis Urgent or Emergent?

81

Jonathan L. Hansen

Pearls and Pitfalls
- In adults, surgery for uncomplicated acute appendicitis may be delayed 12–24 h in patients without significant risk of appendiceal perforation or other complications.
- In children, short delays are also permissible for uncomplicated appendicitis, although some authors recommend no longer than 9 h.
- An extended duration of symptoms from onset to presentation may have a stronger relationship with appendiceal perforation and thus may warrant more timely intervention.
- "Outpatient appendectomy" is a viable treatment option for postoperative care.

Traditionally, emergent surgical resection was the mainstay treatment for acute appendicitis, as progression to appendiceal perforation was felt to be inevitable over time. This dogma has been challenged recently, particularly in uncomplicated appendicitis, with increased recognition that short delays in time to appendectomy may offset risks associated with "after-hours" work, including limited resources and surgeon fatigue [1].

Questions regarding the expediency of surgical treatment have focused mostly on uncomplicated cases, without signs of peritonitis or perforation, as consensus remains that more timely intervention is required for these more complex situations [1]. Optimal timing for surgical care of appendiceal abscess and phlegmon has been studied and will be discussed in greater detail in the next chapter.

In adults, several studies have shown a permissible delay between presentation and surgical intervention for uncomplicated appendicitis. Two large cohort studies found no increased risk of perforation when surgery was performed within 24–48 h of presentation, but the risk of surgical site infection and other postoperative complications rose when surgery was delayed more than 48 h [1, 2]. Similarly, a meta-analysis of 11 nonrandomized studies encompassing 8858 patients showed that delays between 12 and 24 h did not increase the risk of complications [1].

Similar results have been noted in the pediatric population, but with shorter delays recommended between initial evaluation and operative intervention. A retrospective case review of 248 children revealed that no patient experienced appendiceal perforation if surgery was performed within 9 h of presentation. The rate of perforation rose to 21% if surgery occurred between 9 and 24 h, and 41% if surgery occurred after 24 h [3]. Conversely, another retrospective cohort study of 484 patients found no difference in perforation or other surgical complications based on timing, although most patients went to the operating room within 12 h of arrival and very few patients (1.7%) experienced delays greater than 24 h [4]. Most recently, a prospective multicenter, cross-sectional study of 955 children showed no relationship between timing and perforation, although it should also be noted that patients with delays over 24 h were excluded [5].

Given the apparent lack of relationship between hospital presentation and development of appendiceal perforation, other potentially pertinent factors have been explored. Duration of symptoms has been associated with perforation in both the adult and pediatric populations, with some authors recommending that appendectomy occur within 36 h of symptom onset [5, 6]. Other factors associated with perforation include advancing age, male gender, lack of insurance, and the presence of three or more comorbid conditions including coronary artery disease, asthma, diabetes mellitus,

J. L. Hansen
MedStar Franklin Square Medical Center, Baltimore, MD, USA

Georgetown University School of Medicine, Washington, DC, USA
e-mail: jonathan.hansen@me.com

© Springer Nature Switzerland AG 2019
A. Graham, D. J. Carlberg (eds.), *Gastrointestinal Emergencies*, https://doi.org/10.1007/978-3-319-98343-1_81

human immunodeficiency virus infection, and elevated serum creatinine [7].

In summary, short in-hospital delays, up to 24 h for most patients, are permissible in appropriately selected patients presenting with uncomplicated appendicitis. Some studies indicate that shorter delays may be more appropriate for pediatric patients. Other factors, such as duration of symptoms and comorbid conditions, should be considered when planning for surgical care.

Finally, the duration and setting of postoperative care has also been the subject of recent research. "Outpatient appendectomy" has been proposed as a viable treatment strategy, although it should be emphasized that "outpatient" refers to the location of care after appendectomy. Still, the astute physician should be aware of this treatment option, as it is associated with low morbidity, low readmission rates, and significantly lower costs for both adult and pediatric patients [8–10].

Suggested Resource
- Bhangu A, Søreide K, Di Saverio S, Assarsson H, Thurston Drake F. Acute appendicitis: modern understanding of pathogenesis, diagnosis, and management. Lancet. 2015;386:1278–87.

References

1. Bhangu A. Safety of short, in-hospital delays before surgery for acute appendicitis: multicentre cohort study, systematic review, and meta-analysis. Ann Surg. 2014;259:894–903.
2. Fair BA, Kubasiak JC, Janssen I, et al. The impact of operative timing on outcomes of appendicitis: a national surgical quality improvement project analysis. Am J Surg. 2015;209:498–502.
3. Bonadio W, Brazg J, Telt N, et al. Impact of in-hospital timing to appendectomy on perforation rates in children with appendicitis. J Emerg Med. 2015;49(5):597–604.
4. Gurien LA, Wyrick DL, Smith SD, et al. Optimal timing of appendectomy in the pediatric population. J Surg Res. 2016;202:126–31.
5. Stevenson MD, Dyan PS, Dudley NC, et al. Time from emergency department evaluation to operation and appendiceal perforation. Pediatrics. 2017;139(6):e20160742.
6. Kim M, Kim SJ, Cho HJ. Effect of surgical timing and outcomes for appendicitis severity. Ann Surg Treat Res. 2016;91(2):85–9.
7. Drake FT, Mottey NE, Farrokhi ET, et al. Time to appendectomy and risk of perforation in acute appendicitis. JAMA Surg. 2014;149(8):837–44.
8. Litz CN, Stone L, Alessi R, et al. Impact of outpatient management following appendectomy for acute appendicitis: An ACS NSQIP-P analysis. J Pediatr Surg. 2017; https://doi.org/10.1016/j.jpedsurg.2017.06.023. [Article In Press].
9. Frazee R, Burlew CC, Regnar J, et al. Outpatient laparoscopic appendectomy can be successfully performed for uncomplicated appendicitis: a Southwestern Surgical Congress multicenter trial. Am J Surg. 2017; https://doi.org/10.1016/j.amjsurg.2017.08.029. [Article In Press].
10. Gurien LA, Burford JM, Bonasso PC, et al. Resource savings and outcomes associated with outpatient laparoscopic appendectomy for nonperforated appendicitis. J Pediatr Surg. 2017; https://doi.org/10.1016/j.jpedsurg.2017.03.039. [Article In Press].

Does Ruptured Appendicitis with Abscess Warrant Urgent Operative Intervention?

82

Kerrie Lind

> **Pearls and Pitfalls**
> - Abscess formation occurs in up to 10% of appendicitis.
> - Conservative management is generally safe, especially when interventional radiology is available.
> - Because urgent operative intervention may be associated with increased morbidity, it is generally reserved for when IR is unavailable, the patient is imminently sick, there is an extraluminal appendicolith, or there is a large ill-defined abscess.
> - More studies comparing operative intervention and conservative management of appendicitis with abscess are required.

Ruptured appendicitis with abscess accounts for 2–10% of appendicitis cases [1–4]. While urgent operative intervention is generally considered the standard management for uncomplicated appendicitis, patients with ruptured appendicitis and abscess who undergo acute operative intervention risk complications including delayed wound healing, sepsis, and adhesions [2].

While studies regarding management of appendicitis-related intra-abdominal abscess do not provide conclusive evidence regarding timing of operative intervention, they trend toward favoring initial non-operative management. Many authors suggest initial management with intravenous antibiotics and percutaneous drainage by interventional radiology (IR). These patients generally receive interval appendectomy weeks later [5–7]. Patients with peritonitis, extraluminal appendicolith, or large ill-defined abscess may have stronger indications for early appendectomy [5].

Three recent studies showed no appreciable difference between early appendectomy and delayed appendectomy in patients with appendiceal perforation and abscess. Duggan et al. showed no difference in adverse outcomes or readmission rates in a meta-analysis comparing early appendectomy and interval appendectomy in children [8]. Using the Cochrane Database, Cheng et al. compared outcomes with early versus delayed appendectomy and found no clear difference in length of stay, return to normal activities, or quality of life [1]. Kim et al. did not find a difference between treatment outcomes and postsurgical complications when comparing patients who underwent emergent appendectomy and interval appendectomy [2].

Other studies, however, have found benefit with initial non-operative management and interval appendectomy. Jamieson et al. and Marin et al. both reported successful treatment rates of ~90% for appendiceal abscesses treated with CT-guided drainage and IV antibiotics [9, 10]. Erdogan et al. evaluated children with ruptured appendicitis and found the complication rate for emergency surgery reached 26% [11]. Complications with acute surgical intervention arise from the potential to spread a walled-off infection, creation of secondary fistulas, spread of inflammation to other parts of the abdominal cavity, and intraoperative technical difficulties due to anatomic changes from inflammation [2, 12].

One study did find benefit with early surgical intervention in that it yielded fewer readmissions and interventions while producing a comparable hospital stay [13].

Overall, the general trend of the literature is toward conservative management initially with antibiotics and/or percutaneous drainage followed by interval appendectomy. Appropriate antibiotics should cover both aerobic Gram-negative bacteria and anaerobic bacteria [12].

Multiple factors play into the decision between ultrasound (US)- and CT-guided percutaneous abscess drainage. US avoids ionizing radiation and allows real-time observation throughout the procedure. CT is preferred if the abscess is near or obscured by vital structures. It is also preferred for smaller abscesses [5].

More studies comparing operative intervention and conservative management followed by interval appendectomy are required.

K. Lind
Medstar Southern Maryland Hospital Center, Department of Emergency Medicine, Clinton, MD, USA

© Springer Nature Switzerland AG 2019
A. Graham, D. J. Carlberg (eds.), *Gastrointestinal Emergencies*, https://doi.org/10.1007/978-3-319-98343-1_82

Suggested Resources

- Emergency medicine cases: appendicitis controversies. Episode 43. https://emergencymedicinecases. com/episode-43-appendicitis-controversies/.
- EM:RAP: EMA January 1999 Abstract 23. Perforated Appendicitis: is it truly a surgical urgency?

References

1. Cheng Y, Xiong X, Lu J, Wu S, Zhou R, Cheng N. Early versus delayed appendicectomy for appendiceal phlegmon or abscess. Cochrane Database Syst Rev. 2017;2:6. https://doi.org/10.1002/14651858.CD011670.pub2.
2. Kim J, Ryoo S, Oh H, Kim J, Shin R, Choe E, Jeong S, Park K. Management of Appendicitis Presenting with abscess or mass. J Korean Soc Coloproctology. 2010;26(6):413–9. https://doi.org/10.3393/jksc.2010.26.6.413.
3. Sartelli M. The management of intra-abdominal infections from a global perspective: 2017 WSES guidelines for management of intra-abdominal infections. World J Emerg Surg. 2017;12:29. https://doi.org/10.1186/s13017-017-0141-6.
4. Andersson R, Petzold M. Nonsurgical treatment of appendiceal abscess or phlegmon: a systematic review and meta-analysis. Ann Surg. 2007;246(5):741–8.
5. Amin P, Cheng D. Management of complicated appendicitis in the pediatric population: when surgery doesn't cut it. Semin Intervent Radiol. 2012;29(3):231–6. https://doi.org/10.1055/s-0032-1326934.
6. Craig S. Appendicitis treatment and management. Medscape [Internet] 2017, January 19. Available from: http://emedicine.medscape.com/article/773895-treatment.
7. Marin D, Ho M, Barnhart H, Neville M, White R, Paulson E. Percutaneous abscess drainage in patients with perforated acute appendicitis: effectiveness, safety, and prediction of outcome. AJR Am J Roentgenol. 2010;194(2):422–9. https://doi.org/10.2214/AJR.09.3098.
8. Duggan E, Marshall A, Weaver K, St Peter S, Tice J, Wang L, Choi L, Blakely M. A systematic review and individual patient data meta-analysis of published randomized clinical trials comparing early versus interval appendectomy for children with perforated appendicitis. Pediatr Surg Int. 2016;32(7):649–55. https://doi.org/10.1007/s00383-016-3897-y.
9. Jamieson D. Interventional drainage of appendiceal abscesses in children. AJR Am J Roentgenol. 1997;169(6):1619–22.
10. Marin D. Percutaneous abscess drainage in patients with perforated acute appendicitis: effectiveness, safety, and prediction of outcome. AJR Am J Roentgenol. 2010;194(2):422–9.
11. Erdogan D. Comparison of two methods for the management of appendicular mass in children. Pediatr Surg Int. 2005;21(2):81–3.
12. Salari A. Perforated appendicitis, current concepts in colonic disorders. INTECH. 2012. Available from: http://www.intechopen.com/books/current-concepts-incolonic-disorders/perforated-appendicitis. ISBN: 978-953-307-957-8.
13. Mentula P, Sammalkorpi H, Leppaniemi A. Laparoscopic surgery or conservative treatment for appendiceal abscess in adults? A randomized controlled trial. Ann Surg. 2015;262(2):237–42. https://doi.org/10.1097/SLA.0000000000001200.

Consultant Corner: Appendicitis

83

Shawna Kettyle and Patrick G. Jackson

Pearls and Pitfalls
- Malignancy-associated appendiceal disease is generally associated with more prolonged subacute symptoms compared to classic appendicitis. Leukocytosis may not be present.
- Over half of children under 6 years old with acute appendicitis present with appendiceal perforation.
- While all patients should be resuscitated and started on empiric antibiotics, patients with phlegmon/abscess should be treated nonsurgically with antibiotics and percutaneous drainage if appropriate. Patients with generalized purulent peritonitis with sepsis require prompt surgical exploration following resuscitation.
- Nonsurgical management of appendicitis has been hotly debated, and an understanding of its optimal application is still evolving.
- Children who present with perforation should undergo interval appendectomy. In adults interval appendectomy carries a significant rate of morbidity, so many surgeons recommend appendectomy only with recurrent appendicitis.

Introduction

Patrick G. Jackson, MD, FACS, is board certified in general surgery and is program director of the Georgetown University Hospital/Washington Hospital Center General Surgery Residency. He is the chief of the Division of General Surgery at MedStar Georgetown University Hospital. Dr. Jackson has completed fellowships in both research and advanced laparoscopic surgery. Shawna Kettyle, MD, is a senior surgical resident at MedStar Washington Hospital Center. Dr. Jackson and Dr. Kettyle each practice in a large, urban tertiary referral hospital in Washington, DC, and evaluate acute care surgical patients on a regular basis.

Answers to Key Clinical Questions

1. When do you recommend consultation with a surgeon and in what time frame?
Surgical consultation should be pursued early in the workup when there is high clinical suspicion for acute appendicitis. While recent literature has shown that appendicitis is an urgent surgical disease (as opposed to an emergent surgical disease), requiring surgery in the 12–24 h time frame [1–3], delays in surgical consultation and intervention of more than 12–18 h from the time of emergency department presentation have been associated with a greater incidence of advanced disease [4], a longer length of stay, and higher costs [5, 6].

2. What pearls can you offer emergency care providers when evaluating a patient with appendicitis?
Despite the fact that appendectomy is the most common emergent surgical procedure performed worldwide, it remains a diagnostic and management challenge, particularly in its early stages. Diagnosis hinges on the history and physical examination findings.

An Alvarado score of less than 5 may be beneficial to rule out appendicitis, especially in men. It may be less useful in women and children [7]. If using the Alvarado score to rule out appendicitis, patients should be given close follow-up and strict return precautions.

Women may have gynecologic pathologies which mimic acute appendicitis, such as adnexal torsion, pelvic inflammatory disease, and ectopic pregnancy. These should be ruled out to minimize the nontherapeutic appendectomy rate.

S. Kettyle
MedStar Washington Hospital Center, Washington, DC, USA
e-mail: Shawna.Kettyle@medstar.net

P. G. Jackson (✉)
MedStar Washington Hospital Center, Washington, DC, USA

MedStar Georgetown University Hospital, Washington, DC, USA
e-mail: PGJ5@gunet.georgetown.edu

© Springer Nature Switzerland AG 2019
A. Graham, D. J. Carlberg (eds.), *Gastrointestinal Emergencies*, https://doi.org/10.1007/978-3-319-98343-1_83

3. What concepts do you think are key to managing a patient with appendicitis?

All patients with appendicitis should be initially managed with fluid resuscitation and antibiotics with empiric coverage of Gram-negative and anaerobic organisms. This should be closely followed by surgical evaluation.

4. What complications are you concerned about in this patient population?

Patients with a delayed presentation or significant delay to operative intervention risk appendiceal perforation, which can lead to either local peritonitis with phlegmon/abscess formation or generalized purulent peritonitis with sepsis (less common). While all patients should be resuscitated and started on empiric antibiotics, patients with phlegmon/abscess should be treated nonsurgically with antibiotics and percutaneous drainage if appropriate. Patients with generalized purulent peritonitis with sepsis require prompt surgical exploration following resuscitation.

Sepsis and septic shock may be the initial presentation of acute appendicitis, especially in high-risk populations such as the elderly and those with immunocompromise. These patients should be treated as any other patient presenting in septic shock, with fluid resuscitation and broad-spectrum antibiotics. They may be more likely to need operative exploration if the diagnosis is unclear.

Occult malignancy may be present in patients whose disease process follows a subacute course. This may complicate both operative intervention and the postoperative course.

5. What patients will have an "atypical" presentation for appendicitis and what are those presentations?

Pregnancy, especially approaching term, makes the diagnosis of appendicitis more difficult because the gravid uterus displaces the appendix out of its typical anatomic location. Physiologic leukocytosis is also common in pregnancy. Pregnant patients may present with heartburn, bowel irregularity, flatulence, malaise, and/or diarrhea [8, 9]. Delay of surgical intervention for more than 24 h after symptom onset increases the risk of perforation, which in turn increases the risk of fetal loss and early delivery [10].

Patients with congenital anomalies of the midgut, such as midgut malrotation and situs inversus may present with atypical symptoms of appendicitis because the appendix is typically located in the left abdomen rather than in the right lower quadrant [11, 12].

Rarely, patients with appendiceal malignancy may present with abdominal pain and CT findings of a dilated appendix. Malignancy-associated appendiceal disease is generally associated with more prolonged subacute symptoms compared to classic appendicitis. Leukocytosis may not be present.

6. Radiation: when can patients be spared CT scan? Alvarado score? Ultrasound?

Younger male patients with classic history and physical examination findings may be spared exposure to ionizing radiation while maintaining a low nontherapeutic appendectomy rate. The Alvarado scoring system helps identify patients who have a high likelihood of having appendicitis. These patients may be candidates for appendectomy without any imaging.

Ultrasound should be considered as the preferred initial imaging exam in children, who have a higher cancer risk per unit dosing of ionizing radiation and a longer lifetime to manifest the effects [13, 14].

7. MRI: gold standard or emerging technology with limited role?

MRI continues to have a limited role in the diagnosis of acute appendicitis. While it spares the patient ionizing radiation and may have comparable diagnostic accuracy to CT, it is not readily available and is more time-consuming and costly than ultrasound or CT. Additionally, there is less experience overall with MRI, which may contribute to non-visualization of 20–40% of normal appendices [15].

8. What about appendicitis and pregnancy? Is there a systematic approach to save time, reduce radiation and make everyone happy?

Ultrasound may be useful if a thick-walled noncompressible appendix can be identified; however, non-visualization is of the appendix common in pregnant patients. MRI can be used as the next step and has high sensitivity and specificity in pregnant women [16]. If MRI is not available and the diagnosis remains unclear, low-dose CT can be performed with low risk for adverse fetal effects [17].

It is important to note that nontherapeutic appendectomy during pregnancy increases the risk of early delivery and fetal death, as does delayed diagnosis. Accurate and expedient identification or exclusion of appendicitis is beneficial for both mother and fetus.

9. What about kids and appendicitis? Small adults or different approach?

Appendicitis is the most common indication for emergent abdominal surgery in childhood and presents most frequently in the second decade of life. Over half of children under 6 years old present with perforation, most likely as a result of nonspecific symptoms [18]. The differential diagnosis in children should include volvulus (secondary to midgut malrotation) and intussusception, both of which are less common in adults. It should also include ovarian and testicular torsion, bowel obstruction, and ectopic pregnancy.

The approach to managing pediatric appendicitis is virtually the same as it is in adults, including fluid resuscitation, antibiotics, and early surgery for patients with non-perforated disease.

10. Is there a role for medical management of appendicitis?

Nonsurgical management of appendicitis has been hotly debated and an understanding of its optimal application is still evolving. A Cochrane review was inconclusive, but it did show that patients treated with antibiotics alone were less likely to be cured at 2 weeks post-diagnosis and had higher rates of recurrence [19]. However, the studies reviewed were of low to moderate quality.

Patients may decide to accept a higher rate of treatment failure and recurrence with initial antibiotic therapy, hoping for a reasonable chance of avoiding surgery altogether.

11. Does ruptured appendicitis with abscess warrant urgent operative intervention?

No, typically ruptured appendicitis is treated nonoperatively with antibiotics and percutaneous abscess drainage if appropriate. Immediate surgical intervention is associated with a threefold increase in morbidity, including conversion to open procedure, more extensive bowel resection, and postoperative infection compared to nonsurgical management.

Rarely, rupture will be associated with generalized peritonitis and sepsis, which should be treated with exploration.

Children who present with perforation should undergo interval appendectomy. In adults interval appendectomy remains controversial but carries a significant rate of morbidity, so many surgeons recommend appendectomy only with recurrent appendicitis [20, 21].

References

1. Yardeni D, et al. Delayed versus immediate surgery in acute appendicitis: do we need to operate during the night? J Pediatr Surg. 2003;39(3):464–9.
2. Rajendra S, Feargal Q, Prem P. Is it necessary to perform appendicectomy in the middle of the night in children? BMJ. 1993;306(6886):1168.
3. Ingraham AM, et al. Effect of delay to operation on outcomes in adults. Arch Surg. 2010;145(9):886–92.
4. Ditillo MF, Dziura JD, Rabinovici R. Is it safe to delay appendectomy in adults with acute appendicitis. Ann Surg. 2006;244:656–60.
5. Eko FN, et al. Ideal timing of surgery for acute uncomplicated appendicitis. N Am J Med Sci. 2013;5:22–7.
6. Jeon BG, et al. Appendectomy: should it be performed so quickly? Am Surg. 2016;82(1):65–74.
7. Ohle R, et al. The Alvarado score for predicting acute appendicitis: a systematic review. BMC Med. 2011;9:139–52.
8. Pates JA, et al. The appendix in pregnancy: confirming historical observations with a contemporary modality. Obstet Gynecol. 2009;114(4):805–8.
9. Mahmoodian S. Appendicitis complicating pregnancy. South Med J. 1992;85(1):19–24.
10. McGory ML, et al. Negative appendectomy in pregnant women is associated with a substantial risk of fetal loss. J Am Coll Surg. 2007;205(4):534–40.
11. Birnbaum DJ, et al. Left side appendicitis with midgut malrotation in an adult. J Surg Tech Case Rep. 2013;5(1):38–40.
12. Akbukut S, et al. Left-sided appendicitis: review of 95 published cases and a case report. World J Gastroenterol. 2010;16(44):5598–602.
13. Kessler N, et al. Appendicitis: evaluation of sensitivity, specificity, and predictive values of US, Doppler US, and laboratory findings. Radiology. 2004;230(2):472–8.
14. Keyzer C, et al. Comparison of US and unenhanced multi-detector row CT in patients suspected of having acute appendicitis. Radiology. 2005;236(2):527–34.
15. Barger RL, Nandalur KR. Diagnostic performance of magnetic resonance imaging in the detection of appendicitis in adults: a meta-analysis. Acad Radiol. 2010;17(10):1211–6.
16. Burke LM, Bashir MR, et al. Magnetic resonance imaging of acute appendicitis in pregnancy: a 5-year multiinstitutional study. Am J Obstet Gynecol. 2015;213(5):693.e1–6.
17. Hurwitz LM, et al. Radiation dose to the fetus from body MDCT during early gestation. Am J Roentgenol. 2006;186(3):871–6.
18. Rothrock SG, Pagane J. Acute appendicitis in children: emergency department diagnosis and management. Ann Emerg Med. 2000;36(1):39–51.
19. Wilms IM, et al. Appendectomy versus antibiotic treatment for acute appendicitis. Cochrane Database Syst Rev 11. 2011;
20. Quartey B. Interval appendectomy in adults: a necessary evil? J Emerg Trauma Shock. 2012;5(3):213–6.
21. Sakorafas GH, et al. Interval routine appendectomy following conservative treatment of acute appendicitis: is it really needed. World J Gastrointest Surg. 2012;4(4):83–6.

Diagnosing Diverticulitis: Balancing Cost, Efficiency, and Safety. Can I Make This Diagnosis by Clinical Assessment Alone? What Is the Role of Imaging?

Elaine Bromberek and Autumn Graham

Pearls and Pitfalls
- The three strongest predictors of acute diverticulitis are direct tenderness only in the left lower quadrant of abdomen, the absence of vomiting, and C-reactive protein >50 mg/L.
- The high misdiagnosis rates and reliance of CT confirmation for risk assessment, treatment, and disposition translate into low adoption of clinical decision tools and reliance on clinical diagnosis.

Diverticulitis is a common discharge diagnosis from the emergency department (ED). Analysis of the Nationwide Emergency Department Sample (NEDS), the largest publicly available emergency department all-payer database, found that diverticulitis accounted for over 360,000 ED visits in 2013, a 34% increase in visits compared to 2006 [1]. During this same time period (2006–2013), a decrease in admissions from the emergency department (from 58% to 47%), cases managed surgically (decreased by 11%), and deaths per 100,000 admitted patients (decreased by 42%) were documented [1]. In 2013, the aggregate national cost of diverticulitis-related ED visits was over $1.6 billion [1]. The magnitude and shifting management of acute diverticulitis emphasizes the need to develop a nuanced understanding of this disease to provide efficient and safe care.

Can I Make This Diagnosis by Clinical Assessment Alone?

Accuracy of Clinical Assessment

Diverticulitis typically presents with left lower quadrant abdominal pain that may be associated with a change in bowel habits (both diarrhea and constipation are described), fever, loss of appetite, nausea, and urinary frequency due to irritation of the bladder (Table 84.1). In patients of Asian descent or those with a redundant sigmoid colon, right-sided abdominal pain may predominate [4]. On physical examination, left-sided abdominal tenderness, fever, abdominal distention, or a tender palpable mass may be present. Laboratory tests often reflect leukocytosis, an elevated CRP, or sterile pyuria [4].

The American Society of Colon and Rectal Surgeons' (ASCRS) clinical guidelines (2014) state "the diagnosis of acute diverticulitis can often be made following a focused history and physical examination, especially in patients with recurrent diverticulitis whose diagnosis has been previously confirmed" [5]. However, literature on the accuracy of clinical diagnosis alone is limited and the studies that have been published reflect high misdiagnosis rates. Early studies estimated the misdiagnosis rate to be between 34% and 67% [2]. Several studies published in the last decade confirm that the clinical diagnosis of diverticulitis has a low sensitivity rate, but higher specificity.

- Laurell et al. (2007) reported that a clinical diagnosis alone had a sensitivity of 64% but specificity of 97%, after studying 145 admitted patients with suspected diverticulitis compared to 1145 patients admitted with nonspecific abdominal pain. Malignancy, appendicitis, gynecologic etiologies, urinary tract infections, and aortic aneurysm were alternate final diagnoses [2].
- Toorenvliet et al. (2010) prospectively evaluated 802 consecutive patients with abdominal pain that presented to an emergency department. Fifty seven patients had a final diagnosis of diverticulitis. Again, clinical diagnosis alone

E. Bromberek (✉)
MedStar Washington Hospital Center, MedStar Georgetown University Hospital, Washington, DC, USA

A. Graham
Department of Emergency Medicine, MedStar Washington Hospital Center, MedStar Georgetown University Hospital, Washington, DC, USA

© Springer Nature Switzerland AG 2019
A. Graham, D. J. Carlberg (eds.), *Gastrointestinal Emergencies*, https://doi.org/10.1007/978-3-319-98343-1_84

Table 84.1 Diverticulitis signs and symptoms compared with nonspecific abdominal pain

Laurell et al. (2007)			Andeweg et al. (2011)	
Sign/symptom	Diverticulitis ($n = 145$)	NSAP ($n = 1142$)	Sign/symptom	Odd ratio (95% CI)
Mean age	62 years	37 years	Age 41–50	2.08 (0.85–5.11)
			Age >50	3.99 (1.99–8.03)
Previous episodes	54%	40%	One or more previous episodes	7.60 (3.72–15.52)
Duration (hours)	49 h	35 h	Duration >4 days	1.58 (0.81–3.07)
Left abdominal tenderness	37%	7%	Left lower quadrant pain	3.43 (1.98–5.92)
Right abdominal tenderness	7%	19%	Right lower quadrant pain	0.25 (0.11–0.61)
Generalized abdominal tenderness	12%	19%	Diffuse abdominal pain	1.00 (reference)
			Aggravation with movement	2.97 (1.83–4.83)
			Anorexia	0.71 (0.44–1.13)
Vomiting	14%	27%	Vomiting	0.49 (0.59–0.86)
Diarrhea	17%	14%	Diarrhea	1.35 (0.76–2.40)
Constipation	26%	12%		
Temperature	37.7	37.2	Fever >38.5	2.00 (1.06–3.78)
Rebound tenderness	45%	24%	Rebound tenderness	2.92 (1.80–4.74)
Leukocytes ($\times 10^9$/L)	12.1	10.1	WBC 10–12 ($\times 10^9$/L)	2.53 (1.32–4.85)
			WBC 10–12 ($\times 10^9$/L)	2.45 (1.26–4.76)
CRP (mg/L)	73	20	CRP > 50 mg /L	3.78 (1.92–7.43)

Adapted from Refs. [2, 3]

NSAP nonspecific abdominal pain

had a low sensitivity of 68% but high specificity of 98%. The positive predictive value (PPV) of clinical diagnosis for diverticulitis was 0.65, with a negative predictive value (NPV) of 0.98. With the addition of computed tomography (CT), the PPV increased to 0.95 and the NPV was 0.99 [6].

- Andweg et al. (2011) evaluated 1290 hospitalized patients who presented with abdominal pain during a 4-year period. Of the 287 patients with suspected diverticulitis on initial evaluation, 124 patients (43%) had CT-confirmed diverticulitis and 163 patients (57%) had another final diagnosis [3].

Can a Clinical Decision Rule for Diverticulitis Help Me Confirm the Diagnosis and Safely Disposition Patients?

Several clinical decision rules have been described to help clinicians clinically diagnose acute diverticulitis.

Andweg et al. identified seven independent predictors of acute diverticulitis. These predictors included (1) age greater than 50 years, (2) a prior episode of diverticulitis, (3) left lower quadrant abdominal pain, (4) left lower quadrant abdominal tenderness, (5) worsening of symptoms with movement, (6) CRP > 50 mg/L, and (7) the absence of vomiting (Table 84.1). While independently they were not able to accurately predict acute diverticulitis, in combination, these seven predictors demonstrated an accuracy rate of 86% (84% after internal validation) [3].

Lameris et al. developed a clinical decision rule utilizing the three strongest predictors of acute diverticulitis: direct tenderness only in the left lower quadrant of abdomen, the absence of vomiting, and C-reactive protein >50 mg/L. In a prospective study of 1021 patients with acute abdominal pain in the emergency department, 112 patients were diagnosed with diverticulitis. Of those 112 patients, the combination of all 3 predictors were found in 24% of patients and correlated with a 97% likelihood of diverticulitis diagnosis. "Of the 96 patients without all 3 features, 45 (47%) did not have diverticulitis" [7].

While these clinical predictors likely account for the high specificity of clinical assessment in the diagnosis of acute diverticulitis, the high misdiagnosis rates and reliance of CT confirmation for risk assessment, treatment, and disposition translate into low adoption of these decision tools.

What Is the Role of Imaging?

Imaging is a useful tool for risk stratification, treatment, and disposition of diverticulitis patients. Computed tomography (CT), ultrasound, and magnetic resonance imaging (MRI) can all diagnose diverticulitis but do not provide identical information [8, 9]. The diagnosis of acute diverticulitis can be accomplished by colonoscopy, but due to the risk of perforation in acute episodes, it is not recommended. Furthermore, colonoscopy cannot identify abscesses or extensive areas of pericolic stranding and inflammation, decreasing the ability to risk stratify patients [8, 9].

Computed Tomography (CT)

CT is easy to obtain and provides important information not obtained with other imaging modalities, including the degree and location of inflammation, abscess formation, and micro-/macro-perforations [8, 9]. Regardless of contrast strategy, CT remains highly accurate in diagnosis acute diverticulitis. In one study, the sensitivity and specificity of CT for diverticulitis were 97% and 98%, respectively [10]. This is consistent with CT's overall accuracy rate of 99% [11]. The American College of Radiology Appropriateness Criteria recommends CT abdomen and pelvis with IV contrast but adds the caveat "oral and/or colonic contrast may be helpful for bowel luminal visualization" [11]. However, a retrospective review found no significant difference in the ability to diagnosis acute intraabdominal processes with contrast versus non-contrast CT imaging. This included acute diverticulitis. The most common contrast strategy is IV contrast alone as it may help identify diverticulitis complications better than non-contrast studies [12]. Low-dose radiation strategies have been explored and have documented sensitivities and specificities similar to standard-dose CT imaging, but more research would be needed before broad adoption as other diagnoses are often considered when imaging patients with suspected diverticulitis [11].

Ultrasonography

Ultrasonography is accurate in diagnosing diverticulitis in a subset of patients but provides less information regarding complications of diverticulitis. Overall, graded compression sonography has a reported sensitivity between 77% and 98% and a specificity between 80% and 99% [11]. In a meta-analysis comparing ultrasonography to computed tomography to diagnose diverticulitis, ultrasound had a combined sensitivity and specificity of 92% and 90%, respectively, versus 94% and 99% for CT [13]. However, ultrasound identified an alternate diagnosis in 33–78% of cases, while CT identified alternate diagnosis in 50–100% cases [13].

Magnetic Resonance Imaging

MRI provides similar information to CT and provides great detail of the soft tissue structures involved in diverticulitis but is time-consuming. Patients with specific pacemakers and metal implants will not be able to complete this study [4]. Studies suggest that MRI has sensitivities of 86–94% and specificities of 88–92% in patients with left lower quadrant abdominal pain being evaluated for diverticulitis [11].

> **Suggested Resources**
> - FOAMcast, episode 45 – Diverticulitis, foamcast.org/2016/03/04/episode-45-diverticulitis/.
> - McNamara, M. and Panel of Gastrointestinal Imaging (2014). ACR appropriateness criteria. [online] American College of Radiology. Available at: https://www.acr.org/Clinical-Resources/ACR-Appropriateness-Criteria. Accessed 20 Jan 2018.

References

1. Bollom A, Austrie J, Hirsch W, Friedlander D, Ellingson K, Cheng V, Lembo A. Emergency department burden of diverticulitis in the USA, 2006 – 2013. Dig Dis Sci. 2017;62:2694–703. [PMID: 28332105]
2. Laurell H, Hansson LE, Gunnarsson U. Acute diverticulitis—clinical presentation and differential diagnostics. Color Dis. 2007;9:496–501.
3. Andeweg C, Knobben L, Hendricks J, Bleichrodt R, van Goor H. How to diagnose left sided colonic diverticulitis: proposal for a clinical scoring system. Ann Surg. 2011;253(5):940–6.
4. Deery SA, Hodin RA. Management of diverticulitis in 2017. J Gastroinest Surg. 2017; https://doi.org/10.1007/s11605-017-3404-3.
5. Feingold D, Steele S, Lee S, Kaiser A, Boushey R, Buie D, Rafferty J. Practice parameters for the treatment of sigmoid diverticulitis. Dis Colon Rectum. 2014;57:284–94.
6. Toorenvliet BR, Bakker RF, Breslau PJ, et al. Colonic diverticulitis: a prospective analysis of diagnostic accuracy and clinical decision making. Color Dis. 2009;12(3):179–86.
7. Lameris W, van Randen A, van Gulik T, et al. A clinical decision rule to establish the diagnosis of acute diverticulitis at the emergency department. Dis Colon Rectum. 2010;53(6):896–904.
8. Feurstein J, Falchuk K. Diverticulosis and diverticulitis. Mayo Clin Proc. 2016;1(8):1094–104.
9. Stollman N, Smalley W, Hirano I, AGA Institute Clinical Guidelines Committee. American Gastroenterological association institute guideline on the management of acute diverticulitis. Gastroenterology. 2015;149:1944–9. http://www.gastro.org/guidelines/acute-diverticulitis#sec1.10.
10. Werner A, Diehl SJ, Farag-Soliman M, Duber C. Multi-slice spiral CT in routine diagnosis of suspected acute left-sided colonic diverticulitis: a prospective study of 120 patients. Eur Radiol. 2003;13(12):2596–603.
11. McNamara, M. and Panel of Gastrointestinal Imaging (2014). ACR appropriateness criteria. [online] American College of Radiology. Available at: https://www.acr.org/Clinical-Resources/ACR-Appropriateness-Criteria. Accessed 20 Jan 2018.
12. Hill BC, Johnson SC, Owens EK, Gerber JL, Senagore AJ. CT scan for suspected acute abdominal process: impact of combinations of IV, oral, and rectal contrast. World J Surg. 2010;34(4):699–703.
13. Lameris W, van Randen A, Bipat S, Bossuyt P, Boermeester M, Stoker J. Graded compression ultrasonography and computed tomography in acute colonic diverticulitis: meta-analysis of test accuracy. Eur Radiol. 2008;18(11):2498–511.

Medical Management: How Do I Optimize My Treatment Regimen for Uncomplicated Diverticulitis? Am I Ready to Ditch Antibiotics?

85

Traci Thoureen and Sara Scott

> **Pearls and Pitfalls**
> - Chronic nonsteroidal anti-inflammatory or opiate use has been associated with bowel perforation on presentation.
> - An unrestricted diet does not seem to impact treatment or duration of symptoms for acute diverticulitis.
> - Multiple studies have shown no increase in complications when antibiotic therapy is withheld from patients with acute uncomplicated diverticulitis.

Diverticulosis is a common condition as patients age, with a prevalence of 10–66% through the ninth decade [1]. Of those patients with asymptomatic diverticulosis, as many as one quarter will progress to symptomatic diverticulitis [2].

Classically, diverticulitis is divided into uncomplicated or complicated disease. This is likely an oversimplification given there are half a dozen classification systems for staging diverticulitis (e.g., Hinchey, modified Hinchey, Ambrosetti, Hansen/Stock, Koehler, Siewert, etc.). Ultimately, the severity of disease is categorized based on clinical exam and radiologic testing. Uncomplicated diverticulitis is defined radiologically by colonic wall thickening and pericolic inflammatory changes, which may include phlegmon or small abscesses. Conversely, complicated diverticulitis is associated with large or distant abscesses, sepsis, bowel obstruction, strictures, fistulas, or perforated viscous [3]. Of the patients admitted with diverticulitis, 80% are uncomplicated [4]. In a patient who is tolerating oral intake, uncomplicated diverticulitis can be managed in an outpatient setting.

Medical Management: How Do I Optimize My Treatment Regimen for Uncomplicated Diverticulitis?

Traditionally, medical management incorporates antibiotics, bowel rest, and analgesia.

Analgesia

Chronic analgesia use, including nonsteroidal anti-inflammatory drugs (OR 4.0) and opioids (OR 1.8), has been associated with bowel perforation on presentation [5, 6]. However, no evidence exists of adverse effects on disease course once diverticulitis has been diagnosed [7].

Diet

A lack of consensus exists regarding diet during acute diverticulitis episodes. The common adage of clear fluids and bowel rest has little evidential basis. The Netherlands' clinical guidelines state "there is no evidence that bed rest, dietary restrictions or laxatives positively influence the treatment outcome of acute colonic diverticulitis" [7]. Based on a prospective cohort study of 86 patients discharged after acute diverticulitis diagnosis, an unrestricted diet was deemed safe. The study found 8% of patients who resumed a normal diet within 3 days of diagnosis experienced an adverse event (e.g., admission and/or surgery). There were no deaths. The rates of complications with outpatient management range up to 10%, comparable to rates found in this study [8].

T. Thoureen (✉)
Division of Emergency Medicine, Duke University Medical Center, Durham, NC, USA
e-mail: traci.thoureen@duke.edu

S. Scott
Department of Surgery and Perioperative Care, University of Texas at Austin Dell Medical School, Austin, TX, USA
e-mail: sara.scott1@austin.utexas.edu

© Springer Nature Switzerland AG 2019
A. Graham, D. J. Carlberg (eds.), *Gastrointestinal Emergencies*, https://doi.org/10.1007/978-3-319-98343-1_85

Antibiotics

Antibiotics have been the mainstay of acute diverticulitis management. The Infectious Diseases Society of America (IDSA) recommends broad-spectrum antibiotics that cover gram-negative and anaerobic bacteria. Commonly isolated bacteria include *Escherichia coli*, *Bacteroides*, and *Clostridia* [9] (see Table 85.1 for antibiotic recommendations).

Clinical guidelines from IDSA and the Surgical Infection Society recommend continuation of antimicrobial therapy until cessation of "clinical signs" (e.g., pain, normalization of fever, and leukocytosis) [9]. While treatment courses of 7–10 days have traditionally been recommended, recent studies of hospitalized patients suggest a shorter duration may be appropriate. A study of admitted patients receiving IV ertapenam reported that a 4-day course of IV antibiotics was as effective as a 7-day course [10]. With continued research and emphasis on antibiotic stewardship, antibiotic treatment duration will likely shorten to 4–5 days and continuation to 7–10 days if symptoms or signs of infection persist.

Am I Ready to Ditch Antibiotics?

Recently, a paradigm shift in the pathogenesis of diverticulitis, as a predominantly inflammatory disease rather than infectious process, has decreased the need for antibiotics [11]. In 2015, the American Gastroenterological Association (AGA) suggested that antibiotic use for diverticulitis should be selective, rather than routine [12]. The quality of the

Table 85.1 Summary of antibiotic therapy

Uncomplicated acute diverticulitis oral antibiotics (5–7 days)	Complicated acute diverticulitis intravenous antibiotics
Ciprofloxacin (500 mg oral, three times daily) + metronidazole (500 mg oral, three times daily)	Ciprofloxacin + metronidazole
Amoxicillin-clavulanate (875 mg oral, twice daily)	Piperacillin-tazobactam (3.375–4.5 g IV every 6 h)
Moxifloxacin (400 mg oral, daily)	Imipenem-cilastatin (500 mg IV every 6 h)
Cefoxitin	Levofloxacin (500 mg IV every 24 h) + metronidazole (500 mg IV every 8 h)
Cephalosporin (cefazolin, cefuroxime) + metronidazole	Ceftriaxone (1 g IV every 24 h) + metronidazole (500 mg IV every 8 h)
Levofloxacin + metronidazole	Cefotaxime + metronidazole
	Ceftazidime + metronidazole
	Ticarcillin – clavulanate

Recommended by Infectious Diseases Society of America (IDSA) and Surgical Infection Society (SIS). Table courtesy of Brandon Ruderman and Sreeja Natesan

evidence supporting this recommendation was deemed low. It was based on only two randomized controlled trials, which had a high risk of bias and imprecision, as well as two retrospective studies [13].

The AVOD (Antibiotika Vid Okomplicerad Divertikulit) study was the sole, fully published RCT cited by the AGA in their 2015 recommendations. This multicenter study of 623 admitted patients with CT confirmed uncomplicated diverticulitis concluded there was no difference in resolution of pain or fever at 48 h, symptoms at 30-day follow-up, or length of stay in patients with antibiotics compared to patients treated without antibiotics [14]. The complication rate for both groups was low: 1% for the antibiotic group (e.g., three perforations) and 2% for the non-antibiotic group (e.g., three perforations, three abscesses) [14]. In follow-up analysis, antibiotic therapy did not prevent surgery for symptomatic diverticular disease (six patients in non-antibiotic group, two patients in antibiotic group) or recurrence rates. The authors point out that their study was powered for superiority, but not sufficiently powered to discern a statistically significant difference between the two groups. Additionally, the study was not blinded and lacked stringent enforcement of patient enrollment, which resulted in failure to enroll all eligible patients. This may have been due to clinician discretion and potentially have created a selection bias in the patient cohort that was studied [14].

The other RCT referenced in the 2015 AGA recommendations was only available in abstract form at the time of publication of the AGA paper, but has subsequently been fully published and strengthens the level of evidence. The DIABOLO (diverticulitis: antibiotics or close observation) trial was a prospective, multicenter randomized control trial of 522 acute diverticulitis patients that reported noninferiority of close observation versus antibiotics. No significant differences were reported between the observational and antibiotic group in recovery time (14 versus 12 days), complications (3.8% versus 2.6%), recurrent disease (3.4% versus 3.0%), surgery (3.8% versus 2.3%), adverse events (48.5% vs 54%), readmission (18% versus 12%), or mortality (1.1% versus 0.4%) [15]. This study limited enrollment to patients with a first-time episode of mild diverticulitis, defined as modified Hinchey stage Ia–Ib and Ambrosetti classification of mild diverticular disease. It is unclear how generalizable these results would be for patients with more severe disease because >90% of study patients were Hinchey stage Ia. In fact, the authors of the study suggest that their results not be used to justify altering the current management for patients with small abscesses (modified Hinchey stage Ib) until further evidence becomes available.

There continues to be mounting evidence that antibiotics are not required for all patients with acute uncomplicated diverticulitis. There have been multiple retrospective studies looking at patients with acute uncomplicated diverticulitis that were treated conservatively. A Swedish study in 2016 showed no significant change in readmission rates or recurrence [16]. A retrospective cohort study out of Norway found that patients with uncomplicated diverticulitis who were treated without antibiotics did not have significant increased complication rates; however, they did have an increase in recurrence and management failure as compared to the antibiotic group [17].

This growing body of research has led to an emerging paradigm shift in the way many European countries, such as Denmark [18], Italy [19], Germany [20], and the Netherlands [7], are approaching the treatment of diverticulitis. They have all adopted guidelines that advocate for limitations of antibiotics in uncomplicated diverticulitis. In the future, uncomplicated diverticulitis may be added to the ever-growing list of conditions that no longer require antibiotics.

Suggested Resources
- Diverticulitis 2016 [October 20, 2017]. Available from: http://foamcast.org/2016/03/04/episode-45-diverticulitis/.
- Radecki RP. Antibiotics, Hospital admission may not help uncomplicated diverticulitis 2016. Available from: http://www.acepnow.com/article/antibiotics-hospital-admission-may-not-help-uncomplicated-diverticulitis/3/.
- Shahedi K, Chudasama Y, Dea S, Suraweera D. Diverticulitis. Updated August. 2017;15. Available from: https://emedicine.medscape.com/article/173388-overview. Accessed 20 Oct 2017.

References

1. Unlu C, Korte N, Lidewine D, Consten EC, Cuesta MA, Gerhards M, et al. A multicenter randomized clinical trial investigating the cost-effectiveness of treatment strategies with or without antibiotics for uncomplicated acute diverticulitis (DIABOLO trial). BMC Surg. 2010;10(23):1–10.
2. Jacobs DO. Diverticulitis. N Engl J Med. 2007;357(20):2057–66.
3. Klarenbeek BR, de Korte N, van der Peet DL, Cuesta MA. Review of current classifications for diverticular disease and a translation into clinical practice. Int J Color Dis. 2012;27(2):207–14.
4. Anaya DA, Flum DR. Risk of emergency colectomy and colostomy in patients with diverticular disease. Arch Surg. 2005;140(7):681–5.
5. Morris CR, Harvey IM, Stebbings WS, Speakman CT, Kennedy H. Anti-inflammatory drugs, analgesics and the risk of perforated colonic diverticular disease. Br J Surg. 2003;90:1267–72.
6. Wilson RG, Smith AN, Macintyre IM. Complications of diverticular disease and non-steroidal anti-inflammatory drugs: a prospective study. Br J Surg. 1990;77:1103–4.
7. Andeweg CS, Mulder IM, Felt-Bersma RJ, Verbon A, van der Wilt GJ, van Goor H, et al. Guidelines of diagnostics and treatment of acute left-sided colonic diverticulitis. Dig Surg. 2013;30(4–6):278–92.
8. Stam M, Draaisma W, van de Wall B, Bolkenstein H, Consten C, Broeders I. An unrestricted diet for uncomplicated diverticulitis is safe: results of a prospective diverticulitis diet study. Color Dis. 2016;19:372–7.
9. Solomkin JS, Mazuski JE, Bradley JS, et al. Diagnosis and management of complicated intra-abdominal infection in adults and children: guidelines by the Surgical Infection Society and the Infectious Diseases Society of America. Clin Infect Dis. 2010;50:133.
10. Basoli A, Chirletti P, Cirino E, D'Ovidio N, Giulini S, Malizia A, Taffurelli M, Petrovic J, Ecari M. A prospective, double blinded, multicenter, randomized trial comparing ertapenem 3 versus > 5 days in community acquired intraabdominal infection. J Gastrointest Surg. 2008;12:592–600.
11. Floch M. A hypothesis: is diverticulitis a type of inflammatory bowel disease? J Clin Gastroenterol. 2006;40(Suppl 3):S121–S5.
12. Strate LL, Peery AF, Neumann I. American Gastroenterological Association Institute technical review on the management of acute diverticulitis. Gastroenterology. 2015;149(7):1950–76. e12
13. Stollman N, Smalley W, Hirano I. American Gastroenterological Association Institute guideline on the management of acute diverticulitis. Gastroenterology. 2015;149(7):1944–9.
14. Chabok A, Pahlman L, Hjern F, Haapaniemi S, Smedh K, Group AS. Randomized clinical trial of antibiotics in acute uncomplicated diverticulitis. Br J Surg. 2012;99(4):532–9.
15. Daniels L, Unlu C, de Korte N, van Dieren S, Stockmann HB, Vrouenraets BC, et al. Randomized clinical trial of observational versus antibiotic treatment for a first episode of CT-proven uncomplicated acute diverticulitis. Br J Surg. 2017;104(1):52–61.
16. Isacson D, Andreasson K, Nikberg M, Smedh K, Chabok A. No antibiotics in acute uncomplicated diverticulitis: does it work? Scan J Gastroenterol. 2014;49:1–6.
17. Brochmann ND, Schultz JK, Jakobsen GS, Oresland T. Management of acute uncomplicated diverticulitis without antibiotics: a single-centre cohort study. Color Dis. 2016;18(11):1101–7.
18. Andersen JC, Bundgaard L, Elbrond H, Laurberg S, Walker LR, Stovring J. Danish national guidelines for treatment of diverticular disease. Dan Med J. 2012;59(5):C4453.
19. Cuomo R, Barbara G, Pace F, Annese V, Bassotti G, Binda GA, et al. Italian consensus conference for colonic diverticulosis and diverticular disease. United European Gastroenterol J. 2014;2(5):413–42.
20. Kruis W, Germer CT, Leifeld L. Diverticular disease: guidelines of the german society for gastroenterology, digestive and metabolic diseases and the german society for general and visceral surgery. Digestion. 2014;90(3):190–207.

Consultation and Disposition of Acute Diverticulitis: Which Patients with Acute Diverticulitis Require Admission or Surgical Consultation?

86

Brandon Ruderman and Sreeja Natesan

Pearls and Pitfalls
- About 12.5% of patients with CT-diagnosed uncomplicated acute diverticulitis who are discharged will require readmission.
- All patients with complicated diverticulitis should be admitted for intravenous antibiotics and observation.
- About 6% of ED patients with diverticulitis will require surgery, typically laparoscopic.
- Emergent surgical consultation is indicated for signs of peritonitis, severe sepsis, perforation, or abscess formation.

Diverticulitis is a frequently encountered diagnosis in the emergency department, accounting for over 150,000 hospital admissions annually in the United States [1, 2]. Management varies widely from outpatient medical management to hospitalization and operative intervention. In recent years, ED admission rates and surgical rates for acute diverticulitis have been declining [3]. A recent study suggested that uncomplicated diverticulitis can be safely discharged home [2]. Furthermore, a randomized trial demonstrated no significant difference in treatment failure rates between uncomplicated diverticulitis patients discharged home with oral antibiotics and those who were admitted for intravenous (IV) antibiotics (4.5% vs 6.1%, respectively). Total healthcare costs were reduced for discharged patients [4].

Admission Criteria (Table 86.1)

Hinchey Classification: Complicated Versus Uncomplicated Diverticulitis

Multiple classification systems and criteria have been developed to grade the severity of diverticulitis [9, 10]. The Modified Hinchey classification (Fig. 86.1) and corresponding CT findings can help differentiate between uncomplicated (0, Ia) and complicated (1b, II–IV) diverticulitis [11].

High-Risk Clinical Features and Laboratory Abnormalities

Important clinical factors have been shown to impact the decision to hospitalize a patient, including age >70, inability to tolerate oral intake, presence of comorbidities, immunocompromised state, signs of sepsis, or inability to care for self at home [12]. In addition to these clinical factors and imaging findings, laboratory findings such as C-reactive protein (CRP) and white blood cell (WBC) count can help predict complicated diverticulitis and need for admission. Average CRP levels among patients with complicated diverticulitis are approximately 186 mg/L, while average WBC is 14.4×10^9/L [13]. On average, meta-analyses have demonstrated that about 79% of patients will present with uncomplicated diverticulitis compared to 21% with complicated diverticulitis [13].

B. Ruderman (✉) · S. Natesan
Duke University Medical Center, Durham, NC, USA
e-mail: brandon.ruderman@duke.edu; sreeja.natesan@duke.edu

© Springer Nature Switzerland AG 2019
A. Graham, D. J. Carlberg (eds.), *Gastrointestinal Emergencies*, https://doi.org/10.1007/978-3-319-98343-1_86

CT Predictors of Progression to Complicated Diverticulitis

CT findings can also help predict those patients that are at greatest risk for progression from uncomplicated to complicated diverticulitis. The "spilled feces" sign, which is defined as an amorphous extraluminal mass with gas bubbles resembling feces, is significantly associated with need for surgery [14]. Peri-colonic fluid collections, fistulas, bowel obstruction, and a longer inflamed segments of colon (86 mm vs 65 mm) are all associated with progression to complicated diverticulitis [15, 16].

Table 86.1 Disposition

Appropriate for outpatient management +/− antibiotics
CT-confirmed, uncomplicated diverticulitis
Mild to moderate signs and symptoms
No associated abdominal distention
No vomiting, able to tolerate fluids and take medications
Able to control pain with oral medications
Able to follow up with physician in 2–3 days
Able to care for self at home

Inpatient management
Complicated diverticulitis (phlegmon, abscess, perforation, fistula, stricture, obstruction)
High-risk patients

High risk of complications and treatment failure

Clinical risk factors	Diagnostic risk factors	CT imaging risk factors for progression to complicated diverticulitis
Age > 70 years	Generalized	Free fluid or
Fever	abdominal pain/	fluid collections
Vomiting/inability to	tenderness versus	(frequently
tolerate PO	localized to left	anterior to
Poor follow-up or inability	lower quadrant	rectum)
to care for self at home	Leukocytosis –	Greater length of
Multiple comorbid	(WBC 11 × 10⁹/L	inflamed colon
conditions (ASA >/= 2)	sensitivity 82%,	(85 mm vs
Immunocompromised	specificity 45%)	65 mm)
Corticosteroid use	CRP > 90 mg/L	Inflamed
Malnutrition	(sensitivity 88%,	diverticulum
Active malignancy	specificity 75%)	greater than 2 cm
Chronic opiate use	Signs of sepsis	

Bolkenstein et al. [5]; Lorimer and Doumit [6]; Van Diijk et al. [7]; Etzioni et al. [8]; Adapted by Autumn Graham, MD from Chap. 87

Surgical Consultation

Surgical intervention is relatively rare, occurring in only about 6% of patients according to recent retrospective data [17, 18]. Indications for urgent surgery and thus surgical consultation include perforation, severe sepsis, diffuse peritonitis, or failure to improve with initial resuscitation. There has been a recent trend toward trials of medical therapy even in severe, complicated diverticulitis given the significant morbidity associated with urgent surgery for acute complicated diverticulitis. The average postoperative complication rate for complicated diverticulitis is about 18% and includes anastomotic leaks, wound infections, and acute kidney injury [19].

Of patients admitted with acute complicated diverticulitis, about 20% will usually present with an abscess [20]. For patients presenting with smaller abscesses (less than 4–5 cm), conservative treatment with antibiotics is usually successful in up to 73% of cases [21]. However, multiple studies have suggested that percutaneous drainage should be attempted for patients with abscesses larger than 5 cm, as the risk of failure of conservative treatment is significantly higher [20, 21]. Ultimately, about 22% of patients with an abscess will require an urgent resection when compared to conservative treatment failure rates of about 7% in uncomplicated diverticulitis without an abscess or perforation [20].

Perforated sigmoid diverticulitis is a life-threatening condition associated with a 2.6–7.3% mortality rate and requires emergent surgical intervention, traditionally a Hartmann procedure [22, 23]. There is increasing evidence as well that laparoscopic surgery for both emergent and elective colectomies results in lower mortality and complication rates with this becoming the more common approach [22–24]. Recurrence rates of diverticulitis within the subsequent 5 years following the initial diagnosis can approach 20% [17]. Therefore, the recommendation from the American Society of Colon and Rectal Surgeons is to offer elective sigmoid colectomy on an individual basis after uncomplicated diverticulitis, while elective colectomy is usually recommended after a patient recovers from a complicated episode [25, 26].

Fig. 86.1 Modified Hinchey classification; 0 mild clinical diverticulitis; Ia confined pericolic inflammation or phlegmon; Ib pericolic or mesocolic abscess; II pelvic, distant intra-abdominal, or retroperitoneal abscess; III generalized purulent peritonitis; IV generalized fecal peritonitis (Illustrated by Megan Llewellyn, MSMI; copyright Duke University; with permission under a CC BY-ND 4.0 license)

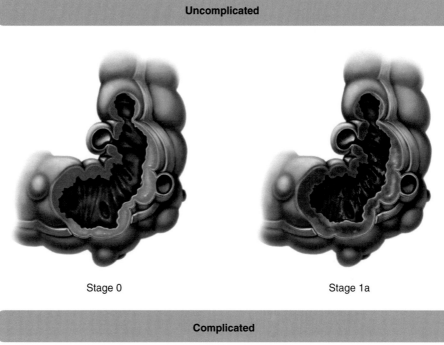

Uncomplicated

Stage 0   Stage 1a

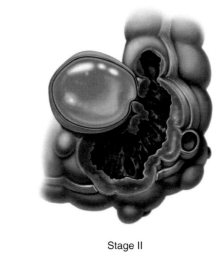

Complicated

Stage 1b   Stage II

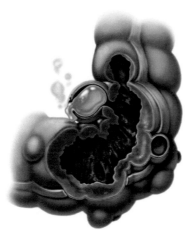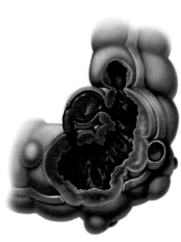

Stage III   Stage IV

Suggested Resources

- EM@3AM: diverticulitis. Sept 2017. http://www. emdocs.net/em3am-diverticulitis/.
- EMDocs: diverticulitis – questioning current clinical practice. Apr 2015. http://www.emdocs.net/ diverticulitis-questioning-current-practice/.
- Chabok A, Pahlman L, Hjern F, et al. Randomized clinical trial of antibiotics in acute uncomplicated diverticulitis. Br J Surg. 2012;99:532–9.
- Core EM: Antibiotics vs observation in uncomplicated diverticulitis. (December 2016: https:// coreem.net/journal-reviews/abx-in-diverticulitis/).
- Horn AE, Ufberg JW. Appendicitis, diverticulitis, and colitis. Em Med Clin North Am. 2011;29:347–68.
- Stollman N, Smalley W, Hirano I, et al. American gastroenterology association institute guidelines on management of acute diverticulitis. Gastroenterology. 2015;149:1944–9.

References

1. Etzioni D, Mack T, Beart R, Kaiser A. Diverticulitis in the United States: 1998–2005. Ann Surg. 2009;249(2):210–7.
2. Sirany A, Gaertner W, Madoff R, Kwaan M. Diverticulitis diagnosed in the emergency room: is it safe to discharge home? J Am Coll Surg. 2017;225(1):21–5.
3. Greenwood-Ericksen M, Havens J, Ma J, Weissman J, Schuur J. Trends in hospital admission and surgical procedures following ED visits for diverticulitis. West J Emerg Med. 2016;17(4):409–17.
4. Biondo S, Golda T, Kreisler E, Espin E, Vallribera F, Oteiza F, et al. Outpatient versus hospitalization management for uncomplicated diverticulitis: a prospective, multicenter randomized clinical trial (DIVER trial). Ann Surg. 2014;259(1):38–44.
5. Bolkenstein HE, Van de Wall BJ, Consten E, Broeders A, Draaisma W. Risk factors for complicated diverticulitis: systemic review and meta-analysis. Int J Colorectal Dis. 2017;32:1375–83.
6. Lorimer JW, Doumit G. Comorbidity is a major determinant of severity in acute diverticulitis. Am J Surg. 2007;193:681. [PMID: 17512276].
7. Van Dijk S, Daniels L, Nio C, Somers I, Van Geloven A, Boermeester M. Predictive factors on CT imaging for progression of uncomplicated into complicated acute diverticulitis. Int J Colorectal Dis. 2017;32:1693–8.
8. Etzioni D, Chiu Y, Cannom R, et al. Outpatient treatment of acute diverticulitis: rates and predictors of failure. Dis Colon Rectum. 2010;53:861–5.
9. Jacobs D. Diverticulitis. N Engl J Med. 2007;357:2057–66.
10. Sartelli M, Catena F, Ansaloni L, Coccolini F, Griffiths E, Abu-Zidan F, et al. WSES guidelines for the management of acute left sided colonic diverticulitis in the emergency setting. World J Emerg Surg. 2016;11(37):1–15.
11. Klarenbeek B, de Korte N, van der Peet D, Meijerink W, Cuesta M. Review of current classifications for diverticular disease and a translation into clinical practice. Int J Color Dis. 2012;27(4):207–14.
12. Jackson J, Hammond T. Systematic review: outpatient management of acute uncomplicated diverticulitis. Int J Color Dis. 2014;29(7):775–81.
13. Bolkenstein H, van de Wall B, Consten E, Broeders A, Draaisma W. Risk factors for complicated diverticulitis: systematic review and meta-analysis. Int J Color Dis. 2017;32(10):1375–83.
14. Kim D, Kim H, Jang S, Yeon J, Shin K. CT predictors of unfavorable clinical outcomes of acute right colonic diverticulitis. AJR. 2017;209:1263–71.
15. Van Dijk S, Daniels L, Nio C, Somers I, van Geloven A, Boemeester M. Predictive factors on CT imaging for progression of uncomplicated into complicated acute diverticulitis. Int J Color Dis. 2017;32:1693–8.
16. Bates D, Fernandez M, Ponchiardi C, von Plato M, Teich J, Narsule C, et al. Surgical management in acute diverticulitis and its association with multi-detector CT, modified Hinchey classification, and clinical parameters. Abdom Radiol. 2017:1–6.
17. Stollman N, Smalley W, Hirano I, AGA Institute Clinical Committee. American Gastroenterology Association Institute guidelines on management of acute diverticulitis. Gastroenterology. 2015;149:1944–9.
18. Schneider E, Singh A, Sung J, Hassid B, Selvarajah S, Fang S, et al. Emergency department presentation, admission, and surgical intervention for colonic diverticulitis in the United States. Am J Surg. 2015;210(2):404–7.
19. Rosen D, Hwang G, Ault G, Ortega A, Cologne K. Operative management of diverticulitis in a tertiary care center. Am J Surg. 2017;214(1):37–41.
20. Kaiser A, Jiang J, Lake J, Ault G, Artinyan A, Gonzalez-Ruiz C, et al. The management of complicated diverticulitis and the role of computed tomography. Am J Gastroenterol. 2005;100:910–7.
21. Andeweg C, Mulder I, Felt-Bersma R, Verbon A, van der Wilt G, van Goor H, et al. Guidelines of diagnostic and treatment of acute left-sided colonic diverticulitis. Dig Surg. 2013;30:278–92.
22. Stocchi L. Current indications and role of surgery in the management of sigmoid diverticulitis. World J Gastroenterol. 2010;16(7):804–17.
23. Biondo S, Lopez Borao J, Millan M, Kreisler E, Jaurrieta E. Current status of the treatment of acute colonic diverticulitis: a systematic review. Color Dis. 2012;14(1):e1–e11.
24. Klarenbeek B, Veenhof A, Bergamaschi R, van der Peet D, van den Broek W, de Lange E, et al. Laparoscopic sigmoid resection for diverticulitis decreases major morbidity rates: a randomized controlled trial. Ann Surg. 2009;249(1):39–44.
25. Feingold D, Steele S, Lee S, Kaiser A, Boushey R, Buie W, et al. Practice parameters for the treatment of sigmoid diverticulitis. Dis Colon Rectum. 2014;57(3):284–94.
26. Deery S, Hodin R. Management of diverticulitis in 2017. J Gastrointest Surg. 2017;21:1732–41.

Who Can Safely Be Discharged Home with Diverticulitis? What Discharge Instructions Do I Give Patients with Diverticulitis?

Elaine Bromberek and Autumn Graham

Pearls and Pitfalls
- Low-risk patients without abscess or complications on CT can be discharged home with close follow-up.
- Outpatient antibiotics include ciprofloxacin and metronidazole or trimethoprim/sulfamethoxazole. A "watch and wait" may be done in the appropriate patient population.
- Improvement in symptoms is expected in 3–4 days.
- Patients need a colonoscopy after resolution of acute disease if high-quality examination of the colon has not been recently performed.
- The American Gastroenterological Association does not recommend either fiber or probiotics.

Can Patients Be Safely Discharged Home?

In studies comparing patients receiving inpatient or outpatient care for acute diverticulitis, there was no statistically significant difference in complications, pain, fever, or need for surgical intervention. Outpatient management of acute diverticulitis was proven to be safe with comparable rates of treatment failure [1–3].

In one retrospective study of 693 diverticulitis patients in the Kaiser Permanente system who were discharged home, 94% were treated successfully as an outpatient. Management consisted of 10–13 days of antibiotic treatment with a fluoroquinolone and metronidazole. Thirty-nine patients (6%) were categorized as treatment failures (a repeat evaluation in an emergency department or nonelective admission for a related complaint). Of note, 88% of CTs demonstrated phlegmons associated with diverticulitis episode. Free fluid in the abdomen on imaging was associated with treatment failure. However, concern for selection bias affected broad adoption [3].

The DIVER trial was a multicenter, prospective randomized controlled trial of 132 patients assigned to hospitalization or discharge home. All patients received the first dose of antibiotics intravenously in the emergency department. Six patients (three hospitalization groups, three outpatient groups) experienced a treatment failure. The authors concluded that "outpatient treatment is safe and effective in selected patients with uncomplicated acute diverticulitis." Of note, 49 patients refused enrollment due to concern for being treated at home. Thus patient engagement is key to outpatient management [1].

Checklist for Discharging the Patient with Acute, Uncomplicated Diverticulitis

- ☐ CT-confirmed, uncomplicated diverticulitis
- ☐ Mild to moderate symptoms with minimal findings on physical exam
- ☐ No associated abdominal distention
- ☐ Able to tolerate fluids and take medication
- ☐ Able to manage pain with oral medications
- ☐ Able to follow up with physician in 2–3 days for re-evaluation
- ☐ Able to care for self at home
- ☐ Lack of significant high-risk features for disease progression or severe course of disease

High-Risk Features

Those patients with uncomplicated diverticulitis that should be admitted include those that are immunocompromised, elderly patients, and those with severe infection, inability to

E. Bromberek (✉)
MedStar Washington Hospital Center, MedStar Georgetown University Hospital, Washington, DC, USA

A. Graham
Department of Emergency Medicine, MedStar Washington Hospital Center, MedStar Georgetown University Hospital, Washington, DC, USA

© Springer Nature Switzerland AG 2019
A. Graham, D. J. Carlberg (eds.), *Gastrointestinal Emergencies*, https://doi.org/10.1007/978-3-319-98343-1_87

tolerate oral intake, and significant comorbidity [4]. Patients without social support and without follow-up should be considered for inpatient care. Patients requiring admission should be treated with fluid resuscitation and antibiotics, as well as monitoring to ensure no progression of disease including worsening pain, fever, or leukocytosis. In the case that these signs and symptoms develop, repeat imaging is needed to evaluate for complications, including abscess formation or perforation, as these may require surgical intervention [2, 5].

General Discharge Instructions

Typically patients are given a course of amoxicillin/clavulanate, ciprofloxacin with metronidazole, moxifloxacin, or alternatively trimethoprim/sulfamethoxazole. In selective patients with mild symptoms and CT-confirmed, uncomplicated diverticulitis, a trial of "wait and see" without antibiotics may be appropriate [6–9]. Clinical improvement is expected within 3–4 days of beginning treatment [5, 10, 11].

Patients discharged home require strict return precautions, including return for persistent fever, worsening pain, inability to tolerate PO, or overall worsening symptoms. In these instances, complicated diverticulitis may develop, and the patient may require inpatient hospitalization, antibiotics, and complication-directed interventions. When these patients return to the emergency department, care must be taken to identify the exact symptoms that prompted their return, and repeat imaging should be considered [5].

Dietary Recommendations

There is little evidence regarding dietary modifications in patients discharged from the emergency department. Effects of high-fiber diets in causation of diverticulosis as well as episodes of acute diverticulitis have not been proven [12]. There are studies with conflicting information but little convincing evidence [10]. No evidence has suggested causation between nut, seed, and popcorn intake and acute diverticulitis. In fact, increased nut intake has been correlated with fewer episodes of diverticulitis than in patients with less nut intake [13–15].

Probiotics

There is little convincing evidence regarding probiotics in patients following an episode of acute uncomplicated diverticulitis. Small studies have shown no statistically significant difference in recurrence rates of diverticulitis with use of probiotics [16, 17]. The American Gastroenterological Association recommends against the use of probiotics in uncomplicated diverticulitis, although it recognizes that further study is needed in this area [18]. Guidelines from the Netherlands recommend a combination of probiotics and anti-inflammatory medication over probiotics alone [19].

Outpatient Colonoscopy

AGA Guidelines

The AGA recommends that colonoscopy be considered in appropriate candidates following resolution of acute diverticulitis. If patients have not recently had a high-quality examination of the colon, screening for neoplasm is necessary to avoid misdiagnosis [18]. Although CT may have been performed for diagnosis of acute diverticulitis, this is not sufficient to rule out colonic neoplasm. In a systematic review, 1 in 67 patients was found to have an underlying neoplasm when colonoscopy was performed after a diagnosis of diverticulitis and was often in the same region as the diverticulitis [20].

Ideal timing has not been formally recommended, but often colonoscopy occurs 6–8 weeks after the resolution of disease. Severity and length of recent illness should be taken into consideration when scheduling and planning colonoscopy.

Netherlands Guidelines

Although colonoscopy is not routinely recommended after acute episode of diverticulitis, it is often performed approximately 6 weeks after resolution of an episode [19]. Risk of colonic neoplasm is approximately 5%, and not believed to be higher following acute uncomplicated diverticulitis, and routine colonoscopy did not find a large number of alternate diagnoses [21–23] (Table 87.1).

Table 87.1 Disposition

Appropriate for outpatient management +/− antibiotics
CT-confirmed, uncomplicated diverticulitis
Mild to moderate signs and symptoms
No associated abdominal distention
No vomiting, able to tolerate fluids and take medications
Able to control pain with oral medications
Able to follow up with physician in 2–3 days
Able to care for self at home

Inpatient management
Complicated diverticulitis (phlegmon, abscess, perforation, fistula, stricture, obstruction)
High-risk patients

High risk of complications and treatment failure

Clinical risk factors	Diagnostic risk factors	CT imaging risk factors for progression to complicated diverticulitis
Age > 70 years	Generalized	Free fluid or
Fever	abdominal pain/	fluid collections
Vomiting/inability to	tenderness versus	(frequently
tolerate PO	localized to left	anterior to
Poor follow-up or inability	lower quadrant	rectum)
to care for self at home	Leukocytosis –	Greater length of
Multiple comorbid	(WBC 11×10^9/L	inflamed colon
conditions (ASA >/= 2)	sensitivity 82%,	(85 mm vs
Immunocompromised	specificity 45%)	65 mm)
Corticosteroid use	CRP > 90 mg/L	Inflamed
Malnutrition	(sensitivity 88%,	diverticulum
Active malignancy	specificity 75%)	greater than 2 cm
Chronic opiate use	Signs of sepsis	

Adapted by Autumn Graham, MD

> **Suggested Resource**
> - Diverticulitis podcast. http://foamcast.org/2016/03/04/episode-45-diverticulitis/.

References

1. Paolillo C, Spallino I. Is it safe to send home an uncomplicated diverticulitis? DIVER Trial Intern Emerg Med. 2015;10:193–4. https://doi.org/10.1007/s11739-014-1162-8.
2. Sirany AM, Gaertner W, Madoff R, KWaan M. Diverticulitis diagnosed in the emergency room: is it safe to discharge home? J Am Coll Surg. 2017;225(1):21–5. https://doi.org/10.1016/j.jamcollsurg.2017.02.016.
3. Etzioni D, Chiu Y, Cannom R, Burchette RJ, Haigh PI, Abbas MA. Outpatient treatment of acute diverticulitis: rates and predictors of failure. Dis Colon Rectum. 2010;53:861–5.
4. Joliat GR, Emery J, Demartines N, Hubner M, Yersin B, Hahnloser D. Antibiotic treatment for uncomplicated and mild complicated diverticulitis: outpatient treatment for everyone. Int J Color Dis. 2017;32:1313–9.
5. Morris A, Regenbogen S, Hardiman K, Hendren S. Sigmoid diverticulitis: a systematic review. JAMA. 2014;311(3):287–97. https://doi.org/10.1001/jama.2013.282025.
6. Deery SA, Hodin RA. Management of diverticulitis in 2017. J Gastroinest Surg. 2017;21(10):1732–41. https://doi.org/10.1007/s11605-017-3404-3.
7. Lue A, Laredo V, Lanas A. Medical treatment of diverticular disease: antibiotics. J Clin Gastroenterol. 2016;50:S57–9.
8. Chabok A, Pahlman A, Hjern R, Haapaniemi S, Smedh K, AVOD Study Group. Randomized clinical trial of antibiotics in acute uncomplicated diverticulitis. Br J Surg. 2012;99(4):532–9.
9. Daniels L, Unlu C, de Korte N, et al. Dutch diverticular disease (3D) collaborative study group. Randomized clinical trial of observational versus antibiotic treatment for a first episode of CT-proven uncomplicated acute diverticulitis. Br J Surg. 2017;104:52–61.
10. Stollman N, Smalley W, Hirano I, AGA Institute Clinical Guidelines Committee. American Gastroenterological Association Institute guideline on the management of acute diverticulitis. Gastroenterology. 2015;149:1944–9.
11. Feurstein J, Falchuk K. Diverticulosis and diverticulitis. Mayo Clin Proc. 2016;1(8):1094–104.
12. Carabotti M, Annibale B, Severi C, Lahner E. Role of fiber in symptomatic uncomplicated diverticular disease: a systematic review. Nutrients. 2017;9:161. https://doi.org/10.3390/nu9020161.
13. Tursi A. Dietary pattern and colonic diverticulosis. Curr Opin Clin Nutr Metab Care. 2017;20:409–13. https://doi.org/10.1097/MCO.0000000000000403.
14. Strate L, Liu Y, Syngal S, Aldoori WH, Giovannucci EL. Nut, corn, and popcorn consumption and the incidence of diverticular disease. JAMA. 2008;300(8):907–14. https://doi.org/10.1001/jama.300.8.907.
15. Strate L, Keeley B, Cao Y, Wu K, Giovannucci EL, Chan AT. Western dietary pattern increases, and prudent dietary pattern decreases, risk of incident diverticulitis in a prospective cohort study. Gastroenterology. 2017;152:1023–30.
16. Dughera L, Serra AM, Battaglia E, Tibaudi D, Navino M, Emanuelli G. Acute recurrent diverticulitis is prevented by oral administration of a polybacterial lysate suspension. Minerva Gastroenterol Dietol. 2004;50:149–53.
17. Tursi A, Brandimarte G, Daffina R. Long-term treatment with mesalazine and rifaximin versus rifaximin alone for patients with recurrent attacks of acute diverticulitis of colon. Dig Liver Dis. 2002;34:510–5.
18. Strate LL, Peery AF, Neumann I. American Gastroenterological Association Institute technical review on the management of acute diverticulitis. Gastroenterology. 2015;149(7):1950–76.
19. Andeweg CS, Mulder IM, Felt-Bersma RJF, Verbon A, van der Wilt GJ, van Goor H, et al. Guidelines of diagnostics and treatment of acute left-sided colonic diverticulitis. Dig Surg. 2013;30:278–92.
20. Daniels L, Unlu C, de Wijkerslooth TR, Dekker E, Boermeester MA. Routine colonoscopy after left-sided acute uncomplicated diverticulitis: a systematic review. Gastrointest Endosc. 2014;79:378–98.
21. Krones CJ, Klinge U, Butz N, Junge K, Stumpf M, Rosch R, et al. The rare epidemiologic coincidence of diverticular disease and advanced colonic neoplasia. Int J Color Dis. 2006;21:18–24.
22. Stefánsson T, Ekbom A, Sparèn P, Påhlman L. Association between sigmoid diverticulitis and left-sided colon cancer: a nested, population-based, case control study. Scand J Gastroenterol. 2004;39:743–7.
23. Meurs-Szojda MM, Terhaar sive Droste JS, Kuik DJ, Mulder CJ, Felt-Bersma RJ. Diverticulosis and diverticulitis form no risk for polyps and colorectal neoplasia in 4,241 colonoscopies. Int J Color Dis. 2008;23:979–84.

Consultant Corner: Diverticulitis

Sandeep Nadella and Zone-En Lee

Pearls and Pitfalls Table
- Diverticulitis must be differentiated from other causes of acute abdominal pain.
- The initial management of diverticulitis revolves around differentiating complicated from uncomplicated diverticulitis.
- Multidisciplinary consultation is essential to the management of complicated diverticulitis.
- Complications of diverticulitis are uncommon, but their early identification is essential.
- Mild uncomplicated, acute diverticulitis can be managed conservatively.

Brief Introduction of Consultant Including Their Practice Setting

Dr. Nadella is a gastroenterology fellow with the MedStar Georgetown University Hospital. As a part of his fellowship, he cares for patients across three different hospitals: MedStar Georgetown University Hospital (MGUH), MedStar Washington Hospital Center (MWHC), and DC Veterans Affairs Medical Center (DCVAMC). MGUH is 609-bed, academic, tertiary care center with centers of excellence including oncology, gastroenterology, transplant, and vascular diseases. MWHC is a 912-bed, academic, tertiary care center with centers of excellence in cardiovascular care, trauma, and others. DCVAMC is a 175-bed, level 1a hospital which provides care only to veterans. Dr. Nadella's scholarly activities include clinical research pertaining to pancreatitis and basic science research focused on pancreatic cancer, nanoparticles, and dietary fat.

Dr. Lee is an attending gastroenterologist at MedStar Washington Hospital Center, the largest academic tertiary care center in Washington, D.C. Dr. Lee is an assistant program director for the combined Georgetown University Gastroenterology Fellowship Program. Her academic interests include gastrointestinal bleeding, women's gastrointestinal health, and colorectal cancer screening. Dr. Lee has an active outpatient gastroenterology practice as well as a busy inpatient consultative service that is a part of the gastroenterology fellowship.

S. Nadella (✉)
Division of Gastroenterology, MedStar Georgetown University Hospital, Washington, DC, USA
e-mail: Sandeep.nadella@gunet.georgetown.edu

Z.-E. Lee
Division of Gastroenterology, MedStar Georgetown University Hospital, Washington, DC, USA

MedStar Georgetown University Hospital, Washington, DC, USA
e-mail: Zone-en.Lee@gunet.georgetown.edu

Answers to Key Clinical Questions

1. When do you recommend consultation with a gastroenterologist/surgeon and in what time frame?

Consultation with a gastroenterologist is recommended in all cases of acute diverticulitis. The time frame for consultation depends on the clinical severity of presentation. Once the diagnosis is established or suspected, patients with complicated diverticulitis such as those with abscess, fistula, obstruction, perforation, or presence of severe clinical signs such as SIRS criteria should undergo a multidisciplinary evaluation by a gastroenterologist and surgeon as soon as possible. This multidisciplinary team ideally manages these complicated patients with intravenous antibiotics but also serves to determine ideal candidates for procedural intervention. Those patients with uncomplicated diverticulitis and mild clinical symptoms can be referred to a gastroenterologist for a non-urgent consultation and follow-up colonoscopy in 1–3 months after the acute episode to rule out underlying colon lesions [1, 2].

2. Can the diagnosis of diverticulitis be made on clinical assessment alone? What is the role of imaging?

The diagnosis of diverticulitis is based on the presence of typical clinical features of LLQ abdominal pain, fever, and leukocytosis; however clinical misdiagnosis can vary from 34% to 68% [2]. Radiologic evaluation can thus help with establishing the diagnosis, identifying complications, and guiding management. Computerized tomography with oral and IV contrast is the ideal test of choice, with sensitivity around 97% [3].

3. What complications are you concerned about in diverticulitis patients?

Although 80% of patients with diverticulitis present with uncomplicated diverticulitis [4], complications of acute diverticulitis can occur. The most common are abscess, fistula, obstruction, and free perforation. Abscess formation can occur in up to 15% of patients with acute diverticulitis [5]. Abscesses can be localized (phlegmon, Hinchey Stage I) or distant (Hinchey Stage II) or can be further complicated by rupture (Hinchey Stage III) and perforation resulting in fecal peritonitis (Hinchey Stage IV) [6]. When a local abscess ruptures into an adjacent organ, a fistula can result. Less than 5% of patients with acute diverticulitis present with fistula, and a minority (20%) are present in those who require surgery for diverticulitis. Colo-vesicular fistulae followed by colo-vaginal fistulas are the most common, less so are colo-enteric, colo-uterine, colo-uterine, and colo-cutaneous fistulas [6]. During an attack of diverticulitis, inflammation of the colon can lead to luminal narrowing and result in partial colonic obstruction. Complete obstruction is unusual. Surgical intervention may be necessary for persistent obstruction. Free perforation caused by diverticulitis is an emergency which shouldn't be missed. Early identification is critical, and CT scan can confirm the cases in ambiguous cases. Early administration of antibiotics and supportive resuscitative measures have led to decrease in mortality from this condition.

4. What is the optimal medical management of diverticulitis? Can you treat diverticulitis without antibiotics at this time?

Once diagnosed, general management of acute diverticulitis depends on the patient's clinical condition and includes supportive care, IV antibiotics which cover colonic flora and inpatient admission. Patients with severe abdominal pain requiring IV pain medications, with peritonitis, unable to tolerate oral intake, and with excessive vomiting, fever, or failure to respond to outpatient therapy should be admitted to the ward [2].

Early identification of complicated diverticulitis and administration of antibiotics to the critically ill are essential concepts in the management of acute diverticulitis.

Failure to tolerate oral intake, excessive vomiting, fever, and failure to improve with outpatient therapy are indications for hospitalizations. Patients without these clinical features can be managed in the outpatient setting with success rates of up to 97% [7]. Patients should be advised bowel rest and oral antibiotic course of 7–10 days directed against gram-negative and anaerobic bacteria [2]. A multicentered, randomized controlled trial from 2012 revealed no differences in hospital stay and recurrent diverticulitis in patients treated with or without antibiotics [8]. Similar findings were obtained from a more recent trial from the Netherlands which evaluated utility of no antibiotics for uncomplicated, primary, left-sided diverticulitis. No differences in the primary endpoint of recovery time to 6 months or the secondary endpoints of readmission rate, ongoing and recurrent diverticulitis, sigmoid resection, and mortality were found [9]. This suggests that selected patients with uncomplicated diverticulitis might be able to undergo close observation.

5. Which patients should be admitted to surgery and which patients are best served with a medicine admission with gastroenterology consultation?

The determination of patient's ideal location in the hospital depends on their comorbidities. Patients with multiple medical comorbidities that will need to be managed concurrently which can include but not limited to diabetes mellitus, advanced age, delirium, and sepsis will ideally need to be managed by the medical team. Additionally, geriatric patients should be admitted to the medicine service. Those patients with complicated diverticulitis such as a large abscess and perforation will benefit from urgent surgical consultation and if they undergo an operative procedure should be admitted to the surgical ward.

6. What discharge instructions do you give your diverticulitis patients? Do all patients with diverticulitis need to follow up with gastroenterology or require an outpatient colonoscopy?

Patients with diverticulitis who are sent home with antibiotics should be educated about possible complications of antibiotic use such as *Clostridium difficile* colitis or interactions with their other medications. Approximately 20% of patients with diverticulitis will experience recurrent diverticulitis within the next 5 years (American Gastroenterological Association guidelines) [1]. Patients with diverticulitis should be made aware of their ongoing risk of diverticulitis and risk of underlying colon lesions which might have precipitated this pain. All patients after an initial episode of diverticulitis should undergo colonoscopy 1–3 months after the episode to evaluate for underlying colon lesions. Patients with recurrent episodes of uncomplicated diverticulitis should be referred for surgical evaluation since they will benefit from resection of the affected colonic segment.

References

1. Stollman N, Smalley W, Hirano I, Committee AGAICG. American Gastroenterological Association Institute guideline on the management of acute diverticulitis. Gastroenterology. 2015;149:1944–9.
2. Feingold D, Steele SR, Lee S, et al. Practice parameters for the treatment of sigmoid diverticulitis. Dis Colon Rectum. 2014;57:284–94.
3. Rao PM, Rhea JT, Novelline RA, et al. Helical CT with only colonic contrast material for diagnosing diverticulitis: prospective evaluation of 150 patients. AJR Am J Roentgenol. 1998;170:1445–9.
4. Stollman NH, Raskin JB. Diagnosis and management of diverticular disease of the colon in adults. Ad Hoc Practice Parameters Committee of the American College of Gastroenterology. Am J Gastroenterol. 1999;94:3110–21.
5. Bahadursingh AM, Virgo KS, Kaminski DL, Longo WE. Spectrum of disease and outcome of complicated diverticular disease. Am J Surg. 2003;186:696–701.
6. Taft P, Bhuket NHS. Diverticular disease of the colon. In: MFLS F, Brandt LJ, editors. Sleisinger and Fordtran's gastrointestinal and liver disease. 10th ed. Philadelphia: Saunders, Elsevier; 2016. p. 2123–38.
7. Abbas MA, Cannom RR, Chiu VY, et al. Triage of patients with acute diverticulitis: are some inpatients candidates for outpatient treatment? Color Dis. 2013;15:451–7.
8. Chabok A, Pahlman L, Hjern F, Haapaniemi S, Smedh K, Group AS. Randomized clinical trial of antibiotics in acute uncomplicated diverticulitis. Br J Surg. 2012;99:532–9.
9. Daniels L, Unlu C, de Korte N, et al. Randomized clinical trial of observational versus antibiotic treatment for a first episode of CT-proven uncomplicated acute diverticulitis. Br J Surg. 2017;104:52–61.

Who Needs Imaging and What Modality?

89

Richard T. Griffey

Pearls and Pitfalls
- Imaging is rarely indicated in ulcerative colitis patients.
- Alternatives to computed tomography are preferred in stable inflammatory bowel disease patients when feasible, as many patients receive recurrent imaging with ionizing radiation.
- Magnetic resonance enterography is an ideal imaging study for suspected small bowel disease in Crohn's disease (CD).
- Ultrasound and magnetic resonance imaging are useful for suspected perianal abscess in CD.

Imaging plays a central role in the diagnosis and assessment of inflammatory bowel disease (IBD). In part due to an early age at diagnosis, IBD patients undergo numerous imaging studies over a lifetime. Repeat imaging, often with computerized tomography (CT), results in increased exposure to ionizing radiation. Substantial subsets of patients receive cumulative-effective doses in excess of 75 mSv [1–10]. The widely used unadjusted risk model from the Biological Effects of Ionizing Radiation VII (BEIR VII) conference estimates that a typical abdominopelvic CT (~10 mSv of radiation) increases one's lifetime attributable risk of cancer by 1/1000 [11]. This risk compounds an already increased baseline risk of intestinal luminal cancers and lymphomas associated with IBD and immune modulators used in treatment [12, 13].

Critical decisions in the acute evaluation of IBD include whether to perform imaging, usually with CT, to determine whether an urgent intervention is indicated. In ED-based studies, the yield of CT for detecting obstruction, perforation, abscesses, and non-IBD-related emergencies (OPAN)

ranges from 32.1% to 38.7% [14–17]. However, given the risks posed by multiple radiation exposures, providers should [1] thoughtfully select who receives CT imaging and [2] choose imaging modalities that do not deliver radiation if feasible.

Though risk stratification schemes based on disease severity and phenotype (age at diagnosis, predominant disease location, and behavior) can help inform clinical decision-making, none of these predicts OPAN in the acute setting. Although phenotype (particularly location) is relatively stable in the short term, Crohn's disease (CD) tends to develop into stricturing or penetrating disease within 5–20 years [18–21], requiring surgical intervention in up to two thirds of patients [22]. Both immune-modulating and immunosuppressive therapies can limit the value of physical examination, history, and laboratory evaluation.

When an acute abdomen is present or clinical suspicion for OPAN is high, patients should undergo urgent imaging in the ED, usually with CT. For CD patients without an acute abdomen in whom imaging can be delayed for hours, magnetic resonance imaging (MRI) is a reasonable alternative. Magnetic resonance enterography (MRE) is an excellent imaging modality to evaluate CD. MRE requires oral contrast, so other modalities may be better when obstruction is suspected. Graded compression ultrasonography has potential value in detecting and diagnosing small bowel involvement [23–25] and small bowel obstruction [26, 27]. It is less reliable than CT and MR, and it has a more limited scope in identifying alternative diagnoses [28, 29]. Sometimes patients can be admitted for endoscopy, sparing ED imaging.

The evaluation and management of perianal CD pose specific challenges. Symptoms include pain with defecation or sitting, increased drainage, and, rarely, hematochezia. MRI, ultrasound, and examination under anesthesia are useful to evaluate for perianal abscesses and fluid collections, which are typically chronic developments and often do not require acute interventions. Ultrasound may provide real-time imaging guidance for drainage. MRI provides detailed information

R. T. Griffey
Washington University School of Medicine, St. Louis, MO, USA
e-mail: griffeyr@wustl.edu

© Springer Nature Switzerland AG 2019
A. Graham, D. J. Carlberg (eds.), *Gastrointestinal Emergencies*, https://doi.org/10.1007/978-3-319-98343-1_89

about fistulae and their relationships with the sphincter complex. This information may aid in long-term management.

Because of the mucosal-predominant distal disease pattern observed in ulcerative colitis (UC), these patients are unlikely to present with perforation or abscess formation as a result of their disease. Imaging in this population is often low yield and should be reserved for cases in which a complication or other cause of pain (e.g., perforation, toxic megacolon) is likely. Endoscopic evaluation is preferred for determining colonic disease burden.

Table 89.1 Imaging studies for various clinical presentations of IBD

Clinical scenario	Imaging considerations	Take-home points
UC patient presenting to ED with worsening symptoms	Endoscopic evaluation best for assessing disease severity	Symptoms not accurate for determining flares Perforation/abscess uncommon
CD patient presenting to ED with symptoms of obstruction	MRE (or CTE) if stable Routine CT if unstable	Obstructive symptoms may respond to IV steroids/conservative measures Surgery should be avoided if possible
CD patient presenting with nonspecific symptoms/pain Consistent with flare	MRE (or CTE) if stable Routine CT if unstable	Imaging in ED may yield change in management in up to 1/3 of patients Avoidance of radiating studies is suggested if possible
CD patient presenting with perianal pain and concern for abscess	US or MRI pelvis Routine CT if other options not available	The main goal of imaging these patients in the ED is to evaluate for drainable collection Characterization of a fistula is best done with MRI in non-urgent setting
CD or UC patient presenting with acute abdomen	Routine CT	CT is still the best imaging modality for unstable patients or those with acute/possible surgical abdomen
CD or UC patient presenting with worsening diarrhea or change in bowel habits	Imaging may not be appropriate in the acute setting MRE is a good option for disease surveillance and monitoring response in outpatient setting	Patient education about disease process and symptoms is essential to help direct care
Pregnant patient with CD presents with abdominal pain	US to assess fetus MRI or MRE to evaluate bowel and exclude alternative diagnosis	MRI can safely be performed without contrast during pregnancy

Reproduced from Griffey et al. [30] with automatic permission from Elsevier under the STM signatory guidelines

Table 89.1 describes potential clinical scenarios in IBD patients that may require imaging, the preferred imaging modalities, and pertinent management pearls.

Suggested Resources

- Kerner C, Carey K, Baillie C, et al. Clinical predictors of urgent findings on abdominopelvic CT in emergency department patients with Crohn's disease. Inflamm Bowel Dis. 2013;19(6):1179–85.
- Kerner C, Carey K, Mills AM, et al. Use of abdominopelvic computed tomography in emergency departments and rates of urgent diagnoses in Crohn's disease. Clin Gastroenterol Hepatol. 2012;10(1):52–7.
- Griffey RT, Fowler KJ, Theilen A, Gutierrez A. Considerations in imaging among emergency department patients with inflammatory bowel disease. Ann Emerg Med. 2017;69(5):587–99.
- Satsangi J, Silverberg MS, Vermeire S, Colombel JF. The montreal classification of inflammatory bowel disease: controversies, consensus, and implications. Gut. 2006;55:749–53.

References

1. Desmond AN, O'Regan K, Curran C, et al. Crohn's disease: factors associated with exposure to high levels of diagnostic radiation. Gut. 2008;57:1524–9.
2. Palmer L, Herfarth H, Porter CQ, Fordham LA, Sandler RS, Kappelman MD. Diagnostic ionizing radiation exposure in a population-based sample of children with inflammatory bowel diseases. Am J Gastroenterol. 2009;104:2816–23.
3. Levi Z, Fraser E, Krongrad R, et al. Factors associated with radiation exposure in patients with inflammatory bowel disease. Aliment Pharmacol Ther. 2009;30:1128–36.
4. Peloquin JM, Pardi DS, Sandborn WJ, et al. Diagnostic ionizing radiation exposure in a population-based cohort of patients with inflammatory bowel disease. Am J Gastroenterol. 2008;103:2015–22.
5. Chatu S, Poullis A, Holmes R, Greenhalgh R, Pollok RCG. Temporal trends in imaging and associated radiation exposure in inflammatory bowel disease. Int J Clin Pract. 2013;67:1057–65.
6. Chatu S, Subramanian V, Pollok RC. Meta-analysis: diagnostic medical radiation exposure in inflammatory bowel disease. Aliment Pharmacol Ther. 2012;35:529–39.
7. Kroeker KI, Lam S, Birchall I, Fedorak RN. Patients with IBD are exposed to high levels of ionizing radiation through CT scan diagnostic imaging: a five-year study. J Clin Gastroenterol. 2011;45:34–9.
8. Hou JSTHM. Effect of age, gender, and ethnicity on radiation exposure among a multi-ethnic IBD population of low socioeconomic status. San Antonio: American College of Gastroenterology Annual Meeting; 2010.
9. Israeli E, Ying S, Henderson B, Mottola J, Strome T, Bernstein CN. The impact of abdominal computed tomography in a ter-

tiary referral Centre emergency department on the management of patients with inflammatory bowel disease. Aliment Pharmacol Ther. 2013;38:513–21.

10. Magro F, Coelho R, Guimaraes LS, et al. Ionizing radiation exposure is still increasing in Crohn's disease: who should be blamed? Scand J Gastroenterol. 2015;50:1214–25.

11. Committee to Assess Health Risks from Exposure to Low Levels of Ionizing Radiation; National Research Council. Health risks from exposure to low levels of ionizing radiation: BEIR VII, phase 2. Washington, DC: The National Academies Press; 2006.

12. Hemminki K, Li X, Sundquist J, Sundquist K. Cancer risks in Crohn disease patients. Annals Oncol. 2008;20:574–80.

13. Siegel CA, Marden SM, Persing SM, Larson RJ, Sands BE. Risk of lymphoma associated with combination anti-tumor necrosis factor and immunomodulator therapy for the treatment of Crohn's disease: a meta-analysis. Clin Gastroenterol Hepatol. 2009;7:874–81.

14. Fishman EK, Wolf EJ, Jones B, Bayless TM, Siegelman SS. CT evaluation of Crohn's disease: effect on patient management. AJR Am J Roentgenol. 1987;148:537–40.

15. Jung YS, Park DI, Hong SN, et al. Predictors of urgent findings on abdominopelvic CT in patients with Crohn's disease presenting to the emergency department. Dig Dis Sci. 2015;60:929–35.

16. Kerner C, Carey K, Mills AM, et al. Use of abdominopelvic computed tomography in emergency departments and rates of urgent diagnoses in Crohn's disease. Clin Gastroenterol Hepatol. 2012;10:52–7.

17. Kerner C, Carey K, Baillie C, et al. Clinical predictors of urgent findings on abdominopelvic CT in emergency department patients with Crohn's disease. Inflamm Bowel Dis. 2013;19:1179–85.

18. Satsangi J, Silverberg MS, Vermeire S, Colombel JF. The Montreal classification of inflammatory bowel disease: controversies, consensus, and implications. Gut. 2006;55:749–53.

19. Cosnes J, Cattan S, Blain A, et al. Long-term evolution of disease behavior of Crohn's disease. Inflamm Bowel Dis. 2002;8:244–50.

20. Magro F, Rodrigues-Pinto E, Coelho R, et al. Is it possible to change phenotype progression in Crohn's disease in the era of immunomodulators? Predictive factors of phenotype progression. Am J Gastroenterol. 2014;109:1026–36.

21. Chow DK, Leong RW, Lai LH, et al. Changes in Crohn's disease phenotype over time in the Chinese population: validation of the Montreal classification system. Inflamm Bowel Dis. 2008;14:536–41.

22. Steele SR. Operative management of Crohn's disease of the colon including anorectal disease. Surg Clin North Am. 2007;87:611–31.

23. Rigazio C, Ercole E, Laudi C, et al. Abdominal bowel ultrasound can predict the risk of surgery in Crohn's disease: proposal of an ultrasonographic score. Scand J Gastroenterol. 2009;44:585–93.

24. Novak KL, Wilson SR. The role of ultrasound in the evaluation of inflammatory bowel disease. Semin Roentgenol. 2013;48:224–33.

25. Fraquelli M, Colli A, Casazza G, et al. Role of US in detection of Crohn disease: meta-analysis. Radiology. 2005;236:95–101.

26. Taylor MR, Lalani N. Adult small bowel obstruction. Acad Emerg Med Off J Soc Acad Emerg Med. 2013;20:528–44.

27. Carpenter CR, Pines JM. The end of X-rays for suspected small bowel obstruction? Using evidence-based diagnostics to inform best practices in emergency medicine. Acad Emerg Med Off J Soc Acad Emerg Med. 2013;20:618–20.

28. Panes J, Bouhnik Y, Reinisch W, et al. Imaging techniques for assessment of inflammatory bowel disease: joint ECCO and ESGAR evidence-based consensus guidelines. J Crohns Colitis. 2013;7:556–85.

29. Parente F, Greco S, Molteni M, et al. Role of early ultrasound in detecting inflammatory intestinal disorders and identifying their anatomical location within the bowel. Aliment Pharmacol Ther. 2003;18:1009–16.

30. Griffey RT, Fowler KJ, Theilen A, Gutierrez A. Considerations in imaging among emergency department patients with inflammatory bowel disease. Ann Emerg Med. 2017;69(5):587–99.

What Are the Complications of Home IBD Medications?

90

Kathryn Voss

Pearls and Pitfalls
- Side effects of glucocorticoids are generally dose-dependent, and even low doses are associated with adverse effects when they are used long term.
- Fluoroquinolones may cause QT prolongation and predispose to life-threatening cardiac dysrhythmias. Ciprofloxacin prolongs the QT interval less than other fluoroquinolones.
- While side effects occur with both sulfasalazine and mesalamine, they are more common with sulfasalazine. 20–25% of patients will discontinue sulfasalazine use due to significant side effects.
- Anti-TNF medications should be used with extreme caution in patients with preexisting demyelinating disease or heart failure.

Inflammatory bowel disease (IBD) medications are vital for both managing acute exacerbations and decreasing long-term morbidity. They have wide-ranging and significant side effects that clinicians must consider both when initiating these medications and when evaluating patients who are already on them. Many of these side effects are class specific (Table 90.1).

Glucocorticoids

Systemic steroids play an important role in the management of IBD and are generally used when patients have severe symptoms or have not responded to other treatments. Side effects are generally dose-dependent, and even low doses are associated with adverse effects when they are used long term

Table 90.1 Adverse reactions of common IBD medications

Drug class	Significant adverse reactions
Steroids[a]	Immune deficiency Endocrine abnormalities, including hyperglycemia and adrenal suppression Osteopenia
Antibiotics[b]	Peripheral neuropathy QT prolongation *Clostridium difficile*
Aminosalicylates	Idiosyncratic reactions Paradoxical worsening Gastrointestinal effects Central nervous system effects Hematologic effects
Immunomodulatory agents	Hepatotoxicity Nephrotoxicity Neurotoxicity Malignancy Infection Bone marrow suppression Gastrointestinal effects
Anti-TNF biologics	Infection Anaphylactoid reactions Anaphylactic reactions Serum sickness-like reaction Pulmonary fibrosis Hepatotoxicity Cutaneous reactions

aSee Table 90.2 for a more complete list of steroid side effects
bSee Table 90.3 for a more complete list of antibiotic side effects

[1]. Glucocorticoids produce a broad range of side effects in various organ systems, many of which are shown in Table 90.2.

Side effects decrease when topical glucocorticoids (rectal foams and enemas) are substituted for systemic steroids. Patients with distal bowel symptoms are candidates for these topical glucocorticoids.

K. Voss
MedStar Georgetown University and Washington Hospital Center, Washington, DC, USA
e-mail: Kathryn.voss@medstar.net

© Springer Nature Switzerland AG 2019
A. Graham, D. J. Carlberg (eds.), *Gastrointestinal Emergencies*, https://doi.org/10.1007/978-3-319-98343-1_90

Table 90.2 Glucocorticoid side effects

Systemic glucocorticoid side effects	
Organ system	Side effects
Skin	Skin thinning, purpura, skin cancer
Eye	Cataracts, glaucoma
Cardiovascular	Ischemic heart disease, heart failure
Gastrointestinal	Gastritis, ulcers, gastrointestinal bleeding
Musculoskeletal	Osteopenia, muscle weakness
Central nervous system/psychiatric	Mood disorders, psychosis, memory decline
Endocrine	Hyperglycemia, adrenal suppression
Immune system	Immune deficiency, leukocytosis, neutrophilia
Genitourinary	Fluid retention, decreased fertility

Table 90.3 Side effects of commonly used antibiotics in IBD patients

Antibiotic	Side effects
Ciprofloxacin	Gastrointestinal effects CNS effects Tendinopathy QT prolongation
Metronidazole	Gastrointestinal effects Peripheral neuropathy
Rifaximin	Peripheral neuropathy Ascites
Clarithromycin	Gastrointestinal effects

Antibiotics

Patients with IBD are frequently treated with antibiotics, most commonly ciprofloxacin, metronidazole, rifaximin, and clarithromycin. Table 90.3 summarizes the side effects of these medications.

Ciprofloxacin and other fluoroquinolone antibiotics most commonly produce mild gastrointestinal (GI) side effects, including anorexia, nausea, and abdominal discomfort. Central nervous system (CNS) side effects also occur, including headache, dizziness, and peripheral neuropathy [2]. Ciprofloxacin predisposes to tendon rupture. Fetal cartilage defects may occur if given during pregnancy [3]. Fluoroquinolones may cause QT prolongation and predispose to life-threatening cardiac dysrhythmias. Ciprofloxacin prolongs the QT interval less than other fluoroquinolones [4].

Metronidazole produces many GI side effects, including anorexia, nausea, altered taste, and disulfiram-like reactions. Metronidazole has also been associated with a 4.3-fold increased risk of permanent peripheral neuropathy [5].

Rifaximin is a broad-spectrum antibiotic which most commonly causes peripheral neuropathy, dizziness, nausea, fatigue, and ascites.

Clarithromycin's most common side effects are gastrointestinal.

Importantly, antibiotics increase the risk of *Clostridium difficile* infection because they disrupt the normal intestinal flora and allow this bacterium to proliferate and increase toxin production. Many antibiotics predispose to *C. difficile*, including ciprofloxacin and metronidazole [6].

Aminosalicylates

Aminosalicylates (5-ASAs), including sulfasalazine and mesalamine, are well tolerated in the majority of patients. Mesalamine is an unconjugated aminosalicylate. Sulfasalazine includes a sulfapyridine group, which accounts for many of its side effects. While side effects occur with both drugs, they are more common with sulfasalazine. In fact, 20–25% of patients will discontinue sulfasalazine use due to significant side effects [7].

Idiosyncratic reactions are an important class of reactions to aminosalicylates, and they occur due to either hypersensitivity or immune-related reactions. They include skin rash, hepatitis, pancreatitis, pneumonitis, interstitial nephritis, agranulocytosis, and aplastic anemia. When these occur, the drug must be stopped, and other aminosalicylates should be avoided. While agranulocytosis is a rare and life-threatening side effect, most leukopenias with these medications are mild, are transient, and occur during the first 3 months of treatment [8].

A small number of patients on oral 5-ASAs will have paradoxical worsening of their abdominal pain, bleeding, and/or diarrhea. These patients should be considered allergic, and the medication should be stopped [9].

Dose-related effects of sulfasalazine include gastrointestinal, central nervous system, and mild hematologic toxicities. The most common symptoms include nausea, headache, fever, and rash.

Immunomodulatory Agents

Immunomodulatory agents commonly used to treat inflammatory bowel disease include azathioprine, 6-mercaptopurine, methotrexate, and tacrolimus.

6-Mercaptopurine is a metabolite of azathioprine, and both are classified at thiopurines. These two drugs produce side effects in 9–15% of patients, usually during the first month. The most common side effects are nausea, vomiting, and anorexia. Dose-dependent adverse reactions include bone marrow suppression in 1–2% and liver dysfunction in 0.3%. Other dose-independent reactions include pancreatitis, allergic reactions, nausea, and pneumonitis [10]. Importantly, patients taking thiopurines are at increased risk of cancers: mostly lymphomas but also lymphoproliferative disorders and non-melanoma skin cancers [11].

The most common side effects of methotrexate include nausea and vomiting. Hepatotoxicity may occur and is related to both the dose and duration of treatment [12].

Tacrolimus and cyclosporine may occasionally be used in refractory inflammatory bowel disease. Their side effects are similar and include nephrotoxicity, hypertension, neurotoxicity, infections, and malignancies. Nephrotoxicity manifests as either an acute reversible creatinine increase or a chronic progressive disease [13]. Hypertension is caused by renal vasoconstriction and sodium retention, and it usually responds to dose reduction [14]. A variety of reversible neurologic side effects have been described, including tremor, headache, seizure, mutism, and pain syndromes [15]. Patients taking cyclosporine and tacrolimus are at increased risk of bacterial, viral, and fungal infections [16]. Both drugs are also associated with an increased risk of developing squamous cell skin cancers and lymphoproliferative disorders [17].

Biologic Therapies

Biologic therapies are generally reserved for severe inflammatory bowel disease.

The most commonly used subclass of medications within the biologics are the antitumor necrosis factor (TNF) antibodies, including infliximab, adalimumab, and certolizumab pegol.

Patients on anti-TNF therapy are thought to be at increased risk for infection, particularly pneumonia, herpes zoster, tuberculosis, and opportunistic pathogens; however, this risk appears to be greatly affected by additional medications and comorbidities [18].

Both acute (within 24 h) and delayed (1–14 days) infusion reactions may occur. Acute reactions are mostly anaphylactoid, but some are anaphylactic, and the treatment of both is the same. Delayed reactions are less common and include fever, rash, myalgias, and fatigue. These delayed reactions resemble serum sickness [19].

While mild neutropenia is not uncommon, pancytopenia and aplastic anemia are rare [20].

TNF inhibitors carry a small but serious risk of pulmonary fibrosis and hepatotoxicity.

Multiple cutaneous reactions occur with TNF inhibitors, including autoimmune dermatologic conditions and cutaneous malignancies [21].

Demyelinating diseases and heart failure have been suggested to occur with anti-TNF medications, but the data remains inconclusive. However, these drugs should be used with extreme caution in patients with preexisting demyelinating disease or heart failure [22, 23].

Suggested Resources

- Overview of inflammatory bowel disease. Merck manual: professional version. http://www.merckmanuals.com/professional/gastrointestinal-disorders/inflammatory-bowel-disease-ibd/overview-of-inflammatory-bowel-disease.
- Management of inflammatory bowel disease flares in the emergency department. EB medicine. Nov 2017. https://www.ebmedicine.net/topics.php?paction=showTopic&topic_id=559.
- Bernstein CN. Treatment of IBD: where we are and where we are going. Am J Gastroenterol. 2015; 110:114–26.

References

1. Curtis J. Population-based assessment of adverse events associated with long-term glucocorticoid use. Arthritis Rheum. 2006;55(3):420–6.
2. Etminan M. Oral fluoroquinolone use and risk of peripheral neuropathy: a pharmacoepidemiologic study. Neurology. 2014;83(14):1261.
3. Khaliq Y. Fluoroquinolone-associated tendinopathy: a critical review of the literature. Clin Infect Dis. 2003;36(11):1404.
4. Kang J. Interactions of a series of fluoroquinolone antibacterial drugs with the human cardiac K+ channel HERG. Mol Pharmacol. 2001;59(1):122–6.
5. Carroll M. Efficacy and safety of metronidazole for pulmonary multidrug-resistant tuberculosis. Antimicrob Agents Chemother. 2013;57(8):3903–9.
6. Deshpande A. Community-associated clostridium difficile infection and antibiotics: a meta-analysis. J Antimicrob Chemother. 2013;68(9):1951.
7. Box SA. Sulphasalazine in the treatment of rheumatoid arthritis. Br J Rheumatol. 1997;36(3):382–6.
8. Farr M. Side effect profile of 200 patients with inflammatory arthritides treated with sulphasalazine. Drugs. 1986;32(Suppl 1):49–53.
9. Schroeder K. Is mesalamine safe? Gastroenterol Hepatol (NY). 2007;3(11):878–9.
10. Chaparro M. Safety of thiopurine therapy in inflammatory bowel disease: long-term follow-up study of 3931 patients. Inflamm Bowel Dis. 2013;19(7):1404–10.
11. Beaugerie L. Lymphoproliferative disorders in patients receiving thiopurines for inflammatory bowel disease: a prospective observational cohort study. Lancet. 2009;374(9701):1617–25.
12. Te HS. Hepatic effects of long-term methotrexate use in treatment of inflammatory bowel disease. Am J Gastroenterol. 2000;95(11):3150.
13. Burdmann EA. Cyclosporine nephrotoxicity. Semin Nephrol. 2003;23(5):465–76.
14. Hoorn EJ. The cacineurin inhibitor tacrolimus activates the renal sodium chloride cotransporter to cause hypertension. Nat Med. 2011;17(10):1304–9.
15. Eidelman BH. Neurologic complications of FK 506. Transplant Proc. 1991;23(6):3175–8.
16. Randomized trial comparing tacrolimus (FK506) and cyclosporin in prevention of liver allograft rejection. European FK506 Multicentre Liver Study Group. Lancet. 1994;344(8920):423–8.

17. Hojo M. Cyclosporine induces cancer progression by a cell-autonomous mechanism. Nature. 1999;397(6719):530–4.

18. Strangfield A. Treatment benefit or survival of the fittest: what drives the time-dependent decrease in serious infection rates under TNF inhibition and what does this imply for the individual patient? Ann Rheum Dis. 2011;70(11):1914–20.

19. Cheifetz A. The incidence and management of infusion reactions to infliximab: a large center experience. Am J Gastroenerol. 2003;98(6):1315–24.

20. Hastings R. Neutropenia in patients receiving anti-tumor necrosis factor therapy. Arthritis Care Res (Hoboken). 2010;62(6):764.

21. Cleynen I. Characteristics of skin lesions associated with anti-tumor necrosis factor therapy in patients with inflammatory bowel disease: a cohort study. Ann Intern Med. 2016;164(1):10–22.

22. Gabriel SE. Tumor necrosis factor inhibition: a part of the solution or a part of the problem of heart failure in rheumatoid arthritis? Arthritis Rheum. 2008 Mar;58(3):637–40.

23. Dreyer L. Risk of multiple sclerosis during tumour necrosis factor inhibitor treatment for arthritis: a population-based study from DANBIO and the Danish multiple sclerosis registry. Ann Rheum Dis. 2016;75(4):785–6.

What Is the Utility of ESR and CRP in the Evaluation of Acute IBD Presentations?

91

Richard T. Griffey

Pearls and Pitfalls
- Though C-reactive protein and erythrocyte sedimentation rate (ESR) are associated with inflammation in inflammatory bowel disease (IBD), normal values do not exclude complications or disease flares.
- Though ESR is part of a classic risk stratification model used for defining severe ulcerative colitis, its use for excluding disease requiring admission is limited.
- Risk stratification models from emergency department-based studies have attempted to use biomarkers in addition to other variables to predict complications of IBD, but these models are based on retrospective data with limited performance, and none has been prospectively validated.

Erythrocyte sedimentation rate (ESR) and C-reactive protein (CRP) are acute phase reactants whose levels rise with inflammation but also with other conditions.

ESR is the rate at which red blood cells clump together and precipitate out of solution under specific conditions. CRP is a pentameric protein made by the liver under certain conditions including (but not limited to) inflammation.

CRP may be more sensitive than ESR and correlates better with disease activity in inflammatory bowel disease (IBD). Both may be more useful in Crohn's disease (CD) than in ulcerative colitis (UC). CRP and ESR are sometimes used to track disease activity, but normal ESR and CRP values do not exclude complications of IBD or flares of disease [1–6].

ESR >30 mm/hr is one element in a classic index originally proposed by Truelove and Witts in 1955 defining severe UC mandating admission [7]. This is the best validated and most widely used index, but it and other more recently developed classification schemes have a number of considerations limiting their use for decision-making in the acute setting [8–11].

A number of emergency department (ED)-based studies have attempted to use these acute phase reactants alone or in combination with other variables to predict complications including disease flares and/or obstruction, perforation, and non-IBD-related emergencies (OPAN). These studies were all retrospective and have limitations including missing laboratory data. None has been prospectively validated.

- *Yarur et al.* identified a CRP >5 mg/dL, history of IBD surgery, black race, and low body mass index as predictive of OPAN [12].
- *Jung et al.* studied CD patients in 11 EDs in Korea over an 11-year period and identified a history of stricturing or penetrating disease, lack of biologic agent use, heart rate >100 beats/min, WBC >10,000, and CRP >2.5 mg/dL to be associated with OPAN [13].
- *Govani et al.* created a decision tool using ESR and CRP values to predict the need for CT in CD patients. While they report an ability to spare >40% of patients from radiation exposure, the retrospective data used for derivation and validation are missing either ESR or CRP ~21% of the time [14–16].

As further decision instruments are developed and current decision instruments are validated, the utility of ESR and CRP in the acute evaluation IBD may become clearer.

R. T. Griffey
Washington University School of Medicine, St. Louis, MO, USA
e-mail: griffeyr@wustl.edu

© Springer Nature Switzerland AG 2019
A. Graham, D. J. Carlberg (eds.), *Gastrointestinal Emergencies*, https://doi.org/10.1007/978-3-319-98343-1_91

References

1. Fagan EA, Dyck RF, Maton PN, et al. Serum levels of C-reactive protein in Crohn's disease and ulcerative colitis. Eur J Clin Investig. 1982;12:351–9.
2. Vermeire S, Van Assche G, Rutgeerts P. Laboratory markers in IBD: useful, magic, or unnecessary toys? Gut. 2006;55:426–31.
3. Alper A, Zhang L, Pashankar DS. Correlation of erythrocyte sedimentation rate and C-reactive protein with pediatric inflammatory bowel disease activity. J Pediatr Gastroenterol Nutr. 2017;65:e25–e7.
4. Poullis AP, Zar S, Sundaram KK, et al. A new, highly sensitive assay for C-reactive protein can aid the differentiation of inflammatory bowel disorders from constipation- and diarrhoea-predominant functional bowel disorders. Eur J Gastroenterol Hepatol. 2002;14:409–12.
5. Shine B, Berghouse L, Jones JE, Landon J. C-reactive protein as an aid in the differentiation of functional and inflammatory bowel disorders. Clin Chim Acta. 1985;148:105–9.
6. Cappello M, Morreale GC. The role of laboratory tests in crohn's disease. Clin Med Insights Gastroenterol. 2016;9:51–62.
7. Truelove SC, Witts LJ. Cortisone in ulcerative colitis; final report on a therapeutic trial. Br Med J. 1955;2:1041–8.
8. Vilela EG, Torres HO, Martins FP, Ferrari Mde L, Andrade MM, Cunha AS. Evaluation of inflammatory activity in Crohn's disease and ulcerative colitis. World J Gastroenterol. 2012;18:872–81.
9. Kornbluth A, Sachar DB, Practice Parameters Committee of the American College of G. Ulcerative colitis practice guidelines in adults: American College of Gastroenterology, Practice Parameters Committee. Am J Gastroenterol. 2010;105:501–23. quiz 24
10. Dignass A, Eliakim R, Magro F, et al. Second European evidence-based consensus on the diagnosis and management of ulcerative colitis part 1: definitions and diagnosis. J Crohns Colitis. 2012;6:965–90.
11. Travis SP, Stange EF, Lemann M, et al. European evidence-based consensus on the management of ulcerative colitis: current management. J Crohns Colitis. 2008;2:24–62.
12. Yarur AJ, Mandalia AB, Dauer RM, et al. Predictive factors for clinically actionable computed tomography findings in inflammatory bowel disease patients seen in the emergency department with acute gastrointestinal symptoms. J Crohns Colitis. 2014;8:504–12.
13. Jung YS, Park DI, Hong SN, et al. Predictors of urgent findings on abdominopelvic CT in patients with crohn's disease presenting to the emergency department. Dig Dis Sci. 2015;60:929–35.
14. Govani SM, Guentner AS, Waljee AK, Higgins PD. Risk stratification of emergency department patients with Crohn's disease could reduce computed tomography use by nearly half. Clin Gastroenterol Hepatol. 2014;12:1702–7. e3
15. Abegunde AT. Computerized tomography of patients with Crohn's disease in the emergency department: the more you look, the less you see. Clin Gastroenterol Hepatol. 2015;13:1706.
16. Govani SM, Waljee AK, Kocher KE, Swoger JM, Saul M, Higgins PD. Validation of a tool predicting important findings on computed tomography among Crohn's disease patients. United European Gastroenterol J. 2017;5:270–5.

IBD: Who Can Go Home? Who Should Be Admitted?

92

Mariana Martinez and Emily Rose

Pearls and Pitfalls

- Acute inflammatory bowel disease (IBD) flares are often difficult to distinguish from disease complications.
- Patients who are well appearing and tolerating oral intake are typically stable for discharge with prompt follow-up.
- Indications for admission include acute severe IBD flares, acute infectious complications, medication reactions, and surgical emergencies. Patients in need of acute immunomodulatory medication infusions also generally require admission.
- Surgical consultation is indicated in patients with an acute abdomen, clinical or radiologic concern of perforation, toxic megacolon, and/or abscess.

The management of acute inflammatory bowel disease (IBD) poses many challenges, including determining which patients require admission and which ones are stable for discharge with specialist follow-up. In making this decision, acute care providers should attempt to differentiate among the multiple potential sources of these patients' symptoms. Patients may present due to a disease flare, disease complication, infection, adverse drug reaction, and/or extra-intestinal

M. Martinez
Department of Emergency Medicine, Los Angeles County + USC Medical Center, Los Angeles, CA, USA
e-mail: marianam@usc.edu

E. Rose (✉)
Department of Emergency Medicine, Los Angeles County + USC Medical Center, Los Angeles, CA, USA

Keck School of Medicine of the University of Southern California, Department of Emergency Medicine, Los Angeles County + USC Medical Center, Los Angeles, CA, USA
e-mail: emilyros@usc.edu

manifestation. Symptoms of these various presentations frequently overlap. Infectious colitis, toxic megacolon, bowel obstruction, and perforation all may mimic a disease flare. Patients may also demonstrate more than one presentation simultaneously. For example, a disease flare may occur concurrently with a bowel obstruction. The frequent use of immunosuppressants and immunomodulators may mask infectious complications, increasing the complexity of disposition decisions. Extra-intestinal complications and medication side effects may be life-threatening. Acute care providers should have a low threshold for involving appropriate specialists in the management and disposition of these complex patients.

The largest determinant of disposition for both ulcerative colitis (UC) and Crohn's disease (CD) patients is the severity of presentation, determined by history, vital signs, physical exam, laboratory results, and imaging results (if obtained). Patients with mild to moderate flares who can tolerate oral intake (PO) and have normal vital signs, reassuring bloodwork, and nonconcerning imaging (if obtained) are candidates for discharge. Decisions regarding medication changes and/or additions should be made in discussion with the patient's gastroenterologist. Acute severe flares usually require admission for medical intervention with immunomodulators such as intravenous corticosteroids. Complications frequently require admission and may require intravenous antibiotics and/or surgical intervention. An awareness of unique presentations and complications of each disease aids in the disposition of patients with IBD.

Ulcerative Colitis

Bloody diarrhea is the most common UC flare symptom. Those presenting with mild/moderate flares, as indicated by <6 bloody stools per day, and no signs of systemic toxicity should be safe for discharge with close outpatient gastroenterology follow-up [1].

© Springer Nature Switzerland AG 2019
A. Graham, D. J. Carlberg (eds.), *Gastrointestinal Emergencies*, https://doi.org/10.1007/978-3-319-98343-1_92

Signs of systemic toxicity include:

1. Abnormal vital signs (most commonly tachycardia or fever)
2. Abnormal examination findings (significant tenderness or signs of peritonitis)
3. Laboratory evidence of inflammatory changes or anemia

White blood cell count, C-reactive protein, and erythrocyte sedimentation rate may help guide medical decision-making and may indicate disease exacerbation and/or infection.

An acute severe flare requires inpatient management with IV corticosteroids and frequent monitoring for development of surgical disease. Early, aggressive management significantly decreases mortality in patients with acute UC flares [2]. Those with more advanced or refractory disease may require treatment with other immunomodulators during their inpatient stay [3]. Other important interventions during hospitalization include restoration of fluid and electrolyte balance. Additionally, withdrawal of medications such as opioids that promote colonic dilation should be considered, particularly in patients at risk for toxic megacolon [4]. Patients with significant systemic toxicity or suspected infection should receive antibiotics. Patients admitted for severe disease should have gastroenterology consultation when available and surgical consultation as needed.

UC puts patients at risk for toxic megacolon and bowel perforation. Toxic megacolon is a nonobstructive colonic dilation with associated systemic toxicity that is an acute surgical emergency. Patients usually present ill-appearing with severe abdominal pain. Transverse colon dilation ≥6 cm is diagnostic and may be visualized on plain radiograph. Prompt surgical consultation and initiation of broad-spectrum antibiotics are indicated when toxic megacolon is suspected.

Crohn's Disease

Given the diverse array of presentations with CD, assessment of flare severity can be more complicated. Various grading systems have been developed to define severity, but they are of limited clinical utility [5, 6]. Providers can employ the patient's disease phenotype (age at diagnosis, predominant disease location, and disease behavior) in their decision-making. The most common presentations of CD are abdominal pain, diarrhea, nausea, and abdominal distention. In general, those who are tolerating PO, well appearing, and hemodynamically stable have a mild or moderate flare and are usually safe for discharge with gastroenterology follow-up. Admission is indicated for unstable patients, those unable to tolerate PO, and those with acute surgical complications [7].

The transmural nature CD makes these patients particularly prone to fistula, stricture, and abscess formation, which may require urgent surgical management and colorectal surgery consultation [2]. Sometimes these complications can be managed in the outpatient setting.

CD patients frequently develop bowel obstructions, which may require surgical intervention if conservative measures fail.

Medication Side Effects and Extra-Intestinal Symptoms

Acute care providers must consider extra-intestinal or medication-related symptoms in IBD patients. Many of these complications, such as uveitis and pathologic fractures, are not life-threatening and can be evaluated, treated, and discharged. IBD patients have higher rates of biliary disease, pulmonary embolism, deep vein thrombosis, and coronary artery disease than the general population [8].

Providers should note that IBD patients with presentations seemingly unrelated to IBD often have worse outcomes than other patients. For example, IBD patients with urinary calculi are more likely to have associated sepsis, renal failure, and UTI than non-IBD patients [9].

Careful consideration must be taken when evaluating and discharging IBD patients presenting with extra-intestinal symptoms.

The acute management of IBD is a complicated and controversial topic with clinical challenges for both acute care providers and experienced specialists. Due to the potential morbidity and mortality of IBD, providers should have a low threshold to involve consultants in the management of these patients.

Suggested Resources
- Burg MD, Riccoboni ST. Management of inflammatory bowel disease flares in the emergency department. Emerg Med Pract. 2017;19(11):1–20.
- Carlberg DJ, Lee SD, Dubin JS. Lower abdominal pain. Emerg Med Clin North Am. 2016;34(2):229–49.
- Huang M, Rose E. Pediatric inflammatory bowel disease in the emergency department: managing flares and long-term complications. Pediatr Emerg Med Pract. 2014;11(7):1–16.

References

1. Truelove SC, Witts LJ. Cortisone in ulcerative colitis; final report on a therapeutic trial. Br Med J. 1955;2:1041e8.
2. Mowat C, Cole A, Windsor A, et al. Guidelines for the management of inflammatory bowel disease in adults. Gut. 2011;60:571.
3. Burger D, Travis S. Conventional medical management of inflammatory bowel disease. Gastroenterology. 2011;140:1827–37.
4. Kedia S, Ahuja V, Tandon R. Management of acute severe ulcerative colitis. World J Gastrointest Pathophysiol. 2014;5(4):579–88.
5. Lichtenstein GR, Hanauer SB, Sandborn WJ, Practice Parameters Committee of American College of Gastroenterology. Management of Crohn's disease in adults. Am J Gastroenterol. 2009;104:465.
6. Harvey RF, Bradshaw JM. A simple index of Crohn's-disease activity. Lancet. 1980;1:514.
7. Carlberg DJ, Lee SD, Dubin JS. Lower abdominal pain. Emerg Med Clin North Am. 2016;34(2):229–49.
8. Burg MD, Riccoboni ST. Management of inflammatory bowel disease flares in the emergency department. Emerg Med Pract. 2017;19(11):1–20.
9. Varda BK, McNabb-Baltar J, Sood A, Ghani KR, Kibel AS, Letendre J, Menon M, Sammon JD, Schmid M, Sun M, Trinh QD, Bhojani N. Urolithiasis and urinary tract infection among patients with inflammatory bowel disease: a review of US emergency department visits between 2006 and 2009. Urology. 2015;85(4):764–70.

Steroids? Antibiotics? Biologics? Immunomodulators? What Are the Optimal Discharge Medications for an IBD Flare?

Jonathan Wagner and Daniel Eum

Pearls and Pitfalls
- Ulcerative colitis and Crohn's disease are different disease entities and are treated differently.
- A thorough past medication history may be the most important determinant of discharge medications.
- If discharge medications are modified without discussion with a gastroenterologist, close gastroenterology follow-up and strict return precautions are recommended.

Inflammatory bowel disease (IBD), encompassing ulcerative colitis (UC) and Crohn's disease (CD), affects 1.5 million Americans [1]. Since diagnosis requires endoscopy and biopsy, every patient with diagnosed IBD has seen a gastroenterologist. Many IBD patients present to acute care setting with flares, sometimes after being lost to follow-up. This chapter focuses on managing patients who are safe for discharge but need to be medically optimized. The information presented will help frame discussions with gastroenterology (GI) regarding discharge medications. It will also aid in discharge medication management when discussion with GI is not feasible.

IBD is a phenotypically diverse condition, and therefore, the efficacy of medications will vary across patients. Most with IBD have suffered from previous flares, and many patients know which medication regimens have worked well in the past. Knowledge of prior successful treatment modalities will allow a provider to tailor a patient's medication regimen to his or her physiologic milieu and help increase the likelihood of successful flare management. Refer to Table 93.1.

Mesalamine

Mesalamine, a 5-aminosalicylate (5-ASA), is used as maintenance therapy in UC, but it is also a first-line treatment for UC flares. However, when mesalamine is used to treat a flare, patients may not see improvement until 6 weeks into treatment.

Mesalamine is rapidly absorbed into the bloodstream from the small intestine, rendering it ineffective. Therefore, mesalamine is typically coated, which allows it to reach the colon, where it is poorly absorbed. It remains in the colonic lumen and exerts its anti-inflammatory effects on the adjacent mucosa [2].

Certain patients with UC may see improvement when direct topical therapy via mesalamine enema or suppository is added to an oral mesalamine regimen [3]. However, enemas and suppositories are not as effective when mucosal inflammation extends more proximally.

The dose of mesalamine is mainly limited by its gastrointestinal side effects, but its efficacy is also dose dependent.

Table 93.1 Common medications used for acute IBD flares

Mesalamine	Steroids	Antibiotics	Biologics and immunomodulators
- Used for UC, not CD - PO and topical best - Up to 4 g daily total	- Avoid if potential acute infectious etiologies - Budesonide 9 mg QD (fewer side effects) - Prednisone 40 mg QD (more effective)	- Admit if suspicious for acute infectious etiology - Rifaximin 800 mg PO BID for patients with CD - Not recommended in UC	Rarely warranted in the acute care setting and only in consultation with a gastroenterologist

J. Wagner · D. Eum (✉)
Keck School of Medicine of the University of Southern California,
Los Angeles County/ University of Southern California
(LAC+USC) Department of Emergency Medicine,
Los Angeles, CA, USA
e-mail: jwagner@usc.edu; deum@dhs.lacounty.gov

© Springer Nature Switzerland AG 2019
A. Graham, D. J. Carlberg (eds.), *Gastrointestinal Emergencies*, https://doi.org/10.1007/978-3-319-98343-1_93

While there have been case reports of mesalamine exacerbating IBD flares, most gastroenterologists recommend its use in mild to moderate flares. During a flare, mesalamine should be increased to the maximum dose of 4 g per day, split between the oral and rectal routes.

Mesalamine has little utility in the management of CD because lesions occur proximal to the colon. Evidence suggests that it is no more efficacious than placebo for these patients [4].

Steroids

Budesonide is the steroid of choice in treating IBD flares. It has extensive first-pass hepatic metabolism (90%), which decreases systemic exposure and leads to fewer adverse effects compared to prednisone [2, 5]. However, prednisone has been associated with higher overall remission rates [5]. Providers should consider budesonide in patients who cannot tolerate higher doses of prednisone (e.g., uncontrolled hyperglycemia, osteopenia, or history of adrenal suppression). Prednisone should be used in those who have failed budesonide.

Budesonide is typically dosed at 9 mg by mouth (PO) daily for 8 weeks, while prednisone is typically dosed at 40 mg PO daily for 8 weeks. These medications should be tapered in the outpatient setting by a gastroenterologist. The daily dose of prednisone may range from 20 to 60 mg depending on the minimum dose needed for efficacy and the degree of side effects experienced in the past.

Antibiotics

As mentioned previously, only nontoxic patients should be considered for discharge. When a significant acute infectious process is suspected, parenteral antibiotics should be started in conjunction with admission and GI consultation. That said, antibiotics have historically been used to treat both CD and UC since an abnormal response to gut flora may play a role in IBD pathophysiology [6]. Colitis models in rats do not show intestinal inflammation in the absence of gut bacteria [6].

The current evidence suggests that rifaximin 800 mg PO twice daily (BID) improves induction rates in CD [6]. The data for UC is less convincing, and antibiotics are not recommended.

Biologics

Infliximab and adalimumab are tumor necrosis factor (TNF) inhibitors that are relatively new medications used for induction and maintenance in patients with IBD. They are effective steroid-sparing medications [7, 8]. However, they are parenteral medications that are administered over

several weeks. They should not be initiated in the acute care setting.

Immunomodulators

Methotrexate

Methotrexate is commonly used, but it is typically dosed parenterally for the treatment of IBD, so outpatient regimens are not initiated in the acute care setting [2].

Thiopurines

Azathioprine and 6-mercaptopurine are typically used in patients with IBD. However, these medications are associated with multiple complexities that make them suboptimal to initiate in the acute care setting. Many gastroenterologists will screen for tuberculosis, hepatitis B, and hepatitis C prior to initiation to avoid reactivation of these pathogens. Furthermore, due to various genetic polymorphisms involved in the metabolism of these compounds, certain patients may be at increased risk for toxicity (i.e., myelosuppression and hepatotoxicity) [2]. Finally, these substances have a slow onset and are not recommended for acute flares [2].

Conclusion

After determining that a patient with an IBD flare is safe for discharge, it is important to take a careful medication history and learn which regimens have worked in the past and which have not. This information may help optimize outpatient management.

For patients with UC, mesalamine should be maximized to a dose of 4 g per day (split between oral and rectal routes), as tolerated by the patient. If needed, providers should consider adding budesonide at 9 mg PO daily. Antibiotics are not recommended to control acute flares of UC if the patient is nontoxic.

For CD patients, providers should start budesonide at 9 mg PO daily. If budesonide has previously failed, prednisone should be used instead. Doses may range from 20 to 60 mg PO daily, and the minimum dose needed previously should be used. Providers should consider adding rifaximin at 800 mg PO BID if the patient has previously been refractory to steroids. Mesalamine is not recommended to treat acute flares of CD.

Suggested Resources

- Carter MJ, Lobo AJ, Travis SPL. Guidelines for the management of inflammatory bowel disease in adults. Gut. 2004;53(Suppl 5(suppl_5)):v16. (9).
- Chang S, Hanauer S. Optimizing pharmacologic management of inflammatory bowel disease. Expert Rev Clin Pharmacol. 2017;10(6):595–607.
- Gomollón F, Dignass A, Annese V, et al. 3rd european evidence-based consensus on the diagnosis and management of crohn's disease 2016: part 1: diagnosis and medical management. J Crohns Colitis. 2017;11(1):3–25. (10).

References

1. Ananthakrishnan AN. Epidemiology and risk factors for IBD. Nat Rev Gastroenterol Hepatol. 2015;12(4):205–17.
2. Chang S, Hanauer S. Optimizing pharmacologic management of inflammatory bowel disease. Expert Rev Clin Pharmacol. 2017;10(6):595–607.
3. Ford AC, Khan KJ, Achkar J, Moayyedi P. Efficacy of oral vs. topical, or combined oral and topical 5-aminosalicylates, in ulcerative colitis: systematic review and meta-analysis. Am J Gastroenterol. 2012;107(2):176. author reply 177.
4. Moja L, Danese S, Fiorino G, Del Giovane C, Bonovas S. Systematic review with network meta-analysis: comparative efficacy and safety of budesonide and mesalazine (mesalamine) for Crohn's disease. Aliment Pharmacol Ther. 2015;41(11):1055–65.
5. Ford AC, Bernstein CN, Khan KJ, Abreu MT, Marshall JK, Talley NJ, et al. Glucocorticosteroid therapy in inflammatory bowel disease: systematic review and meta-analysis. Am J Gastroenterol. 2011;106(4):599. quiz 600
6. Khan KJ, Ullman TA, Ford AC, Abreu MT, Abadir A, Abadir A, et al. Antibiotic therapy in inflammatory bowel disease: a systematic review and meta-analysis. Am J Gastroenterol. 2011;106(4):661–73.
7. Rutgeerts P, Sandborn WJ, Feagan BG, Reinisch W, Olson A, Johanns J, et al. Infliximab for induction and maintenance therapy for ulcerative colitis. N Engl J Med. 2005;353(23):2462–76.
8. Sandborn WJ, van Assche G, Reinisch W, Colombel J, D'Haens G, Wolf DC, et al. Adalimumab induces and maintains clinical remission in patients with moderate-to-severe ulcerative colitis. Gastroenterology. 2012;142(2):265.e3.

When Should I Suspect Undiagnosed Inflammatory Bowel Disease in the Acute Care Setting? How Should I Manage a Suspected New Diagnosis of Inflammatory Bowel Disease?

94

Ghady Rahhal and Mark Levine

> **Pearls and Pitfalls**
> - Clinicians should have a high index of suspicion for undiagnosed inflammatory bowel disease (IBD) in patients presenting with concerning chronic and/or episodic symptoms, including abdominal pain, diarrhea, and fatigue.
> - When clinicians have a high suspicion for undiagnosed IBD, it may be beneficial to calculate a Mayo score and/or determine the Montreal classification, as these may help guide additional treatment.
> - Beyond history and physical exam, evaluating patients with suspected IBD often requires multiple diagnostic tests such as inflammatory markers, imaging, and endoscopy.

When Should I Suspect Undiagnosed Inflammatory Bowel Disease in the Acute Care Setting?

Abdominal pain, vomiting, diarrhea, and bloating are all common symptoms in the acute care setting. While all of these complaints are nonspecific, they may represent undiagnosed inflammatory bowel disease (IBD) in a subset of patients; thus, care providers should keep undiagnosed IBD in their differential diagnosis for these complaints.

The epidemiology of ulcerative colitis (UC) and Crohn's disease (CD) may lead providers to suspect IBD in certain patients. UC presents more commonly in men and nonsmokers, and CD presents more commonly in women and smokers. Both UC and CD typically present in young adults; however, UC has a bimodal distribution peaking between the ages of 15–30 and 50–70 [1, 2].

Specific complaints that increase suspicion for undiagnosed IBD include chronic diarrhea, recurring diarrhea, chronic abdominal pain, recurring abdominal pain, and fatigue. Additionally, low-grade fever and bloody stool may suggest IBD, but these also occur in higher-priority diagnoses such as infectious diarrhea and ischemic bowel disease. While many IBD symptoms are nonspecific, certain historical and exam findings may increase the likelihood of undiagnosed IBD, including aphthous ulcers, odynophagia, and gallstones. Presence or history of extraintestinal findings such as migratory polyarthritis, erythema nodosum, pyoderma gangrenosum, and uveitis should further increase the suspicion for IBD. Patients with a family history of IBD are more likely to develop IBD [3].

Sometimes computed tomography (CT) may suggest the possibility of IBD. Findings may be subtle, such as:

1. Colonic inflammation from the rectum and extending proximally
2. Focal enteritis in one loop of small bowel

Often these CT findings are read as "infectious vs inflammatory" by a radiologist. CT findings may also be highly suggestive, including active inflammation in one or more small bowel loops with structuring in one or more locations. Terminal ileitis, fistula, unexplained phlegmon, and/or unexplained abscess may also be suggestive.

How Should I Manage a Suspected New Diagnosis of Inflammatory Bowel Disease?

Because IBD is such a challenging and complex chronic disease, making a definitive diagnosis in the acute care setting is not necessary. In many ways, the goals of evaluating and managing IBD-related symptoms overlap with the evaluation and management of other acute abdominal complaints. Acute care physicians should provide symptomatic relief

G. Rahhal (✉) · M. Levine
Washington University School of Medicine, St. Louis, MO, USA
e-mail: grahhal@wustl.edu; levinem@wustl.edu

© Springer Nature Switzerland AG 2019
A. Graham, D. J. Carlberg (eds.), *Gastrointestinal Emergencies*, https://doi.org/10.1007/978-3-319-98343-1_94

while working to identify disease processes requiring acute intervention.

When suspicion for undiagnosed IBD is high, clinicians can attempt to determine disease severity, as it may help guide further management. While there is no generally accepted consensus on the definitions of mild, moderate, and severe IBD, common severity classifications include the Mayo score for UC (Table 94.1) and the Montreal classification for both UC (Table 94.2) and CD (Table 94.3) [4, 5]. As a rule of thumb, patients with normal physical examinations have mild IBD, and those with abnormal exams and systemic symptoms have moderate or severe disease.

Laboratory Testing

Laboratory workup is likely useful. A complete blood count assesses for anemia and elevated white blood cell count, and a basic metabolic panel assesses for electrolyte abnormalities. Erythrocyte sedimentation rate and

Table 94.1 Mayo score/disease activity index (DAI) for ulcerative colitis

Measure	Scoring	Interpretation
Stool frequency (per day)	0 1 2 3	Normal number of stools for patient 1–2 more stools than normal 3–4 more stools than normal 5+ more stools than normal
Rectal bleeding	0 1 2 3	No blood seen Streaks of blood with stool less than 50% of time Obvious blood with stool most of time Passes blood without stool
Findings on endoscopy	0 1 2 3	Normal or inactive disease Mild disease Moderate disease Severe disease
Physician's global assessment	0 1 2 3	Normal Mild disease Moderate disease Severe disease

A score of 0–2 suggests remission, 3–5 suggests mild disease, 6–10 suggests moderate disease, and 11–12 suggests severe disease

Table 94.2 Montreal classification for ulcerative colitis

Severity	Definition
S0 – Clinical remission	Asymptomatic
S1 – Mild UC	Passage of four or fewer stools per day, absence of systemic illness, normal erythrocyte sedimentation rate (ESR)
S2 – Moderate UC	Passage of more than four stools per day, minimal signs of systemic illness
S3 – Severe UC	Passage of at least six bloody stools per day, pulse >90 per minute, temperature ≥37.5, Hb <10.5, ESR ≥30

Table 94.3 Montreal classification for Crohn's disease

Measure	Definition
Age at diagnosis	A1 16 years or younger A2 between 17 and 40 years A3 above 40 years
Location	L1 ileal L2 colonic L3 ileocolonic L4 isolated upper disease
Behavior	B1 non-stricturing, non-penetrating B2 stricturing B3 penetrating p perianal disease modifier

A patient receives a grade for each category: age at diagnosis, location, and behavior. For example, a patient would be classified as A2, L3, or B2p

C-reactive protein measure systemic inflammation and are frequently elevated in acute IBD flares. While elevation of these may be suggestive, they neither rule in nor rule out IBD. Other labs may also be included as indicated by the clinical situation to assess for extraintestinal manifestations, such as a liver function panel (to assess for hepatobiliary pathology, including primary sclerosing cholangitis), D-dimer (due to increased risk of thromboembolisms in IBD), and vitamin B12 level (due to risk of B12 deficiency in CD). *Clostridium difficile* testing should be considered in patients with diarrhea and suspected UC.

Imaging

Imaging should be ordered based on presenting symptoms. Imaging with the sole intent of evaluating for possible IBD is not indicated, but imaging to evaluate for complications of suspected IBD may be warranted in certain situations. A plain radiograph may help evaluate for bowel obstruction, perforation, and toxic megacolon. Routine CT to evaluate patients presenting with IBD should generally be limited to patients with suspected complications that would require intervention, as the majority of patients do not have acutely intervenable complications and a subset of IBD patients will receive many CTs throughout their lifetimes [6, 7]. UC patients are unlikely to present with perforation or abscess, and imaging will likely only demonstrate the extent of inflammation. Potential intervenable CD complications demonstrated by CT include obstruction, mass, infection, inflammation, and abscess [8]. CT to evaluate for other potential disease processes (e.g., appendicitis) may be indicated.

Management

When undiagnosed IBD is suspected, treatment should include hydration and electrolyte replacement as needed.

One retrospective study showed preoperative narcotic use in Crohn's patients was associated with a longer hospitalization and postoperative complications [9].

Empiric antibiotics may be warranted in patients with bloody diarrhea, as this is a frequent presentation of infectious colitis. While it was previously believed that antibiotics played a beneficial role in managing IBD, controlled trials have cast doubt on this belief [10].

Starting IBD-specific medications (steroids, immunomodulators) in the patient with undiagnosed but presumed IBD should probably be avoided in the acute care setting and deferred to the gastroenterologist who will follow up with the patient.

Generally patients with mild symptoms, normal vital signs, benign physical exams, and reassuring blood work are safe for discharge with planned follow-up and appropriate precautions. Acute care providers should refer moderate- to high-risk patients to gastroenterology for further workup and definitive diagnosis. Low-risk patients can follow up with primary care providers who can monitor their symptoms and refer to gastroenterology as necessary.

Patients who present with the acute complications of peritonitis, bowel obstruction, bowel perforation, toxic megacolon, or hemorrhage should be admitted and receive appropriate consultation.

Suggested Resources
- Berg DF, Bahadursingh AM, Kaminski DL, Longo WE. Acute surgical emergencies in inflammatory bowel disease. Am J Surg. 2002;184:45–51.
- El-Chammas K, Majeskie A, Simpson P, Sood M, Miranda A. Red flags in children with chronic abdominal pain and Crohn's disease-a single center experience. J Pediatr. 2013;162:783–7.

- Griffey RT, Fowler KJ, Theilen A, et al. Considerations in imaging among emergency department patients with inflammatory bowel disease. Ann Emerg Med. 2017;69:587–99.

References

1. Epidemiology of the IBD. Centers for disease control and prevention, centers for disease control and prevention, 31 Mar 2015. www.cdc.gov/ibd/ibd-epidemiology.htm.
2. Cioffi M, et al. Laboratory markers in ulcerative colitis: current insights and future advances. World J Gastrointest Pathophysiol. 2015;6(1):13. https://doi.org/10.4291/wjgp.v6.i1.13.
3. Khor B, Gardet A, Xavier RJ. Genetics and pathogenesis of inflammatory bowel disease. Nature. 2011;474:307–17.
4. Peyrin-Biroulet L, Panés J, Sandborn WJ, Vermeire S, Danese S, Feagan BG, et al. Defining disease severity in inflammatory bowel diseases: current and future directions. Clin Gastroenterol Hepatol. 2016;14(3):458–354.
5. Satsangi J, Silverberg MS, Vermeire S, Colombel JF. The Montreal classification of inflammatory bowel disease: controversies, consensus, and implications. Gut. 2006;55(6):749–53. https://doi.org/10.1136/gut.2005.082909.
6. Gashin L, Villafuerte-Galvez J, Leffler DA, Obuch J, Cheifetz AS. Utility of CT in the emergency department in patients with ulcerative colitis. Inflamm Bowel Dis. 2015;21(4):793–800.
7. Govani SM, Guentner AS, Waljee AK, Higgins PD. Risk stratification of emergency department patients with Crohn's disease could reduce computed tomography use by nearly half. Clin Gastroenterol Hepatol. 2014;12(10):1702–7.
8. Griffey RT, Fowler KJ, Theilen A, et al. Considerations in imaging among emergency department patients with inflammatory bowel disease. Ann Emerg Med. 2017;69(5):587–99.
9. Srinath AI, Walter C, Newara MC, Szigethy EM. Pain management in patients with inflammatory bowel disease: insights for the clinician. Ther Adv Gastroenterol. 2012;5(5):339–57.
10. Travis S, Stange E, Lémann M, Øresland T, Bemelman W, Chowers Y, et al. European evidence-based consensus on the management of ulcerative colitis: current management. J Crohns Colitis. 2008;2(1):24–62.

Nidhi Malhotra and I. David Shocket

Pearls and Pitfalls

- Emergencies in inflammatory bowel disease are uncommon but sometimes life-threatening.
- Fulminant colitis and toxic megacolon are the two most common surgical emergencies in ulcerative colitis.
- Abscess formation (intra-abdominal or perianal), intestinal perforation, and intestinal obstruction are the three most common emergencies in Crohn's disease.
- Patients with more than six bloody bowel movements a day, fever, tachycardia, hemoglobin less than 10gm/dl, and C-reactive protein greater than 10 mg/L should be considered for hospital admission.
- An intra-abdominal abscess can be difficult to differentiate from a CD exacerbation, as both can present with abdominal pain, nausea, leukocytosis, and low-grade fever. However, fever above 101.5 °F is usually associated with an intra-abdominal abscess.
- Recurrent incision and drainage of perianal abscesses can lead to chronic incontinence. Consultation with a surgeon with IBD expertise in this situation may decrease this risk.

Introduction to Consultant

Nidhi Malhotra, MD, and I. David Shocket, MD, both practice gastroenterology at MedStar Washington Hospital Center. Dr. Malhotra has completed subspecialty training in inflammatory bowel disease (IBD). She is actively involved in fellow training as well as research in IBD. Dr. Shocket serves as Section Director of Gastroenterology at MedStar Washington Hospital Center, and his clinical expertise also involves treating IBD patients. Both teach extensively on the topic. MedStar Washington Hospital Center is a large, urban tertiary referral hospital in Washington, DC.

Answers to Key Clinical Questions

1. What pearls can you offer emergency care providers when evaluating an inflammatory bowel disease patient with a potential complication?

Inflammatory bowel disease (IBD) patients are typically under the care of a gastroenterologist but will often present for emergency care with complaints ranging from trivial to complex. It is imperative to differentiate patients who can be safely discharged from those requiring urgent medical or surgical consultation and hospital admission. Identifying this group of patients can be a challenge, as emergent complications are uncommon. However, these complications may lead to end-organ injury and are often life-threatening [1].

2. What complications are you concerned about in inflammatory bowel disease patients, and what are key concepts in managing these patients?

Ulcerative Colitis

Fulminant colitis, toxic megacolon, and refractory bleeding are the most common emergencies in ulcerative colitis (UC).

Fulminant colitis is the initial presentation of UC in up to 30% of cases, with an overall incidence of about 10% [3]. In fulminant colitis, inflammation extends beyond the colonic mucosa, potentially triggering the systemic inflammatory response syndrome (SIRS). Fulminant colitis may present with signs of SIRS in addition to the common symptoms of a disease flare, which include abdominal pain, bloody diarrhea, rectal urgency, and tenesmus. Fulminant colitis patients require close monitoring with urgent gastroenterology and

N. Malhotra (✉) · I. D. Shocket
MedStar Washington Hospital Center, Washington, DC, USA
e-mail: nidhi.malhotra@gunet.georgetown.edu; ira.d.shocket@gunet.georgetown.edu

© Springer Nature Switzerland AG 2019
A. Graham, D. J. Carlberg (eds.), *Gastrointestinal Emergencies*, https://doi.org/10.1007/978-3-319-98343-1_95

surgery consultations. If computed tomography (CT) is not performed, plain radiographs of the abdomen should be obtained to exclude toxic megacolon. Stool studies, including *Clostridium difficile* testing, should be sent. Once infection has been excluded, attempts to induce remission are initiated with intravenous cyclosporine, infliximab, or steroids. However, these patients often fail medical therapy and require a sub-total colectomy.

Toxic megacolon is defined as colonic dilation, either segmental or complete, noted on imaging. Advanced toxic megacolon, which features pneumatosis coli, peritoneal signs, obstruction, and metabolic acidosis, may require urgent surgery [4]. Antidiarrheal agents are contraindicated in toxic megacolon patients, and some gastroenterologists advise avoiding opiates as they may mask the development of peritonitis. Urgent consultation with a surgeon with expertise in IBD is imperative to assess if and/or when proctocolectomy is necessary. Intestinal perforation, peritonitis, refractory bleeding, and persistent dilation of the colon on imaging are indications for urgent colectomy.

Crohn's Disease

Abscess formation (intra-abdominal or perineal) with sepsis, intestinal perforation, and intestinal obstruction are the most common emergencies in Crohn's disease (CD) and often require surgical intervention [2].

Up to 25% of CD patients with perforating or fistulizing disease will present with an intra-abdominal abscess at some point in their clinical course [5]. An intra-abdominal abscess can be difficult to differentiate from a CD exacerbation, as both can present with abdominal pain, nausea, leukocytosis, and low-grade fever. However, fever above 38.6 °C is usually associated with an intra-abdominal abscess. Steroid use may blunt the typical response to infection.

While CD-related complications often require CT for diagnosis, patients should be spared ionizing radiation when possible. For example, when managing a perianal abscess, providers may consider obtaining surgical consultation before imaging, as MRI or rectal endoscopic ultrasound (EUS) will better delineate an abscess without the risks of radiation.

Abscesses in CD often require drainage, antibiotics, and admission to the hospital. Most large intra-abdominal abscesses are amenable to percutaneous drainage by interventional radiology. Abscesses smaller than 2 cm can often be managed medically [5]. However, more than 50% of patients initially managed medically will eventually require surgical resection of the affected bowel, since an abscess most likely results from an intestinal perforation.

Perianal abscesses require adequate drainage and also frequently require seton placement. A seton is a piece of silk or latex string that is placed into the perianal fistula tract to allow long-term drainage of the associated abscess and help heal the fistulous tract from inside out. Perianal abscesses are often amenable to drainage in the acute care setting with a plan for outpatient antibiotics and close follow-up.

Recurrent incision and drainage of perianal abscesses can lead to incontinence, with potentially devastating lifelong quality-of-life implications. In this circumstance, consultation with a surgeon with IBD expertise may decrease the risk.

Perianal fistulas may require drainage and antibiotic administration. They are often an indication for initiation biologic therapy by a gastroenterologist.

Perforation is a surgical emergency. Free perforation in CD is rare, occurring in about 1–3% of patients [6]. The ileum is the most common site of intestinal perforation, followed by the colon [6]. Jejunal perforations are less common, and upper gastrointestinal perforations are even rarer [6, 7]. Most perforations in CD tend to occur slowly and present with entero-enteric fistulae and intra-abdominal abscesses. When feasible, fistulae and abscesses are usually treated initially with medical therapy followed by interval intestinal resection, but the presence of free air and/or sepsis suggests the need for urgent surgical intervention [8]. A primary anastomosis is often not possible in these situations, and an end or diverting ileostomy is required.

Intestinal obstruction is the most common complication in Crohn's disease, occurring in as many as 50% of patients. Obstruction often results from acute inflammation superimposed on some degree of preexisting underlying fibrostenotic disease. The initial management of an obstruction is usually medical therapy with initiation of steroids to reduce acute inflammation. However, surgical management is the only definitive treatment of a stricture. If performed, surgical resection should be followed postoperatively by initiation of medical therapy (biologics, immunomodulators, or combination therapy with the goal of avoiding long-term steroids) [9].

3. IBD: Who can go home? Who should be admitted?

Patients with more than six bloody bowel movements a day, fever, tachycardia, hemoglobin less than 10gm/dl, and C-reactive protein greater than 10 mg/L should be considered for hospital admission. UC patients with fulminant colitis or toxic megacolon should be admitted, as should CD patients with abscess formation (intra-abdominal or perineal) with sepsis, intestinal perforation, or intestinal obstruction.

Patients with mild symptoms can be safely discharged if they can eat and drink, control their pain, and follow up with an appropriate gastroenterologist within 1 week.

4. Steroids? Antibiotics? Biologics? Immunomodulators? What are the optimal discharge medications for an IBD flare?

IBD patients discharged home should often be prescribed a short course of budesonide for mild flares or prednisone for mild to moderate flares. Antibiotics are generally not indicated for IBD patients being discharged unless there is a documented infection.

5. When should I suspect undiagnosed inflammatory bowel disease in the acute care setting? How should I manage a suspected new diagnosis of inflammatory bowel disease?

When providers suspect undiagnosed IBD in patients being discharged, a stool culture, *Clostridium difficile* assay, and fecal calprotectin level should be sent to aid the gastroenterologist who will see the patient in follow-up. Patients with suspected but undiagnosed IBD with findings of ileitis or colon inflammation on CT should be prescribed antibiotics, but not steroids upon discharge, as many prove to have an infectious cause rather than IBD.

Suggested Resources

- Colombel JF, Mahadevan U. Inflammatory bowel disease 2017: innovations and changing paradigms. Gastroenterology. 2017;152:309–12.
- Maddu KK, Mittal P, Shuaib W, Tewari A, Ibraheem O, Khosa F. Colorectal emergencies and related complications: a comprehensive imaging review-imaging of colitis and complications. AJR Am J Roentgenol. 2014;203(6):1205–16.
- Nguyen GC, Seow CH, Maxwell C, et al. The Toronto consensus statements for the management of inflammatory bowel disease in pregnancy. Gastroenterology. 2016;150(3):734–57.

References

1. Cheung O, Regueiro MD. Inflammatory bowel disease emergencies. Gastroenterol Clin N Am. 2003;32(4):1269–88.
2. Berg DF, Bahadursingh AM, Kaminski DL, Longo WE. Acute surgical emergencies in inflammatory bowel disease. Am J Surg. 2002;184:45–51.
3. Roy MA. Inflammatory bowel disease. Surg Clin North Am. 1997;77:1419–31.
4. Knechtle SJ, Davidoff AM, Rice RP. Pneumatosis intestinalis: surgical management and clinical outcome. Ann Surg. 1990;212(2):160.
5. Cellini C, Safar B, Fleshman J. Surgical management of pyogenic complications of Crohn's disease. Inflamm Bowel Dis. 2010;16(3):512–7.
6. Bundred NJ, Dixon JM, Lumsden AB, Gilmour HM, Davies GC. Free perforation in Crohn's colitis: a ten year review. Dis Colon Rectum. 1985;28:35–7.
7. Katz S, Schulman N, Levin L. Free perforation in Crohn's disease: a report of 33 cases and review of literature. Am J Gastroenterol. 1986;81(1):38–43.
8. Ananthakrishnan AN, McGinley EL. Treatment of intra-abdominal abscesses in Crohn's disease: a nationwide analysis of patterns and outcomes of care. Dig Dis Sci. 2013;58(7):2013–8.
9. Mao R, Chen BL, He Y, Cui Y, Zeng ZR, Chen MH. Factors associated with progression to surgery in Crohn's disease patients with endoscopic stricture. Endoscopy. 2014;46(11):956–62.

How Do I Approach the Patient with Diarrhea? Key History, Physical Examination, and Diagnostic Considerations

96

Alexa R. Gale and Matthew Wilson

Acute gastroenteritis accounts for 179 million outpatient visits, approximately 500,000 hospitalizations, and >5000 deaths in the United States each year [1]. The evaluation of diarrhea begins with a thorough history to determine potential causes to customize initial diarrheal illness management, followed by a careful physical examination to assess the patient's level of dehydration, determine supportive care requirements, and refine the diagnostic workup. We recommend asking five questions as outlined by Sweetser et al. in 2012 [2] to help narrow the differential diagnosis for diarrhea.

Table 96.1 Clinically significant clinical and physical examination findings for patient's with diarrhea

Historical features	Clinical implication
Duration	Acute <14 days Persistent >14 days but <4 weeks Chronic >4 weeks
Epidemiology	History of travel Recent epidemics/outbreaks Rural or urban home environment Source of drinking water
Iatrogenic factors	Drugs – acid-reducing agents, antacids (e.g., magnesium), antibiotics, anti-inflammatory agents, herbal products, colchicine, theophylline Radiation Surgery
Systemic diseases	Diabetes HIV/AIDS Collagen vascular Neoplastic lymphoma
Volume of diarrhea	Frequent, small, painful stool – left (distal) colon Painless, large volume stool – small intestines or right colon etiology
Character of stool	Watery – osmotic or secretory process Fatty – lactose intolerance, celiac disease, biliary atresia, Crohn's disease Bloody – invasive bacterial infection, inflammatory bowel disease, or malignancy Excessive flatus – poorly absorbed carbohydrates in the small intestine
Physical exam findings	Hyperpigmentation – Addison's disease Lymphadenopathy – HIV, lymphoma, cancer Muscle wasting, edema – malnutrition
High-risk factors	Extremes of age Immunocompromised Recent travel or antibiotic use Occupational exposures, e.g., day care, healthcare Untreated water

Schiller L, Sellin J. Diarrhea. Sleisenger and Fordtran's Gastrointestinal and Liver Disease. Chapter 16, 221–241.e5

A. R. Gale (✉) · M. Wilson
Georgetown University School of Medicine, MedStar Washington Hospital Center, Department of Emergency Medicine, Washington, DC, USA
e-mail: alexa.r.gale@medstar.net; Mdw12@medstar.net

© Springer Nature Switzerland AG 2019
A. Graham, D. J. Carlberg (eds.), *Gastrointestinal Emergencies*, https://doi.org/10.1007/978-3-319-98343-1_96

"Simplified 5-Question Approach from Sweetser 2012" [2] + Risk Assessment

Does My Patient Have Diarrhea?

Diarrhea is defined as up to three or more stools per day or greater than 250 g of stool per day. Patients may confuse increased stool frequency with fecal incontinence or impaction, with leaking of stool around impaction site [3].

Rule Out Medications as Cause of Diarrhea

Drug-induced diarrhea is common. Determining a temporal relationship between the initiation of a medication and frequent stools is key. Common medications that cause diarrhea include caffeine, herbal/vitamin supplements, and antacids, especially those containing magnesium [2]. Both antibiotics and acid-suppressing medications such as proton pump inhibitors are associated with *C. difficile* infections due to colonic bacterial flora alteration. Nonsteroidal anti-inflammatory medications cause diarrhea by inciting intestinal inflammation. Chemotherapeutic agents cause diarrhea by damaging intestinal and colonic crypts as well as impairing water absorption.

Acute Versus Chronic?

Acute diarrhea is less than 14 days [3], whereas *persistent diarrhea* is increased stool frequency lasting longer than 14 days. Diarrhea continuing more than 30 days is referred to as *chronic diarrhea* [4]. The vast majority of acute diarrheal illnesses occur from self-limited, viral etiologies, requiring little evaluation or treatment. By analyzing stool cultures, the Centers for Disease Control and Prevention (CDC) confirms that bacteria such as *salmonella* (16.1 cases per 100,000 population), *campylobacter* (13.4 cases per 100,000 population), *shigella* (10.3 cases per 100,000 population), *Escherichia coli* O157:H7 (1.7 cases per 100,000 population), and cryptosporidium (1.4 cases per 100,000 population) are rarely the source of diarrheal illness [3]. However, *cryptosporidiosis* cases have risen from increased exposure in community swimming pools [5]. Chronic diarrhea warrants an evaluation with outpatient, gastroenterology consultation to methodically evaluate its broad differential diagnosis.

Inflammatory, Fatty, Watery?

Watery diarrhea is attributed to either osmotic or secretory etiologies. Osmotic diarrhea is caused by poor absorption of osmotically active substances (e.g., lactulose) and can be differentiated from the more commonly encountered secretory diarrheal illnesses by a patient's response to eating. Secretory diarrhea occurs when electrolyte absorption is impaired in the intestines from bacterial toxins, reduced absorptive surface area (e.g., bowel resection), laxatives, drugs, and compromised intestinal function [6]. Patients will continue to have diarrhea during fasting periods although the amount of stool output may decrease due to decreased endogenous secretions. Patients with osmotic diarrhea will have a resolution of symptoms with fasting [6]. Electrolyte absorption is not impaired in osmotic diarrhea, while secretory diarrhea has impaired absorption of sodium and potassium with accompanying anions [6].

Inflammatory diarrhea typically presents with frequent, small-volume, blood-tinged stool. Fever, abdominal pain, and tenesmus may also be present. Inflammatory diarrhea suggests damaged mucosa, and its differential diagnosis includes ischemic colitis, inflammatory bowel disease (e.g., Crohn's disease, ulcerative colitis), and invasive infectious infections (e.g., *C. difficile*, *Entamoeba histolytica*, *E. coli*). Patients with suspected inflammatory diarrhea may warrant antibiotics and elective colonoscopy.

Fatty stools are often characterized by a history of weight loss, greasy or bulky stools, or oil in the toilet bowl. Floating stools are not associated with steatorrhea but usually indicate increased gas production by colonic bacteria [7]. Fat malabsorption occurs from celiac disease, pancreatic exocrine insufficiency (e.g., pancreatitis, pancreatic mass), small intestinal bacterial overgrowth (SIBO), or cirrhosis. Further outpatient evaluation may include Sudan stain to evaluate for excess fecal fat, endoscopy with small bowel biopsies, computed tomography to appraise the anatomy of the pancreas and liver, and hydrogen breath test (SIBO). Small intestinal bacterial overgrowth (SIBO) occurs with excessive bacteria in the small intestine and presents with chronic diarrhea, malabsorption with nutritional deficiencies, osteoporosis, and weight loss [6].

Factitious Diarrhea: Laxative Ingestion?

Laxatives fall in five major classes:

- Bulk-forming agents (e.g., fiber, psyllium) which have been shown to improve the frequency of stools when compared to placebo.
- Stimulants (e.g., senna, bisacodyl) engage the myoenteric plexus, thus stimulating peristalsis. Side effects include abdominal discomfort, cramping, and, in some instances, electrolyte abnormalities. It is unlikely to cause "cathartic colon" based on available evidence [8].
- Osmotic laxatives (e.g., lactulose, polyethylene glycol (PEG), glycerin, sorbitol) are widely available. Studies

suggest PEG (Miralax) has a greater efficacy than lactulose with fewer side effects such as flatulence and bloating [8].

- Stool softeners (e.g., docusate) are commonly prescribed but not a highly effective constipation treatment.
- Pro-secretory (e.g., lubiprostone, linaclotide) work by stimulating pathways regulated by prostaglandin E1 or guanylate cyclase 2c agonists.

Risk Assessment

Historical risk factors for an invasive bacterial cause or a complicated disease course include extremes of age (>65 years of age); immunocompromised; recent international travel or antibiotic use, associated with severe abdominal pain, fever, blood-tinged stool, and known or suspected inflammatory bowel disease; occupational exposures (e.g., day care, raw meat/dairy, healthcare); or untreated water exposure [4]. These high-risk patients should be considered for empiric antimicrobial therapy. For example, a pregnant woman with *listeria* may require antibiotics as well as admission for consultations with multiple specialties.

Diagnostic Considerations

There are no required laboratory tests for the evaluation of uncomplicated acute diarrheal illness. In the absence of clinical concern for dehydration or electrolyte derangement, it is unlikely that basic metabolic panel findings would affect disposition. BUN monitoring has been used to assess volume status, but it is neither sensitive nor specific for predicting dehydration in children. Specific gravity testing in urinalysis is also not accurate for assessing the degree of dehydration from diarrhea [9]. However, serum bicarbonate levels have been shown to predict clinical course. A normal serum bicarbonate level suggests a child is not currently dehydrated, with a likelihood ratio between 0.18 (95% CI, 0.08–0.37) and 0.22 (95% CI, 0.12–0.43) [8]. A serum bicarbonate level of less than 13 mEq per L suggests a pediatric patient will likely fail outpatient rehydration [10, 11].

Stool testing is recommended by the Infectious Diseases Society of America (IDSA) for patients with "diarrhea accompanied by fever, bloody or mucoid stools, severe abdominal cramping or tenderness, or signs of sepsis" but may take time to result and thus require close outpatient follow-up [4]. For community-acquired or traveler's diarrhea with fever or blood in the stool, stool cultures for *Salmonella*, *Shigella*, *Campylobacter*, *E. coli* O157:H7, and *C. difficile* may be helpful. For hospital-acquired or recent antibiotics/chemotherapy test, *C. difficile* toxin testing may be indicated; and for persistent diarrhea (>14 days), stool testing for

parasites (*Giardia, Cryptosporidium, Cyclospora, Isospora belli*) may direct care [4]. Because these results may ultimately be managed by a patient's primary care doctor, referral for stool studies with a primary care physician may be appropriate for acute care providers.

The CDC recommends notification of public health authorities if the following bacterial diarrheal illnesses are strongly suspected or definitively diagnosed: *cholera, enterohemorrhagic E. coli, listeria, salmonella,* and *shigella*.

For typical diarrheal illnesses, there is no indication for radiological imaging, although a chief complaint of diarrhea may be a component of a constellation of signs or symptoms suggesting an overarching acute surgical process. These conditions are usually accompanied by systemic findings (fever, bleeding, or weight loss), abdominal pain, and tenderness on physical examination. These presentations are the true impetus for radiologic examination. Abdominal radiographs or commuted tomography imaging may be performed to identify bowel obstruction, fecal impaction, ischemic bowel, malabsorption following gastric bypass, or mass.

Suggested Resources

- FoodNet – CDC surveillance of foodborne diseases. https://www.cdc.gov/foodnet/surveillance.html.
- National Outbreak Reporting System (NORS) – web based platform used by local, state, and territorial health departments to report waterborne and foodborne disease outbreaks and enteric disease outbreaks. https://www.cdc.gov/nors/index.html.
- Schiller LR, Sellin JH. Diarrhea. In: Feldman M, Friedman LS, Brandt LJ, editors. Sleisenger and Fordtran's gastrointestinal and liver disease. Philadelphia: Saunders Elsevier; 2010. p. 211–32.
- Shane A, Mody R, Crump J, Tarr P, Steiner T, Kotloff K, et al. 2017 Infectious Diseases Society of America clinical practice guidelines for the diagnosis and management of infectious diarrhea. Clin Infect Dis. 2017;65(12):e45–80.
- Thielman NM, Guerrant RL. Acute infectious diarrhea. N Engl J Med. 2004;350:38–47.

References

1. Scallan E, Griffin PM, Angulo FJ, Tauxe RV, Hoekstra R. Foodborne illness acquired in the United States – unspecified agents. Emerg Infect Dis. 2011;17:16–22.
2. Sweetser S. Evaluating the patient with diarrhea: a case based approach. Mayo Clin Proc. 2012;87(6):596–602.
3. Thielman NM, Guerrant RL. Acute infectious diarrhea. N Engl J Med. 2004;350:38–47.

4. Guerrant RL, Van Gilder T, Steiner TS, Thielman NM, Slutsker L, Tauxe RV, et al. Practice guidelines for the management of infectious diarrhea. Clin Infect Dis. 2001;32:331–50.

5. Crawford C. Cryptosporidiosis outbreaks on the rise, CDC warns [document on the Internet]. AAFP News, American Academy of Family Physicians; 2015 July 1. Available from: https://www.aafp.org/news/health-of-the-public/20150701cryptooutbreaks.html.

6. Schiller LR, Sellin JH. Diarrhea. In: Feldman M, Friedman LS, Brandt LJ, editors. Sleisenger and Fordtran's gastrointestinal and liver disease. Philadelphia: Saunders Elsevier; 2010. p. 211–32.

7. Bardhan PK, Beltinger J, Beltinger RW, Hossain A, Mahalanabis D, Gyr K. Screening of patients with acute infectious diarrhoea: Evaluation of clinical features, faecal microscopy, and faecal occult blood testing. Scan J Gastroenterol. 2000;3591:54–60.

8. Rhodes F, Carty E. Laxatives: a rational approach to prescribing. Br J Hospital Med. 2014;75(8):C114–8.

9. Churgay CA, Aflab Z. Gastroenteritis in children: part I. Diagn Am Fam Physician. 2012;85(11):11.

10. Steiner MJ, DeWalt DA, Byerley JS. Is this child dehydrated? JAMA. 2004;291(22):2746–54.

11. Teach SJ, Yates EW, Feld LG. Laboratory predictors of fluid deficit in acutely dehydrated children. Clin Pediatr (Phila). 1997;36(7):395–400.

Antibiotic Stewardship in the Patient with Diarrhea: Who Needs Antibiotics? And Which Antibiotics Do I Prescribe?

Alexa R. Gale and Matthew Wilson

Pearls and Pitfalls

- Bacterial stool cultures are rarely positive.
- In developed countries, *Campylobacter* accounts for 3% of cases. *Salmonella* causes 2% of cases, and other bacterial etiologies (ETEC, other *E. coli*, *Shigella*, and *V. cholerae*) are each found in less than 0.2% of cases.
- Shiga toxin-producing *E. coli* (STEC) is associated with hemolytic-uremic syndrome (HUS) after antibiotic treatment of *Escherichia coli* O157:H7, *Shigella*, or *Campylobacter* containing the O157:H7 phage.
- Antibiotic treatment can be instituted as recommended by the IDSA, based on historical or exam findings that suggest an invasive, bacterial disease.
- Empiric antibiotics should be directed at common etiologies or most likely bacterial causes based on individual risk.

Who Needs Antibiotics?

Most diarrheal illnesses do not benefit from antibiotics and they should not be prescribed for uncomplicated cases lasting less than 5 days. Bacterial stool cultures are rarely positive [1]. In developed countries, *Campylobacter* accounts for 3% of cases. *Salmonella* causes 2% of cases, and other

bacterial etiologies (ETEC, other *E. coli*, *Shigella*, and *V. cholerae*) are each found in less than 0.2% of cases [2]. The majority of acute diarrheal illnesses are viral. Specifically, noroviruses are a common source of acute diarrhea and have been implicated in cruise ship and daycare/school outbreaks. Rotavirus is also a common viral etiology. The frequency and severity of seasonal outbreaks have decreased with the adoption of the *Rotavirus* vaccine [3].

Patients can be advised that not only do empiric antibiotics not benefit most cases of acute diarrhea but they have detrimental short- and long-term effects on the intestinal microbiome [4]. Serious side effects of antibacterial agents include the development of antimicrobial resistance, medication cost, eradication of normal intestinal flora, and the induction of the Shiga toxin phage by quinolones [1].

Even when a bacterial source is identified, antibiotics may have limited value. Several studies have demonstrated a mildly decreased duration of symptoms of *Campylobacter* infections with antibiotics. A meta-analysis of these studies showed a 1-day symptom improvement in those given antibiotics (fluoroquinolone or azithromycin) versus placebo. Symptoms were self-limited in both groups [5]. *Salmonella* proven diarrheal infections have no proven benefit with antimicrobial treatment [5].

Shiga toxin-producing *E. coli* (STEC) is associated with hemolytic-uremic syndrome (HUS) after antibiotic treatment of *Escherichia coli* O157:H7, *Shigella*, or *Campylobacter* containing the O157:H7 phage. In a prospective evaluation of risk factors, antibiotics were independently associated with the development of HUS [6]. Hemolytic-uremic syndrome results in microangiopathic hemolytic anemia, acute kidney injury, and thrombocytopenia. The vascular endothelial damage can be fatal or result in acute kidney injury requiring dialysis. Intravenous fluids during the diarrheal phase have been shown to reduce the risk of acute kidney injury in children [5]. STEC typically

A. R. Gale · M. Wilson (✉)
Georgetown University School of Medicine, MedStar Washington Hospital Center, Department of Emergency Medicine, Washington, DC, USA
e-mail: alexa.r.gale@medstar.net, Mdw12@medstar.net

© Springer Nature Switzerland AG 2019
A. Graham, D. J. Carlberg (eds.), *Gastrointestinal Emergencies*, https://doi.org/10.1007/978-3-319-98343-1_97

presents with afebrile, bloody diarrhea, with only 10% developing HUS without history of bloody diarrhea [5]. Approximately 65% patients with STEC will have leukocytosis >10,000 cells/uL [5]. Although PCR has been used in research for rapid diagnosis of the Shiga toxin phage, it is not widely available, and STEC O157 and Shiga toxin tests are recommended. Clinicians have to exercise caution with any antimicrobial treatment prior to definitive bacterial identification.

And Which Antibiotics Do I Prescribe?

The specific causal agent is usually not cultured in time for acute decision-making and management in the acute setting. Antibiotic treatment can be instituted as recommended by the IDSA based on historical or exam findings that suggest an invasive, bacterial disease. Empiric antibiotics should be directed at common etiologies or most likely bacterial agent based on individual risk (Table 97.1).

Table 97.1 Suspected bacterial etiology and suggested antibiotic regimen

Clinical scenario	Causative etiology	Treatment

Suspected bacterial etiology	Unknown	• Ciprofloxacin 500 mg PO BID × 1–3 days
		• Levofloxacin 500 mg PO daily × 1–3 days
		• Azithromycin 500 mg PO daily × 3 days
		• Bactrim DS PO BID × 5 days
		
		Infants <3 months –
		  • Third-generation cephalosporin (weight-based dosing)
		  • Azithromycin (weight-based dosing)
		
		Campylobacter suspected
		  • Azithromycin 500 mg PO daily × 3 days

Traveler's diarrhea: international travel with acute diarrhea; often with abdominal cramping, tenesmus, nausea, vomiting	*ETEC, Norovirus, Rotavirus, Salmonella, Campylobacter, Shigella, Aeromonas, Bacteroides,* and *Vibrio*	• Azithromycin 1000 mg PO single dose • Ciprofloxacin 500 mg PO BID × 3 days • Bactrim DS PO BID × 3 days Treatment may reduce duration by 2–3 days
Febrile/invasive: severe dysentery with fever/bloody diarrhea; very contagious	*Campylobacter, Salmonella, Shigella,* and *Yersinia*	• Ciprofloxacin 500 mg PO BID × 3 days • Bactrim DS PO BID × 3 days Treatment may reduce duration of bacterial shedding
Persistent diarrhea after untreated water exposure	Giardia	• Metronidazole 500 mg PO TID for 7–10 days
Bloody diarrhea, pain, lack of fever	Suspected *STEC*	• No antimicrobial agents as they may worsen the risk of HUS and do not ameliorate O157 illness
"Rice-water diarrhea"; severely dehydrating secretory diarrhea from cholera enterotoxin; only endemic in the USA along Gulf Coast	*Cholera*	• Doxycycline 300 mg PO single dose • Bactrim DS PO BID × 3 days or • Ciprofloxacin 500 mg PO × 3 days • Azithromycin 1000 mg PO single dose
Severe dysentery with fever/bloody diarrhea; very contagious	*Shigella*	• Bactrim DS PO BID × 3 days • Ciprofloxacin/Levofloxacin 500 mg PO BID × 3 days Treatment may reduce bacterial elimination and shorten duration of disease
Acute watery diarrhea; associated with "pseudo-appendicitis"	*Yersinia*	• Antibiotics usually only needed in immunocompromised
Acute watery diarrhea; poultry reservoir; associated with Guillain-Barre, reactive arthritis and IBD	*Campylobacter*	• Erythromycin 500 mg PO BID × 5 days
Food-borne, travelers, or childhood diarrhea in developing countries; multiple strains	*E. coli*	ETEC: • Bactrim DS PO BID × 3 days or • Ciprofloxacin/levofloxacin 500 mg PO BID for 3 days
Systemic (fever, body aches, neck stiffness); transmitted from human to human (typhoid type)	*Salmonella*	• Not routinely recommended unless immunocompromised, extremes of age, valvular heart disease, or persistent symptoms • Bactrim DS PO BID × 5–7 days or • Ciprofloxacin/levofloxacin 500 mg PO BID × 5–7 days
Mild systemic symptoms (fever, body aches); severe invasive disease in pregnancy or immunocompromised	*Listeria*	• Not routinely recommended unless immunocompromised or pregnant in which case ampicillin should be used

Adapted from Guerrant (Ref. [1]), Lubbert (Ref. [4]), Shane (Ref. [5])

Empiric Antibiotics

IDSA Recommendations [5]

(a) Infants <3 months of age with suspicion of bacterial etiology

(b) Ill immunocompetent people with fever documented in medical setting, abdominal pain, bloody diarrhea, and bacillary dysentery (frequent scant bloody stool, fever, abdominal cramps, tenesmus) presumptively from Shigella

(c) People who have recently traveled internationally with body temperatures greater than or equal to 38.5° Celsius

(d) Signs of sepsis (patients with enteric fever should also have blood cultures sent)

High-Risk Patients Determine the need for empiric antibiotics while awaiting stool testing results based on clinical presentation.

- Immunocompromised
- Extremes of age
- Visible blood in stool or hemoccult-positive stool (higher likelihood of bacterial source)
- High-risk exposure (local outbreak data, occupational exposure, untreated water source)

Suggested Resources
- Shane AL, Mody RK, Crump JA, Tarr PI, Steiner TS, Kotloff K, Langley JM, Wanke C, Warren CA, Cheng AC, Cantey J, Pickering LK. 2017 Infectious Diseases Society of America clinical practice guidelines for the diagnosis and management of infectious diarrhea. Clin Infect Dis. 2017;65(12):e45–80. https://doi.org/10.1093/cid/cix669

References

1. Guerrant RL, Van Gilder T, Steiner TS, Thielman NM, Slutsker L, Tauxe RV, et al. Practice guidelines for the management of infectious diarrhea. Clin Infect Dis. 2001;32:331–50.
2. Fletcher SM, McLaws ML, Ellis JT. Prevalence of gastrointestinal pathogens in developed and developing countries: systematic review and meta-analysis. J Public Health Res. 2013;2(1):42–53.
3. Centers for disease control and prevention. Reduction in rotavirus after vaccine introduction – United States, 2000–2009. MMWR Morb Mortal Wkly Rep. 2009;58(41):1146–9.
4. Lübbert C. Antimicrobial therapy of acute diarrhoea: a clinical review. Expert Rev Anti-Infect Ther. 2016;14(2):193–206. https://doi.org/10.1586/14787210.2016.1128824.
5. Shane AL, Mody RK, Crump JA, Tarr PI, Steiner TS, Kotloff K, et al. 2017 infectious diseases society of America clinical practice guidelines for the diagnosis and management of infectious diarrhea. Clin Infect Dis. 2017;65(12):1963–73. https://doi.org/10.1093/cid/cix669.
6. Wong CS, Jelacic S, Habeeb RL, Watkins SL, Tarr PI. The risk of the hemolytic-uremic syndrome after antibiotic treatment of Escherichia coli O157:H7 infections. N Engl J Med. 2000;342(26):1930.

What Discharge Instructions Should I Give? Oral Rehydration, Zinc Supplementation, Diet, Probiotics, and Antimotility Medications

Alexa R. Gale and Matthew Wilson

Pearls and Pitfalls (Table 98.1)

- Oral rehydration therapy (ORT) was designed to correct dehydration and metabolic acidosis and is recommended for mild to moderate dehydration from diarrheal illness.
- Sodas and fruit juices with their high sugar content may worsen diarrhea and dehydration.
- Zinc supplementation in children <5 years of age may decrease the duration of diarrhea.
- Early initiation of age-appropriate diet is encouraged.
- Probiotics reduce the duration of diarrhea.

Oral Rehydration Therapy

Because most diarrheal illnesses will last 7–14 days, repletion of water, electrolytes, and nutrients is key. For mild to moderate dehydration, oral rehydration therapy (ORT) is recommended, providing a safe and cost-effective replacement of fluids and electrolytes. ORT was developed 40 years ago with the goal of providing an alternative to sterile intravenous hydration for the overwhelming number of patients affected by cholera outbreaks in developing countries. ORT is an "iso-osmolar, glucose-electrolyte solution with added base (e.g. citrate in World Health Organization (WHO) -ORT) that was designed to correct dehydration and metabolic acidosis" [1]. Composed of sodium, dextrose, and bicarbonate in a ratio that does not overwhelm hyperactive bowels, ORT is concentrated enough to replace electrolyte loss [2].

Standard WHO-ORT (osmolarity 311 mmol/L) has limitations, including the inability to reduce the severity of diarrhea and risk of hypernatremia in non-cholera diarrhea. In 2002, the WHO recommended a hypotonic oral rehydration solution with an osmolarity <250 mmol/L. A meta-analysis of children comparing standard WHO-ORT to hypotonic oral rehydration solution (ORS) demonstrated reduced stool output and decreased vomiting in the hypotonic ORS group [3]. However, a combined analysis of children and adults found higher rates of hyponatremia but no serious outcome differences [4].

In a meta-analysis of 16 studies of 1545 children in 11 countries, oral rehydration was associated with fewer major adverse events (relative risk 0.36, 95% confidence interval, 0.14–0.89) and shorter hospital stays (mean 21 h; 95% CI, 8–35 h) compared to IV hydration. The failure rate of oral rehydration was 4% (95 CI, 3–5%) [5]. A subsequent Cochrane review in 2006 confirmed there was no difference in failure to rehydrate, total fluid intake in 24 h, rates of hyponatremia/hypernatremia, or duration of diarrhea between IV hydration and oral rehydration [6].

In the United States, oral rehydration solutions include Pedialyte, Infalyte, or WHO oral rehydration solutions. Gatorade with its high sugar content is acceptable but should be used with caution in children under 2 years of age. Sodas and fruit juices with their high sugar content may worsen diarrhea and dehydration [7]. Clear liquids (e.g., water, sodas, chicken broth, and apple juice) should also be avoided because they are hypo-osmolar and do not adequately replace potassium and sodium [2].

In 2004, WHO and United Nation's Children fund (UNICEF) recommended zinc supplementation for acute diarrhea in children <5 years of age. A systematic literature review of children < age 5 analyzed 18,822 cases of diarrhea, of which 9460 received zinc and 9353 did not receive zinc. Studies reported "decreased episode duration, stool output, stool frequency, hospitalization duration, and proportion of episodes lasting beyond three to seven days" [8]. An overall 26% reduction in duration of diarrhea beyond 3–7 days was

A. R. Gale · M. Wilson (✉)
Georgetown University School of Medicine, MedStar Washington Hospital Center, Department of Emergency Medicine, Washington, DC, USA
e-mail: alexa.r.gale@medstar.net; Mdw12@medstar.net

found in children receiving zinc supplementation. Zinc dosing did not seem to impact results significantly [8].

Diet

Patients should no longer be limited to bananas, rice, applesauce, and toast as has been promoted in the past, but instead a healthy diet should be encouraged to promote enterocyte recovery. In RCT trials comparing early refeeding (<12 h) to late refeeding (>12 h) after rehydration initiation, there was no difference between early and late refeeding groups in vomiting, development of persistent diarrhea, need for IV fluids, or hospital length of stay. Both groups had wide variations in duration of diarrhea, and no conclusions were reached regarding refeeding strategy on duration of diarrhea [9]. Lactose-containing foods may be difficult to digest because of the transient lactose intolerance that often follows diarrhea. However, IDSA guidelines recommend that "human milk feeding should be continued in infants and children throughout the diarrheal episode and resumption of an age-appropriate usual diet is recommended during or immediately after the rehydration process is completed" [10].

Probiotics

Probiotics reduce the duration of diarrhea. Based on a recent Cochrane review with 63 studies, the use of probiotics in acute diarrhea reported no adverse events and a reduction in the duration of diarrhea (mean difference 24.76 h; 95% confidence interval 15.9–33.6 h; n = 4555, trials = 35) [11]. Ultimately, encouraging continued attention to electrolyte-based fluid resuscitation followed by gradual transition back to a normal diet as tolerated promotes ongoing enterocyte recovery as an outpatient.

Antimotility

Loperamide (Imodium) is an opioid receptor agonist that acts locally in the bowel to decrease motility of the intestinal wall as well as inhibiting fluid and electrolyte secretion. It is indicated for nonspecific diarrhea, mild traveler's diarrhea, irritable bowel syndrome, chronic diarrhea from bowel resection or inflammatory bowel disease, and chemotherapy-induced diarrhea. Loperamide is contraindicated in children <2 years of age and should be used with caution in children <12 years old.

Loperamide is safe at therapeutic doses but has been associated with adverse cardiac events in high doses. Of the 48 cases reported, most were associated with intentional misuse

for self-treatment of opioid withdrawal or euphoric effects. ECG abnormalities including QT prolongation, QRS interval widening, and ventricular dysrhythmias have been described [12].

Studies show that loperamide reduces diarrhea at both 24 h and 48 h after initiation of treatment and reduced duration of symptoms [10]. Use of concomitant antimotility treatment with antibiotics for traveler's diarrhea has been well established. Studies demonstrate that loperamide in traveler's diarrhea reduces stool volume and duration of symptoms with no increase in adverse events [13].

Based largely on animal and observational reports, antimotility agents were discouraged if suspicion of invasive pathogens, such as *Salmonella*, *Shigella*, and invasive *E. Coli*. However, this edict has been questioned based on multiple studies demonstrating symptomatic improvement with loperamide use in traveler's diarrhea without adverse effects. Specific concerns continue to exist regarding *Clostridium perfringens* because of the risk of toxic megacolon and STEC (*Shigella* toxin *E. Coli*) because of the risk of HUS (hemolytic uremic syndrome). In one analysis of 20 reports of antimotility agents and *Clostridium difficile* infections which included 55 patients, patients who "experienced complications or died were given antimotility agents initially alone without appropriate antibiotics" [14]. Patients who received metronidazole or vancomycin with antimotility agents reported no complications [14]. Based on these observations, the authors concluded that their "systemic review of the literature provided little support for the hypothesis that antimotility agents used to treat C. difficile diarrhea and colitis worsen clinical illness by increasing local toxin effects secondary to intestinal stasis and organism localization" [14]. However, given consensus recommendations and case reports of worsening clinical course with use of antimotility agents and *Clostridium difficile*, use of loperamide in *C. difficile* infections or invasive infections should be avoided.

Table 98.1 Summary of treatment recommendations for diarrhea

Category	Recommendations
Rehydration, electrolytes, nutrients	Pedialyte, Infalyte, WHO-ORT hypotonic solution Zinc supplementation
Diet	Initiation of normal diet early Continue dairy for infants and children Limit dairy for adults because concern for transient lactose intolerance
Probiotics	Yes, can't hurt and may help
Antimotility	Yes, in traveler's diarrhea and secretory diarrhea Maybe, in invasive diarrhea With caution if suspect *C. difficile* or STEC

References

1. Binder HJ, Brown I, Ramakrishna BS, Young GP. Oral rehydration therapy in the second decade of the twenty-first century. Curr Gastroenterol Rep. 2014;16(3):376.
2. Churgay CA, Aftab Z. Gastroenteritis in children: part I. Diagn Am Fam Physician. 2012;85(11):1059–62.
3. Hahn S, Kim S, Garner P. Reduced osmolarity oral rehydration solution for treating dehydration caused by acute diarrhea in children. Cochrane Database Sys Rev. 2002;1:CD002847.
4. Muskiwa A, Vomink J. Oral rehydration salt solution for treating cholera: <270 mOsm/L solutions vs > 310 mOsm/L solutions. Cochrane Database Sys Rev. 2009;2:CD003754.
5. Fonseca BK, Holdgate A, Craig JC. Enteral vs intravenous rehydration therapy for children with gastroenteritis: a meta-analysis of randomized controlled trials. Arch Pediatr Adolesc Med. 2004;158(5):483–90.
6. Hartling L, Bellemare S, Wiebe N, Russell K, Klassen TP, Craig W. Oral versus intravenous rehydration caused by acute diarrhea in children. Cochrane Database Syst Rev. 2006;3:CD004390.
7. Pillow MT, Porter E, Hostetler MA, ACEP. Now focus on: current management of gastroenteritis in children. ACEP News. 2008:9.
8. Lamberti LM, Walker CL, Chan KY, Jian WY, Black RE. Oral zinc supplementation for the treatment of acute diarrhea in children: a systematic review and meta-analysis. Nutrients. 2013;5(11):4715–40.
9. Gregorio G, Dans L, Silvestre M. Early versus delayed refeeding for children with acute diarrhea. Cochrane Database Sys Rev. 2011;7:CD007296.
10. Shane AL, Mody RK, Crump JA, Tarr PI, Steiner TS, Kotloff K, Langley JM, et al. 2017 Infectious Diseases Society of America clinical practice guidelines for the diagnosis and management of infectious diarrhea. Clin Infect Dis. 2017;65(12):e45–80.
11. Allen SJ, Martinez EG, Gregorio GV, Dans LF. Probiotics for treating acute infectious diarrhoea. Cochrane Database Syst Rev. 2010;11:CD003048.
12. Wu PE, Juurlink DN. Clinical Review: loperamide toxicity. Ann Emerg Med. 2017;70(2):245–52.
13. Riddle MS, Connor BA, Beeching NJ, DuPont HL, Hamer DH, Kozarsky P, et al. Guidelines for the prevention and treatment of travelers' diarrhea: a graded expert panel report. J Travel Med. 2017;24(suppl_1):S63–80.
14. Koo HL, Koo DC, Musher DM, DuPont HL. Antimotility agents for the treatment of *Clostridium difficile* diarrhea and colitis. Clin Infect Dis. 2009;48(5):598–605.

Traveler's Diarrhea

99

Alexa R. Gale and Matthew Wilson

Pearls and Pitfalls

- Mild traveler's diarrhea does not interfere with the patient's life and is treated symptomatically without antibiotics.
- Moderate traveler's diarrhea interferes with patient's normal daily activities and is treated with antimotility agents and antibiotics.
- Severe traveler's diarrhea is distressing to the patient, and antibiotics are first-line therapy.
- Persistent traveler's diarrhea may be protozoan or parasitic in origin.

The world is now a smaller place, where international travel is feasible and accessible to a large population. Traveler's diarrhea (TD) is a clinical syndrome of diarrhea, abdominal pain, fever, vomiting, and bloody diarrhea within 2 weeks of travel. The CDC estimates that TD affects 30–70% of travelers [1]. The highest-risk areas for TD are Asia, the Middle East, Africa, Mexico, Central America, and South America. Bacterial pathogens are responsible for 80–90% of TD cases [1]. Epidemiologically, the incidence of traveler's diarrhea is the same across gender and age; however, infants and toddlers may experience a more severe clinical course and require hospitalization [2]. While most cases of traveler's diarrhea are self-limited, the clinical course can be complicated by long-term sequelae, such as Guillain-Barre syndrome, reactive arthritis, irritable bowel syndrome, and chronic diarrhea [1].

A. R. Gale (✉) · M. Wilson
Georgetown University School of Medicine, MedStar Washington Hospital Center, Department of Emergency Medicine, Washington, DC, USA
e-mail: alexa.r.gale@medstar.net; Mdw12@medstar.net

A good history and physical exam is the first step to managing traveler's diarrhea. TD is largely characterized by the functional impact of symptoms on activities of daily living. Red flags, such as abdominal distention or severe abdominal pain, should prompt a broader differential diagnosis. It is important to document the patient's travel history, vaccinations prior to departure, and types of food consumed. For instance, while most traveler's diarrhea is bacterial in origin, patients who travel on cruise ships have a higher incidence of *Norovirus*. The most common bacterial pathogens are ETEC (enterotoxigenic *Escherichia coli*), enteroaggregative *E. Coli*, diffusely adherent *E. Coli*, *Norovirus*, *Rotavirus*, *Salmonella* species, *Campylobacter jejuni*, *Shigella*, *Aeromonas* species, *Bacteroides fragilis*, and *Vibrio* species [2].

After managing dehydration, treatment is determined by severity of disease and duration of symptoms. Categorization of the severity of TD is based on the functional impact of diarrhea rather than amount of diarrhea (Table 99.1). Persistent diarrhea, symptoms greater than 14 days, should trigger additional work-up and treatment.

Mild Traveler's Diarrhea

Definition Diarrhea that is tolerable, is not distressing, and does not interfere with planned activities.

For mild TD, loperamide without antibiotics is recommended. In a study of 310 adults with TD, patients were randomly assigned to receive rifaximin 200 mg 3 times a day for 3 days, loperamide 4 mg initially followed by 2 mg after each unformed stool, or a combination of rifaximin and loperamide. Rifaximin alone and loperamide alone performed similarly with 6.2 and 6.7 unformed stools, respectively. The group receiving a combination of rifaximin and loperamide reported 4.0 unformed stools during the TD episode. In this study, loperamide alone had a longer duration of diarrhea

© Springer Nature Switzerland AG 2019
A. Graham, D. J. Carlberg (eds.), *Gastrointestinal Emergencies*, https://doi.org/10.1007/978-3-319-98343-1_99

347

Table 99.1 Major Categories of Traveler's Diarrhea

Traveler's diarrhea category	Treatment recommendations
Prophylaxis	Antimicrobial prophylaxis for travelers with high risk of complications Rifaximin 200 mg PO TID × 3 days recommended for prophylaxis Fluoroquinolones *NOT* recommended for prophylaxis Bismuth subsalicylate (high level of evidence)
Mild Diarrhea that is tolerable, is not distressing, and does not interfere with planned activities	Antibiotic treatment *NOT* recommended Loperamide 4 mg PO initially then 2 mg after each unformed stool to max 16 mg/day OR Bismuth subsalicylate 2 tabs or 30 mL PO q30 to 60 min up to 8 doses/day for up to 2 days
Moderate Diarrhea that is distressing or interferes with planned activities	Azithromycin 1 gm PO single dose (high level of evidence) Levaquin 500 mg PO single dose Ciprofloxacin 500 mg PO single dose Fluoroquinolones (note: resistance in Asia, adverse dysbiotic sequelae, and musculoskeletal consequences) Loperamide adjunct therapy or monotherapy without antibiotics (high level of evidence)
Severe Diarrhea that is incapacitating or completely prevents planned activities; all dysentery is considered severe.	Antibiotics should be used (high level of evidence) Azithromycin is preferred antibiotic agent (moderate level of evidence) Fluoroquinolones may be used to treat severe, nondysenteric TD Rifaximin may be used to treat severe, nondysenteric TD Single-dose antibiotic regimens may be used (high level of evidence)

Connor [8], Mark et al. [9]

(69 h) compared to either rifaximin alone (33 h) or rifaximin-loperamide combination (27 h). None of the patients receiving loperamide alone required antibiotics. No difference in outcome was found for patients in each treatment group [3].

Moderate Traveler's Diarrhea

Definition Diarrhea that is distressing or interferes with planned activities.

For moderate TD, antibiotics reduce duration of diarrhea to approximately 1.5 days, and with addition of loperamide

to 0.5 days [4]. Single-dose regimens have proven effective and are well tolerated. The Trial Evaluating Ambulatory Therapy of Traveler's Diarrhea (TrEAT TD) study published in 2017 compared US and UK service members with acute watery diarrhea who were randomized to single-dose azithromycin (500 mg), levofloxacin (500 mg), or rifaximin (1650 mg) in combination with loperamide. Clinical cure at 24 h was comparable among the groups: levofloxacin (81%), azithromycin (78%), and rifaximin (75%). Compared with levofloxacin, azithromycin was not inferior ($P = 0.01$). At 48 and 72 h, all regimens reported similar efficacies (91% and 96%, respectively). Treatment failure was low in all groups: azithromycin (3.8%), levofloxacin (4.4%), and rifaximin (1.9%) [5].

In travelers from Southeast Asia, azithromycin is a better treatment option as patients may have been exposed to a fluroquinolone-resistant species of *Camplyobacter* [6]. There is also growing concern of fluoroquinolone-associated peripheral neuropathy, musculoskeletal issues, and cardiotoxic effects which has prompted changing antibiotic recommendations for TD. Antibiotics for TD have also been linked to colonization with ESBL-PE (extended spectrum beta-lactamase-producing *Enterobacteriaceae*) in asymptomatic patients [7].

Severe Traveler's Diarrhea

Definition Diarrhea that is incapacitating or completely prevents planned activities; all dysentery is considered severe.

First-line therapy with azithromycin (1 gm PO single dose or 500 mg daily × 3 days) is superior to levofloxacin (500 mg PO daily × 3 days) in achieving clinical cure, especially in Asia with increased likelihood of fluoroquinolone-resistant *Campylobacter* and limited efficacy against *Shigella*, enteroinvasive *E Coli*, and *Yersinia enterocolitica* [6].

Persistent Traveler's Diarrhea

Persistent traveler's diarrhea (>14 days of diarrhea) is usually attributed to persistent infection, coinfection with a second organism, or post-infectious process. Most bacterial infections last 3–7 days, while viral diarrhea lasts on average 2–3 days. Protozoan parasites have an incubation period of 1–2 weeks and symptoms persist for weeks. The most common protozoan infection is *Giardia*, and suspicion should remain high when upper gastrointestinal symptoms are predominant. Other parasitic pathogens of TD are *Cryptosporidium*, *Cyclospora cayetanensis*, and *Entamoeba histolytica*. Antimicrobial therapy may be useful for treating parasitic infections. Tropical sprue and Brainerd diarrhea may also be considered but are rare and will likely require consultation with infectious disease specialists to make a diagnosis [1].

Suggested Resource
• Binder HJ, Brown I, Ramakrishna BS, Young GP. Oral rehydration therapy in the second decade of the twenty-first century. Curr Gastroenterol Rep. 2014;16:376.

References

1. Connor B. Travelers' health [document on internet]. 2017 June 13 [cited 2018 January 16]. Available from https://wwwnc.cdc.gov/travel/yellowbook/2018/the-pre-travel-consultation/travelers-diarrhea.
2. Steffen R, Hill DR, Dupont HL. Traveler's diarrhea. A clinical review. JAMA. 2015;313(1):71–80.
3. Dupont HL, Jiang ZD, Belkind-Gerson J, Okhuysen PC, Ericsson CD, Ke S, et al. Treatment of traveler's diarrhea: randomized trial comparing rifaximin, rifaximin plus loperamide and loperamide alone. Clin Gastroenterol Hepatol. 2007;5(4):451–6.
4. Dupont HL, Ericsson C, Farthing M, Gorbach S, Pickering LK, Rombo L, et al. Expert review of the evidence base for self-therapy of traveler's diarrhea. J Travel Med. 2009;16(3):161–71.
5. Riddle MS, Connor P, Fraser J, Porter CK, Swierczewski B, Hutley EJ, et al. Trial evaluating ambulatory therapy of travelers' diarrhea (TrEAT TD) study: a randomized controlled trial comparing 3 single-dose antibiotic regimens with loperamide. Clin Infect Dis. 2017;65(12):2008–17.
6. Tribble DR, Sanders JW, Pang LW, Mason C, Pitarangsi C, Bagar S, et al. Traveler's diarrhea in Thailand: randomized, double-blind trial comparing single-dose and 3-day azithromycin- based regimens with a 3-day levofloxacin regimen. Clin Infect Dis. 2007;44(3):338–46.
7. Woerther P, Andremont A, Kantele A. Travel acquired ESBL-producing enterobacteriaceae: impact of colonization at individual and community level. J Travel Med. 2017;24(1):S29–34.
8. Connor B. Travelers' Health. 2017. Retrieved January 16, 2018, from https://wwwnc.cdc.gov/travel/yellowbook/2018/the-pre-travel-consultation/travelers-diarrhea.
9. Riddle MS, Connor BA, Beeching NJ, DuPont HL, Hamer DH, Kozarsky P, Libman M, Steffen R, Taylor D, Tribble DR, Vila J, Zanger P, Charles D. Ericsson; Guidelines for the prevention and treatment of travelers' diarrhea: a graded expert panel report. J Travel Med. 2017;24(suppl_1):S63–80. https://doi-org.proxy.library.georgetown.edu/10.1093/jtm/tax026

Chronic Diarrhea

100

Alexa R. Gale and Matthew Wilson

Pearls and Pitfalls
- Persistent diarrhea is defined as symptoms lasting more than 2 weeks, while chronic diarrhea lasts longer than 30 days.
- *Giardia lamblia* is the most common parasitic cause of chronic diarrhea.
- Patients who have traveled to countries with poor sanitation are susceptible to intestinal amoebiasis.

Persistent or chronic diarrhea can be a challenging diagnosis in the acute care setting. Persistent diarrhea is defined as symptoms lasting more than 2 weeks, while chronic diarrhea lasts longer than 30 days. The evaluation should be initiated in coordination with primary care and gastroenterology follow-up to ensure definitive diagnosis. Management is primarily alleviation of symptoms until definitive diagnosis can be determined.

General Considerations

Chronic diarrhea can be divided into several subgroups including surgical, endocrine, HIV, bacterial, parasitic, chronic conditions and medications. Acute surgical conditions that could present as chronic diarrhea include ischemic bowel, partial bowel obstruction, fecal impaction, and cancer. These presentations would require prompt surgical evaluation. Postoperative sequelae can be seen in patients

A. R. Gale · M. Wilson (✉)
Georgetown University School of Medicine, MedStar Washington Hospital Center, Department of Emergency Medicine, Washington, DC, USA
e-mail: alexa.r.gale@medstar.net; Mdw12@medstar.net

who have malabsorption syndromes from bowel resections or in weight reduction surgeries such as gastric bypass. Secretory diarrhea from endocrine abnormalities prove a challenging diagnosis because most mimic other more common etiologies. For example, Addison's disease can have an initial presentation of vague abdominal pain and diarrhea. These nonspecific symptoms make it challenging for clinicians to address the underlying systemic disease. While a definitive diagnosis of Addison's disease, VIPomas, or hyperthyroidism may not be achieved in the acute care setting, clinicians can arrange for additional testing and outpatient follow-up.

Parasitic Disease

There are numerous parasitic causes of chronic diarrhea, including *Cryptosporidium*, *Giardia*, and *Entamoeba*. A detailed history of the patient's recent travels or preexisting conditions may help to narrow the potential causes. For example, outbreaks of *Cryptosporidium* have been associated with international travel to Nepal and Russia, as well as local sources, such as daycares and waterparks [1, 2].

Cryptosporidium is a protozoal infection that causes up to 60,000 cases of diarrhea per year in the United States [3, 4]. Outbreaks can be attributed to poor sanitation. In 2012, there were almost 2000 cases and 95 hospitalizations reported to the CDC from *Cryptosporidium* contracted at a recreational water facility [2]. The protozoa are extremely resistant to conventional water treatments, such as chlorine [2]. In addition, an outbreak may be hard to pinpoint due to its long incubation period (7–10 days) [2]. Symptoms include watery diarrhea, malabsorptive states, severe dehydration, and electrolyte abnormalities [3–5]. While most cases are self-limited, patients that have sustained diarrhea may be treated with rehydration and nitazoxanide (100–500 mg depending on age, twice daily for 3 days) [6, 7]. Patients susceptible to

A. Graham, D. J. Carlberg (eds.), *Gastrointestinal Emergencies*, https://doi.org/10.1007/978-3-319-98343-1_100

more serious infections and thus requiring closer monitoring include young, pregnant, and HIV-positive patients.

Giardia lamblia is the most common parasitic cause of chronic diarrhea [8]. The cyst form of *Giardia* is resistant to treatment and highly infectious as it is easily transmitted through infected food and water. Inflammation at the gut's epithelial border in response to the parasite causes a malabsorptive diarrhea which results in the giardiasis syndrome – classic triad of bloating, abdominal cramping, and steatorrhea. Symptoms can be so severe that patients have profound weight loss [9, 10]. Treatment includes metronidazole (500 mg TID for 7–10 days). Some patients may require admission to treat the underlying dehydration and electrolyte abnormalities associated with *Giardia* [11].

Chronic Diarrhea Associated with International Travel

Patients who have traveled to countries with poor sanitation are susceptible to intestinal amoebiasis. *Entamoeba histolytica* is transmitted through contaminated water and food. It predominantly affects children in developing countries with 35–50 million cases recorded annually [12]. In Spain, *Entamoeba histolytica* is emerging as a sexually transmitted disease in the men who have sex with men and especially in HIV-positive patients [13]. Diagnosis requires stool samples taken on 3 consecutive days for confirmation [1]. The parasite is cytotoxic and, like *Giardia*, treated with a course of metronidazole.

Autoimmune

While infectious etiologies are more likely in underdeveloped nations, autoimmune conditions (e.g., celiac disease) have increased in developing countries. In the United States, more than 2 million people have been diagnosed with celiac disease [9]. Most patients present with chronic diarrhea and weight loss. Subsequent laboratory investigations show electrolyte derangements and vitamin deficiencies (iron, folic acid, B12, and fat-soluble vitamins) [14]. Gluten, found in wheat, barley, and rye, causes an inflammatory response in the gut leading to malabsorptive diarrhea. The gold standard for diagnosis is transglutaminase or endomysial antibodies found in intestinal biopsy.

Medication Related

Finally, patients experience chronic diarrhea due to the side effects of medications. Laxative abuse presents with diarrhea. In addition to *C. difficile* overgrowth, antibiotic-associated diarrhea is common. Other medications linked to diarrhea include nonsteroidal anti-inflammatory drugs (NSAIDs), protease inhibitors, metformin, and antineoplastic medications.

> **Suggested Resource**
> • Juckett G, Trivedi R. Evaluation of chronic diarrhea. Am Fam Physician. 2011;84:10.

References

1. DuPont AU. Guidelines on acute infectious diarrhea in adults. The Practice Parameters Committee of the American College of Gastroenterology. Am J Gastroenterol. 1997;92(11):1962.
2. Crawford, C. Cryptosporidiosis outbreaks on the rise, CDC Warns [document on the Internet]. Home, American Academy of Family Physicians; 1 July 2015. Available from: www.aafp.org/news/health-of-the-public/20150701cryptooutbreaks.html.
3. Dikman AE, Schonfeld E, Srisarajivakul NC, Poles MA. Human immunodeficiency virus-associated diarrhea: still an issue in the era of antiretroviral therapy. Dig Dis Sci. 2015;60(8):2236–45.
4. Scallan E, Hoekstra RM, Angulo FJ, Tauxe RV, Hoekstra RM. Foodborne illness acquired in the United States—major pathogens. Emerg Infect Dis. 2011;17(1):7–15.
5. Lew EA, Poles MA, Dieterich DT. Diarrheal diseases associated with HIV infection. Gastroenterol Clin N Am. 1997;26(2):259–90.
6. Treatment. Centers for disease control and prevention, centers for disease control and prevention [document on the Internet]. 2015 February 20. Available from: www.cdc.gov/parasites/crypto/treatment.html.
7. Parasites – Cryptosporidium (Also Known as 'Crypto')." Centers for disease control and prevention, centers for disease control and prevention, 20 Feb 2015. Available from: https://www.cdc.gov/parasites/crypto/index.html.
8. Juckett G, Trivedi R. Evaluation of chronic diarrhea. Am Fam Physician. 2011;84(10):1119–26.
9. Bartelt LA, Sartor RB. Advances in understanding Giardia: determinants and mechanisms of chronic sequelae. F1000Prime Rep. 2015;7:62.
10. Buret AG. Mechanisms of epithelial dysfunction in giardiasis. Gut. 2007;56(3):316–7.
11. Guerrant RL, Van Gilder T, Steiner TS, Thielman NM, Slutsker L, Tauxe RV, et al. Practice guidelines for the management of infectious diarrhea. Clin Infect Dis. 2001;32(3):331–50.
12. Ralston KS, Petri WA. Tissue destruction and invasion by Entamoeba histolytica. Trends Parasitol. 2011;27(6):254–63.
13. Escolà-Vergé, L, Arando M, Vall M, Rovira R, Espasa M, Sulleiro E, et al. Eurosurveillance – view article. Eurosurveillance banner, European centre for disease prevention and control2.2017 July 27. Available from: www.eurosurveillance.org/ViewArticle.aspx?ArticleId=22843.
14. Murray JA, Rubio-Tapia A. Diarrhoea due to small bowel diseases. Best Pract Res Clin Gastroenterol. 2012;26(5):581–600.

Clostridium Difficile

101

Alexa R. Gale and Matthew Wilson

Center for Disease Control (CDC) data in 2011 found the incidence of *Clostridium difficile* was approximately 500,000, with 29,000 deaths attributed to *C. difficile* infections (CDI). One third (66%) were healthcare associated [1]. In part, the morbidity and mortality of CDI have been attributed to emerging virulent strains, such as NAP1/027/BI, which are associated with higher recurrence rates and increased mortality [2]. The prevalence of asymptomatic colonization of *C. difficile* in healthy individuals is unclear. However, approximately 21–48% of neonates, infants, and young children are colonized with *C. difficile*. This is believed to fall off in adulthood. Hospitalized patients have been found to have colonization rates of 4–23%, with geographic variation noted [3].

Risk Factors

Initially thought to occur following clindamycin use [4], it is now understood that most antibiotics contribute to its colonization and overgrowth, due to disruption of normal intestinal flora. Approximately 85% of CDI patients report antibiotic use within 1 month of diarrhea [5]. *C. difficile* infections are strongly associated with second-/third-generation cephalosporins, B-lactam/B-lactamase inhibitors, clindamycin, and quinolones [5]. Risk factors for progression to symptomatic illness include proton pump inhibitors [6], advancing age (>65 years), antibiotic use, chemotherapeutic agents, and healthcare exposure.

Immunocompromised patients are at a greater risk of CDI and a severe clinical course. Inflammatory bowel disease, especially ulcerative colitis, is associated with a higher incidence of CDI, as well as increased severity and higher mortality. The likelihood of CDI within 5 years of diagnosis of ulcerative colitis is >3%, and UC patients are 33% more likely to develop a recurrence [7]. Solid organ transplant recipients have an overall prevalence of 7.4% of CDI. Multiple solid organ transplants have the greatest risk of CDI, followed by the lung, liver, intestine, kidney, and pancreas [7]. Patients with chronic kidney disease and end-stage renal disease have a 2–2.5-fold increased risk of CDI with a 1.5-fold increase in severe course compared to general hospitalized patients [7].

In recent years, a changing epidemiology of CDI has been emerging with greater community-acquired CDI. In community-acquired *C. difficile* (CA CDI), healthcare exposure is still a significant risk with 82% of patients with CDI versus 58% of control patients reporting outpatient healthcare setting exposure within 12 weeks of CDI diagnosis, especially emergency department visits (adjusted matched odds ratio 17.37; 95% CI, 1.99–151.22) [8]. In another study of CA CDI, 36% reported no antibiotic exposure in the preceding 3 months. Of those without antibiotic exposure, 31% were taking a proton pump inhibitor prior to CDI diagnosis,

A. R. Gale (✉) · M. Wilson
Georgetown University School of Medicine, MedStar Washington Hospital Center, Department of Emergency Medicine, Washington, DC, USA
e-mail: alexa.r.gale@medstar.net; Mdw12@medstar.net

© Springer Nature Switzerland AG 2019
A. Graham, D. J. Carlberg (eds.), *Gastrointestinal Emergencies*, https://doi.org/10.1007/978-3-319-98343-1_101

likely highlighting the importance of a healthy intestinal bacterial flora in disease prevention [9].

Presentation and Complications

Typically, patients present with large volume, watery, diarrhea 7–10 days after starting antibiotics or exposure to a healthcare setting. Crampy abdominal pain and low-grade fevers are common [10]. Leukocytosis greater than 15,000/mL, renal insufficiency, and elevated lactate levels predict severe CDI, with increased morbidity and mortality [11]. Colonoscopy classically shows pseudomembranous colitis, yellow plaques concentrated in the right colon. Severe cases of *C. difficile* may develop toxic megacolon, which presents as severe abdominal pain and distention. Toxic megacolon has been associated with advanced age >70 years, leukocytosis >15,000/mL, creatinine greater than 1.5 times baseline, or albumin less than 3 g/dL. These patients require surgical consultation because they often do not respond to medical management and bowel perforation is common [11].

Management

As with all causes of diarrhea, it is important to assess the patient's level of dehydration. This can either be done with physical examination (i.e., skin turgor) or with laboratory data (if warranted based on patient's clinical presentation). Intravenous fluid resuscitation may be needed to keep pace with copious diarrhea. Unnecessary antibiotics that may have triggered CDI should be discontinued [12].

However, the cornerstone of *C. difficile* treatment is antibiotic therapy (Table 101.1). Antibiotic recommendations are based on classification of CDI as mild/moderate and severe; however, little guidance is available on what consti-

tutes severe disease. Poor prognostic features have been described and are summarized in Table 101.2 [12].

The first-line choice of antibiotic has evolved with recent research. While initial studies demonstrated no differences between metronidazole or vancomycin treatment, recent randomized controlled trials have shown that oral vancomycin is more efficacious than oral metronidazole. In one study, vancomycin had a 97% clinical cure rate compared to metronidazole with an 84% clinical cure rate [7]. Fidaxomicin was introduced as a treatment for CDI in 2011, and its use has been limited based on cost and unclear efficacy. Recent studies, however, suggest that it may be cost-effective, especially in recurrent cases of CDI and even in primary cases due to its impact on environmental transmission [12]. Two RCTs have compared oral vancomycin treatment to fidaxomicin. Of 1105 patients enrolled, both vancomycin and fidaxomicin had similar rates of resolution of diarrhea, 86% and 88%, respectively. Patients who had been treated with fidaxomicin (71%) had a lower 25-day recurrence rate compared with vancomycin (57%) [7].

Guidelines vary on empiric antibiotic treatment for suspected CDI without microbiological confirmation. ESCMID (European Society for Clinical Microbiology and Infectious Diseases) recommends a 48 h "wait and see" policy after causative antibiotic cessation for mild illness, whereas the ACG (American College of Gastroenterology) recommends immediate treatment initiation and completion of full course of antibiotics if strong suspicion (even if negative microbiologic studies). False-negative microbiologic testing occurs in 14% of tests after 1 day and 45% of tests after 3 days [12].

Most patients will have clinical resolution of symptoms with a 10-day antibiotic course, but in those patients with persistent symptoms, especially if taking metronidazole, an extension of treatment to 14 days may improve response to treatment [7].

Table 101.1 Antibiotic regimens for C difficile

	Mild disease	Severe disease
Initial episode	(1) Vancomycin 125 mg PO q6h for 10 days[a] (2) Fidaxomicin 200 mg PO q12h for 10 days[b] *Alternate regimen:* (3) Metronidazole 500 mg PO/IV q8h for 10 days	(1) Vancomycin 125 mg PO q6h for 10 days Consider adding vancomycin 500 mg PR in 100–500 mL of normal saline via enemas q6h if oral antibiotics cannot reach a segment of the colon (2) Fidaxomicin 200 mg PO q12h. for 10 days *Alternate regimen:* (3) Metronidazole 500 mg PO/IV q8h for 10 days
Severe fulminant *Ie ileus, sepsis, hypotension, shock*	Vancomycin 500 mg PO/NGT q6h PLUS Metronidazole 500 mg IV q8h PLUS Vancomycin 500 mg PR enemas q6h	
Pediatric	Metronidazole 7.5 mg/kg/dose PO q8h for 10 days (max 500 mg QID) Vancomycin 10 mg/kg/dose PO q6h for 10 days (max 125 mg QID)	Vancomycin 10 mg/kg/dose PO/PR q6h for 10 days (max 125 mg QID) +/− Metronidazole 7.5 mg/kg/dose IV q8h for 10 days (max 500 mg QID)
First relapse Recurrence is relapse of symptoms within 8 weeks of initial treatment	Vancomycin 125 mg PO q6h for 10 days if metronidazole used previously Fidaxomicin 200 mg PO q12h for 10 days if vancomycin used previously IDSA/SHEA/WSES recommend same as initial episode	
Second relapse	Fidaxomicin 200 mg PO q12h for 10 days Pulsed dose of vancomycin (1) 125 mg PO q6h for 7–14 days (2) 125 mg PO q12h for 7 days (3) 125 mg PO q24h for 7 days (4) 125 mg PO q every other day for 7 days (5) 125 mg PO q every 3 days for 14 day 3 Recurrences or severe disease – consider intestinal microbiota transplant	

Adapted from: Feher and Mensa [12], Clifford McDonald et al. [13]

[a]Multiple sources recommend vancomycin as first-line medication especially in patients with high risk of recurrence

[b]Since release in 2011, expensive

IDSA Infectious Disease Society of America, *SHEA* Society for Healthcare Epidemiology of America, *ACG* American College of Gastroenterology, *ESCMID* European Society of Clinical Microbiology and Infectious Diseases, *ASID* Australasian Society for Infectious Diseases

Table 101.2 High risk for complicated clinical course of C. difficile

Severe Clostridium difficile infection			
Signs and symptoms	Laboratory red flags	Complications	Mitigating factors
Fever >38.5 Celsius Rigors Abdominal tenderness Mental status changes Respiratory failure Hemodynamic instability	WBC > 15,000/mL Creatinine >1.5 times baseline value (renal failure) Albumin <30 g/L Lactate >2.2 mmol/L	Ileus Colonic wall thickening Pericolonic fat stranding Peritonitis Bowel perforation Pseudomembranous colitis Toxic megacolon	ICU admission Need for surgery Advanced age Serious comorbidities Immunocompromised Chronic renal disease Malignancy Diabetes mellitus Inflammatory bowel disease (IBD) Liver cirrhosis Cardiopulmonary conditions

Adapted from: Feher and Mensa [12]

Suggested Resources

- Bartlett J. Clostridium difficile infection. Infect Dis Clin N Am. 2017;31:489–95.
- Clifford McDonald L, Gerding DN, Johnson S, Bakken JS, Carroll KC, Coffin SE, Dubberke ER, Garey KW, Gould CV, Kelly C, Loo V, Sammons JS, Sandora TJ, Wilcox MH. Clinical practice guidelines for Clostridium difficile infection in adults and children: 2017 update by the Infectious Diseases Society of America (IDSA) and Society for Healthcare Epidemiology of America (SHEA). Clin Infect Dis. 2018 https://doi.org/10.1093/cid/cix1085

References

1. Lessa FC, Bamberg WM, Beldavs ZF, et al. Burden of clostridium difficile infection in the United States. NEJM. 2015;372:825–34.
2. Warny M, Pepin J, Fang A, Killgore G, Thompson A, Brazier J, et al. Toxin production by an emerging strain of Clostridium difficile associated with outbreaks of severe disease in North America and Europe. Lancet. 2005;366:1079–84.
3. Hung Y, Lee J, Lin H, Liu H, Wu Y, Tsai P, et al. Clinical impact of Clostridium difficile colonization. J Microbiol Immunol Infect. 2015;48:241–8.
4. Bartlett JG. Narrative review: the new epidemic of clostridium difficile–associated enteric disease. Ann Intern Med. 2006;145:758–64.
5. Shane AL, Mody RK, Crump JA, Tarr PI, Steiner TS, Kotloff K, et al. 2017 Infectious Diseases Society of America clinical practice guidelines for the diagnosis and management of infectious diarrhea. Clin Infect Dis. 2017;65(12):1963–73.
6. Trifan A, Stanciu C, Girleanu I, Stoica OC, Singeap AM, Maxim R, et al. Proton pump inhibitors therapy and risk of Clostridium difficile infection: systematic review and meta-analysis. World J Gastroenterol. 2017;23(35):6500–15.
7. McDonald LC, Gerding DN, Johnson S, Bakken JS, Carroll KC, Coffin SE, et al. Clinical practice guidelines for Clostridium difficile infection in adults and children: 2017 update by the Infectious Diseases Society of America (IDSA) and Society for Healthcare Epidemiology of America (SHEA). Clin Infect Dis. 2018;66(7):987–94.
8. Guh A, Adkins SH, Li Q, Bulens SN, Farley MM, Smith Z, et al. Risk factors of community-associated Clostridium difficile infection in adults: a case control study. Open Forum Infect Dis. 2017;4(4):1–8. https://doi.org/10.1093/ofid/ofx171.
9. Chitnis A, Holzbauer S, Belflower R, Winston LG, Bamberg WM, Lyons C, et al. Epidemiology of community associated Clostridium difficile infection, 2009–2011. JAMA Intern Med. 2013;173(14):1359–67.
10. Hensgens MP, Goorhuis A, Dekkers OM, Kuijper EJ. Time interval of increased risk for Clostridium difficile infection after exposure to antibiotics. J Antimicrob Chemother. 2012;67(3):742–8.
11. Bartlett J. Clostridium difficile infection. Infect Dis Clin N Am. 2017;31:489–95.
12. Feher C, Mensa J. A comparison of current guidelines of five international societies on Clostridium difficile infection management. Infect Dis Ther. 2016;5(3):207–30.
13. Clifford McDonald L, Gerding DN, Johnson S, Bakken JS, Carroll KC, Coffin SE, Dubberke ER, Garey KW, Gould CV, Kelly C, Loo V, Sammons JS, Sandora TJ, Wilcox MH. Clinical practice guidelines for *Clostridium difficile* infection in adults and children: 2017 update by the Infectious Diseases Society of America (IDSA) and Society for Healthcare Epidemiology of America (SHEA). Clin Infect Dis. 2018 https://doi.org/10.1093/cid/cix1085

Diarrhea and AIDS

Alexa R. Gale and Matthew Wilson

Pearls and Pitfalls
- Protease inhibitors decrease the risk of infectious diarrhea.
- Cryptosporidiosis is a difficult condition to manage in HIV/AIDS patients.
- Patients, who do not have an infectious etiology, can also be treated with anti-motility and anti-secretory agents for symptom management.

HIV and AIDS affect over 30 million people worldwide, and diarrhea affects 28–60% of HIV-positive patients [1, 2]. Patients who have low CD4 counts (less than 350) are highly susceptible to a range of opportunistic infections. Approximately half of HIV/AIDS patients presenting with diarrhea have an infectious etiology. Noninfectious causes include medication side effects from antiretroviral (ART) therapy, enteropathy from depletion of CD4 T-cell lymphocytes in the gastrointestinal lymphoid tissue, malabsorption from their chronic illness, and malignancies due to the progression of HIV to AIDs [2–7]. Due to the destruction of the CD4 T lymphocytes, patients are more susceptible to severe dehydration and malabsorption.

Infectious Considerations for HIV Patients with Diarrhea

Common bacterial etiologies of diarrhea in HIV-positive patients include *Campylobacter*, *Shigella*, *Salmonella*, *Escherichia coli*, and *Clostridium difficile*. While often the cause of diarrhea in non-HIV-positive patients, the clinical course can be prolonged and more severe for HIV patients. A brief synopsis of common infectious causes of diarrhea in the HIV population and their treatment is found in Table 102.1.

Cryptosporidiosis is a difficult condition to manage in HIV/AIDS patients. Nitazoxanide has demonstrated no benefit compared to placebo [14]. Though a higher dose and longer treatment course may produce benefit, the drug has not been approved by the FDA in high doses [14]. A Cochrane review supports its use as an option alone or in combination with other antimicrobials as well as emphasizes the importance of immune reconstitution with HAART for curative therapy [15].

Treatment for Noninfectious Causes of Diarrhea

Patients, who do not have an infectious etiology, can also be treated with anti-motility (e.g., loperamide, diphenoxylate, opiates) and anti-secretory agents. However, it is important to counsel patients who are suffering from diarrhea from protease inhibitors that they should continue their medication. Protease inhibitors decrease the risk of infectious diarrhea from 53% to 13% [9, 10]. Patients with chronic diarrhea from HAART should be managed in close consultation with their infectious disease doctor to help mitigate side effects.

A. R. Gale (✉) · M. Wilson
Georgetown University School of Medicine, MedStar Washington Hospital Center, Department of Emergency Medicine, Washington, DC, USA
e-mail: alexa.r.gale@medstar.net; Mdw12@medstar.net

Table 102.1 Common Causes of Diarrhea in HIV/AIDs Patients

Common causes	
Lymphogranuloma venereum	Can lead to severe proctocolitis with ensuing perirectal abscesses, strictures, and fistulas Treatment: doxycycline 100 mg PO BID × 21 days
Clostridium difficile	Most common cause of diarrhea in advanced AIDS [8] Risks: antibiotic use and prophylactic treatment of PCP pneumonia [9] Treatment: vancomycin PO
Cytomegalovirus	Most common viral GI infection in AIDS patients [10, 11] Symptoms: rectal bleeding, abdominal pain, fever, and weight loss [10, 12] Treatment: ganciclovir, foscarnet, and valganciclovir [13]
Cryptosporidium	Protozoa infection that causes 60,000 cases per year in the USA [10] Risks: poor sanitation Symptoms: watery diarrhea, malabsorption, severe dehydration, electrolyte abnormalities [10, 12] Treatment: supportive measures and treatment with nitazoxanide or rifampin [13]
Microsporidium	Protozoa that affects small intestine [10] Symptoms: causes a malabsorptive state in immunocompetent patients [10] Treatment: albendazole associated with treatment failure; other potential therapies include metronidazole, azithromycin, and doxycycline
Entamoeba histolytica	Symptoms: colitis, ulceration, hematochezia, and toxic megacolon [10] Treatment: metronidazole
Mycobacterium avium complex (MAC)	Found throughout our environment Transmission via inhalation or ingestion Symptoms: fever and weight loss [10] Treatment: combination of clarithromycin and azithromycin [13]. Additional treatments include amikacin and streptomycin in severely immunocompromised patients (CD4 <50)

Suggested Resource
- Logan C, Beadsworth M, Beeching N. HIV and diarrhea: what is new? Curr Opin Infect Dis. 2016;29(5):486–94.

References

1. Logan C, Beadsworth M, Beeching N. HIV and diarrhea: what is new? Curr Opin Infect Dis. 2016;29(5):486–94.
2. Nwachukwu CE, Okebe JU. Antimotility agents for chronic diarrhoea in people with HIV/AIDS. Cochrane Database Syst Rev. 2008;4:CD005644.
3. O'Brien ME, Clark RA, Besch CL, Myers L, Kissinger P. Patterns and correlates of discontinuation of the initial HAART regimen in an urban outpatient cohort. J Acquir Immune Defic Syndr. 2003;34(4):407–14.
4. Carcamo C, Hooton T, Wener MH, Weiss NS, Gilman R, Arevalo J, et al. Etiologies and manifestations of persistent diarrhoea in adults with HIV-1 infection: a case-control study in Lima. Peru J Infect Dis. 2005;191(1):11–9.
5. Silverberg MJ, Gore ME, French AL, Gandhi M, Glebsy MJ, Kovacs A, et al. Prevalence of clinical symptoms associated with highly active antiretroviral therapy in the women's interagency HIV Study. Clin Infect Dis. 2004;5(1):19–24.
6. Moyle GJ, Youle M, Higgs C, Monaghan J, Prince W, Chapman S, et al. Safety, pharmacokinetics and antiretroviral activity of the poten, specific human immunodeficiency virus protease inhibitor nelfinavir: results of a phase I/II trial and an extended follow-up in patients infected with human immunodeficiency virus. J Clin Pharmacol. 1998;38:736–43.
7. Carr A, Cooper DA. Adverse effects of antiretroviral therapy. Lancet. 2000;356:1423–30.
8. DuPont AU, Guidelines on acute infectious diarrhea in adults. The Practice Parameters Committee of the American College of Gastroenterology. Am J Gastroenterol. 1997;92(11):1962.
9. Call SA, Heudebert G, Saag M, Wilcox CM. The changing etiology of chronic diarrhea in HIV infected patients with CD4 cell counts less than 200 cells/mm3. Amer J Gastroenterol. 2000;95(11):3142–6.
10. Dikman AE, Schonfeld E, Srisarajivakul NC, Poles MA. Human immunodeficiency virus-associated diarrhea: still an issue in the era of antiretroviral therapy. Dig Dis Sci. 2015;60(8):2236–45.
11. Cello JP, Day LW. Idiopathic AID enteropathy and treatment of gastrointestinal opportunistic pathogens. Gastroenterology. 2009;136:1952–65.
12. Lew EA, Poles MA, Dieterich DT. Diarrheal diseases associated with HIV infection. Gastroenterol Clin N Am. 1997;26:259–90.
13. Thoden J, Potthoff A, Bogner JR, et al. Therapy and prophylaxis of opportunistic infections in HIV-infected patients: a guideline by the German and Austrian AIDS societies (DAIG/ÖAG) (AWMF 055/066). Infection. 2013;41(Suppl 2):91–115.
14. Fox LM, Saravolatz LD. Nitazoxanide: a new thiazolide antiparasitic agent. Clin Infect Dis. 2005;40(8):1173–80.
15. Abubakar I, Aliyu SH, Arumugam C, Hunter PR, Usman NK. Prevention and treatment of cryptosporidiosis in immunocompromised patients. Cochrane Database Syst Rev. 2007;1:CD004932.

Ahnika Kline and Krishna Dass

Pearls and Pitfalls

Pearls:

- Fluoroquinolones will treat most infectious causes of diarrhea.
- Remember to think about and include *Listeria* treatment in pregnant women with diarrhea and fever.
- New rapid diagnostics can help identify the cause of diarrhea and will likely increase the number of organisms identified.

Pitfalls:

- There is no evidence of benefit and a possible risk of precipitating hemolytic uremic syndrome with antibiotic therapy for enterohemorrhagic *E. Coli*.
- In toxigenic diarrheas (*Clostridium difficile* and Shiga toxin), antimotility agents can prolong the diarrhea.

Do not forget to consider reporting diarrheal illness to your state or county health department. Do not assume the laboratory will report.

Introduction

Ahnika Kline, MD, PhD is an Infectious Disease Fellow at the National Institutes of Health. Many of the patients she sees at the NIH are severely immunocompromised and prone to unusual infections and atypical presentations of diarrhea.

Krishna Dass, MD is a Board-certified Infectious Disease specialist serving as private consultant at MedStar Washington Hospital Center, a large, urban tertiary referral hospital in Washington, DC; MedStar National Rehabilitation Hospital, a subacute rehabilitation hospital; and Bridgepoint Hospital – a subacute nursing facility. He is the chairman for infection control at Bridgepoint Hospital, won numerous awards for teaching medical students and residents, has been voted the top doctor in *Washingtonian* magazine, and has authored many research papers.

Answers to Key Clinical Questions

1. When do you recommend a consultation with an infectious disease specialist in the acute care setting and in what time frame?

Generally, infectious disease consults are not indicated for patients presenting with acute diarrhea in the emergency department. Though there are often cases where infectious diseases can and should be consulted for assistance (such as immunocompromised individuals or pregnant women with possible listeriosis), the consult can often wait until after the patient has been admitted. The exception, of course, comes from diarrhea in certain returning travelers.

At your individual facility, you may need to contact ID faculty for antibiotic approvals and/or for clarification of isolation precautions. Your ID consultant can also assist you with reportable diseases. Many diarrheal diseases require mandatory reporting to local departments of health and sometimes to the CDC. The assumption that the laboratory will report the disease and that you as a treating physician are not also required to report is a false one. Suspected cholera is just one example of a reportable diarrheal disease that requires immediate reporting in many jurisdictions.

A. Kline
National Institute of Health, Bethesda, MD, USA
e-mail: ahnika.kline@nih.gov

K. Dass (✉)
MedStar Washington Hospital Center, Department of Infectious Disease, Washington, DC, USA
e-mail: Krishna.Dass@medstar.net

© Springer Nature Switzerland AG 2019
A. Graham, D. J. Carlberg (eds.), *Gastrointestinal Emergencies*, https://doi.org/10.1007/978-3-319-98343-1_103

2. What high-risk diarrheal infections should you consider in returning travelers?

Diarrhea and vomiting can be the presenting symptoms in patients with malaria, especially in children. Identifying the likely species of malaria, the parasite burden, and classifying the illness as severe or not is critical early in management. Infectious disease physicians can be useful in this setting to help coordinate with the hematology lab to evaluate the parasite burden and species as well as assist with pharmacy coordination with the CDC if artesunate is needed for severe malaria. Importantly, do not delay the administration of quinidine therapy (10 mg/kg loading dose over 1–2 h followed by 0.02 mg/kg/min continuous infusion) with either doxycycline (100 mg IV or PO q12h) or clindamycin (10 mg/kg IV loading dose followed by 5 mg/kg q8h) while waiting for artesunate to arrive.

Ebola virus often presents 9–11 days after exposure, first with a nonspecific prodrome of fevers, chills, malaise, and myalgias, followed usually by watery diarrhea and vomiting. Discussion with infectious disease as well as your hospital's infectious control officer should be initiated immediately if there is concern that a patient has Ebola virus disease. The CDC no longer recommends routine screening of all patients for Ebola virus disease in all healthcare settings but does recommend that all returning travelers with fever be questioned about the countries they recently visited at triage. Ebola virus should be thought about in any patient returning from West Africa, specifically Guinea, Liberia, or Sierra Leone.

3. What pearls can you offer emergency care providers when evaluating immunocompromised patients with diarrhea?

Immunocompromised patients often have unusual causes of diarrhea. Depending on the nature and severity of immune compromise, potential etiologies include parasites, persistent viruses, or medication side effects. In patients who have received organ transplants, mycophenolate is a common cause of diarrhea. In this patient population, the clinician is often tasked with determining whether this is CMV-mediated diarrhea or a side effect of the medication. These patients will often require admission for an EGD to identify the cause of their HIV.

4. What pearls can you offer emergency care providers when evaluating HIV patients with diarrhea?

In HIV, especially in patients who have CD4 counts less than 200 cells/ml (AIDS), there are a number of unusual causes of diarrhea including *Microspora*, *Isospora*, and *Cryptosporidium*. Patients who perform receptive anal intercourse may have diarrhea secondary to proctitis from

Shigella, and receptive oral sex can put partners at increased risk of *Giardia* infection.

5. What concepts do you think are key to diagnosis and management of patients with diarrhea?

The critical component to the diarrhea workup is a detailed exposure history including travel, exposure to unusual foods or unsanitary water, as well as medications the patient is taking. For instance, a posttransplant patient who drinks well water will generate a different differential than a healthy person who has recently returned from travel abroad or a healthy person who has developed an acute toxigenic diarrheal illness from a not risky source.

6. What complications are you concerned about in immunocompromised patients with diarrhea?

There are some causes of immune compromise that can make the evaluation of diarrhea more difficult. For example, a patient who is neutropenic should not have a rectal exam due to the concern about translocation of bacterial organisms. Additionally, some immunodeficiencies can cause chronic diarrhea. Examples of this include *Cryptosporidium* in HIV patients, for whom it appears no amount of nitazoxanide can treat the infection until immune reconstitution has been achieved. Certain rare immunodeficiencies (e.g., GATA2 deficiency and chronic granulomatous disease) predispose patients to chronic norovirus infection. In general, an immunocompromised patient with diarrhea and any other systemic inflammatory symptoms (leukocytosis, tachycardia, or fever) may require admission for further workup.

7. What are future advances in the diagnostic workup for diarrhea?

The diagnosis of diarrhea is changing. Rapid diagnostic tools are becoming more commonplace, albeit they can be costly. There are three commercial, FDA-cleared, multiplex assays for the detection of gastrointestinal pathogens. The Luminex x-tag GPP was first approved by the FDA in 2013 and identifies six bacteria, two bacterial toxins, three viruses, and three parasites in stool samples. It was followed by the FilmArray by BioFire Diagnostics which identifies 11 bacteria, 2 bacterial toxins, 5 viruses, and 4 parasites. Also in 2014, the Verigene Nanosphere received FDA approval and identifies five bacteria, two bacterial toxins, and two viruses. These rapid diagnostics have some clear advantages: results return in a matter of hours allowing for targeted treatment, and they have a high sensitivity. One disadvantage of these rapid diagnostics comes from identification of a number of organisms that have not been routinely tested for in the past, such as *Sapovirus*, enteropathogenic *E. coli*, and enteroaggregative

E. coli. Because we did not previously routinely identify these organisms in standard laboratories, the standard of care has not been established

If a clinician suspects *Yersinia*, *Campylobacter*, or *Vibrio*, they should discuss with the microbiology lab, as these organisms are not identified in standard stool culture and are reportable illnesses. That can signify outbreaks of foodborne or waterborne disease.

Suggested Resource

- Danila RN, Laine ES, Livinston F, Como-Sabetti K, Lamers L, Johnson K, Barry AM. Legal authority for infectious disease reporting in the United States: case study of the 2009 H1N1 influenza pandemic. Am J Public Health. 2015;105(1):13–8.

Part XIV

Abdominal Pain and the Pregnant Patient

What Are the Chances of Developing a Non-obstetric Abdominal Emergency During Pregnancy? What Risks Do Abdominal Emergencies Pose to the Developing Pregnancy?

Elizabeth Pontius

Pearls and Pitfalls

- Up to 1 in 500 pregnant women develop an acute abdomen, and up to 1% of women need an operation during pregnancy for a non-obstetric abdominal emergency.
- Normal anatomic and physiologic changes during pregnancy can alter typical presentations of non-obstetric abdominal emergencies.
- Appendicitis is the most common non-obstetric surgical abdominal emergency during pregnancy.
- Non-obstetric abdominal emergencies during pregnancy may result in increased maternal and fetal morbidity and mortality, especially if treatment is delayed.

What Are the Chances of Developing a Non-obstetric Abdominal Emergency During Pregnancy?

The differential diagnosis of abdominal pain in pregnancy is large, encompassing both obstetric and non-obstetric causes. Up to 1 in 500 pregnant women will develop an acute abdomen, and 0.2–1% of women will need an operation during pregnancy for a non-obstetric abdominal emergency [1–3].

Several factors may hamper the clinician's ability to diagnose various abdominal emergencies. Physiologic and anatomic changes in pregnancy can change clinical presentations of various diseases, and clinicians often hesitate to perform radiographic tests because of risks from ionizing radiation.

E. Pontius
Georgetown University School of Medicine, Washington, DC, USA

Department of Emergency Medicine, MedStar Georgetown University Hospital and MedStar Washington Hospital Center, Washington, DC, USA

Delays in diagnosis, however, may harm both mothers and fetuses [1].

Non-obstetric abdominal emergencies in pregnancy may originate from the gastrointestinal, genitourinary, and gynecologic systems [2, 3].

Anatomic and physiologic changes in pregnancy should be considered when evaluating pregnant women with abdominal pain. As the gravid uterus grows, it displaces abdominal organs, such as the appendix, from their typical locations, leading to atypically localized pain. Peritoneal signs can be masked or delayed as the abdominal wall musculature is stretched [1, 3]. Using an elevated white blood cell count as a marker of pathology is unreliable, due to the physiologic leukocytosis of pregnancy [2, 3].

Gastrointestinal Causes

Gastrointestinal causes of acute abdominal pain range from heartburn and constipation to diverticulitis and worsening inflammatory bowel disease to surgical emergencies such as appendicitis and cholecystitis [1, 2, 4]. Decreased gastric motility and compression of hollow viscous structures by the uterus cause heartburn and constipation to occur more commonly during pregnancy. Gastroesophageal reflux disease affects 30–85% of pregnant women, and constipation affects up to 40% of pregnant women [2–4].

Appendicitis is the most common non-obstetric surgical emergency in pregnancy and affects between 1 in 500 and 1 in 3000 pregnancies. It is responsible for one-quarter of the non-obstetric surgeries performed during pregnancy [1–4]. Appendicitis is most common in the second trimester, with 40% of cases occurring during this time [1, 2, 4, 5]. The incidence of appendicitis in pregnancy is identical to the incidence in nonpregnant women. A ruptured appendix, however, is two to four times more common in pregnant women [2, 4, 5]. A perforated appendix increases fetal mortality from 0–1.5% to 20–35% [1, 2, 5]. Delaying operative intervention leads to maternal complications such as septic shock, peritonitis, and venous thromboembolism [2].

Cholecystitis affects approximately 1 in 1600 to 1 in 10,000 pregnancies. It is the second most common non-obstetric surgical emergency in pregnancy [1–3, 5]. Bile stasis occurs because of increased estrogen and progesterone levels during pregnancy. The incidence of cholelithiasis and cholecystitis is higher in pregnant women [1, 2, 5]. Cholecystitis may be managed conservatively with hydration and antibiotics; however, this increases the rate of spontaneous abortion from 0 to 2% with surgical management to 0–12% with conservative management [2, 3].

Intestinal obstruction occurs in 1 in 1500 to 1 in 16,000 pregnancies [1–3]. Obstruction may be caused by adhesions, intussusception, hernia, carcinoma, or sigmoid volvulus. It may also be caused by the rapidly growing uterus [1, 2]. Average maternal mortality is 6%, but it can be as high as 20% in the third trimester. Fetal mortality is 26% [1]. Some cases may be managed conservatively, while other cases many require operative intervention, especially if perforation, bowel necrosis, or peritonitis is present [2]. Obstruction is the third most common cause of non-obstetric surgical emergency during pregnancy [3].

Pancreatitis occurs in 1 in 1000 to 1 in 3300 pregnancies, with more than 50% of cases occurring in the third trimester [2, 3]. Pancreatitis is caused by gallstones in two-thirds of pregnant patients [2]. Supportive care, including intravenous hydration, bowel rest, and analgesia, is the mainstay of management [1, 2]. Gallstone pancreatitis recurs in 70% of pregnant patients, as opposed to 20–30% of nonpregnant patients, so surgical consultation should be considered [2]. Gallstone pancreatitis can lead to fetal death in 10–20% of cases [5].

Urinary Tract Causes

In the urinary tract, patients may suffer from urinary tract infection (UTI) and urolithiasis. UTI in pregnancy ranges from asymptomatic bacteriuria to cystitis to pyelonephritis. Asymptomatic bacteriuria can progress to pyelonephritis in 20–30% of pregnant women and should be treated when detected [2]. Pyelonephritis occurs in 0.5–2% of pregnancies, with 80–90% of cases occurring in the second or third trimester [2].

The incidence of urolithiasis in pregnancy is equal to that in the general population. One in 200 to 1 in 2500 pregnancies are affected by urolithiasis, with 80–90% occurring in the second and third trimester [2]. Diagnosis can be difficult, as hydronephrosis is a common finding in normal pregnancy [2]. One potential algorithm for diagnosing urolithiasis is performing an initial renal ultrasound evaluating for unilateral hydronephrosis, followed by MRI or ultra-low-dose CT if the diagnosis is still unclear. Fifty to 80% of women will pass stones with conservative management. Surgery is required if there is intractable pain or persistent obstruction [2].

Gynecologic Causes

Adnexal torsion is the most common non-uterine gynecologic emergency during pregnancy and occurs in up to 1 in 1800 pregnancies, most commonly in the first and second trimester. Assisted reproductive technologies often increase ovarian size. The incidence of torsion increases to 6–16% in these patients [1, 2]. Early operative intervention is crucial for preservation of both the pregnancy and future fertility [2].

Pelvic inflammatory disease (PID) is an inflammation and polymicrobial infection of the upper female genital tract. Acute PID in pregnancy is rare, and it happens most frequently during the first trimester. PID may lead to maternal morbidity, preterm delivery, and fetal demise [2].

Other causes of acute gynecologic abdominal pain during pregnancy include ovarian cysts and fibroids [2].

What Risks Do Abdominal Emergencies Pose to the Developing Pregnancy?

More than 8000 emergent surgical procedures are performed on pregnant patients annually in the United States [6]. A 2009 review article by Cohen-Kerem et al. showed the overall rate of miscarriage following surgery was 5.8%, but the postoperative miscarriage rate during the first trimester was 10.6% [6]. A large observational study of 47,000 patients who underwent non-obstetric surgery during pregnancy showed that surgery led to higher rates of stillbirth and preterm delivery [7]. However, another recent study showed no significant difference in pregnancy outcomes in patients undergoing non-obstetric invasive procedures other than an increased rate of Caesarian delivery [8].

Suggested Resources
- Emergency medicine cases: medical and surgical emergencies in Pregnancy (August 2010: https://emergencymedicinecases.com/episode-7-medical-and-surgical-emergencies-in-pregnancy/).
- Emergency medicine clinics of North America: nonobstetric abdominal pain and surgical emergencies in pregnancy. Emerg Med Clin N Am. 2012;30:885–901.

References

1. Diegelmann L. Nonobstetric abdominal pain and surgical emergencies in pregnancy. Emerg Med Clin N Am. 2012;30:885–901.
2. Shasteen M, Pontius E. Non-obstetric abdominal pain in pregnancy. In: Borhart J, editor. Emergency department management of obstetric complications. Switzerland: Springer International Publishing AG; 2017.
3. Bouyou J, Gaujoux S, Marcellin L, Leconte M, Goffinet F, Chapron C, Dousset B. Abdominal emergencies during pregnancy. J Visc Surg. 2015;152:S105–15.
4. Longo SA, Moore RC, Canzoneri BJ, Robichaux A. Gastrointestinal conditions during pregnancy. Clin Colon Rectal Surg. 2010;23(2):80–9.
5. Barber-Millet S, Lledo JB, Castro PG, Gavara IG, Pla NB, Dominguez RG. Update on the management of non-obstetric acute abdomen in pregnant patients. Cir Esp. 2016;94(5):257–65.
6. Cohen-Kerem R, Railton C, Oren D, Lishner M, Koren G. Pregnancy outcome following non-obstetric surgical intervention. Am J Surg. 2005;190:467–73.
7. Aylin P, Bennett P, Bottle A, Brett S, Sodhi V, Rivers A, Balinskaite V. Estimating the risk of adverse birth outcomes in pregnant women undergoing non-obstetric surgery using routinely collected NHS data: an observational study. Health Serv Deliv Res. 2016;29(4):1–76.
8. Schwarzman P, Baumfeld Y, Bar-Niv Z, Baron J, Mastrolia SA, Sheiner E, Mazor M, Hershkovitz R, Weintraub AY. The effect of non-obstetric invasive procedures during pregnancy on perinatal outcomes. Arch Gynecol Obstet. 2015;292:603–8.

What Are the Risks of Ionizing Radiation to a Developing Fetus?

Diana Ladkany and Kerri Layman

Pearls and Pitfalls
- Ionizing radiation exposure is dependent on the type of study and the anatomic location being studied.
- Fetal exposure to ionizing radiation should be limited as much as possible, following the "as low as reasonably achievable" principle.
- The most vulnerable period for the fetus is 8–15 weeks gestation.
- Fetal loss or teratogenesis has not been shown after radiation exposure of <50 mSv.
- Ultrasound and MRI are the imaging modalities of choice for pregnant patients and should be used if the clinical scenario allows.

Ionizing radiation is commonly used in medical imaging, most frequently in the form of plain radiographs (X-ray) and computed tomography (CT). Studies that utilize ionizing radiation during pregnancy expose both the mother and the fetus. The degree of radiation exposure is dependent on the type of study and several other factors including the proximity of the uterus to the anatomic location of the scan plane, patient size, study technique, and use of protective mechanisms such as lead to shield the abdomen and pelvis.

Ionizing radiation has various clinical effects on the fetus depending on gestational age. In very early pregnancy (less than 4 weeks), the embryo is partially protected from the effects of ionizing radiation due to the totipotent nature of the cells [1]. At this early stage, radiation exposure tends to result in death of the embryo or have no consequence. Between 4 and 8 weeks gestation, there is risk to the developing fetal genitals, organs, and the skeleton. The most vulnerable period for the fetus is between 8 and 15 weeks gestation [2]. During this period of organogenesis, higher doses of radiation may cause more significant complications, including fetal demise and microcephaly [3].

The amount of radiation also determines the clinical effect on the fetus. Above 100 mSv there is risk of teratogenesis and pregnancy loss; however, medical diagnostic studies deliver radiation doses far below this threshold. Neither fetal anomalies nor fetal loss has not been reported below 50 mSv [4]. X-ray is the most common form of ionizing radiation used in pregnancy. Most X-ray studies are very low-dose examinations (<0.1 mSv) and pose essentially no risk to the fetus. The highest exposure to radiation comes from CT, particularly chest, abdomen, and pelvis scans (Table 105.1). Still, the radiation dose for most of these studies is well below 50 mSv.

The risk of future malignancy as a result of in utero exposure to ionizing radiation is unknown but thought to be very small. When performing diagnostic imaging studies that utilize ionizing radiation, doses should be kept as low as reasonably achievable (ALARA principle).

Ultrasonography and magnetic resonance imaging are the imaging modalities of choice for pregnant patients, as these studies are not associated with ionizing radiation risk. However, The American College of Obstetricians and Gynecologists emphasizes that a necessary diagnostic test should not be withheld from a pregnant patient, even if the test utilizes ionizing radiation [5].

D. Ladkany (✉) · K. Layman
Department of Emergency Medicine, MedStar Washington Hospital Center & MedStar Georgetown University Hospital, Washington, DC, USA

© Springer Nature Switzerland AG 2019
A. Graham, D. J. Carlberg (eds.), *Gastrointestinal Emergencies*, https://doi.org/10.1007/978-3-319-98343-1_105

Table 105.1 Fetal radiation doses associated with common radiologic examinations

Type of examination	Fetal absorbed dose (mSv)[a]
Very low dose (<0.1 mSv)	
Cervical spine X-ray (AP and lateral)	< 0.001
Any extremity X-ray	< 0.001
Chest X-ray (two views)	0.0005–0.01
Low to moderate dose (0–10 mSv)	
Radiographs	
Thoracic spine X-ray	0.003
Abdominal X-ray	0.1–3
Lumbar spine X-ray	1–10
CT	
Head, neck, or extremity CT[b]	0–10
Chest CT or CT pulmonary angiography	0.01–0.66
Higher dose (10–50 mSv)	
Abdominal CT	1.3–35
Pelvic CT	10–50
Abdomen and pelvis CT	13–25
Aortic angiography of chest, abdomen, and pelvis with or without contrast agent	6.7–56
Coronary artery angiography	0.1–3
Non-enhanced CT of abdomen and pelvis to evaluate for nephrolithiasis	10–11

Adapted from Ladkany and Layman [6]

[a]Fetal dose varies with gestational age, maternal body habitus, and exact acquisition parameters

[b]Most authors report fetal dose from head, neck, or extremity CT close to zero (negligible scatter)

CT computed tomography

Suggested Resources

- Masselli G. Evaluating the acute abdomen in the pregnant patient. Radiol Clin N Am. 2015;53:1309.
- McCollough C, Schueler BA. Radiation exposure and pregnancy: when should we be concerned? Radiographics. 2007;27:909–17.
- McGahan J. Imaging non-obstetrical causes of abdominal pain in the pregnant patient. Appl Radiol. 2010;39:10–25.

References

1. Goodman R. Medical imaging radiation safety for the female patient: rationale and implementation. Radio Graphics. 2012;32:1829–37.
2. Gomes M. Risks to the fetus from diagnostic imaging during pregnancy: review and proposal of a clinical protocol. Pediatr Radiol. 2015;45:1916–29.
3. Baysinger CL. Imaging during pregnancy. Anesth Analg. 2010;110:863–7.
4. American College of obstetricians and gynecologists. Committee opinion no. 656: guidelines for diagnostic imaging during pregnancy and lactation. Obstet Gynecol. 2016;127:e75–80.
5. American College of obstetricians and gynecologists. Committee opinion no. 723: guidelines for diagnostic imaging during pregnancy and lactation. Obstet Gynecol. 2017;130:e210–6.
6. Ladkany D, Layman K. Imaging considerations in pregnancy. In: Borhart J, editor. Emergency department management of obstetric complications. 1st ed. Gewerbestrasse (Switzerland): Springer International; 2017. p. 159–68.

What Are the Risks of Doppler Ultrasound in Pregnancy?

106

Maria Dynin and Joelle Borhart

> **Pearls and Pitfalls**
> - Ultrasound is safe and considered an imaging modality of choice for pregnant patients.
> - Ultrasound waves do not produce ionizing radiation, but they do emit heat.
> - There is a theoretical risk of thermal damage to fetal tissue if acoustic output is too high.
> - B-mode and M-mode ultrasound waves are recommended over Doppler waves for fetal assessment whenever possible.

Ultrasound is a safe, effective, and readily available tool for the assessment pregnant patients. It is often the only imaging tool used to diagnose unstable pregnancy conditions such as ruptured ectopic pregnancy. It is also the first-line modality for determining the location and assessing the viability of an early pregnancy.

Ultrasound uses high-frequency sound waves to produce images. Sound waves do not produce ionizing radiation but do emit heat, which can theoretically cause thermal damage to tissues if the acoustic output is too high. Although standard B-mode ultrasound waves have potential to cause thermal injury, Doppler imaging requires a higher acoustic output and therefore confers a higher risk of thermal damage.

In addition, Doppler imaging confers a potential risk of mechanical effects on fetal tissue. A pulsed Doppler ultrasound wave can produce contraction or cavitation of bubbles in the fetal lungs or bowels, which can theoretically damage fetal organs or disrupt loosely tethered embryonic tissues [1].

Despite these theoretical concerns, no studies have documented adverse fetal effects from Doppler imaging [2]. That said, multiple professional societies, including the American Institute of Ultrasound Medicine and the International Society of Ultrasound in Obstetrics and Gynecology, recommend against the routine use of Doppler imaging in pregnancy [3–5].

It is important to mention that there are some cases where Doppler imaging in pregnancy is necessary. Ovarian torsion is an emergency diagnosis with high morbidity, and pregnancy is a risk factor for ovarian torsion. Pelvic ultrasound with color Doppler is the imaging modality of choice to diagnose ovarian torsion, as it helps determine the presence of blood flow to the ovary [6, 7].

Ultrasound is safe and considered the imaging modality of choice for the pregnant patient. B-mode and M-mode ultrasound waves are recommended over Doppler waves for fetal assessment whenever possible.

> **Suggested Resources**
> - Gynecologists, The American College of Obstetricians and. Committee opinion no. 656: guidelines for diagnostic imaging during pregnancy and lactation. Committee opinion. Obstet Gynecol. 2016;127:e75–80.
> - Ladkany D, Layman K. Imaging considerations in pregnancy. In: Borhart J, editor. Emergency department management of obstetric complications. 1st ed. Gewerbestrasse (Switzerland): Springer International; 2017. p. 159–68.
> - Stratmeyer ME, Greenleaf JF, Dalecki D, Salvesen K. Fetal ultrasound: mechanical effects. J Ultrasound Med. 2008;27:597–605.

M. Dynin · J. Borhart (✉)
Department of Emergency Medicine, MedStar Washington Hospital Center & MedStar Georgetown University Hospital, Washington, DC, USA

© Springer Nature Switzerland AG 2019
A. Graham, D. J. Carlberg (eds.), *Gastrointestinal Emergencies*, https://doi.org/10.1007/978-3-319-98343-1_106

References

1. Church CC, Carstensen EL, Nyborg WL, Carson PL, Frizzell LA, Bailey MR. The risk of exposure to diagnostic ultrasound in postnatal subjects: nonthermal mechanisms. J Ultrasound Med. 2008;27:565–92.
2. Gynecologists, The American College of Obstetricians and. Committee opinion no. 656: guidelines for diagnostic imaging during pregnancy and lactation. Committee opinion. Obstet Gynecol. 2016;127:e75–80.
3. American Institute of Ultrasound in Medicine. Official statement: statment on measurement of fetal heart rate. Approved Nov 5, 2011; Reapproved Oct 30, 2016. https://www.aium.org/officialStatements/43. Accessed Aug 27, 2018.
4. American Institute of Ultrasound in Medicine. Official statement: statment on the safe use of Doppler during the 11-14 week scans (or earlier in pregnancy). Approved 4/18/2011; Revised 3/21/16, 10/30/106. https://www.aium.org/officialStatements/42. Accessed Aug 27, 2018.
5. Salvesen K, Lees C, Abramowicz J, Brezinka C, Ter Har G, Marsal K. ISUOG statement on the safe use of Doppler in the 11 to 13+6-week fetal ultrasound examination. Ultrasound Obstet Gynecol. 2011;37:628.
6. Zucchini S, Marra E. Diagnosis of emergencies/urgencies in gynecology and during the first trimester of pregnancy. J Ultrasound. 2014;17(1):41–6.
7. Tsai H, Kuo T, Chung M, Lin M, Kang C, Tsai Y. Acute abdomen in early pregnancy due to ovarian torsion following successful in vitro fertilization treatment. Taiwan J Obstet Gynecol. 2015 Aug;54(4):438–41.

107

What Are the Implications of Abdominal Pain in Preeclampsia and HELLP Syndrome?

Joelle Borhart and Caroline Massarelli

Pearls and Pitfalls

- Preeclampsia and HELLP syndrome are major causes of morbidity and mortality in pregnant patients.
- Abdominal pain in a pregnant patient greater than 20 weeks gestation should raise suspicion for preeclampsia and/or HELLP syndrome.
- In patients with preeclampsia or HELLP syndrome, abdominal pain is an ominous sign signifying end-organ damage.
- Immediate obstetric consultation should be obtained in any pregnant patient with signs and symptoms of preeclampsia or HELLP syndrome, especially when presenting with abdominal pain.

Table 107.1 Signs/symptoms of end-organ damage and severe features of preeclampsia

Severe persistent right upper quadrant or epigastric pain unresponsive to medication
Impaired liver function (LFTs twice normal)
Thrombocytopenia (platelet count <100,000/microL)
Renal insufficiency (creatinine >1.1 mg/dL or doubling of creatinine in the absence of other renal diseases)
Pulmonary edema
New-onset cerebral or visual disturbances
Systolic blood pressure >160 mmHg or diastolic >110 mmHg

Adapted from the American College of Obstetricians and Gynecologists' Task Force on Hypertension in Pregnancy [11] and Olsen-Chen and Seligman [12]
LFTs Liver Function Tests

Table 107.2 Diagnosis of HELLP syndrome

Evidence of hemolysis
Schistocytes on peripheral smear
Lactate dehydrogenase >600 IU/L
Total bilirubin >1.2 mg/dL
Thrombocytopenia (platelets <100,000/microL)
Elevated aspartate aminotransferase (>70 IU/L)

Adapted from Olsen-Chen and Seligman [12]

Definitions

Preeclampsia and HELLP syndrome are two leading causes of maternal and perinatal morbidity and mortality, and the incidence is rising [1]. Preeclampsia is defined by the presence of new onset hypertension (systolic blood pressure ≥140 mmHg and/or diastolic ≥90 mmHg) after 20 weeks gestation with either proteinuria or other signs or symptoms of end-organ damage, listed in Table 107.1.

While the exact mechanism is still unclear, recent research suggests that abnormalities of early placentation can lead to placental insufficiency, triggering endothelial dysfunction and the resulting symptoms of preeclampsia [2]. HELLP syndrome, an acronym for its characteristic features of hemolysis, elevated liver enzymes, and low platelets, is a syndrome related to preeclampsia but can be present with or without coexisting hypertension [3]. Diagnostic criteria for HELLP syndrome are listed in Table 107.2.

Implications

Abdominal pain in the setting of preeclampsia can be an ominous sign. Persistent right upper quadrant or epigastric abdominal pain is a sign of end-organ damage. In HELLP syndrome, patients will often present with right upper quadrant or epigastric pain as well as nausea and vomiting [4]. One study of women with HELLP syndrome reported that 90% had epigastric or right upper quadrant abdominal pain

J. Borhart (✉)
Department of Emergency Medicine, MedStar Washington Hospital Center & MedStar Georgetown University Hospital, Washington, DC, USA

C. Massarelli
Georgetown University School of Medicine, Washington, DC, USA
e-mail: com6@georgetown.edu

© Springer Nature Switzerland AG 2019
A. Graham, D. J. Carlberg (eds.), *Gastrointestinal Emergencies*, https://doi.org/10.1007/978-3-319-98343-1_107

[5]. The abdominal pain in HELLP syndrome is thought to be due to periportal necrosis, microthrombi, and fibrin deposits in the sinusoids, causing inflammation of the liver and subsequently stretch of Glisson's capsule. The pain can be intense and unremitting [6].

Diagnosis

Any pregnant patient greater than 20 weeks gestational age presenting with epigastric or right upper quadrant abdominal pain should be evaluated for preeclampsia and HELLP syndrome. Minimum laboratory testing includes complete blood count, complete metabolic panel, and urinalysis or urine protein/creatinine ratio. These tests evaluate for signs of end-organ damage associated with preeclampsia and HELLP syndrome. If the clinical picture or labs suggest possible HELLP syndrome (anemia, elevated liver enzymes, thrombocytopenia), lactate dehydrogenase can be included to assess for the possibility of hemolysis.

Treatment

Emergency department treatment of preeclampsia is aimed at controlling blood pressure, initiating seizure prophylaxis to limit progression to eclampsia, and obtaining emergent obstetric consultation.

Blood pressure should be slowly stabilized around 140/90 mmHg rather than rapidly normalized. The most commonly used antihypertensive agents include labetalol, hydralazine, and nifedipine. All are considered first-line therapy and are safe in pregnancy [7].

Prophylaxis against seizures should be given to any woman with preeclampsia and abdominal pain, as this constitutes a presentation of preeclampsia with severe features. Magnesium sulfate is the drug of choice and is given at a suggested dose of 4 g IV over 5 min, followed by a 1 g/h infusion. This treatment has been shown to decrease the risk of eclampsia by 50% [8]. If seizures develop, further magnesium administration is indicated with an additional 2–4 g IV over 5 min followed by a 2 g/h infusion [9].

Since the only definitive treatment for both preeclampsia and HELLP syndrome is delivery, emergent obstetric consultation should be obtained. Patients with preeclampsia and HELLP syndrome can deteriorate rapidly and may require high level, multidisciplinary care. If the care setting is not equipped to handle both a patient with preeclampsia with severe features and a potentially preterm neonate, transfer to another facility should be considered [10].

Suggested Resources
- Olsen-Chen C, Seligman NS. Hypertensive emergencies in pregnancy. Crit Care Clin. 2016;32:29–41.
- Core EM—Preeclampsia and Eclampsia. https://coreem.net/core/preeclampsia-and-eclampsia/.
- Sherman W, Descallar E, Borhart J. Hypertensive disorders of pregnancy. In: Borhart J, editor. Emergency department management of obstetric complications. 1st ed. Gewerbestrasse (Switzerland): Springer International; 2017. p. 41–51.

References

1. Wallis AB, Saftlas AF, Hsia J, et al. Secular trends in the rates of preeclampsia, eclampsia, and gestational hypertension, United States, 1987–2004. Am J Hypertens. 2008;21:521–6.
2. Redman C. Preeclampsia: a complex and variable disease. Pregnancy Hypertens. 2014;3:241–2.
3. Haram K, Svendsen E, Abildgaard U. The HELLP syndrome: clinical issues and management: a review. BMC Pregnancy Childbirth. 2009;9:8.
4. Kennedy A. Assessment of acute abdominal pain in the pregnant patient. Semin Ultrasound CT MR. 2000;21(1):64–77.
5. Sibai BM, Ramadan MK, Usta I, Salama M, Mercer BM, Friedman SA. Maternal morbidity and mortality in 442 pregnancies with hemolysis, elevated liver enzymes, and low platelets (HELLP syndrome). Am J Obstet Gynecol. 1993;169:1000–6.
6. Dekker GA, Sibai BM. Etiology and pathogenesis of preeclampsia: current concepts. Am J Obstet Gynecol. 1998;179:1359–75.
7. American College of Obstetricians and Gynecologists. Committee opinion no 623: emergent therapy for acute-onset, severe hypertension during pregnancy and the postpartum period. Obstet Gynecol. 2015;125:521–5.
8. Duley L, Gulmezoglu AM, Henderson-Smart DJ, et al. Magnesium sulfate and other anticonvulsants for women with preeclampsia. Cochrane Database Syst Rev. 2010;11:CD000025.
9. Mol BW, Roberts CT, Thangaratinam S, et al. Preeclampsia. Lancet. 2016;387(10022):999–1011. https://doi.org/10.1016/S0140-6736(15)00070-7.
10. Repke JT, Norwitz ER. Management of eclampsia. In: Heazell A, Norwitz ER, Kenny LC, et al., editors. Hypertension in pregnancy. New York: Cambridge University Press; 2011. p. 141–58.
11. American College of Obstetricians and Gynecologists, Task Force on Hypertension in Pregnancy. Hypertension in pregnancy. Report of the American College of Obstetricians and Gynecologists' task force on hypertension in pregnancy. Obstet Gynecol. 2013;122:1122–11.
12. Olsen-Chen C, Seligman NS. Hypertensive emergencies in pregnancy. Crit Care Clin. 2016;32:29–41.

What Is Acute Fatty Liver of Pregnancy?

108

Jessica Palmer and Joelle Borhart

Pearls and Pitfalls
- Acute fatty liver of pregnancy (AFLP) is rare but associated with high morbidity and mortality for both the mother and the fetus.
- Three percent of pregnant women will develop some sort of liver dysfunction.
- There is significant overlap between preeclampsia; eclampsia; the syndrome of hemolysis, elevated liver enzymes, and low platelets; and AFLP.
- Emergency department management of AFLP is maternal stabilization and emergent obstetric consultation. Definitive management is delivery.

Acute fatty liver of pregnancy (AFLP) is a rare complication with high morbidity and mortality for both mother and fetus. It tends to occur in the third trimester, typically between 30 and 38 weeks gestation [1, 2].

In AFLP, there is microvesicular fatty infiltration of liver hepatocytes. Several genetic defects have been found that predispose women to AFLP, most commonly long-chain 3-hydroxyacyl-coenzyme A dehydrogenase (LCHAD), an autosomal recessive genetic inborn error of metabolism [3]. Usually, women who are heterozygous for this disorder are asymptomatic until becoming pregnant. However, these women may be at increased risk for developing AFLP, especially if they carry a fetus that is homozygous for LCHAD. When the fetus is homozygous for LCHAD, it has reduced ability to oxidize long-chain fatty acids in the liver. The unoxidized fatty acids from the fetus are then transferred through the placenta to the mother. This leads to a buildup of toxic metabolites in the maternal liver [4]. These toxic metabolites, in addition to the metabolic stress of the third trimester and environmental stressors such as a high-fat diet, can lead to AFLP. There are cases of AFLP that occur in the absence of LCHAD defects, suggesting another possible etiology [5, 6].

The presentation of AFLP ranges from non-specific symptoms such as anorexia, malaise, nausea, vomiting, and abdominal pain to fulminant liver failure including hypoglycemia, coagulopathy, jaundice, and encephalopathy [2, 4, 6]. With progression of disease, patients can develop ascites, pleural effusions, renal failure, and respiratory failure [2]. The reported maternal mortality is 18%, while the reported fetal mortality is 23% [1].

Approximately 3% of pregnant women will develop some sort of liver dysfunction [7]. There is significant clinical overlap between the various liver complications of pregnancy including preeclampsia; eclampsia; the syndrome of hemolysis, elevated liver enzymes, and low platelets (HELLP); and AFLP, and distinguishing between these complications is challenging. The Swansea criteria can be used to aid in diagnosis of AFLP [8] [Table 108.1].

Table 108.1 Swansea criteria for the diagnosis of acute fatty liver of pregnancy [8]

Six or more of the following, in the absence of other diagnoses
Vomiting
Abdominal pain
Polydipsia/polyuria
Encephalopathy
Elevated bilirubin
Hypoglycemia
Elevated uric acid
Leukocytosis
Ascites or bright liver on ultrasound
Elevated transaminases
Elevated ammonia
Renal impairment
Coagulopathy
Microvesicular steatosis on liver biopsy

J. Palmer · J. Borhart (✉)
Department of Emergency Medicine, MedStar Washington Hospital Center & MedStar Georgetown University Hospital, Washington, DC, USA
e-mail: Jessica.l.palmer@medstar.net

© Springer Nature Switzerland AG 2019
A. Graham, D. J. Carlberg (eds.), *Gastrointestinal Emergencies*, https://doi.org/10.1007/978-3-319-98343-1_108

For emergency physicians, the management of all four disorders is the same: maternal stabilization and emergent obstetric consultation. The definitive treatment for all four disorders is delivery.

Suggested Resources

- Jawyyed SM, Blanda M, Kubina M. Acute fatty liver of pregnancy. J Emerg Med. 1999;17(4):673–7.
- Martin S. Fatty liver in pregnancy. MDEdge: Emergency Medicine. Accessed 12 Nov 2017. http://www.mdedge.com/emed-journal/dsm/7578/obstetrics/fatty-liver-pregnancy.
- Nickson C. Acute fatty liver of pregnancy. Life in the Fast Lane. Accessed 12 Nov 2017. https://lifein-thefastlane.com/ccc/acute-fatty-liver-of-pregnancy/.

References

1. Ahmed KT, Almashhrawi AA, Rahman RN, et al. Liver diseases in pregnancy: diseases unique to pregnancy. World J Gastroenterol. 2013;19(43):7639–46.
2. Westbrook RH, Dusheiko G, Williamson C. Pregnancy and liver disease. J Hepatol. 2016;64:933–45.
3. Ibdah JA, Bennett MJ, Rinaldo P, et al. Fatty-acid oxidation disorder as a cause of liver disease in pregnant women. N Engl J Med. 1999;340(22):1723–31.
4. Greenes V, Williamson C. Liver disease in pregnancy. Best Pract Res Clin Obstet Gynecol. 2015;29:612–24.
5. Italian Association for the Study of the Liver. AISF position paper on liver disease and pregnancy. Dig Liver Dis. 2016;48(2):120–37.
6. Hammoud GM, Ibdah JA. Preeclampsia-induced liver dysfunction, HELLP syndrome, and acute fatty liver of pregnancy. Clin Liver Dis. 2014;4:69–73.
7. Minakami H, Morikawa M, Yamada T, Yamada T, Akaishi R, Nishida R. Differentiation of acute fatty liver of pregnancy from syndrome of hemolysis, elevated liver enzymes and low platelet counts. J Obstet Gynaecol Res. 2014;40:641–9.
8. Ch'ng CL, Morgan M, Hainsworth I, et al. Prospective study of liver dysfunction in pregnancy in Southwest Wales. Gut. 2002;51:876e80.

109

What Are the Best Management Strategies for Hyperemesis Gravidarum?

Lindsey DeGeorge and Lauren Wiesner

Pearls and Pitfalls
- Early treatment of nausea and vomiting in pregnancy with diet modification and pyridoxine (vitamin B_6) with or without doxylamine can decrease progression to hyperemesis gravidarum (HG).
- Medications for acute HG symptoms include metoclopramide, ondansetron, and diphenhydramine.
- Basic metabolic panel, liver function tests, and urinalysis may be obtained to help quantify disease severity and guide fluid and electrolyte replacement.
- Consider thiamine and folate administration prior to dextrose infusion in cases of severe or prolonged HG.
- Pelvic ultrasound is indicated in patients who have not yet had a confirmatory study to evaluate for multiple gestations or trophoblastic disease.

Nausea and vomiting in pregnancy is common. Treatment in the early stages may prevent more serious complications such as hyperemesis gravidarum (HG). HG represents the most severe form of nausea and vomiting in pregnancy and is estimated to affect between 0.5% and 2% of pregnancies [1]. It is characterized by unrelenting nausea and vomiting. Additional findings that may accompany HG include weight loss greater than 5% of prepregnancy weight, evidence of dehydration, electrolyte disturbance(s), and ketosis [2].

L. DeGeorge (✉)
Department of Emergency Medicine, MedStar Washington Hospital Center, Washington, DC, USA

L. Wiesner
Georgetown University School of Medicine, Department of Emergency Medicine, Washington, DC, USA

MedStar Washington Hospital Center, Washington, DC, USA
e-mail: lauren.m.wiesner@medstar.net

Laboratory testing for patients with HG includes urinalysis to evaluate for elevated specific gravity and ketones and basic metabolic panel to evaluate for hyponatremia, hypochloremia, hypokalemia, acidosis, elevated blood urea nitrogen, and elevated creatinine. Liver function tests may show increased AST, ALT, and/or total bilirubin. If not previously obtained, a pelvic ultrasound should be performed to evaluate for a multiple gestation pregnancy or trophoblastic disease, as these are associated with increased risk of HG [3].

The first step in management of HG is restoration of normal volume status. Most cases of HG require intravenous (IV) fluid resuscitation with dextrose 5% in either normal saline or ½ normal saline. Caution should be taken to prevent overly rapid correction of hyponatremia. Repletion of thiamine and folate prior to dextrose infusion should be considered in cases of severe or prolonged symptoms to prevent Wernicke encephalopathy [4].

The American College of Obstetricians and Gynecologists (ACOG) recommends pyridoxine (vitamin B_6) alone or with doxylamine as the first-line pharmacologic therapy for nausea and vomiting in pregnancy [5]. However, slow onset of action and lack of IV formulation make this therapy impractical for acute symptom control in HG.

Medications frequently used for acute management of HG include dopamine antagonists, selective serotonin inhibitors, and H1 antagonists (Table 109.1).

Dopamine antagonists used for treatment of symptoms in HG include metoclopramide, promethazine, and prochlorperazine. Metoclopramide was evaluated in a large, retrospective cohort study that found no adverse fetal outcomes associated with its use in the first trimester [6].

Ondansetron is a selective serotonin inhibitor. A study comparing ondansetron to metoclopramide found similar efficacy but fewer maternal side effects with ondansetron. Two large retrospective cohort studies have yielded conflicting results regarding fetal safety of ondansetron use. One study found that ondansetron was not associated with an increased risk of abortion, stillbirth, any major birth defect, preterm delivery, or low birth weight [7]. A second large

A. Graham, D. J. Carlberg (eds.), *Gastrointestinal Emergencies*, https://doi.org/10.1007/978-3-319-98343-1_109

Table 109.1 Recommended pharmacologic therapies for treatment of hyperemesis gravidarum

Treatment option	Clinical considerations
Dopamine antagonists: Metoclopramide 10 mg Promethazine 25 mg every 4 h Prochlorperazine 10 mg every 6 h	Metoclopramide: FDA pregnancy category B, preferred dopamine antagonist Promethazine: FDA pregnancy category C, rectal dosing available Prochlorperazine: less well studied *Side effects:* maternal sedation, tardive dyskinesia, acute dystonic reaction
Selective serotonin antagonists: Ondansetron 4 mg every 8 h, maximum 16 mg IV	Ondansetron: FDA pregnancy category B, high efficacy in studies Consider ECG and/or telemetry for IV use, especially if concurrent electrolyte abnormalities or QT-prolonging medications *Side effects:* maternal QT prolongation in IV formulation, may cause fetal cardiac septum malformation
H1 antagonists: Diphenhydramine 25 mg every 6 h Dimenhydrinate 50 mg every 6 h Meclizine 25 mg every 8 h	FDA pregnancy category B *Side effects:* sedation, dry mouth, urinary retention

study concluded that the teratogenic risk of ondansetron is low but that there was a statistically significant increased incidence of fetal cardiac septum defects associated with ondansetron use [8].

H1 antagonists include diphenhydramine, dimenhydrinate, and meclizine [9]. These agents generally cause more maternal sedation and have no proven treatment superiority when compared with metoclopramide and ondansetron. They may be useful adjuncts for persistent symptoms [10].

Use of steroids as part of the management of HG is controversial, and overall evidence supporting its use is lacking. According to ACOG guidelines, use of methylprednisolone should be reserved as a last resort for refractory symptoms based on its risk profile and its association with low birth weight and fetal malformations including cleft lip and palate [5]. The decision to treat HG with steroids should be made in consultation with an obstetrician.

For patients who achieve adequate symptom control and rehydration in the ED, discharge with outpatient obstetrics follow-up is appropriate. They should be educated on lifestyle modifications including eating small, frequent, bland meals and avoiding olfactory stimuli that trigger symptoms. Patients may find symptom relief with non-pharmacologic therapies. Ginger supplements can be given as 250 mg doses four times daily and have shown benefit in several small studies [11]. Though frequently ineffective for the acute treatment of HG, pyridoxine with doxylamine is recommended upon discharge from the acute care setting to reduce recurrent symptoms.

Hospital admission is typically required for patients with persistent nausea and vomiting who remain unable to tolerate oral intake despite treatment in the ED. It is also recommended for those with severe dehydration and lab abnormalities requiring significant correction.

Suggested Resources
- American College of obstetricians and gynecologists practice bulletin summary no. 153. Obstet Gynecol. 2015;126(3):687–8.
- DeGeorge L, Wiesner L. Approach to the patient with nausea and vomiting in pregnancy. In: Borhart J, editor. Emergency department management of obstetric complications. 1st ed. Gewerbestrasse (Switzerland): Springer International; 2017. p. 31–40.
- McParlin C, O'Donnell A, Robson SC, et al. Treatments for hyperemesis gravidarum and nausea and vomiting in pregnancy: a systematic review. JAMA. 2016;316(13):1392–401.

References

1. Sheehan P. Hyperemesis gravidarum – assessment and management. Aust Fam Physician. 2007;36(9):698–701.
2. World Health Organization. International classification of diseases: 10. Version: 2010. 2012. http://tinyurl.com/ctcuekp. Accessed 29 June 2016.
3. Kuscu NK, Koyuncu F. Hyperemesis Gravidarum: current concepts and management. Postgrad Med J. 2002;78(916):76–9.
4. Ismail SK, Kenny L. Review on hyperemesis gravidarum. Clin Gastroenterol. 2007;21(5):755–69.
5. American College of obstetricians and gynecologists practice bulletin summary no. 153. Obstet Gynecol. 2015;126(3):687–8.
6. Matok I, Gorodischer R, Koren G, Sheiner E, Wiznitzer A, Levy A. The safety of metoclopramide use in the first trimester of pregnancy. N Engl J Med. 2009;360(24):2528–35.
7. Pasternak B, Svanström H, Hviid A. Ondansetron in pregnancy and risk of adverse fetal outcomes. N Engl J Med. 2013;368:814–23. Erratum in N Engl J Med 2013;368:2146.
8. Danielsson B, Wikner BN, Källén B. Use of ondansetron during pregnancy and congenital malformations in the infant. Reprod Toxicol. 2014;50:134–7.
9. Abas MN, Tan PC, Azmi N, Omar SZ. Ondansetron compared with metoclopramide for hyperemesis gravidarum: a randomized controlled trial. Obstet Gynecol. 2014;123:1272–9.
10. Magee LA, Mazzotta P, Koren G. Evidence- based view of safety and effectiveness of pharmacologic therapy for nausea and vomiting of pregnancy (NVP). Am J Obstet Gynecol. 2002;186(5 Suppl Understanding):S256–61. 37.
11. Fischer-Rasmussen W, Kiaer SK, Dahl C, Asping U. Ginger treatment of hyperemesis gravidarum. Eur J Obstet Gynecol Reprod Biol. 1991;38(1):19–24.

Consultant Corner: Abdominal Pain and the Pregnant Patient

110

John Davitt, Anna Zelivianskaia, and John David Buek

Pearls and Pitfalls

- As pregnancy progresses, the gravid uterus displaces the viscera and confounds physical exam findings. Patients may have loss of rebound tenderness, and appendicitis pain may not occur at McBurney's point.
- Elevations in progesterone during pregnancy cause smooth muscle to relax, which exacerbates painful symptoms of GERD, bloating, and constipation.
- Progesterone causes ureteral relaxation, and, when coupled with compression by the gravid uterus, the resulting urinary stasis increases the risk of pyelonephritis.
- Pyelonephritis increases the risk of complications during pregnancy, including acute respiratory distress syndrome and preterm labor.
- If the abdominal pain is the result of direct abdominal trauma and the pregnancy is greater than 23 weeks gestation, immediate OB/GYN consultation is warranted.

Introduction

John Davitt, MD, and Anna Zelivianskaia, MD, are completing their residency in obstetrics and gynecology at MedStar Georgetown University Hospital and MedStar Washington Hospital Center. Dr. Zelivianskaia plans to practice as a generalist OB/GYN after completing her training. John D. Buek, MD, is the Residency Program Director of the MedStar Obstetrics and Gynecology Residency Program and is board certified in obstetrics and gynecology. Drs. Davitt,

J. Davitt · A. Zelivianskaia · J. D. Buek (✉)
MedStar Washington Hospital Center, Department of Obstetrics and Gynecology, Washington, DC, USA
e-mail: john.m.davitt@medstar.net; anna.s.zelivianskaia@medstar.net; john.d.buek@medstar.net

Zelivianskaia, and Buek practice in a large, urban tertiary referral hospital in Washington, DC, where they see a variety of OB/GYN patients.

Answers to Key Clinical Questions

1. When do you recommend consultation with an OB/GYN and in what time frame?

For first trimester abdominal pain, especially lower abdominal pain, providers must consider pregnancy complications as a potential cause. The most worrisome early pregnancy-related cause of abdominal pain is ectopic pregnancy. If there is any concern about an extrauterine pregnancy, an immediate consultation with an OB/GYN is necessary. If an intrauterine pregnancy is confirmed, early pregnancy loss may cause abdominal pain. Worrisome causes of pregnancy-related abdominal pain as the pregnancy progresses may include preterm labor and placental abruption. The diagnostic algorithm for potential ectopic pregnancy and the evaluation for other causes of pregnancy-related abdominal pain are beyond the scope of this chapter, but if providers suspect a pregnancy-related emergency, OB/GYN should be consulted.

If the abdominal pain is the result of direct abdominal trauma and the pregnancy is greater than 23 weeks gestation, immediate OB/GYN consultation is also warranted.

2. What pearls can you offer emergency care providers when evaluating a pregnant patient with abdominal pain?

Acute care providers should consider a broad differential diagnosis for abdominal pain, including pregnancy-related pain as well as musculoskeletal, gastrointestinal, urologic, gynecologic, and neuropathic etiologies of pain. It is easy to focus on the pregnancy and neglect other potential causes. Potential etiologies of abdominal pain during pregnancy are listed in Table 110.1.

© Springer Nature Switzerland AG 2019
A. Graham, D. J. Carlberg (eds.), *Gastrointestinal Emergencies*, https://doi.org/10.1007/978-3-319-98343-1_110

Table 110.1 Potential causes of abdominal pain during pregnancy, listed by trimester

First trimester	Second trimester	Third trimester
Early pregnancy loss	Gastroesophageal reflux disease (GERD)	GERD
Incomplete abortion	Round ligament pain	Preterm labor
Ectopic pregnancy	Preterm labor	UTI/
Urinary tract infection (UTI)/	UTI/pyelonephritis	pyelonephritis
pyelonephritis	Preeclampsia	Preeclampsia
Other gastrointestinal (GI) causes	Syndrome of hemolysis, elevated liver enzymes, and low platelets (HELLP)	HELLP
	Other GI causes	Other GI causes

As pregnancy progresses and the gravid uterus occupies a significant amount of the abdominal cavity, displaced viscera will confound typical physical exam findings. Patients may have loss of rebound tenderness, and appendicitis pain may not occur at McBurney's point.

Although ultrasound and magnetic resonance imaging are the preferred methods of diagnostic imaging in pregnancy, radiation from plain radiography, computed tomography, and nuclear medicine is generally well below doses associated with fetal harm.

3. What concepts do you think are key to managing a pregnant patient with abdominal pain?

Elevations in progesterone during pregnancy cause smooth muscle to relax, which exacerbates painful symptoms of GERD, bloating, and constipation, all of which can lead to significant pain; however, all have relatively simple medical solutions.

Progesterone also causes ureteral relaxation, and, when coupled with compression by the gravid uterus, the resulting urinary stasis increases the risk of pyelonephritis, which requires admission and IV antibiotics.

Care should be taken to ensure that pregnancy-specific laboratory reference ranges are used, as maternal physiology changes significantly in pregnancy.

The best way to ensure the health of the pregnancy is to ensure the health of the mother.

4. What complications are you concerned about in this patient population?

Pyelonephritis – Any pregnant patient with pyelonephritis should be admitted for treatment with parenteral antibiotics due to the increased risk of complications in pregnancy, including acute respiratory distress syndrome and preterm labor. Providers should consider a chest x-ray if the patient complains of shortness of breath.

Appendicitis – Acute and severe gastrointestinal causes of abdominal pain can still present during pregnancy. Appendicitis should always be in the differential for the pregnant patient with abdominal pain.

Preeclampsia/HELLP – Hypertensive disorders of pregnancy and HELLP syndrome (hemolysis, elevated liver enzymes, and low platelets) may initially present as benign-appearing epigastric or abdominal pain. Preeclampsia and HELLP can rapidly progress to significant end-organ damage, and a high index of suspicion for these is necessary.

Suggested Resources

- Committee Opinion: Guidelines for Diagnostic Imaging During Pregnancy and Lactation. American College of Obstetrics and Gynecology. Oct 2017. https://www.acog.org/-/media/Committee-Opinions/Committee-on-Obstetric-Practice/co723.pdf?dmc=1&ts=20180127T0150226583.
- Practice Bulletin: Early Pregnancy Loss. American College of Obstetrics and Gynecology. Published May 2015, reaffirmed 2017. https://www.acog.org/Resources-And-Publications/Practice-Bulletins/Committee-on-Practice-Bulletins-Gynecology/Early-Pregnancy-Loss.

An Introduction: Is My Patient Immunocompromised? How Do I Interpret History and Physical Examination Findings in the Immunocompromised Patient? What Does the Work-Up Look Like for an Immunocompromised Patient? What Are the Unique Risks and Potential Pitfalls?

111

Mary Carroll Lee and Jack Perkins

Pearls and Pitfalls
- Patients will have varying levels of immune compromise; this should be considered in the evaluation and management of suspected intra-abdominal pathology.
- Patients with significant intra-abdominal pathology may not exhibit fever, leukocytosis, or even expected abnormalities on abdominal examination.
- Immunocompromised patients with abdominal complaints warrant a thorough investigation and strong consideration of advanced imaging and likely will require admission or observation.

The assessment of the immunocompromised patient with abdominal pain requires a high index of suspicion for severe disease. It is not uncommon for the presentation to underwhelm clinicians even in the presence of surgical disease. Emergency medicine providers (EPs) rely on the first impression, vital signs, physical exam, and laboratory evaluation to determine severity of illness or potential for severe illness. However, in the immunocompromised patient, the EP should expect the unexpected presentation.

This chapter will serve as an introduction to approaching the immunocompromised patient with abdominal pain. We will begin with a discussion on what it means to state that a patient is "immunocompromised" and how this should change the EP's evaluation and management. We then explore some of the pitfalls in the approach to these patients in an effort to change the approach to the immunocompromised patient with abdominal pain. In many ways, the EP should view these patients with the same trepidation and diligence that we have for years approached the neutropenic fever patient who is undergoing chemotherapy.

Is My Patient Immunocompromised?

The initial step is *recognition* of a patient who is immunocompromised (see Table 111.1). While most providers will recognize the inherent risk of a patient with AIDS who has abdominal pain, an EP might overlook the immunocompromised status of a COPD patient who is chronically on steroids. Thus, recognition begins during the initial patient encounter, and it is essential that the EP reflect as to whether the patient is immunocompromised and to what degree?

The second step is assessing the *severity* of immune compromise. Much like sepsis, immune compromise is a spectrum that is associated with varying risks to the patient, in terms of morbidity, mortality, and likelihood of serious pathology. Risk to the patient includes both usual and unusual infectious pathogens, delayed wound healing from surgery, and complications from abdominal pathology which might have a more benign course in a patient with a normal immune system [1]. For example, immunocompromised patients are

M. C. Lee
Virginia Tech Carilion Emergency Medicine Residency, Roanoke, VA, USA
e-mail: mflee@carilionclinic.org

J. Perkins (✉)
Virginia Tech Carilion School of Medicine, Roanoke, VA, USA
e-mail: jcperkins@carilionclinic.org

© Springer Nature Switzerland AG 2019
A. Graham, D. J. Carlberg (eds.), *Gastrointestinal Emergencies*, https://doi.org/10.1007/978-3-319-98343-1_111

Table 111.1 Immunocompromised classification

Mild to moderate immunosuppression
Diabetes
Systemic lupus erythematosus (SLE)
Elderly
HIV with CD4 count >200
Posttransplant on maintenance immunosuppressive therapy
Severe immunosuppression
HIV with CD4 count <200
Organ transplant within 60 days
Neutropenia
Medications
Steroids
Cyclosporin
Tacrolimus
Methotrexate

at higher risk of ruptured diverticulitis, small bowel obstruction associated with colitis, and abscess formation from appendicitis [2]. The important point to remember is that the immunocompromised patient may not manifest expected signs and symptoms of surgical pathology until late in the disease course.

How Do I Interpret History and Physical Examination Findings in the Immunocompromised Patient?

As with any patient, vital signs are highly contributory in assessing disease severity. Unfortunately, immunocompromised patients may have normal or slightly abnormal vital signs despite having moderately advanced pathology. Consequently, meticulous attention to initial vital signs is paramount as a triage heart rate of 102, an oral temperature of 99.9 °F, or a blood pressure of 102/50 mmHg may be abnormal for the patient and forewarn significant illness. We recommend obtaining a core temperature (e.g., rectal if not neutropenic or bladder) in these patients, as oral and axillary are insufficiently sensitive. Furthermore, it is important to obtain more frequent vital signs in these patients as trends in heart rate, blood pressure, or respiratory rate can be helpful in predicting course of illness.

The physical exam in immunocompromised patients can be significantly misleading. Suppression of inflammatory markers blunts symptoms, and physical exam findings are more readily identifiable in immunocompetent hosts [1]. Consequently, immunocompromised patients may be less

likely to experience localized pain. For example, patients with appendicitis may present with generalized abdominal discomfort, and those with colitis may experience non-specific vomiting or diarrhea. Furthermore, immunocompromised patients are more likely to experience complications, such as bowel perforation due to diverticulitis. Despite surgical pathology, the patient may still look and feel relatively well. These patients also have a decreased ability to experience visceral abdominal pain; thus complaints of shoulder pain or flank pain may represent an intra-abdominal surgical process.

What Does the Work-Up Look Like for an Immunocompromised Patient?

All immunocompromised patients with abdominal pain should have some bare minimum labs (e.g., complete blood count, basic metabolic panel, hepatic function tests, lipase) sent upon presentation to the ED. Additional testing such as blood cultures, erythrocyte sedimentation rate (ESR), C-reactive protein (CRP), and urinalysis should be tailored to the suspected pathology. However, lab testing can also be a source for pitfalls in the immunocompromised patient. These patients may have a delayed or nonexistent leukocytosis due to their decreased ability to mount inflammatory responses. Adjunctive inflammatory markers (e.g., ESR and CRP) may be normal or near normal even with significant pathology [3]. Unfortunately, severe disease is not excluded even if all inflammatory markers are normal.

Immunocompromised patients should still be able to exhibit lactic acidosis, but the specificity of this test diminishes as a number of immunocompromised patients may have baseline elevations of lactic acid [4]. For example, patients with cirrhosis and HIV patients taking nucleoside reverse transcriptase inhibitors therapy may have an elevated lactic acid at baseline as a result of their treatment [4].

What Are the Unique Risks and Potential Pitfalls?

Table 111.2 summarizes the unique risks and potential pitfalls for common sources of abdominal pain in immunocompromised patients.

Table 111.2 Risks and potential pitfalls for common sources of abdominal pain in immunocompromised patients

Disease	Immunocompetent host	Immunocompromised host	Pearls
Diverticulitis	Lower risk of complicated course	Higher risk of perforation, abscess formation, sepsis	Lower threshold to admit diverticulitis in immunocompromised patients [5]
Appendicitis	Lower risk for complicated course	Higher risk for need for repeat surgery, prolonged hospitalization, abscess formation, perforation	CMV infection linked to complex appendicitis course in immunocompromised patients
Colitis	Lower risk, usually non-operative	Higher risk for enterocolitis, obstruction, need for laparotomy Infectious pathology from both typical and atypical organisms	Neutropenic enterocolitis is becoming the most common cause of abdominal pain in patients with triad of neutropenia, abdominal pain, and fever after receiving chemotherapy
Mesenteric ischemia	High risk of mortality	Also high risk of mortality; less likely to produce robust leukocytosis	Absence of lactic acidosis doesn't exclude disease [6]
Pyelonephritis	Typically uncomplicated course with oral antibiotics	More likely to have resistant organisms, treatment failure, hematogenous spread, chronic pyelonephritis, renal abscess, and sepsis More likely to have pathology due to non-enteric bacteria, aerobic bacteria, gram-negative rods, and candida	Common in the 2 months post renal transplant secondary to postsurgical vesicoureteral reflux [7]
Pyelonephritis with stone	At risk for complicated course, but could still consider outpatient antibiotics if clinically appropriate	Very high risk for treatment failure, renal abscess, cortical scarring, and sepsis	CT imaging recommend in any septic patient with pyelonephritis to evaluate for stone
Cholecystitis	Usually uncomplicated surgical course	Higher risk from infectious organisms, and may follow infectious gastroenteritis [8]	More likely to have atypical presentations in immunocompromised

Suggested Resources

- McKean J, Ronan-Bentl S. Abdominal pain in the immunocompromised patient—human immunodeficiency virus, transplant, cancer. Emerg Med Clin North Am. 2016;34(2):377–86. https://doi.org/10.1016/j.emc.2015.12.002.
- Spencer SP, Power N. The acute abdomen in the immune compromised host. Cancer Imaging. 2008;8(1):93–101. https://doi.org/10.1102/1470-7330.2008.0013.

References

1. McKean J, Ronan-Bentl S. Abdominal pain in the immunocompromised patient—human immunodeficiency virus, transplant, cancer. Emerg Med Clin North Am. 2016;34(2):377–86. https://doi.org/10.1016/j.emc.2015.12.002.
2. Hardy A. Evaluation of the acute abdomen. In: Todd SR, editor. Common problems in acute care surgery. 1st ed. New York: Springer; 2013. p. 19–31.
3. Liu D, Ahmet A, Ward L, Krishnamoorthy P, Mandelcorn ED, Leigh R, Kim H. A practical guide to the monitoring and management of the complications of systemic corticosteroid therapy. Allergy Asthma Clin Immunol. 2013;9(1):30.
4. Arenas-Pinto A, Grant AD, Edwards S, Weller IV. Lactic acidosis in HIV infected patients: a systematic review of published cases. Sex Transm Infect. 2003;79:340–3.
5. Alby K, Nachamkin I. Gastrointestinal infections. Microbiol Spectr. 2016;4(3) https://doi.org/10.1128/microbiolspec.
6. Van den Heijkant TC, Aerts BA, Teijink JA, Buurman WA, Luyer MD. Challenges in diagnosing mesenteric ischemia. World J Gastroenterol. 2013;19(9):1338–4.
7. Ramakrishnan K, Scheid DC. Diagnosis and management of acute pyelonephritis in adults. Am Fam Physician. 2005;71(5):933–42.
8. Indar AA, Beckingham IJ. Acute cholecystitis. BMJ: Br Med J. 2002;325(7365):639–43.

Who Should I Image and When? CT Negative: Now What?

112

John B. Pierson and Michelle Clinton

Imaging Considerations for Immunocompromised Patients

Most immunocompromised patients who present to the emergency department (ED) with abdominal pain will require cross-sectional imaging (e.g., CT or magnetic resonance imaging). Consideration should be given to the degree to which the patient's immune system is suppressed. Physical examination is unreliable in patients with severe immunosuppression. Waiting for peritonitis or focal tenderness to develop before imaging may significantly delay diagnosis. Opportunistic infections, postsurgical complications, mass effect from cancer, and delayed presentation of typical intra-abdominal pathology such as appendicitis are a few of the considerations when evaluating the immunocompromised patient for which imaging may aid in assessment [1].

Administration of intravenous contrast is indicated in the vast majority of cases as this will help identify intra-abdominal inflammatory changes; particularly in patients without a significant amount of adipose tissue [2]. In patients with significant gastrointestinal (GI) bleeding or known vascular disease, arterial phase acquisition (e.g., CT angiography) may help identify a source for intervention. Oral contrast may help identify bowel thickening and abscesses; however the delay in obtaining CT imaging and potential inability of the patient to tolerate oral intake limit overall usefulness (Table 112.1).

Table 112.1 Indications for various advanced imaging modalities in immunocompromised patients presenting to the ED with abdominal pain

Imaging modality suggested	Suggested indications for this modality of imaging
CTAP without contrast	Anaphylactic contrast allergy Acute kidney injury or chronic kidney disease with GFR <30 Perforation highly suspected Ill patient with critical need for immediate diagnostic data Lack of IV access
CTAP with IV contrast	Infectious etiology suspected Obstruction suspected Graft-versus-host disease suspected with recent bone marrow transplant Gastrointestinal bleeding Vascular etiology suspected
CTAP with IV and oral contrast	Tolerating oral liquids and time to diagnosis less critical Suspect bowel inflammation or partial obstruction Multiple bowel resections (e.g., complex anatomy, bowel altering surgeries)
Magnetic resonance imaging (MRI)	Young patient, ionizing radiation of particular concern Pregnant patient Iodinated contrast allergy Tuberculosis risk factors High index of suspicion of serious intra-abdominal pathology with previous negative imaging
Ultrasound (US)	Biliary pathology suspected Pain localized to right upper quadrant Kidney stones suspected in patient <50 years old Young patient, ionizing radiation is of particular concern

J. B. Pierson (✉) · M. Clinton
Virginia Tech – Carilion Clinic, Department of Emergency Medicine, Roanoke, VA, USA
e-mail: jbpierson@carilionclinic.org

© Springer Nature Switzerland AG 2019
A. Graham, D. J. Carlberg (eds.), *Gastrointestinal Emergencies*, https://doi.org/10.1007/978-3-319-98343-1_112

Opportunistic Infections

Opportunistic infections often are associated with identifiable abnormalities on CT. These infections include disseminated mycobacterial disease, cytomegalovirus (CMV), typhlitis (neutropenic colitis), cryptosporidium, pseudomembranous colitis (PMC), and amebic colitis. One study revealed that 10% of HIV patients who presented to the ED with undifferentiated abdominal pain were diagnosed with an opportunistic infection [3]. Computed tomography is very good in identifying colonic wall thickening, pericolic stranding, and ascites [2, 4]. However, normal imaging does not fully exclude serious intra-abdominal pathology; up to 14% of patients with PMC and 8% of patients with CMV colitis have normal appearing CT scans [4]. Therefore, if a patient appears ill or if clinical gestalt suggests serious intra-abdominal pathology, admission or observation for serial examination and monitoring is appropriate. Further imaging with MRI may be required in the inpatient setting.

Obstruction

Bowel obstruction is most reliably detected by CTAP and can represent a complication of an incarcerated hernia, postsurgical adhesions, or cancer. Additionally, biliary obstruction should be considered in patient with jaundice, elevated total bilirubin, and right upper quadrant tenderness. Initial imaging for suspected biliary pathology should involve US with consideration of CT imaging if the US is nondiagnostic.

Abdominal Tuberculosis

Abdominal tuberculosis (TB) carries high morbidity and mortality and should be considered in HIV and immunocompromised patients presenting with abdominal complaints. This is especially important in endemic areas and in patients with specific risk factors for TB. Both CT and MRI may be used to diagnose abdominal TB with high sensitivity and specificity [5]. However, MRI provides better soft tissue resolution and improved detection of abdominal TB inflammation and lymphadenitis, which is the most common manifestation of abdominal TB. Adenopathy showing peripheral rim enhancement with relative low attenuation centers can suggest a diagnosis of tuberculosis in appropriate clinical settings. Administration of IV contrast improves detection of abdominal TB findings in both CT and MRI.

Graft-Versus-Host Disease

Graft-versus-host disease (GVHD) should be considered as a cause of abdominal pain in patients with a history of bone marrow transplant [4]. Evidence of GVHD on CT includes small bowel wall thickening, mesenteric stranding, ascites, large bowel thickening, or hepatic thrombosis. Veno-occlusive disease may occur in peripheral branches of hepatic veins obstructed by microthrombi in GVHD and produce a Budd-Chiari like syndrome. Duplex Doppler ultrasonography can detect hepatic venous flow abnormalities and heterogeneity of hepatic parenchyma in this condition [6].

Summary

A high index of suspicion for serious intra-abdominal pathology should be maintained in significantly immunocompromised patients with negative imaging. This is especially true in patients who present with a concerning history, symptoms, vital signs, abdominal examination, or laboratory values. It is highly recommended to consider admission or a prolonged ED observation period in these patients to allow for serial abdominal examinations, lab assessment, additional imaging, or specialty consultation as deemed necessary based on the patient's presentation and differential diagnoses (Fig. 112.1).

Fig. 112.1 Imaging algorithm for immunocompromised patients presenting to the emergency department with abdominal pain

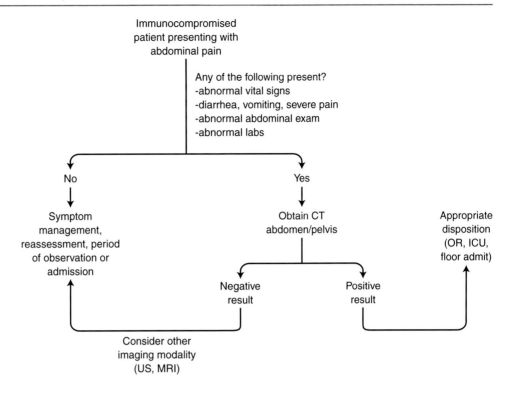

References

1. Abt PL, Abdullah I, Korenda K, Frank A, Peterman H, Stephenson GR, et al. Appendicitis among liver transplant recipients. Liver Transpl. 2005;11(10):1282–4.
2. Tonolini M, Bianco R. Acute HIV-related gastrointestinal disorders and complications in the antiretroviral era: spectrum of cross-sectional imaging findings. Abdom Imaging. 2013;38(5):994–1004.
3. Yoshida D, Caruso JM. Abdominal pain in the HIV infected patient. J Emerg Med. 2002;23(2):111–6.
4. Spencer SP, Power N, Reznek RH. Multidetector computed tomography of the acute abdomen in the immunocompromised host: a pictorial review. Curr Probl Diagn Radiol. 2009;38(4):145–55.
5. Joshi AR, Basantani AS, Patel TC. Role of CT and MRI in abdominal tuberculosis. Curr Radiol Rep. 2014;2:66.
6. Defalque D, Menu Y, Girard PM, Coulaud JP. Sonographic diagnosis of cholangitis in AIDS patients. Gastrointest Radiol. 1989;14(1):143–7.

Who Should Be Admitted? Who Can Be Discharged Safely and with What Instructions?

113

Timothy J. Fortuna and Zachary Shaub

Pearls and Pitfalls
- A large portion of the patients presenting to the emergency department with abdominal pain have some degree of immunosuppression.
- There are many opportunistic infections and iatrogenic complications of treatments that need to be considered, such as cytomegalovirus (CMV) colitis, mycobacterium avium complex (MAC) enteritis, typhlitis, peptic ulceration, pancreatitis, and iatrogenic complications from immunosuppressive therapies.
- Without a clear diagnosis, immunocompromised patients with abdominal pain should be admitted for serial abdominal exams and hemodynamic monitoring.
- The lack of reliable physical exam findings and laboratory markers make a discharge disposition more challenging in this patient population.

Abdominal pain was the most common complaint presenting to the emergency department (ED) based on data from the 2006 National Hospital Ambulatory Care Survey, and a subset of these patients are immunocompromised [1]. The immunocompromised population presents a truly difficult diagnostic dilemma. The "classic" symptoms and physical exam findings of abdominal pain are often absent. Laboratory studies that can typically be helpful in identifying pathology are unreliable in immunocompromised patients. These patients have a unique risk of diseases that are easily overlooked. The combination of a higher likelihood of serious pathology and the lack of reliable clinical signs and laboratory markers markedly increases the risk of morbidity and mortality for these patients. Thus, immunocompromised patients often require admission, unless there is a clear etiology for their abdominal pain that can be safely managed in an outpatient setting [2].

Immunocompromised patients can be immunosuppressed for a variety of reasons, and the extent of suppression can range from mild to severe (Table 113.1). Uncommon opportunistic infections and complications from immunomodulation therapies cause abdominal pain in this population and are not routinely considered in the immunocompetent host (Table 113.2). Because the signs, symptoms, and laboratory markers are unlikely to secure a diagnosis in this patient population, the emergency provider (EP) needs to aggressively consider adjunctive imaging to explore for serious pathology. The majority of immunocompromised patients will be candidates for either (or both) computed tomography (CT) or ultrasonography (US) to search for a diagnosis and guide therapy [3].

Table 113.1 Classification of immunocompromised patients

Mild to moderate immunosuppression
Diabetes
Systemic lupus erythematosus (SLE)
Elderly
HIV with CD4 count >200
Posttransplant on maintenance immunosuppressive therapy
Severe immunosuppression
HIV with CD4 count <200
Organ transplant within 60 days
Neutropenia
Medications
Steroids
Cyclosporin
Tacrolimus
Methotrexate

T. J. Fortuna (✉) · Z. Shaub
Virginia Tech Carilion School of Medicine, Department of Emergency Medicine, Roanoke, VA, USA
e-mail: tjfortuna@carilionclinic.org; zjshaub@carilionclinic.org

© Springer Nature Switzerland AG 2019
A. Graham, D. J. Carlberg (eds.), *Gastrointestinal Emergencies*, https://doi.org/10.1007/978-3-319-98343-1_113

Table 113.2 Causes of acute abdomen in the immunocompromised patient

Opportunistic infections	Pseudomembranous colitis Typhlitis (neutropenic colitis) Cytomegalovirus (CMV) Colitis/esophagitis/gastritis Mycobacterial enteritis *Cryptosporidium* gastritis AIDS-related cholangitis Hepatosplenic abscesses – pyogenic or fungal
Treatment-related conditions	Intestinal graft versus host disease (GVHD) Peptic ulceration – steroids, antimetabolite medications Pancreatitis – steroids Indinavir kidney stones – HIV Hepatic veno-occlusive disease – chemotherapeutic agents Exacerbation of pre-existing inflammatory bowel disease/diverticular disease post-radiotherapy
Complications of primary pathology (*may occur due to lymphadenopathy or AIDS-related neoplasms of the GI tract*)	Bowel obstruction/intussusception Gastrointestinal hemorrhage Biliary tract obstruction

Disposition

The majority of immunocompromised patients presenting to the ED with abdominal pain will be admitted. Even if a diagnosis is not attained in the ED, observation and serial examinations are often the prudent course of action. Any patient who is considered to be a potential candidate for discharge most certainly needs strong consideration of CT/US imaging prior to discharge. Abdominal CT should be performed with intravenous contrast if possible because it is helpful in identifying more unusual pathologies such as typhlitis and intra-abdominal abscesses. Typhlitis or neutropenic enterocolitis is a clinical syndrome in neutropenic patients characterized by fever and abdominal pain, most often in the right lower quadrant [4]. The condition is thought to arise due to a combination of mucosal injury (from leukemic infiltration or cytotoxic drugs), neutropenia, and impaired host defenses to intestinal bacteria [4]. Normal imaging decreases the likelihood of abdominal pathology but does not rule it out.

Discharge Criteria

If the exact etiology of the abdominal pain cannot be determined and the patient is otherwise stable (i.e., normal vital signs, well appearing), shared decision-making can be utilized to identify suitable patients for discharge with close follow-up.

- The patient must be involved in the decision to be discharged home and understand the increased risk given their immunocompromised state.
- All patients being considered for discharge should be able to tolerate liquids and have their nausea (if present) controlled.
- Every effort should be made to contact the patient's physician to ensure agreement on an outpatient plan of care and secure follow-up in an expeditious fashion. We would recommend the patient be re-evaluated within 24 h in these circumstances.

Unfortunately, the typical return precautions, given to the undifferentiated abdominal pain patient being discharged from the ED, are not reliable in the immune-suppressed patient. Indicators such as worsening pain, fever, chills, nausea, and vomiting may be absent, and therefore, a worsening clinical course can go unrecognized. Symptoms like nausea, vomiting, and malaise may already be present from their chemotherapy or other treatments. In the absence of a clear diagnosis or the patient being admitted for continued observation, strong consideration should be given to initiating broad-spectrum antibiotics until the patient is seen in follow-up [5].

Suggested Resources
- McKean J, Ronan-Bentle S. Abdominal pain in the immunocompromised patient—human immunodeficiency virus, transplant, cancer. Emerg Med Clin North Am. 2016;34(2):377–86.
- Spencer SP, Power N. The acute abdomen in the immune compromised host. Cancer Imaging. 2008;8(1):93–101.
- EM:RAP C3 HIV and AIDS – GI (Nov 2017: Chapter 4).

References

1. Pitts SR, Niska RW, Xu J, Burt CW. National hospital ambulatory medical care survey: 2006 emergency department summary. Natl Health Stat Rep. 2008;7:1–38.
2. Spencer SP, Power N. The acute abdomen in the immune compromised host. Cancer Imaging. 2008;8(1):93–101. https://doi.org/10.1102/1470-7330.2008.0013.
3. Chen EH, Mills AM. Abdominal pain in special populations. Emerg Med Clin North Am. 2011;29(2):449–58.
4. Urbach DR, Rotstein OD. Typhlitis. Can J Surg. 1999;42:415–9.
5. McKean J, Ronan-Bentle S. Abdominal pain in the immunocompromised patient—human immunodeficiency virus, transplant, cancer. Emerg Med Clin North Am. 2016;34(2):377–86.

Introduction to the Transplant Patient

114

Robert Loflin and Jack Perkins

Liver and kidney transplant patients presenting to the emergency department with abdominal pain offer unique challenges in diagnosis and management. In addition to the usual abdominal pathologies, the emergency provider must consider unusual causes of pain that stem from anatomical complications related to the transplant procedure itself, the intended and adverse effects of the immunosuppressive medication regimen, and organ rejection. Infection is very common, but presentation can be subtle. The risk of infection due to drug-resistant bacteria, as well as viruses, fungi, and parasites, is much higher in this population. The timing of presentation in relation to the date of transplant is critical to determine as this influences the key considerations in the differential and guides antimicrobial therapy. Finally, early communication with the patient's transplant team or surgeon is crucial to guide appropriate workup and disposition decisions (Table 114.1).

R. Loflin
University of Rochester Medical Center, Rochester, NY, USA
e-mail: Robert_Loflin@urmc.rochester.edu

J. Perkins (✉)
Virginia Tech Carilion School of Medicine, Roanoke, VA, USA
e-mail: jcperkins@carilionclinic.org

© Springer Nature Switzerland AG 2019
A. Graham, D. J. Carlberg (eds.), *Gastrointestinal Emergencies*, https://doi.org/10.1007/978-3-319-98343-1_114

Table 114.1 Common liver and kidney transplant medications and their potential adverse effects

Medication	Mechanism	Adverse effect
Cyclosporine (Sandimmune, generic)	Calcineurin inhibitor, decreasing T-lymphocyte activity and IL-2 function	Acute or chronic nephrotoxicity, electrolyte derangements (hyperkalemia, hypomagnesemia), gout, hemolytic-uremic syndrome, hirsutism, gingival hyperplasia, hypertension, hyperlipidemia
Tacrolimus (Prograf)	Calcineurin inhibitor, inhibiting T-lymphocyte activity and IL-2 function	Similar to cyclosporine above Neurotoxicity (headache, tremor, paresthesias, seizures), hyperkalemia, hair loss instead of hirsutism, less hypertension/hyperlipidemia, no gingival hyperplasia
Azathioprine (Imuran)	Block nucleotide production for immune cell replication	Bone marrow suppression, macrocytosis, anemia, hepatotoxicity, pancreatitis
Mycophenolate mofetil (CellCept)	Cytostatic effect on B and T cells, decreasing proliferation through inhibiting nucleotide synthesis	Abdominal pain, decreased oral intake, nausea, vomiting, diarrhea, anemia, leukopenia, thrombocytopenia
Corticosteroids	Impairs phagocyte function Attenuates production of proinflammatory mediators Decreases T-cell activity Decreases cell signal transduction	Weight gain, cataracts, acne, skin thinning, bruising, osteoporosis, GI bleeding, hyperglycemia, hyperlipidemia, psychologic effects, cushingoid appearance
Sirolimus (Rapamune)	Blocks mTOR receptor and immune cell signal transduction, reducing B- and T-cell activity	Thrombocytopenia, leukopenia/anemia (less common), hyperlipidemia, mucosal irritation, buccal ulceration, diarrhea, interstitial pneumonitis
Polyclonal antibodies (antithymocyte gamma globulin)	Antilymphocyte antibody Used for immunosuppression when nephrotoxic agent is held Used for treatment of corticosteroid-resistant rejection	Fever, serum sickness, anaphylaxis, anemia, thrombocytopenia
Monoclonal antibodies (OKT3, IL-2 receptor antibody)	Antilymphocyte antibody Used for prophylaxis against rejection in early period Used for immunosuppression when nephrotoxic agent is held Used for treatment of corticosteroid-resistant rejection	OKT3: during first 3 days of therapy-may have headache, aseptic meningitis, encephalopathy, seizures, nausea, vomiting, diarrhea, pulmonary edema, nephrotoxicity; after 3 days-low risk of adverse effects IL-2 receptor antibodies have rare adverse effects such as anaphylaxis

Adapted from Table 6 in Long B, Koyfman A. The emergency medicine approach to transplant complications. *Am J Emerg Med.* 2016. with automatic permission from Elsevier through the STM Signatory Guidelines

What Are the Unique Considerations
of Liver Transplant Patients
with Abdominal Pain?

115

Patrick Sandiford and Robert Loflin

Key Concepts/Pearls and Pitfalls
- Fever may indicate mechanical complications, graft rejection, as well as infection in the transplant patient.
- Time from transplant guides the choice of empiric antimicrobial therapy.
- Right upper quadrant ultrasound with Doppler is the best initial test to evaluate vascular complications.
- Cirrhosis can redevelop in transplanted patients based on prior cirrhosis etiology.
- Adverse effects of immunosuppressive drugs can mimic pathology.
- Early communication with the transplant surgeon is vital.

What Are the Unique Considerations of Liver Transplant Patients with Abdominal Pain?

Abdominal pain and fever are the most common complaints in liver transplant patients presenting to emergency departments. The majority of these patients are ultimately diagnosed with an infection or gastrointestinal/genitourinary etiology [1–3]. In addition to the usual concerns in abdominal pain patients, liver transplant patients have distinct

P. Sandiford
Emergency Medicine Residency, University of Rochester Medical Center, Rochester, NY, USA

R. Loflin (✉)
University of Rochester Medical Center, Rochester, NY, USA
e-mail: Robert_Loflin@urmc.rochester.edu

diagnostic issues: (1) subtle infectious presentations, (2) unique anatomic complications arising from the transplant procedure itself, (3) graft rejection, and (4) adverse immunosuppressive medication effects.

Subtle Infectious Presentations

Infection is common in liver transplant patients. The likelihood of a particular pathogen is related to the time from transplantation and degree of immunosuppression (Table 115.1). Unfortunately, fever and leukocytosis cannot be relied upon to herald infection as they may be absent in up to half of transplant patients with serious infections [2]. In addition to blood and urine cultures, further diagnostic testing should be directed by the patient's presentation, postsurgical complications, state of immunosuppression, and elapsed time since orthotopic liver transplantation (OLT).

During the first 6 months posttransplantation, empiric antibiotics target Gram-positive organisms, Gram-negative organisms including *P. aeruginosa*, and anaerobic organisms. For example, vancomycin in combination with piperacillin/tazobactam or cefepime and metronidazole, are reasonable empiric antibiotic regimens. The addition of an echinocandin, such as caspofungin, may be considered for antifungal coverage. Suspicion for nosocomial, resistant organisms (e.g., VRE, MRSA, or ESBL) and viral, fungal, and parasitic infections is important, and treatment may be expanded based on these suspicions [4, 5]. In patients with a remote history of OLT, community-acquired infections emerge, and typical targeted antibiotic therapy is appropriate. Obtaining and reviewing the patient's prior culture data, consulting institutional antibiograms for local antimicrobial sensitivities, and consultation with infectious disease are recommended if available.

A. Graham, D. J. Carlberg (eds.), *Gastrointestinal Emergencies*, https://doi.org/10.1007/978-3-319-98343-1_115

Table 115.1 Potential infectious etiologies in reference to time from transplant [7]

Transplant period	Infection	
Early <30 days posttransplant	*Donor derived*	MRSA (methicillin-resistant *Staph aureus*) VRE (vancomycin-resistant *Enterococcus*) Tuberculosis Fungi (Candida) Parasitic (toxoplasmosis, Chagas disease)
	Nosocomial/ surgery related	Aspiration pneumonia Surgical site infection (SSI) Urinary tract infection Superinfection of graft tissue Vascular access infection Clostridium difficile colitis
Intermediate 1–6 months posttransplant	*Opportunistic infections (highest risk)*	*Pneumocystis jirovecii* Histoplasma *Coccidioides* *Cryptococcus* Hepatitis B/C BK Polyomavirus Kaposi sarcoma *Cytomegalovirus* (CMV) Tuberculosis Epstein-Barr virus (EBV)
	Surgery related	Surgical site infections
	Reactivation of dormant host infections	CMV Herpes zoster virus EBV
Late >6 months posttransplant	*Community- acquired infections*	Respiratory viruses Pneumococcus *Legionella* Listeria Influenza EBV

Unique Anatomic Complications

During an orthotopic liver transplant, there are five key anastomoses performed – suprahepatic IVC, infrahepatic IVC, hepatic artery, portal vein, and bile duct – and pathology can arise directly or indirectly from these areas [6].

- Vascular complications include thrombosis and stenosis of the vascular anastomoses; most importantly hepatic artery thrombosis (HAT) and portal vein thrombosis (PVT). Hepatic artery thrombosis occurs in 5–10% of recipients, leading to graft necrosis, gangrene, and biliary leaks/strictures/biliomas. The best initial diagnostic test is a right upper quadrant ultrasound (RUQ U/S) with Doppler to evaluate the patency of the hepatic artery, hepatic vein, and portal veins.
- Biliary complications include obstruction due to strictures, stones or sludge, as well as leaks and fluid collections. Biliary strictures develop in 10–30% of liver transplantations and should be included in the differential

for patients with graft dysfunction. Studies such as ERCP, MRCP, T-tube studies, or percutaneous transhepatic cholangiogram may be necessary to diagnose and treat biliary strictures, while CT imaging can be used to evaluate for fluid collections and guide percutaneous drainage, if necessary [6] (Table 115.2).

Graft Rejection

Graft rejection is an immune-mediated process and is a serious concern after liver transplantation. Acute rejection occurs in the first 6 months, usually in the first 2 weeks. It may present with nonspecific symptoms that include weakness, jaundice, RUQ pain, and fever or may be asymptomatic with only a mild elevation in the transaminases. Chronic rejection presents similarly but occurs months to years after transplantation. The definitive test for diagnosis of rejection is liver biopsy [6, 7]. LFTs, fractionated bilirubin, and RUQ U/S with Doppler are included in the initial workup.

Adverse Effects from Immunosuppressive Medications

To minimize the risk of graft rejection, all patients receive immunosuppressive therapy. Unfortunately, this results in an increased susceptibility to infection and the potential for adverse drug effects. Epstein-Barr virus-induced posttransplant lymphoproliferative disease (PTLD) is due to the uninhibited growth of EBV-infected B cells with therapeutic immunosuppression after organ transplantation [8]. Its incidence ranges from 3% to 12% in liver transplant patients and presents with fevers, weight loss, cervical lymphadenopathy, pharyngitis, hepatospenomegaly, atypical lymphocytosis, as well organ-specific symptoms, such as hepatitis, pneumonitis, and gastrointestinal symptoms [8]. In liver transplant patients, it is often localized to the liver [8]. Biopsy is the gold standard for diagnosis, but computed tomography can aid in making the initial diagnosis. Treatment begins with reducing immunosuppression.

The most common medications used in liver transplant are tacrolimus (Prograf), cyclosporine (Neoral, Gengraf), mycophenolate mofetil (CellCept, Myfortic), and prednisone. Mycophenolate mofetil is known to cause abdominal pain, nausea, vomiting, and diarrhea, which may lead to poor oral intake and dehydration [9]. Tacrolimus is known to cause hyperglycemia and new-onset diabetes as well as metabolic derangements, such as hyperkalemia and hypomagnesemia, that may contribute to gastrointestinal symptoms in transplant patients. The clinician should inquire about the specific immunosuppressive medications and recent changes to the regimen, as well as any prophylactic antimicrobials (e.g., TMP/SMX),

Table 115.2 Unique causes of abdominal pain in the liver transplant recipient [10]

Diagnosis	Timing	Signs/symptoms	Laboratory tests	Diagnostic Imaging
Hepatic artery thrombosis (HAT)	Most common in first month but anytime in association with rejection	RUQ pain, high fever, jaundice; may progress to liver failure rapidly	Elevated AST/ALT, TB, prolonged INR	1. RUQ Doppler U/S: evaluate artery flow, bile ducts, liver abscess, infarction 2. Equivocal presentation: arteriography
Portal vein thrombosis (PVT)	Most common in first month but anytime in association with rejection	Hematemesis (variceal bleed), abdominal pain, ascites	Nonspecific liver test abnormalities; rarely high liver enzymes	1. RUQ Doppler U/S 2. If positive or negative with high suspicion: arteriography with portal venous phase
Biliary obstruction/ stricture	Anytime, often after T-tube removal	Nonspecific to cholangitis (high fever, jaundice, sepsis); often no abdominal pain	High TB, AP, GGT Less common: elevations in AST/ALT	1. RUQ Doppler U/S: exclude HAT, evaluate bile duct dilation 2. T-tube cholangiogram 3. ERCP or PTC
Biliary leak	Anytime	Abdominal pain, fever, often peritonitis	Nonspecific liver test abnormalities	1. RUQ Doppler U/S 2. Spiral CT
Acute rejection	In first 6 months, especially first 2 weeks, but can occur anytime	Typically, low-grade fever, malaise, jaundice, RUQ pain; sometimes asymptomatic	Early: high AP, GGT; mild AST/ALT Severe: high AST/ALT (usually <1000) and TB	1. RUQ Doppler U/S; exclude HAT, biliary obstruction 2. Liver biopsy
Chronic rejection	Usually >3–6 months after transplant	Generalized abdominal pain, malaise, fevers, diarrhea, progressive jaundice, clay-colored stools, dark urine	Persistently elevated AST/ALT, TB, and prolonged INR	1. RUQ Doppler U/S; exclude HAT, biliary obstruction 2. Liver biopsy

Adapted from Levitsky and Cohen [10]. Permission automatically granted by Elsevier through the STM signatory guidelines
RUQ right upper quadrant, *CT* computed tomography, *AST* aspartate aminotransferase, *ALT* alanine aminotransferase, *TB* total bilirubin, *AP* alkaline phosphatase, *GGT* gamma-glutamyl transferase, *INR* international normalized ratio, *U/S* ultrasound, *ERCP* endoscopic retrograde cholangiopancreatography, *PTC* percutaneous transhepatic cholangiogram

antifungals (e.g., fluconazole), and antivirals (e.g., acyclovir) prescribed. Consultation with an ED pharmacist, if available, is helpful to avoid drug-drug interactions.

Summary

Liver transplant patients presenting to the ED with abdominal pain often require extensive diagnostic testing and hospital admission for complete workup [1–3]. In all cases, early communication with the patient's transplant team or surgeon is crucial to guide appropriate workup and safe disposition.

Suggested Resources

- http://www.emdocs.net/transplant-emergencies-part-i-infection-rejection-and-medication-effects/.
- http://www.emdocs.net/transplant-emergencies-part-ii-organ-specific-complications/.
- http://epmonthly.com/article/fear-rejection-managing-transplant-patient-ed/.

References

1. Turtay MG, Oguzturk H, Aydin C, Colak C, Isik B, Yilmaz S. A descriptive analysis of 188 liver transplant visits to an emergency department. Eur Rev Med Pharmacol Sci. 2012;16(Suppl 1):3–7.
2. Savitsky EA, Votey SR, Mebust DP, Schwartz E, Uner AB, McCain S. A descriptive analysis of 290 liver transplant patient visits to an emergency department. Acad Emerg Med. 2000;7:898–905.
3. Unterman S, Zimmerman M, Tyo C, Sterk E, Gehm L, Edison M, Benedetti E, Orsay EM. A descriptive analysis of 1251 solid organ transplant visits to the emergency department. West J Emerg Med. 2009;10:48–54.
4. Trzeciak S, Sharer R, Piper D, Chan T, Kessler C, Dellinger RP, et al. Infections and severe sepsis in solid-organ transplant patients admitted from a university-based ED. Am J Emerg Med. 2004;22:530–3.
5. O'Shea DT, Humar A. Life-threatening infection in transplant recipients. Crit Care Clin. 2013;29(4):953–73.
6. Savitsky EA, Uner AB, Votey SR. Evaluation of orthotopic liver transplant recipients presenting to the emergency department. Ann Emerg Med. 1998;31:507–17.
7. Long B, Koyfman A. The emergency medicine approach to transplant complications. Am J Emerg Med. 2016;34:2200–8.
8. Nijland ML, Kersten MJ, Pals ST, Bemelman FJ, Ten Berge IJ. Epstein-Barr virus–positive posttransplant lymphoproliferative disease after solid organ transplantation: pathogenesis, clinical manifestations, diagnosis, and management. Transplant Direct. 2015;2(1):e48. https://doi.org/10.1097/TXD.0000000000000557.
9. Moini M, Schilsky ML, Tichy EM. Review on immunosuppression in liver transplantation. World J Hepatol. 2015;7(10):1355–68.
10. Levitsky J, Cohen SM. The liver transplant recipient: what you need to know for long-term care. J Fam Pract. 2006;55:136–44.

What Are the Unique Considerations in Renal Transplant Patients with Abdominal Pain?

116

Kenneth Potter and Jordan B. Schooler

Pearls and Pitfalls
- Mortality and morbidity related to renal transplants are relatively uncommon.
- Maintain a broad differential for abdominal pain in these patients. The transplant may not be the issue.
- Acute kidney injury or oliguria should be evaluated by Doppler ultrasound.
- Immunosuppression may alter presentations and directly cause complications.
- Intravenous contrast may be used in transplanted kidneys, if otherwise indicated.

Since the advent of renal transplantation in 1954, outcomes have steadily improved. The risk of death in the first year after transplant is now as low as 3% [1]. Graft loss in the first year has decreased to 7–12%, depending on whether the transplant was from a living or deceased donor [2]. While acute rejection still occurs in 24% in the first year, the half-life of a transplanted kidney has increased to 19.5 years (cadaveric) or 35.9 years (living). This suggests that many presentations of abdominal pain in the renal transplant patient will be unrelated to the transplant itself. Accordingly, the differential diagnosis for these patients ought to include many of the same diseases as in other patients.

Nevertheless, diagnosis of abdominal pain may be uniquely challenging in the setting of a renal transplant. Immunosuppression may mask symptoms. It also increases the risk of both infectious complications and other medication-related effects. The prevalence of transplant-related complications varies with time from transplant [3, 4].

< 1 Month Post-transplant

The early postoperative period (up to 1 month) will be dominated by surgical complications and hospital-acquired infections. Surgical complications may be vascular, such as graft torsion, renal artery thrombosis, or renal vein thrombosis. These presentations may be painless since the graft is not innervated, and sudden oliguria may be the only sign. Duplex ultrasound of the renal transplant is the best initial imaging modality [5, 6]. Urological complications include anastomotic leak of the ureter and subsequent potential formation of urinoma. This occurs in 1–6.5% of patients and may present with pain, oliguria, or acute kidney injury (AKI) [6]. While a fluid collection may be seen on ultrasound, discriminating between a seroma, hematoma, or lymphocele will usually require sampling of fluid or contrast-enhanced computed tomography (CT) or magnetic resonance imaging (MRI). Early consultation of the transplant team is recommended for any suspected surgical complication.

Infections in the first month are usually hospital acquired and related to the wound, catheters, or other devices [3, 7]. Empiric antimicrobial coverage should incorporate consideration of the potential for methicillin-resistant *Staphylococcus aureus*, vancomycin-resistant *Enterococcus*, and *Candida* species. Viral infections may be transmitted from the donor even though rigorous screening is performed prior to transplant. Rare viral infections such as lymphocytic choriomeningitis, rabies, and West Nile have been reported [3].

> 1 Month Post-transplant

Transplant renal artery stenosis is the most frequent complication overall, usually seen between 3 months and 3 years after transplant [5, 8]. This is found in 1–25% of patients and

K. Potter
Department of Anesthesiology and Perioperative Medicine, Penn State Hershey Medical Center, Hershey, PA, USA
e-mail: kpotter@pennstatehealth.psu.edu

J. B. Schooler (✉)
Department of Anesthesiology and Perioperative Medicine, Penn State Hershey Medical Center, Hershey, PA, USA

Department of Emergency Medicine, Penn State Hershey Medical Center, Hershey, PA, USA
e-mail: jschooler@pennstatehealth.psu.edu

© Springer Nature Switzerland AG 2019
A. Graham, D. J. Carlberg (eds.), *Gastrointestinal Emergencies*, https://doi.org/10.1007/978-3-319-98343-1_116

often presents as graft dysfunction (oliguria or AKI) and refractory hypertension. Ultrasound is the initial imaging modality of choice, but the transplant team should be consulted as acute or chronic rejection can present identically. Other surgical complications in this late period include renal artery aneurysm, ureteral obstruction, or stricture. Ureteral stricture occurs in 2–10% of patients and presents as painless AKI or colicky pain [5, 8].

Infections in the intermediate postoperative period (1 month to 1 year) vary depending on the use of prophylaxis for opportunistic pathogens such as cytomegalovirus (CMV) and PJP. If prophylaxis is given, other viral species such as adenovirus and polyomavirus BK are more frequent. *Cryptococcus*, hepatitis C virus, tuberculosis, and *Clostridium difficile* may also be seen [3].

> 6 Months Post-transplant

After 6 months, immunosuppression regimes are usually stable, and lower doses are employed; consequently, opportunistic infections are more uncommon. Most infections are therefore community acquired [3]. Long-term immunosuppression use itself may cause abdominal pain. Pancreatitis and biliary calculi have been observed with immunosuppression [4]. Mycophenolate is associated with perforated jejunal diverticula [9]. Posttransplant lymphoproliferative disorder (PTLD) is a form of lymphoma occurring in 0.8–2.5% of renal transplant recipients [10]. The pathogenesis is often related to Epstein-Barr virus. The presentation is quite varied and may include constitutional symptoms, single organ failure, or multiple organ failure.

Diagnostic Evaluation

As with the non-transplant patient, the evaluation of abdominal pain should be guided first and foremost by the history and physical exam. Laboratory studies should at the very least include a urinalysis, complete blood count, a basic metabolic panel, liver function tests, and consideration of immunosuppressive medication levels if applicable. Immunosuppression may mask typical responses to infection, and so the threshold for imaging should be lowered. Computed tomography is a highly useful modality. If indicated, intravenous contrast is likely safe in transplant patients with normal renal function [11, 12]. A substantial body of evidence has emerged in the recent years suggesting that contrast nephropathy is an epiphenomenon, with contrast causing a temporary increase in creatinine but no actual renal damage or increased rate of long-term renal failure [13–15]. However, this remains controversial, and at present, it may be wise to avoid contrast administration in patients with reduced renal function unless urgently indicated, such as for suspicion of active bleeding.

Suggested Resources
- Lopez-Ruiz A, Chandrashekar K, Juncos LA. Changing paradigms in contrast nephropathy. J Am Soc Nephrol. 2017;28:397–9.
- Moreno CC, Mittal PK, Ghonge NP, et al. Imaging complications of renal transplantation. Radiol Clin N Am. 2016;54:235–49.

References

1. Farrugia D, Cheshire J, Begaj I, Khosla S, Ray D, Sharif A. Death within the first year after kidney transplantation--an observational cohort study. Transpl Int. 2014;27:262–70.
2. Hariharan S, Johnson CP, Bresnahan BA, Taranto SE, McIntosh MJ, Stablein D. Improved graft survival after renal transplantation in the United States, 1988 to 1996. N Engl J Med. 2000;342:605–12.
3. Fishman JA. Infection in solid-organ transplant recipients. N Engl J Med. 2007;357:2601–14.
4. Fontana F, Gianni C. Acute pancreatitis associated with everolimus after kidney transplantation: a case report. BMC Nephrol. 2016;17:163–6.
5. Haberal M, Boyvat F, Akdur A, Kirnap M, Özçelik Ü, Yarbuğ KF. Surgical complications after kidney transplantation. Exp Clin Transplant. 2016;14:587–95.
6. Moreno CC, Mittal PK, Ghonge NP, Bhargava P, Heller MT. Imaging complications of renal transplantation. Radiol Clin N Am. 2016;54:235–49.
7. Briggs JD. Causes of death after renal transplantation. Nephrol Dial Transplant. 2001;16:1545–9.
8. Dimitroulis D, Bokos J, Zavos G, Nikiteas N, Karidis NP, Katsaronis P, et al. Vascular complications in renal transplantation: a single-center experience in 1367 renal transplantations and review of the literature. Transplant Proc. 2009;41:1609–14.
9. Thongprayoon C, Cheungpasitporn W, Edmonds PJ, Thamcharoen N. Perforated jejunal diverticulum in the use of mycophenolate mofetil. N Am J Med Sci. 2014;6:599–600.
10. Dierickx D, Habermann TM. Post-transplantation lymphoproliferative disorders in adults. N Engl J Med. 2018;378:549–62.
11. Cheungpasitporn W, Thongprayoon C, Mao MA, Mao SA, D'Costa MR, Kittanamongkolchai W, et al. Contrast-induced acute kidney injury in kidney transplant recipients: a systematic review and meta-analysis. World J Transplant. 2017;7(1):81–8.
12. Haider M, Yessayan L, Venkat KK, Goggins M, Patel A, Karthikeyan V. Incidence of contrast-induced nephropathy in kidney transplant recipients. Transplant Proc. 2015;47:379–83.
13. Wilhelm-Leen E, Montez-Rath ME, Chertow G. Estimating the risk of radiocontrast-associated nephropathy. J Am Soc Nephrol. 2017;28:653–9.
14. McDonald RJ, McDonald JS, Carter RE, Hartman RP, Katzberg RW, Kallmes DF, et al. Intravenous contrast material exposure is not an independent risk factor for dialysis or mortality. Radiology. 2014;273:714–25.
15. Hinson JS, Ehmann MR, Fine DM, Fishman EK, Toerper MF, Rothman RE, et al. Risk of acute kidney injury after intravenous contrast media administration. Ann Emerg Med. 2017;69:577–586.e4.

What Clinicians Should Consider When Evaluating the Cancer Patient with Abdominal Pain?

Karin Chase

Pearls and Pitfalls
- Abdominal pain, ascites, and early satiety may be the initial presenting symptoms of a malignancy.
- Up to 50% of patients with undiagnosed cancer present with ascites.
- Malignant bowel obstruction occurs in 3% of cancer patients.
- Neutropenic enterocolitis (typhlitis) is more commonly seen in patients with hematologic malignancies who have profound neutropenia from chemotherapy.

Table 117.1 Causes of abdominal pain in the cancer patient

Direct complications due to the malignant lesion	Complications secondary to treatment of the cancer
Malignant bowel obstruction	Radiation enteritis
Intestinal perforation	Neutropenic enterocolitis
Malignant ascites	Procedural complications
Budd-Chiari syndrome	Medication side effects
Mass effect from malignant lesion	

Up to 40% of patients with malignancy will present to the emergency department (ED) with abdominal pain [1]. It is important to ascertain the type of malignancy, the presence or absence of metastases, and what current or prior treatments the patient has undergone. It is also possible that abdominal pain may be the presenting symptom of a new cancer diagnosis.

When evaluating the patient with abdominal pain and known malignancy, your differential diagnosis can be divided into direct complications from the malignancy and indirect complications secondary to the treatment of the malignancy (Table 117.1).

Direct Complications

Malignant Bowel Obstruction

Malignant bowel obstruction (MBO) is a common cause of morbidity and mortality in cancer patients. It occurs in approximately 3% of cancer patients [2, 3]. This diagnosis is confirmed by evidence of bowel obstruction secondary to either an intra-abdominal primary tumor or a non-intra-abdominal primary tumor with clear intraperitoneal disease [2]. Patients with colon cancer have the highest incidence (25–40%) of MBO, followed by ovarian (16–29%) and gastric cancer (6–19%) [3]. Management of these patients can include medical, surgical, and palliative approaches. In the ED, treatment should focus on symptom control with analgesics and antiemetics, gastrointestinal decompression (e.g., nasogastric tube), and a surgical consultation.

Abdominal Perforations

Abdominal perforations occur by a number of different mechanisms in patients with cancer. Malignant bowel obstruction, tumor erosion, and atypical infections can all lead to devastating consequences [1]. Computed tomography (CT) is the imaging modality of choice if perforation is suspected. Once diagnosed, urgent administration of broad-spectrum antibiotics and a surgical consultation should be initiated. The patient may require more aggressive care while in the ED including IV fluid resuscitation and vasopressor support.

K. Chase
University of Rochester Medical Center, Rochester, NY, USA
e-mail: Karin_chase@URMC.rochester.edu

© Springer Nature Switzerland AG 2019
A. Graham, D. J. Carlberg (eds.), *Gastrointestinal Emergencies*, https://doi.org/10.1007/978-3-319-98343-1_117

Malignant Ascites

Malignant ascites is often the first sign of a malignant intra-abdominal process [4]. Up to 50% of patients with undiagnosed cancer present in this fashion. Concerning signs and symptoms include increasing abdominal girth, pain, bloating, anorexia, and weight loss. Ultrasound at bedside or CT can be used to detect the presence of ascitic fluid. A diagnostic paracentesis evaluates for infection as well as cytologic examination. Ovarian cancer is the most common malignancy to cause ascites and occurs in up to 37% of such patients. Pancreatobiliary, endometrial, breast, gastric, esophageal, and colorectal cancers can also be complicated by ascites [1, 4]. A rare cause of ascites is Budd-Chiari syndrome (BCS). While BCS is often secondary to hypercoagulable states, malignant tumor invasion has been identified as a rare cause. Pathophysiology includes obstruction of the hepatic venous outflow tract leading to hepatocyte necrosis and cirrhosis of the liver [5]. In addition to ascites, these patients present with signs of hepatic necrosis, abdominal pain, and hepatosplenomegaly. In fulminant cases, the patient can progress to liver failure [5].

Indirect Complications

During the work-up and treatment for their malignancy, patients may undergo invasive testing, procedural interventions, chemotherapy, and radiation. It is imperative to know whether your patient is immunosuppressed as this subjects them to a wide variety of complications, most of which are infectious.

Neutropenic Enterocolitis

Neutropenic enterocolitis (typhlitis) is more commonly seen in patients with hematologic malignancies who have profound neutropenia from chemotherapy. The pathogenesis is not precisely known but involves mucosal injury thought to be due to the combination of cytotoxic drugs and concurrent impaired host defenses, leading to invasion of the bowel wall with microorganisms. This infectious catastrophe may lead to bowel wall necrosis and can be life-threatening. In fact, the mortality can be as high as 50% [1, 6, 7]. Patients often present with abdominal pain, fever, and neutropenia. Emergent CT imaging can be helpful, but imaging should not delay broad-spectrum antibiotics covering gram-positive, gram-negative, and anaerobic organisms. Fungal coverage is recommended only if clinical

improvement does not occur within 72 h of antibiotic initiation [6]. In addition to aggressive fluid resuscitation and antibiotics, blood cultures, stool cultures, and *Clostridium difficile* toxin testing should be included in the work-up of these patients. Strict bowel rest is also an important component of treatment.

Radiation Injury

Roughly 70% of all cancer patients receive radiotherapy during the course of their disease, and ionizing radiation injury to the GI tract is a frequent side effect. Radiation injury can present acutely due to mucosal injury and inflammation or months later due to fibrosis and sclerosis [8]. Patients with gynecologic and urologic cancers are particularly susceptible to radiation enteritis because the greatest volume of bowel is located in the pelvis where the radiation is directed [1]. Severe mucositis and radiation-induced enteritis can lead to fever, diarrhea, abdominal pain, dehydration, and severe malnutrition [9, 10].

Invasive Procedures

Invasive procedures including biopsies, endoscopy, colonoscopy, and stenting can lead to complications in the cancer patient presenting as abdominal pain. Perforation, stent migration, bleeding, or infection may occur. A careful history and physical exam can help guide your work- up as timing of these procedures is important when considering potential complications.

Suggested Resources
- Ilgen J, Marr A. Cancer emergencies: the acute abdomen. Emerg Med Clin N Am. 2009;27:381–99.
- Vehreschild M, et al. Diagnosis and management of gastrointestinal complications in adult cancer patients: evidence-based guidelines of the Infectious Diseases working Party (AGIHO) of the German Society of Hematology and Oncology (DGHO). Ann Oncol. 2013;24:1189–202.

References

1. Ilgen J, Marr A. Cancer emergencies: the acute abdomen. Emerg Med Clin N Am. 2009;27:381–99.
2. Alese O, Kim S, Chen Z, Owonikoko T, El-Rayes B. Management patterns and predictors of mortality among US patients with

cancer hospitalized for malignant bowel obstruction. Cancer. 2015;121:1772–8.

3. Hirst B, Regnard C. Management of intestinal obstruction in malignant disease. Clin Med. 2003;3:311–4.

4. Adam R, Adam Y. Malignant ascites: past, present, and future. J Am Coll Surg. 2004;198(6):999–1011.

5. Menon K, Shah V, Kamath P. The Budd-Chiari syndrome. N Engl J Med. 2001;350:578–85.

6. Rodrigues F, Dasilva G, Wexner S. Neutropenic enterocolitis. World J Gastroenterol. 2017;23(1):42–7.

7. Vehreschild M, Vehreschild K, Hubel M, Hentrich M, Schmidt-Hieber M, Christopeit M, et al. Diagnosis and management of gastrointestinal complications in adult cancer patients: evidence-based guidelines of the Infectious Diseases working Party (AGIHO) of the German Society of Hematology and Oncology (DGHO). Ann Oncol. 2013;24(5):1189–202.

8. Shadad A, Sullivan F, Martin J, Egan L. Gastrointestinal radiation injury: prevention and treatment. World J Gastroenterol. 2013;19(2):199–208.

9. Grabenbauer G. Management of radiation and chemotherapy related acute toxicity in gastrointestinal cancer. Best Pract Res Clin Gastroenterol. 2016;30:655–64.

10. Shadad A, Sullivan F, Martin J, Egan L. Gastrointestinal radiation injury: symptoms, risk factors and mechanisms. World J Gastroenterol. 2013;19(2):185–98.

Can I Do a Rectal Exam in a Neutropenic Patient?

Chad Mosby and Matthew P. Borloz

Pearls and Pitfalls
- Patients with neutropenia have <1.5 × 10^9 neutrophils/L, while severe neutropenia indicates <0.5 × 10^9 neutrophils/L, exposing the patient to increased risk of infection
- The conventional recommendation for decades has been to avoid DRE in neutropenic patients, but no research exists to support this recommendation
- While there are many indications for DRE, many of these indications can be investigated through imaging studies that do not present the same potential risk
- Among febrile neutropenic patients, DRE may be considered to identify an anorectal infection when alternate sources have been excluded and other testing is not readily available

Neutropenia is defined as a neutrophil count less than 1.5 × 10^9 cells/liter (L), while severe neutropenia describes a neutrophil count less than 0.5 × 10^9 cells/L [1]. Most commonly caused by cytotoxic drugs, it may also be present following irradiation and in acute leukemias, among other conditions [2]. The neutropenic state leads to an increased risk for a variety of infectious diseases (particularly bacterial and fungal) and decreases resistance to infection during invasive procedures or with rectal manipulation. Severe neutropenia (<0.5 × 10^9 neutrophils/L) raises the risk even higher [3]. This concern spawned a long-standing recommendation to avoid digital rectal exam (DRE) in this population.

Most consensus recommendations advise against performing DRE in neutropenic patients, with frequent mention of possible bacterial translocation (specifically Gram-negative bacteria) into the bloodstream with manipulation of the rectum. While this theoretical concern is reasonable, the literature is silent on the true risk posed by DRE in neutropenic patients. A 2009 guideline, cosponsored by multiple national and international organizations, such as the American Society for Blood and Marrow Transplant (ASBMT), the Infectious Diseases Society of America (IDSA), and the Centers for Disease Control and Prevention (CDC), states that "the use of rectal thermometers, enemas, or suppositories; internal rectal exams; and sexual practices involving anal penetration are contraindicated among [neutropenic patients] to avoid skin or mucosal breakdown, which can introduce pathogens" [4]. This is labeled a DIII recommendation, indicating "moderate evidence…for adverse outcome supports a recommendation against use," where that evidence is "from opinions of respected authorities based on clinical experience, descriptive studies, or reports of expert committees" [4, 5]. Of note, no societies have published guidelines refuting this recommendation; however, the colorectal surgery literature provides scant evidence that operative management of anorectal disease among patients with severe neutropenia does not worsen outcome [6]. Another small study in the surgical literature cited a 7% rate of bacteremia due to digital exam or instrumentation of the rectum among neutropenic patients [7].

Given the lack of evidence directly addressing whether DRE leads to bacterial translocation, the endoscopy literature was consulted. Interestingly, there are few recommendations regarding lower gastrointestinal (GI) endoscopy in neutropenic patients, which exposes the patient to more extensive mucosal trauma than DRE, and presumably has a corresponding increased risk of bacterial translocation. The American Society for Gastrointestinal Endoscopy (ASGE) notes there is "insufficient evidence to recommend for or against administration of antibiotic prophylaxis before routine endoscopic procedures in patients with severe [neutropenia]… so the decision to use antibiotic prophylaxis in these scenarios must be individualized." [8] Additionally, the Infectious Diseases Society of America does not provide

C. Mosby · M. P. Borloz (✉)
Virginia Tech Carilion School of Medicine, Department of Emergency Medicine, Roanoke, VA, USA
e-mail: cwmosby@carilionclinic.org; mpborloz@carilionclinic.org

© Springer Nature Switzerland AG 2019
A. Graham, D. J. Carlberg (eds.), *Gastrointestinal Emergencies*, https://doi.org/10.1007/978-3-319-98343-1_118

recommendations for or against endoscopy in neutropenic patients.

When treating immunocompetent patients, DRE provides a quick and inexpensive way to evaluate for anorectal pathology, prostatic abnormalities, fecal impaction, and neurologic deficits, among other findings. Additionally, rectal temperatures are favored to temporal, otic, or oral measurements in certain situations, as they provide more accurate results. With respect to neutropenic patients, DRE may help identify anorectal infections, as neutropenic patients are more susceptible to these infections and their attendant morbidity and mortality [6].

Recommendations regarding DRE for neutropenic patients with fever or suspected anorectal infectious conditions are variable. Some experts advise against it due to concern for mucosal trauma and subsequent bacteremia [9], while others assert that the "rectal exam should not be neglected and invasive procedures must be undertaken with the appropriate consideration of the risk of bacterial translocation and disease worsening" [10]. Unfortunately, neither camp is supported by conclusive literature. An accurate and early diagnosis in neutropenic patients with anorectal infectious conditions is particularly important to facilitate prompt antibiotic therapy and, sometimes, source control with operative intervention [6].

While a certain diagnosis is essential in many of the above instances, DRE is but one of many available tools. Most of the relevant conditions may be identified using methods other than DRE, whether by simple visual inspection of the anus or cross-sectional imaging through the pelvis with computed tomography (CT) or magnetic resonance imaging (MRI). Specific to the concern for anorectal infections, CT is readily available in the ED and may be helpful to evaluate the extent of the infection and the presence of a drainable abscess. Additionally, rectal temperatures, which likely confer risks similar to DRE, provide information that can often be obtained through less invasive means. Despite the lack of conclusive evidence demonstrating harm from DRE in neutropenic patients, alternative diagnostic approaches that pose minimal risk are available in most settings.

Final Summary

The conventional recommendation for decades has been to avoid DRE in neutropenic patients, but no research exists to support this recommendation. While there are many indications for DRE, many of these indications can be investigated through imaging studies that do not present the same potential risk as DRE.

References

1. Hsieh MM, Everhart JE, Byrd-Holt DD, Tisdale JF, Rodgers GP. Prevalence of neutropenia in the U.S. population: age, sex, smoking status, and ethnic differences. Ann Intern Med. 2007;146:486–92.
2. Schouten HC. Neutropenia management. Ann Oncol. 2006;17(Suppl 10):x85–9.
3. Dale D, Welte K. Neutropenia and neutrophilia. In: Kaushansky K, Lichtman M, Prchal J, Levi M, Press O, Burns L, et al., editors. Williams hematology. 9th ed. New York: McGraw-Hill; 2016. p. 991–1004.
4. Tomblyn M, Chiller T, Einsele H, Gress R, Sepkowitz K, Storek J, et al. Guidelines for preventing infectious complications among hematopoietic cell transplantation recipients: a global perspective. Biol Blood Marrow Transplant. 2009;15:1143–238.
5. Freifeld AG, Bow EJ, Sepkowitz KA, Boeckh MJ, Ito JI, Mullen CA, et al. Clinical practice guideline for the use of antimicrobial agents in neutropenic patients with cancer: 2010 update by the Infectious Diseases Society of America. Clin Infect Dis. 2011;52:e56–93.
6. Grewal H, Guillem JG, Quan SH, Enker WE, Cohen AM. Anorectal disease in neutropenic leukemic patients. Operative vs. nonoperative management. Dis Colon Rectum. 1994;37:1095–9.
7. Boddie AW, Bines SD. Management of acute rectal problems in leukemic patients. J Surg Oncol. 1986;33:53–6.
8. ASGE Standards of Practice Committee, Khashab MA, Chithadi KV, Acosta RD, Bruining DH, Chandrasekhara V, et al. Antibiotic prophylaxis for GI endoscopy. Gastrointest Endosc. 2015;81:81–9.
9. Smiley S, Almyroudis N, Segal B. Epidemiology and management of opportunistic infections in immunocompromised patients with cancer. Abstr Hematol Oncol. 2005;8:20–30.
10. Perazzoli C, Feitosa MR, de Figueiredo-Pontes LL, da Rocha JJR, Simões BP, Féres O. Management of acute colorectal diseases in febrile neutropenic patients. J Coloproctology. 2014;34:189–92.

Consultant Corner: Abdominal Pain and the Immunocompromised Patient

119

Seema Patil, Sandra Quezada, and Jennifer Wellington

Pearls and Pitfalls

- Immunocompromised patients are particularly susceptible to infections including opportunistic, viral, fungal, and parasitic organisms that are often not identified by initial testing.
- Colitis/enteritis can cause bacterial translocation, intestinal perforation, and abscess.
- Complications of immunosuppressive drugs include diarrhea, pancreatitis, mucosal injury and ulceration, calculous biliary disease, posttransplantation lymphoproliferative disorder, acute graft rejection, and graft-versus-host disease, as well as an increased likelihood of infections.
- Given the low diagnostic value of rectal examination in the acute care setting, the risk of potential bacterial translocation and bleeding (if also thrombocytopenic) likely outweighs the benefit of digital rectal examination.

Introduction

Drs. Patil, Quezada, and Wellington practice at the University of Maryland School of Medicine in Downtown Baltimore. Their patient population is largely urban, although many of their patients also live in rural and suburban settings. Their patients are also as diverse as are the city of Baltimore and the state of Maryland, which are 63% Black or African-American and 9.2% Latino, respectively. They work in both the inpatient and outpatient setting, also serving the veteran population at the Baltimore

VA Medical Center. They treat patients presenting with a variety of gastrointestinal diseases, with a focus on managing inflammatory bowel disease.

Answers to Key Clinical Questions

1. When do you recommend consultation with a gastroenterologist and in what time frame for immunocompromised patients with abdominal pain?

Early involvement of the gastroenterologist or surgeon is important when assessing patients with suspected gastrointestinal (GI) emergencies, in particular, those with:

A. Unstable hemodynamics and need for resuscitation
B. Markedly abnormal laboratory tests such as severe anemia or leukocytosis
C. Abnormal imaging with evidence of either intestinal obstruction or perforation should also receive surgical consultation

2. What unique considerations should clinicians factor into the evaluation of an immunocompromised patient with abdominal pain?

Immunocompromised patients often lack the classic clinical abdominal pain presentations, making the etiology difficult to ascertain. Knowledge of the patient's immunocompromised status, whether it is due to chemotherapy, transplantation, HIV, or autoimmune disease, will help clinicians assess the unique complications that arise in each of these patient populations. Overall, this population is particularly susceptible to numerous infectious, inflammatory, and medication/iatrogenic complications and can present with atypical symptoms. Given the frequency of atypical presentations, clinicians must have a lower threshold to obtain objective data including laboratory and imaging tests to rule out underlying pathology not readily suspected through history.

S. Patil · S. Quezada (✉) · J. Wellington
Division of Gastroenterology and Hepatology,
University of Maryland School of Medicine, Baltimore, MD, USA
e-mail: squezada@som.umaryland.edu

© Springer Nature Switzerland AG 2019
A. Graham, D. J. Carlberg (eds.), *Gastrointestinal Emergencies*, https://doi.org/10.1007/978-3-319-98343-1_119

Suggestions when evaluating the immunocompromised patient with abdominal pain include:

- First consider and rule out infectious etiologies
- Expand differential diagnoses to include a broader range of infectious etiologies
- While GERD also occurs in this population, remember to consider bacterial, viral, or candidal esophagitis in the immunocompromised patient with "GERD-like" symptoms
- Imaging can help identify sources of mid and lower abdominal pain. Radiographic findings such as bowel thickening and stranding would help to identify a potential infectious source of abdominal pain and diarrhea

3. What complications are you concerned about in this patient population?

This population is particularly susceptible to numerous infections including opportunistic, viral, fungal, and parasitic organisms that are often not identified by initial testing. In patients with an immunocompromised status, localized infections can quickly become systemic, and timing of antibiotic administration is crucial. In addition, toxicity to medications such as chemotherapeutics, steroids, antiretroviral, and immunosuppressive agents can cause numerous gastrointestinal abnormalities. Examples of specific complication seen in immunocompromised patients include:

A. Significant diarrhea resulting in dehydration
B. Colitis/enteritis can cause bacterial translocation, intestinal perforation, and abscess
C. Pancreatitis, especially due to HIV therapy, can be severe and life-threatening

4. Who should I image and when? CT negative – now what?

Imaging should be considered when there is a concern for an infectious complication such as abscess or a possible surgical issue such as perforation, small bowel obstruction, or large bowel obstruction. If the CT is negative, a gastroenterology consult may be needed to continue the workup. Whether that workup should be conducted on an inpatient versus outpatient basis depends upon the need for IV pain control, PO tolerance (oral intake), or presence of concerning signs/symptoms such as fever, leukocytosis, or GI bleeding.

5. Who should be admitted? Who can be discharged safely and with what instructions?

A. It is reasonable to admit any immunocompromised patient with:
- Inability to tolerate PO including meds, diet, and hydration
- Significant diarrhea >5 large watery stool in 24 h
- Clinically significant bleeding from GI source
- Fever and leukocytosis
- Inability to manage pain with oral medications
B. Conversely, you can consider discharging any patient with normal labs and imaging studies who also:
- Are able to tolerate PO
- Are afebrile
- Can manage pain at home with oral medication
- Follow up with their primary care provider or specialist that can be established to ensure adequate outpatient management prior to discharge

6. What are the unique considerations in a patient with liver transplant and abdominal pain?

Immunosuppressive agents may mask or alter symptoms; thus, a thorough investigation including labs and imaging should be performed in transplant patients presenting with abdominal pain. Complications of immunosuppressive drugs include diarrhea, pancreatitis, mucosal injury and ulceration, calculous biliary disease, posttransplantation lymphoproliferative disorder, acute graft rejection, and graft-versus-host disease, as well as an increased likelihood of infections [1].

In addition to the increased risk for infection with immune suppression, there are a few unique clinical scenarios that can result in abdominal pain in this patient population. Immediate workup to evaluate for these complications includes LFTs (liver function tests) and RUQ US (right upper quadrant ultrasound) with Dopplers.

A. Acute cellular rejection: typically manifests as liver test abnormalities, but abdominal pain may also be present
B. Bile leak/biliary stenosis: common clinical presentation includes RUQ pain and jaundice and +/− fever
C. Budd-Chiari syndrome (hepatic venous outflow obstruction): presents with RUQ pain, marked hepatomegaly, and ascites
D. Hepatic sinusoidal obstruction syndrome: presents with abdominal pain, liver dysfunction, and sudden weight gain

7. What should clinicians consider when evaluating the cancer patient with abdominal pain?

Pain is obviously a common manifestation of cancer and can be related to the primary cancer, treatment, or immune suppression.

A. Related to primary cancer: small bowel obstruction and mesenteric venous thrombosis
B. Related to treatment: graft-versus-host disease, opioid-induced constipation or narcotic bowel syndrome, adverse effects of chemotherapy, and radiation enteritis
C. Related to immune suppression: CMV and other opportunistic infections and typhlitis in neutropenic patients

8. Can I do a rectal exam in a neutropenic patient?

Given the low diagnostic value of rectal examination in the acute care setting, the risk of potential bacterial translocation and bleeding (if also thrombocytopenic) likely outweighs the benefit of digital rectal examination.

Suggested Resources
- Laine L, Jensen D. Management of patients with ulcer bleeding. Am J Gastroenterol. 2012;107: 345–60.
- Spencer S, Power N. The acute abdomen in the immune compromised host. Cancer Imaging. 2008; 8:93–101.

Reference

1. Helderman H, Goral S. Gastrointestinal complications of transplant immunosuppression. J Am Soc Nephrol. 2002;13:277–87.

Part XVI

Abdominal Pain in the Bariatric Patient

What Are the Different Types of Bariatric Surgeries/Procedures and the Unique, Clinically Relevant Features of Each?

Katrin Takenaka

Pearls and Pitfalls
- Bariatric surgery has been shown to be superior to conventional therapy (i.e., diet, lifestyle modifications, medications) in reducing body mass index (BMI) and reversing comorbidities.
- Bariatric procedures promote weight loss by causing intestinal malabsorption and/or restricting gastric volume. They may also affect hormonal controls for appetite and satiety.
- Combined restrictive/absorptive procedures include Roux-en-Y gastric bypass and biliary pancreatic diversion with or without duodenal switch.
- Purely restrictive procedures include sleeve gastrectomy and laparoscopic adjustable gastric banding.
- Endoscopically placed intragastric balloons are a recently approved bariatric procedure; however, the FDA has issued an alert regarding five unexpected deaths in patients with these balloons.

Obesity is a global epidemic, impacting an increasing number of Americans [1–5]. It has been associated with an increased incidence of comorbid conditions affecting quality of life (e.g., migraines, fertility) as well as those affecting life expectancy (e.g., hyperlipidemia (HLD), hypertension (HTN), type II diabetes (DM2), and cardiovascular disease) [5–7]. Because bariatric surgery has been shown to be superior to conventional therapy (i.e., diet, lifestyle modifications, and medications) in reducing body mass index (BMI) and improving comorbidities, bariatric procedures are being performed more frequently [2, 6]. According to the National Institutes of Health, bariatric surgery may be appropriate for patients who have clinically severe obesity (i.e., BMI >= 40 kg/m^2 or BMI >= 35 kg/m^2 with comorbidities such as HLD, HTN, DM2, or obstructive sleep apnea (OSA)) that have failed other treatment modalities [8].

Bariatric procedures promote weight loss through intestinal malabsorption and/or restricting gastric volume. Malabsorptive procedures bypass some portion of the stomach and small intestine, resulting in decreased food absorption [6, 9]. Procedures that restrict gastric size create a functionally smaller stomach and small gastric outlet, ultimately leading to decreased calorie intake and early satiety. These procedures may also impact hormonal controls for appetite and satiety such as ghrelin, peptide YY (PYY), and glucagon-like peptide 1 (GLP-1) as well as alter intestinal flora [6].

Combination Restrictive/Malabsorptive Procedures

Roux-en-Y Gastric Bypass (RYGB) (Fig. 120.1)

This is currently the most commonly performed bariatric procedure worldwide [3, 6, 10]. With a RYGB, a small proximal gastric pouch (15–50 mL) is created, while the remnant distal stomach is stapled shut. The proximal gastric pouch is anastomosed to a Roux limb of small bowel (30–50 cm distal to the ligament of Treitz). The proximal jejunum (biliary limb) is then connected to the Roux limb via jejunojejunostomy. In simple terms, RYGBs physically restrict the amount of oral intake and additionally bypass the distal stomach and a length of proximal jejunum, leading to incomplete absorption [6, 10]. Furthermore, this procedure may affect levels of PYY, GLP-1, and ghrelin, resulting in appetite suppression and earlier satiety [6].

Success rates for weight loss are as high as 60–80% at 5 years and 54% at 10 years and beyond [6, 10]. Additionally, studies have shown a reversal of comorbidities such as HTN, HLD, DM2, and OSA following RYGB [6, 11]. Reported

K. Takenaka
McGovern Medical School (part of UT Health/The University of Texas Health Science Center at Houston), Houston, TX, USA
e-mail: Katrin.takenaka@uth.tmc.edu

© Springer Nature Switzerland AG 2019
A. Graham, D. J. Carlberg (eds.), *Gastrointestinal Emergencies*, https://doi.org/10.1007/978-3-319-98343-1_120

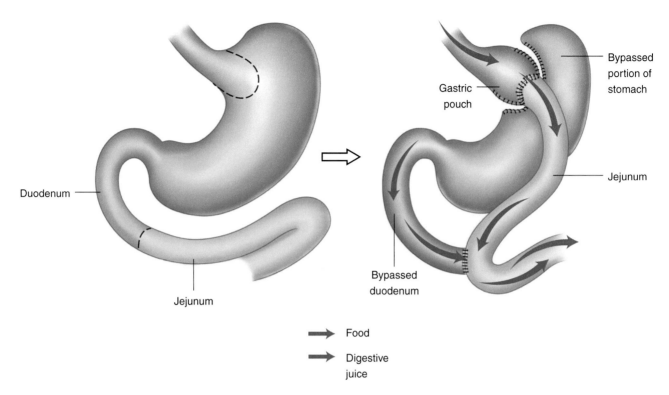

Fig. 120.1 Roux-en-Y gastric bypass (RYGB)

complication rates of RYGB have ranged from 6% to 14% with mortality rates <1% [12, 13].

Key Components
- Malabsorptive/restrictive
- No pylorus (risk of Dumping syndrome)
- Laparoscopic surgical procedure causes defects in mesentery (risk of internal hernias)

Biliary Pancreatic Diversion (BPD) With/ Without Duodenal Switch (DS) (Fig. 120.2)

BPD is a less commonly performed bariatric procedure compared to RYGB [6]. In a BPD, a distal gastrectomy is performed followed by an anastomosis of the distal ileum to the proximal stomach (to create an alimentary limb). The detached proximal ileum (the biliopancreatic limb) is subsequently connected to the alimentary limb proximal to the ileocecal valve. Weight loss results from a combination of decreased gastric size and bypass of the duodenum and jejunum [6, 9, 10]. BPD has been associated with sustained excess weight loss (61–80% at greater than 10 years post-surgery) [6, 9, 11].

A variation is the BPD-DS which consists of a sleeve gastrectomy and anastomosis of the duodenum to the ileum, leaving the pylorus and proximal duodenum intact [6, 9–11]. BPD-DS is associated with a lower incidence of malabsorption complications and stomal ulceration than BPD [6, 9, 10]. Thus, it has become more commonly performed worldwide compared to BPD [6]. Like BPD, BPD-DS has been associated with sustained excess weight loss more than 10 years after surgery [6]. BPD-DS is mostly performed in patients with BMI >= 50 kg/m^2 in two stages as the single combined procedure is associated with higher morbidity and mortality than other bariatric surgeries [14]. Although more recent studies have reported improved morbidity and mortality rates, BPD-DS has historically been associated with higher morbidity and mortality rates than RYGB (morbidity rates up to 16% and a mean mortality rate of 1.1%) [12, 14, 15].

Key Components
- Significant malabsorptive component/restrictive.
- BPD-DS pylorus intact (lower risk of Dumping syndrome).
- BPD/BPD-DS diverts large segment of the small intestine (high risk of vitamin deficiency and malnutrition).
- Higher complications but significant, long-term weight loss as well.

Biliopancreatic diversion

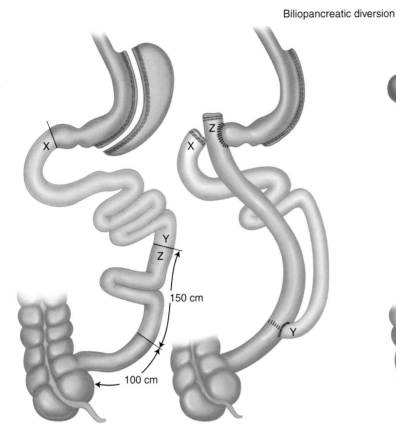

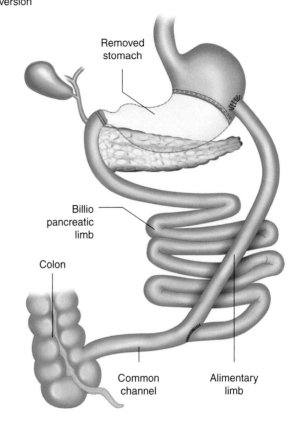

Fig. 120.2   Biliopancreatic diversion

Restrictive Procedures

Sleeve Gastrectomy (SG) (Fig. 120.3)

Although initially performed as a procedure leading to subsequent RYGB or DS in patients with BMI > 60 kg/m², SG has become increasingly popular as an independent surgery [1, 3, 6]. During a SG, a narrow tubular structure is created by resection of the greater curvature of the stomach [3, 6]. In addition to the resultant restriction of gastric size, SG also affects neurohormonal controls of appetite such as ghrelin [3, 5, 6]. Although further studies are currently in progress, excess weight loss of 61–67% has been observed [1, 6]. Reported morbidity rates for SG range from 2.2% to 13% with mean mortality rates <1% [12, 16].

Key Components
- Restrictive
- Pylorus intact (low risk of Dumping syndrome)
- No mesenteric defects with surgical procedure (low risk of internal hernia)

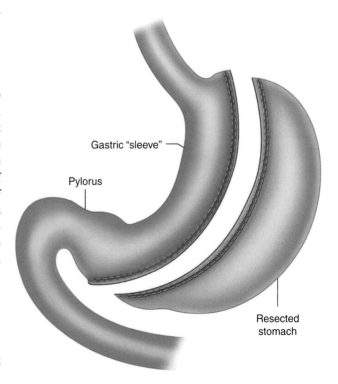

Fig. 120.3   Sleeve gastrectomy (SG)

Laparoscopic Adjustable Gastric Banding (LAGB) (Fig. 120.4)

LAGB provides a less invasive and potentially reversible alternative to other types of bariatric procedures [9–11]. A small gastric pouch is created by the placement of an adjustable silastic band around the upper stomach. The saline-filled band is connected to a subcutaneous port that can be accessed percutaneously to adjust the band size [1, 10, 11]. LAGB also appears to affect appetite/satiety through unknown mechanisms (possibly vagal stimulation) [6]. Excess weight loss at 2 years is modest at approximately 47%; however, weight loss ranges from 47% to 68% over a 10-year period, making it comparable to RYGB [6, 11]. Reported complication rates range from 7.8% to 13% with a mortality rate <1% [16, 17]. However, surgical revision is needed in 30–60% of patients due to complications or inadequate weight loss [17].

Key Components
- Restrictive
- Adjustable and reversible
- High rates of reversal due to intolerance of side effects from procedure

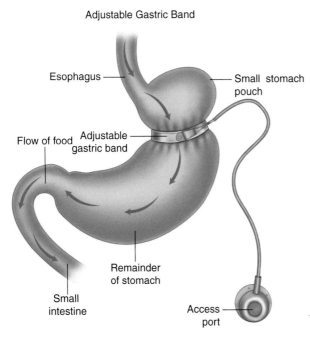

Adjustable Gastric Band

Fig. 120.4 Adjustable gastric band

Intragastric Balloon (IGB) (Fig. 120.5)

Although used outside of the United States for decades, IGBs were only approved by the US Food and Drug Administration (FDA) in 2015 for patients with BMI 30–40 kg/m^2 who have failed conventional weight loss treatment (e.g., diet and exercise) [7]. Two types were approved at that time: a dual balloon system (ReShape) and a single balloon device (Orbera) [6, 18]. The saline-filled balloons are placed endoscopically and removed after 6 months. Both are thought to induce satiety by filling the stomach and delaying gastric emptying [7]. Studies have shown an average weight loss of 10–12%, total body weight at 6 months and an improvement in obesity-related comorbidities such as DM2, HLD, and HTN [7, 18]. The reported incidence of serious complications is about 10%, in some cases necessitating early device removal [19, 20]. The most common complications include balloon rupture and gastric ulceration, and in rare cases, aspiration or bowel obstruction. The saline in the balloon is often stained with methylene blue causing green- or blue-tinted urine if the balloon ruptures. Although IGBs provide a minimally invasive and reversible method of weight loss, the FDA recently issued an alert to healthcare providers due to five unanticipated deaths that were reported in patients with IGBs placed during the preceding month. At this time, the underlying cause of these deaths is unknown [21].

Key Components
- Restrictive
- Temporary
- Unknown long-term weight loss impact or full understanding of risks associated with procedure

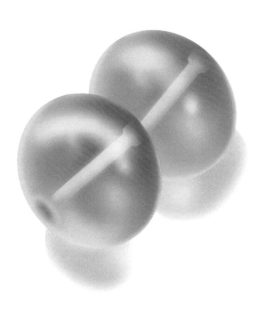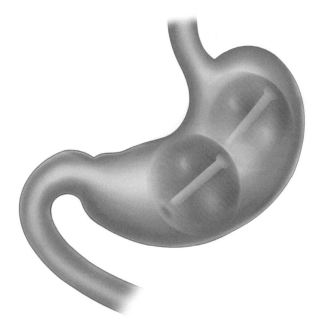

Fig. 120.5 Gastric balloon

Suggested Resource
- American Society for Metabolic and Bariatric Surgery. https://asmbs.org/patients/bariatric-surgery-procedures.

References

1. Gaetke-Udager KWA, Kaza RV, Al-Hawary MM, Maturen KE, Cohan RH. A guide to imaging in bariatric surgery. Emerg Radiol. 2014;21:309–19.
2. Monkhouse SJMJ, Norton SA. Complications of bariatric surgery: presentation and emergency management – a review. Ann R Coll Surg Engl. 2009;91:280–6.
3. Lehnert BMM, Osman S, Khandelwal S, Elojeimy S, Bhargava P, Katz DS. Imaging of complications of common bariatric surgical procedures. Radiol Clin N Am. 2014;52:1071–86.
4. Pernar LILR, McCormack C, Chen J, Shikora SA, Spector D, Tavakkoli A, Vernon AH, Robinson MK. An effort to develop an algorithm to target abdominal CT scans for patients after gastric bypass. Obes Surg. 2016;26:2543–6.
5. Wernick B, Jansen M, Noria S, Stawicki SP, El Chaar M. Essential bariatric emergencies for the acute care surgeon. Eur J Trauma Emerg Surg. 2016;42:571–84.
6. Lewis KDTK, Luber SD. Acute abdominal pain in the bariatric surgery patient. Emerg Med Clin N Am. 2016;34:387–407.
7. Popov VBOA, Schulman AR, Thompson CC. The impact of intragastric balloons on obesity-related co-morbidities: a systematic review and meta-analysis. Am J Gastroenterol. 2017;112:429–39.
8. National Heart B and Lung Institute Obesity Education Initiative. The practical guide: identification, evaluation, and treatment of overweight and obesity in adults 2000 1 October 2017.
9. Luber SDFD, Venkat A. Care of the bariatric surgery patient in the emergency department. J Emerg Med. 2008;34:13–20.
10. Edwards EDJB, Gagner M, Pomp A. Presentation and management of common post-weight loss surgery problems in the emergency department. Ann Emerg Med. 2006;47:160–6.
11. Ellison SRES. Bariatric surgery: a review of the available procedures and complications for the emergency physician. J Emerg Med. 2008;34:21–32.
12. Topart PBG, Ritz P. Comparative early outcomes of three laparoscopic bariatric procedures: sleeve gastrectomy, Roux-en-Y gastric bypass, and biliopancreatic diversion with duodenal switch. Surg Obes Relat Dis. 2012;8:250–4.
13. Sima LVSA, Dan RG, Breaza GM, Cretu OM. Complications of Roux-en-Y gastric bypass. Chirurgia. 2013;108:180–3.
14. Rezvani MSI, Klar A, Bonanni F, Antanavicius G. Is laparoscopic single-stage biliopancreatic diversion with duodenal switch safe in super morbidly obese patients? Surg Obes Relat Dis. 2014;10:427–31.
15. Biertho LS-HF, Marceau S, Lebel S, Lescelleur O, Biron S. Current outcomes of laparoscopic duodenal switch. Ann Surg Innov Res. 2016;10:1.
16. Chang SSC, Song J, Varela E, Eagon CJ, Colditz GA. The effectiveness and risks of bariatric surgery: an updated systematic review and meta-analysis, 2003–2012. JAMA Surg. 2014;149:275–87.
17. Chansaenroj PAL, Lee W, Chen S, Chen J, Ser K. Revision procedures after failed adjusted gastric banding: comparison of efficacy and safety. Obes Surg. 2017;27:2861–7.
18. ORBERA Intragastric Balloon System – P14008 [press release]. 2015.
19. Yorke ESN, Reso A, Shi X, de Gara C, Birch D, Gill R, Karmali S. Intragastric balloon for management of severe obesity: a systematic review. Obes Surg. 2016;26:2248–54.
20. Tate CMGA. Intragastric balloon treatment for obesity: review of recent studies. Adv Ther. 2017;34:1859–75.
21. Administration UFaD. Liquid-filled Intragastric Balloon Systems: letter to healthcare providers – potential risks. https://www.fda.gov/Safety/MedWatch/SafetyInformation/SafetyAlertsforHumanMedicalProducts/ucm570916.htm2017.

Imaging: What Are the Evidence-Based Strategies for Imaging the Bariatric Patient?

121

Christina S. Houser and Julie T. Vieth

> **Pearls and Pitfalls**
> - CT is generally considered the first-line imaging modality; however, it is only necessary to diagnose gastric or anastomotic leak, intra-abdominal infection, or obstruction.
> - Fluoroscopy can be used to assess band slippage, anastomotic narrowing, strictures, pouch dilation, and gastric outlet obstruction.
> - Radiologic evaluations can be used in conjunction with each other as well as endoscopy.
> - Up to 20% of CTs can be falsely [not false] negative when assessing for obstruction in bariatric patients.

Patients who have undergone bariatric surgery are at risk for a myriad of perioperative and postoperative complications that physicians need to be able to efficiently and effectively recognize and diagnose. Each bariatric procedure comes with a set of unique complications, and even vague complaints such as heartburn, nausea, abdominal pain, or failure to lose weight can have a potential lethal etiology; subsequently, prompt imaging studies should always be thoughtfully considered by the clinician [1, 2]. The aforementioned complaints in a postoperative bariatric surgery patient may trigger an instant reflex to order a computed tomography (CT) scan. However, the physician should recognize that plain films, fluoroscopy, and CT each have a role in the evaluation of abdominal pain in a bariatric patient, depending upon the type of bariatric surgery that was performed, the suspected complication, and the resources available at a specific hospital.

Computed Tomography

CT is generally considered the first-line imaging modality for many potential complications from bariatric surgery [3, 4] as it is widely available and can rapidly scan the entire abdomen for the detection of abdominal catastrophes [5]. Specifically, CT is the optimal imaging modality when searching for gastric or anastomotic leak, intra-abdominal infection, and bowel obstruction [6–8]. In recent years, radiologic protocols have eliminated the use of oral contrast for many abdominal CT imaging studies. However, in the bariatric patient, oral contrast is indicated so as to optimize images and the sensitivity of such scans.

Gastric or Anastomotic Leak

Gastric or anastomotic leak is one of the most common complications after Roux-en-Y gastric bypass (RYGB) or sleeve gastrectomy with an incidence estimated to be as high as 6% [7, 9–12]. Moreover, it is also one of the most feared and potentially lethal complications of bariatric surgery [13]. With sleeve gastrectomy, leaks can occur at the staple line or gastroesophageal junction. After Roux-en-Y gastric bypass, leaks can occur at the proximal gastrojejunal anastomosis or the distal jejunojejunal anastomosis. Of note, the majority of leaks occur within the first postoperative week [7, 9]. Studies indicate that persistent tachycardia with a pulse greater than 120 beats per minute in a postoperative bariatric surgery patient should prompt immediate evaluation for a leak [11, 14]. This involves a CT with intravenous (IV) and water-soluble oral contrast and may include an upper gastrointestinal (UGI) series with endoscopy if the CT is negative (Figs. 121.1 and 121.2).

C. S. Houser (✉)
MedStar Washington Hospital Center, MedStar Georgetown University Hospital, Washington, DC, USA
e-mail: Christina.S.Houser@medstar.net

J. T. Vieth (✉)
Canton-Potsdam Hospital, Potsdam, NY, USA
e-mail: jvieth@cphospital.org

© Springer Nature Switzerland AG 2019
A. Graham, D. J. Carlberg (eds.), *Gastrointestinal Emergencies*, https://doi.org/10.1007/978-3-319-98343-1_121

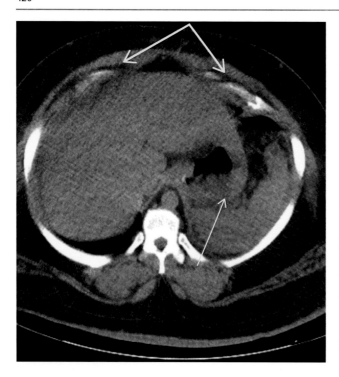

Fig. 121.1 Non-contrast CT of the abdomen and pelvis of patient with abdominal pain 10 days after sleeve gastrectomy. Large arrows, intraperitoneal free air; small arrow, suspected gastric content outside of the stomach, concern for staple line leak

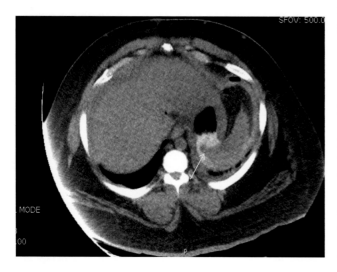

Fig. 121.2 With addition of oral and IV contrast, the gastric leak is illustrated by the yellow arrow

The sensitivity of CT for gastric or anastomotic leak is approximately 56%. When CT is combined with fluoroscopy, the sensitivity only improves to 70% [10]. A negative CT scan for this complication does not rule out the diagnosis and some patients will still require surgical exploration despite negative imaging. The most feared complication of gastric or anastomotic leak is the development of intraabdominal abscess and sepsis. However, intra-abdominal

abscesses may have other etiologies in bariatric patients, including infection of bariatric hardware. If the physician has any suspicion of intra-abdominal infection or abscess, an intravenous and oral contrast-enhanced CT must be obtained [3, 8].

Bowel Obstruction

Bowel obstruction is one of the most common causes of abdominal pain after Roux-en-Y surgery [3], with an incidence of approximately 3–5% [9, 10, 12]. It can also occur after biliopancreatic diversion with duodenal switch. Internal hernias after Roux-en-Y gastric bypass are a potentially devastating cause of bowel obstruction. There are three main types of mesenteric defects with laparoscopic RYGB: Petersens, mesocolic, and jejunojejunal [9, 10, 12, 13, 15], and the incidence of a hernia in this population is 0.9–4.5% [16]. Intravenous and oral contrast-enhanced CT is the preferred method of radiologic evaluation, and a positive scan will often show the classic mesenteric "swirl" or "whirl" sign which is caused by rotation of the mesentery (Fig. 121.1). This has an 83% specificity for a Petersen hernia [17]. Unfortunately, the sensitivity of such a sign is approximately 80% [13]. Thus, a high index of suspicion should be maintained, and patients with symptoms of obstruction should be considered for urgent surgical exploration if negative imaging and concerning signs or symptoms [11, 13] (Fig. 121.3).

Fluoroscopy

Fluoroscopy is indicated when the physician is concerned about pouch dilation, band slippage, stricture, or gastric outlet obstruction [1, 7, 8]). Many physicians also start the evaluation for gastric or anastomotic leak with an UGI series under fluoroscopy, but its sensitivity can be as low as 22–30% [8, 10–12]. Fluoroscopy may not have as widespread availability as CT, which is a significant limitation of its use (Fig. 121.4).

Gastric band surgery may lead to several complications that can be easily diagnosed with fluoroscopy. Strictures and anastomotic narrowing can both be readily diagnosed with fluoroscopy, as can gastric outlet obstruction and pouch dilation [1, 7]. The diagnoses may present with similar complaints, including odynophagia, abdominal pain, vomiting, and regurgitation. Many bariatric physicians routinely obtain fluoroscopic studies in the immediate postoperative period before patient discharge. This can provide easy access to images for comparison when the clinician decides to obtain repeat fluoroscopic studies [6, 13, 15]. Fluoroscopy for this purpose does require that the patient be cooperative and capable of standing [15].

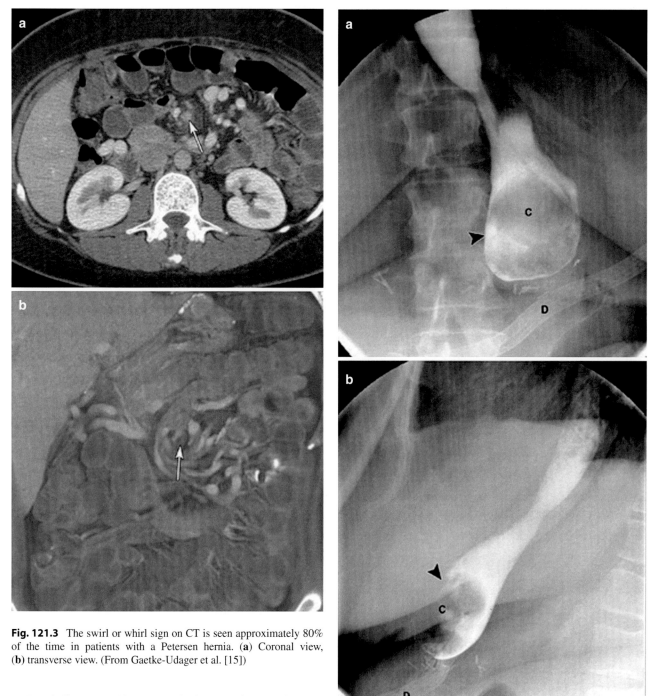

Fig. 121.3 The swirl or whirl sign on CT is seen approximately 80% of the time in patients with a Petersen hernia. (**a**) Coronal view, (**b**) transverse view. (From Gaetke-Udager et al. [15])

Band slippage, which has an incidence of approximately 15% [12], is diagnosed by assessing the phi angle on either plain films or fluoroscopy. This is the angle made by the vertical axis of the spine and the intersection of the long axis of the gastric band [1, 15]. The phi angle should typically be between 4° and 58°; if the angle is less than 4°, the band has slipped posteriorly, and if the angle is greater than 58°, the band has slipped anteriorly [10, 15] (Fig. 121.5).

Fig. 121.4 Obstruction of gastric pouch following Roux-en-Y gastric bypass surgery. (**a**) Frontal and (**b**) right lateral images from an upper GI fluoroscopic image show holdup of water-soluble iodinated contrast in the gastric pouch (*arrowheads*), with a large filling defect (C confirmed as clot on endoscopy) and no discernible gastric emptying. D surgical drain. (From Gaetke-Udager et al. [15])

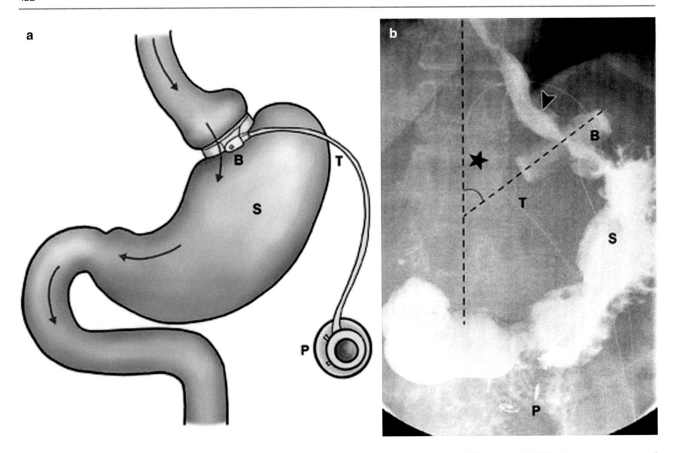

Fig. 121.5 The phi angle can be used to determine band slippage. (**a**) Normal adjustable gastric band placement. (**b**) This demonstrates a normal phi angle of between 4–58° on xray, Abnormal is greater than 58°. (From Gaetke-Udager et al. [15])

Radiation Exposure

With the exception of an abdominal radiograph series, the radiation exposure for the proposed diagnostic modalities is quite similar. Fluoroscopy for an upper gastrointestinal series is around 6 millisieverts, while abdominal and abdominal/pelvic CT scans are approximately 8 and 10 millisieverts, respectively (Table 121.1). The exposure difference between these is minimal, but it is important to remember that bariatric patients will likely be exposed to many radiologic studies over their lifetime. Moreover, many patients may require more than one test, which carries financial implications for the patient.

Summary and Recommendation

Given the availability and efficiency of CT, CT is often the first-line imaging modality for bariatric patients, especially for undifferentiated abdominal pain, fevers, tachycardia, or leukocytosis of unknown origin. However, negative CT scans in patients with concerning features for anastomotic leak, band slippage, obstruction, or infection should prompt further evaluation either with fluoroscopy, endoscopy, or urgent laparoscopy.

Table 121.1 Radiation doses in imaging modalities routinely used in postoperative bariatric imaging

Imaging modality	Estimated radiation exposure (millisieverts)
Abdominal X-ray	0.07 mSv
Upper GI series	6.0 mSv
CT abdomen	8.0 mSv
CT abdomen/pelvis	10.0 mSv

Suggested Resource

- Levine M, Carucci L. Imaging of bariatric surgery: normal anatomy and postoperative complications. Radiology. 2014;270(2):327–41.

References

1. Kurian M. Imaging studies after bariatric surgery. [Internet]. Uptodate.com. 2017 [cited 12 Sept 2017]. Available from: https://www.uptodate.com/contents/imaging-studies-after-bariatric-surgery?csi=c7f71472-51e6-48e6-9b36-786e77107419&source=contentShare.

2. Haddad D, David A, Abdel-Dayem H, Socci N, Ahmed L, Gilet A. Abdominal imaging post bariatric surgery: predictors, usage and utility. Surg Obes Relat Dis. 2017;13(8):1327–36.3.

3. Miao T, Kielar A, Patlas M, Riordon M, Chong S, Robins J, et al. Cross-sectional imaging, with surgical correlation, of patients presenting with complications after remote bariatric surgery without bowel obstruction. Abdom Imaging. 2015;40(8):2945–65.

4. Uppot R. Impact of obesity on radiology. Radiol Clin N Am. 2007;45(2):231–46.

5. Guniganti P, Bradenham C, Raptis C, Menias C, Mellnick V. CT of gastric emergencies. Radiographics. 2015;35(7):1909–21.

6. Chandler R, Srinivas G, Chintapalli K, Schwesinger W, Prasad S. Imaging in bariatric surgery: a guide to postsurgical anatomy and common complications. Am J Roentgenol. 2008;190(1):122–35.

7. Levine M, Carucci L. Imaging of bariatric surgery: normal anatomy and postoperative complications. Radiology. 2014;270(2):327–41.

8. Varghese J, Roy-Choudhury S. Radiological imaging of the GI tract after bariatric surgery. Gastrointest Endosc. 2009;70(6):1176–81.

9. Carucci L, Turner M. Imaging after bariatric surgery for morbid obesity: roux-en-Y gastric bypass and laparoscopic adjustable gastric banding. Semin Roentgenol. 2009;44(4):283–96.

10. Lehnert B, Moshiri M, Osman S, Khandelwal S, Elojeimy S, Bhargava P, et al. Imaging of complications of common bariatric surgical procedures. Radiol Clin N Am. 2014;52(5):1071–86.

11. Lewis K, Takenaka K, Luber S. Acute abdominal pain in the bariatric surgery patient. Emerg Med Clin North Am. 2016;34(2):387–407.

12. Ni Mhuircheartaigh J, Abedin S, Bennett A, Tyagi G. Imaging features of bariatric surgery and its complications. Seminars in Ultrasound, CT and MRI. New York: WB Saunders. 2013;34(4):311–324.

13. Kothari S. Bariatric surgery and postoperative imaging. Surg Clin N Am. 2011;91(1):155–72.

14. Lainas P, Tranchart H, Gaillard M, Ferretti S, Donatelli G, Dagher I. Prospective evaluation of routine early computed tomography scanner in laparoscopic sleeve gastrectomy. Surg Obes Relat Dis. 2016;12(8):1483–90.

15. Gaetke-Udager K, Wasnik A, Kaza R, Al-Hawary M, Maturen K, Cohan R. A guide to imaging in bariatric surgery. Emerg Radiol. 2014;21(3):309–19.

16. de Bakker JK, Budde van Namen YW, Bruin SC, de Brauw LM. Gastric bypass and abdominal pain: think of Petersen hernia. J Soc Laparoendosc Surg. 2012;16(2):311–3.

17. Lockhart ME, Tessler FN, Canon CL, et al. Internal hernia after gastric bypass: sensitivity and specificity of seven CT signs with surgical correlation and controls. AJR Am J Roentgenol. 2007;188:745–50.

Anastomotic Leak, Sepsis, Pulmonary Embolism, and Early Hemorrhage: How Do I Diagnose and Manage Early Complications of Bariatric Surgeries and Procedures?

Katrin Takenaka

Pearls and Pitfalls

- Bariatric patients may not always present with typical signs of severe illness (e.g., peritoneal signs, fever) and often lack the physiologic reserve to compensate for severe illness.
- The complications of bariatric procedures may be described as early (<=1 month post-procedure) or late (>1 month post-procedure).
- Tachycardia should be considered a "red flag" to the presence of significant disease (e.g., dehydration, pulmonary embolus, gastric leak, sepsis). Sustained tachycardia of >120 beats per minute without source may require laparoscopic evaluation.
- Early complications following Roux-en-Y gastric bypass and biliary pancreatic diversion include anastomotic leak, GI obstruction, and dumping syndrome.
- Patients with a sleeve gastrectomy may present with anastomotic leak or gastric stenosis.
- Following a laparoscopic adjustable gastric banding, patients may have esophageal/gastric pouch dilatation, gastric slippage, or gastric injury/necrosis.

Bariatric surgeries have become the second most commonly performed abdominal surgery in the USA [1]. Although the mortality following these procedures is <1%, post-bariatric surgery patients frequently present to emergency departments (EDs) with postoperative concerns [2–4]. The most common chief complaints include nausea, vomiting, diarrhea, dehydration, and abdominal pain [1–3]. Most bariatric patients will not require readmission postoperatively. In one review by Garg et al., only 5.2% were readmitted within a month of their bariatric surgery [3].

Caring for the bariatric patient begins with an initial assessment and, if necessary, stabilization. Intravenous access is often needed for fluids, antiemetics, and pain relief. Additionally, diagnostics such as complete blood count, metabolic profile, lipase, lactate, blood gas, urinalysis, pregnancy test, and electrocardiogram may be helpful [5]. Further imaging and therapeutics depend on the specific diagnoses being considered.

Complications of bariatric surgeries and procedures are categorized as early (<30 days post-procedure) or late (>30 days post-procedure) [refer to Table 122.1]. Some complications can occur following any invasive procedure while others are associated with specific types of bariatric surgeries.

How Do I Diagnose and Manage Early Complications of Bariatric Surgeries and Procedures?

Infection

Infectious complications in bariatric patients are similar to those found in other patients undergoing colorectal surgery. Peritonitis, with or without abscess formation, may result from intraoperative contamination, fistula development after sleeve gastrectomy (2.2%) or gastric bypass surgery (~2%), anastomotic leak, staple line dehiscence, or surgical site infection [9]. However, an absence of clinical signs at the time of diagnosis of peritonitis is reported in 49% of non-ICU patients [9]. Common signs and symptoms include fever (74%), dyspnea (98%), tachycardia (100%), tenderness (30%), pus (33%), and ileus (37%) [9]. Source control and antibiotics are key. In one study comparing bariatric (49 patients) and non-bariatric surgical patients (134 patients),

K. Takenaka
McGovern Medical School (part of UT Health/The University of Texas Health Science Center at Houston), Houston, TX, USA
e-mail: Katrin.takenaka@uth.tmc.edu

© Springer Nature Switzerland AG 2019
A. Graham, D. J. Carlberg (eds.), *Gastrointestinal Emergencies*, https://doi.org/10.1007/978-3-319-98343-1_122

Table 122.1 Early versus late complications of bariatric surgeries [5, 6, 7, 8]

Early (<=1 month post-procedure)
Nonspecific
Surgical site infection
Deep vein thrombosis/pulmonary embolus[a]
Postoperative bleeding
Roux-en-Y gastric bypass or biliary pancreatic diversion
Anastomotic leak
GI obstruction
Dumping syndrome
Sleeve gastrectomy
Anastomotic leak
Gastric stenosis
Laparoscopic adjustable gastric banding
Esophageal/gastric pouch dilatation
Gastric slippage
Gastric injury/necrosis
Late (>1 month post-procedure)
Nonspecific
Cholelithiasis
Roux-en-Y gastric bypass or biliary pancreatic diversion
Stomal stenosis
Internal hernia
Ventral incisional hernia (open procedures)
Small bowel obstruction[a]
Stomal ulcer
Gastroesophageal reflux disease
Nutritional complications
Sleeve gastrectomy
Gastroesophageal reflux disease
Laparoscopic adjustable gastric banding
Band erosion
Esophagitis
Gastroesophageal reflux disease

[a]Note that some complications can occur both early and late

bariatric patients had a 37% higher rate of Gram-positive cocci, a 33% lower rate of Gram-negative bacilli, and a 50% lower rate of anaerobes [10]. Empiric treatment with broad-spectrum antibiotics is appropriate if suspicious of peritonitis.

Surgical Site Infections (SSI)

In bariatric patients who undergo open surgeries, the rate of SSIs can reach as high as 16% and is associated with a two- to threefold increase in risk of death [11]. The rate of SSI drops to approximately 4% with laparoscopic bariatric surgeries [11]. Surgical site infections occur most commonly within 2–3 weeks of surgery [5]. The most frequent etiologic organisms include *Staphylococcus*, *Streptococcus*, and *Enterococcus* species [5, 12]. Early source control (e.g., abscess drainage, operative intervention) and antibiotics are important in the management of SSIs [5, 12].

Port Infections in Laparoscopic Adjustable Gastric Band (LAGB)

Special mention is made of port site infections associated with laparoscopic adjustable gastric band (LAGB). Patients with port infections often present with swelling, erythema, and tenderness over the port site [5, 6, 13]. Because it may be difficult to assess the extent of infection on exam, further diagnostics such as ultrasound (to evaluate for superficial abscess), CT (to rule out deeper abscesses), or endoscopy (to identify band erosion) may be needed [5, 6, 13]. Port infections are treated with systemic antibiotics and may necessitate port removal [5].

In patients presenting 24–48 h after LAGB with peritoneal signs, gastric injury and/or necrosis should be considered. The cornerstones of initial management are IV fluids, broad-spectrum antibiotics, and prompt surgical consultation for expeditious operative exploration [7].

Pulmonary Embolism

Deep vein thrombosis (DVT)/pulmonary embolus (PE) is the second most common cause of death following bariatric surgery, occurring in 1–2% [4, 8, 12]. The diagnostic and therapeutic approach for bariatric patients with suspected and/or confirmed DVT/PE is the same as for other patients [4, 8].

Hemorrhage

Postoperative bleeding is categorized as intraperitoneal bleeding which may present with hypotension, decreasing hemoglobin and hematocrit, or tachycardia and intraluminal bleeding which more commonly presents as a late event with melena, hematemesis, and hematochezia. The prevalence of hemorrhage following gastric bypass surgery is reportedly 1.7% [14]. However, in one study of 4466 patients who had undergone gastric bypass during a 10-year period, less than 1% experienced postoperative bleeding [15]. Bleeding occurred at the staple line, from iatrogenic visceral injury (i.e., liver or splenic injury) or due to mesenteric vessel bleeding, requiring surgical intervention in 43% of cases. Bleeding complications lead to increased morbidity due to sepsis, respiratory compromise, and organ failure; thus, early diagnosis and intervention are critical. Initial management involves volume resuscitation (i.e., IV fluids, blood products), correction of any coagulopathies, and gastric acid suppression [5, 7, 12]. In patients for whom this supportive therapy is not sufficient, endoscopy and/or operative intervention may be needed [5, 7, 12, 16].

Anastomotic Leak

Anastomotic leaks (ALs) occur in up to 5% of RYGB and BPD patients and are associated with significant morbidity and mortality rates as high as 17% [17, 18]. The most common site is the gastrojejunal anastomosis [5–7, 13]. The etiologies of ALs are multifactorial including local tissue ischemia, technical factors, and patient comorbidities that affect wound healing [19]. Masoomi et al. identified the following risk factors for ALs: Medicare payer, open technique, age greater than 50 years, congestive heart failure, chronic lung disease or kidney failure, and male gender [17]. Patients with an AL typically present within 7–10 days of surgery with fever, tachycardia, and/or abdominal pain [5, 8, 12, 13, 20]. Other symptoms may include back pain, hiccups, restlessness, shortness of breath, and unexplained sepsis [5, 7, 8]. In some patients, differentiating between an AL and PE based on clinical presentation may be difficult as sustained tachycardia, tachypnea, and a sense of "impending doom" are described in both processes [19, 21]. In fact, one study found that tachycardia >120 beats/minute and respiratory distress were the most sensitive findings for ALs [19]. There may be a role for C-reactive protein (CRP) levels in the diagnosis of ALs based on a study in which CRP >229 mg/L on postoperative day 2 was almost 100% sensitive (although not specific) for ALs in patients following laparoscopic gastric bypass [22]. Upper GI series and CT may identify ALs [5–8]. However, even combined, these studies only detect about 70% of ALs (30% with upper GI alone, 56% with CT alone) [13, 20]. According to the American Society for Metabolic and Bariatric Surgery, surgical re-exploration is the definitive method to identify ALs with higher sensitivity and specificity than diagnostic imaging [18]. Hemodynamically stable patients may improve with IV fluids, bowel rest, and broad-spectrum antibiotics alone. Endoscopic stenting and percutaneous drainage are additional therapeutic options [12]. However, unstable patients and those with severe symptoms require surgical intervention [7, 12, 20].

In SG patients, ALs usually arise from the proximal 1/3 of the staple line [13, 20]. Clinical presentations resemble those of RYGB or BPD patients with ALs: fever, tachycardia, abdominal pain, and less commonly sepsis [5, 13, 20]. However, the incidence of ALs and the associated mortality may be higher in SG patients than in those who have undergone gastric bypass [23]. Although a quick diagnosis is the key to initiating early therapy, upper GI radiography and CT may both miss detecting the leak. Thus if there is a strong clinical suspicion of an AL, re-exploration should be considered [20]. Similar to RYGB and BPD patients with this diagnosis, treatment options include IV fluids, bowel rest, and IV antibiotics for stable patients and surgical intervention for unstable patients. Percutaneous drainage and endoscopic stenting are other possible modalities of treatment for stable patients [20].

Obstruction

Gastric Bypass

Early GI obstruction is usually caused by distention of the gastric remnant due to edema or blockage at the jejunojejunostomy site [7, 8]. Patients often present with nausea, vomiting, hiccups, abdominal pain, and bloating. It can be diagnosed by a distended gastric pouch with air-fluid levels seen on abdominal imaging, specifically computed tomography [7, 8]. Optimal management includes percutaneous decompression of the gastric remnant or operative management [7, 8].

Sleeve Gastrectomy

Patients with gastric stenosis, an uncommon complication of SG, present with nausea, vomiting, and/or dysphagia [5]. Upper GI radiographs may be diagnostic; however, endoscopy offers an added therapeutic benefit. Early gastric stenosis may be caused by edema or hematoma and, therefore, may be managed with bowel rest and IV fluids. If conservative management is unsuccessful, endoscopic dilation should be considered [5].

Adjustable Gastric Banding

Esophageal/gastric pouch dilatation is may be caused by an overly restrictive band, dietary noncompliance, or excessive vomiting [7]. Presenting symptoms include vomiting, abdominal pain, and dysphagia [5]. The diagnosis can be made with an upper GI series [7]. Initial management involves band deflation. If this is unsuccessful, surgical intervention (e.g., band revision or removal, conversion to RYGB) may be mandated [5].

With gastric slippage, part of the stomach herniates upward through the gastric band, resulting in an enlarged gastric pouch [5, 7]. Although the clinical presentation of these patients is similar to those with gastric pouch dilatation due to an overly restrictive band, band deflation does not relieve the symptoms in patients with gastric slippage [5]. Upper GI radiographs will generally reveal the diagnosis (e.g., eccentric gastric pouch dilation, abnormal location/orientation of the gastric band) [7, 13]. Initial management involves IV hydration, electrolyte repletion, and surgical consultation as early surgical intervention decreases the incidence of further complications [7].

Summary

It can be difficult to identify those with potentially serious complications because they may not present with typical signs or symptoms of severe illness (e.g., peritoneal signs, fever) [4–6, 8]. Furthermore, these patients often lack the physiologic reserve to compensate for severe illness [6]. In bariatric patients, tachycardia should be considered indicative of potential significant disease. A sustained heart rate greater than 120 beats/min may indicate an anastomotic leak, sepsis, hemorrhage, or pulmonary embolism [4, 5, 7, 8].

References

1. Chen J, Mackenzie J, Zhai Y, O'Loughlin J, Kholer R, Morrow E, Glasgow R, Volckmann E, Ibele A. Preventing return to the emergency department following bariatric surgery. Obes Surg. 2017;27:1986–92.
2. Macht R, George J, Ameli O, Hess D, Cabral H, Kazis L. Factors associated with bariatric postoperative emergency department visits. Surg Obes Relat Dis. 2016;12:1826–31.
3. Garg T, Rosas U, Rivas H, Azagury D, Morton JM. National prevalence, causes, and risk factors for bariatric surgery readmissions. Am J Surg. 2016;212:76–80.
4. Kassir R, Debs T, Tiffet O, Blanc P, Caldwell J, Iannelli A, Gugenheim J. Management of complications following bariatric surgery: summary. Int J Surg. 2014;12:1462–4.
5. Lewis KD, Takenaka KY, Luber SD. Acute abdominal pain in the bariatric surgery patient. Emerg Med Clin N Am. 2016;34:387–407.
6. Edwards ED, Jacob BP, Gagner M, Pomp A. Presentation and management of common post-weight loss surgery problems in the emergency department. Ann Emerg Med. 2006;47:160–6.
7. Ellison SR, Ellison SD. Bariatric surgery: a review of the available procedures and complications for the emergency physician. J Emerg Med. 2008;34:21–32.
8. Luber SD, Fischer DR, Venkat A. Care of the bariatric surgery patient in the emergency department. J Emerg Med. 2008;34:13–20.
9. Montavers P, Augustin P, Zapella N, et al. Diagnosis and management of the postoperative surgical and medical complications of bariatric surgery. Anaesth Crit Care Pain Med. 2015;34:45–52.
10. Montravers P, Guglielminotti J, Zappella N, Desmard M, Muller C, Fournier P, et al. Clinical features and outcome of postoperative peritonitis following bariatric surgery. Obes Surg. 2013;23:1536–44.
11. Chopra T, Zhao J, Alangaden G, Wood M, Kaye K. Preventing surgical site infections after bariatric surgery: value of perioperative antibiotic regimens. Expert Rev Pharm Outcomes Res. 2010;10(3):317–28.
12. Monkhouse SJ, Morgan JD, Norton SA. Complications of bariatric surgery: presentation and emergency management – a review. Ann R Coll Surg Engl. 2009;91:280–6.
13. Lehnert B, Moshiri M, Osman S, Khandelwal S, Elojeimy S, Bhargava P, Katz DS. Imaging of complications of common bariatric surgical procedures. Radiol Clin N Am. 2014;52:1071–86.
14. Contival N, Menahem B, Gautier T, Le Roux Y, Alves A. Guiding the non-bariatric surgeon through complications of bariatric surgery. J Visc Surg. 2017;754:1–14.
15. Heneghan H, Meron-Elder S, Yenumula P, Rogula T, Brethauer S, Schauer P. Incidence and management of bleeding complications after gastric bypass surgery in the morbidly obese. Surg Obes Relat Dis. 2012;8:729–35.
16. Hussain A, El-Hasani S. Bariatric emergencies: current evidence and strategies of management. World J Emerg Surg. 2013;8:58.
17. Masoomi H, Kim H, Reavis KM, Mills S, Stamos MJ, Nguyen NT. Analysis of factors predictive of gastrointestinal tract leak in laparoscopic and open gastric bypass. Arch Surg. 2011;146:1048–51.
18. Committee TACI. ASMBS guideline on the prevention and detection of gastrointestinal leak after gastric bypass including the role of imaging and surgical exploration. Surg Obes Relat Dis. 2009;5:293–6.
19. Gonzalez R, Nelson LG, Gallagher SF, Murr MM. Anastomotic leaks after laparoscopic gastric bypass. Obes Surg. 2004;14:1299–307.
20. Wernick B, Jansen M, Noria S, Stawicki SP, El Chaar M. Essential bariatric emergencies for the acute care surgeon. Eur J Trauma Emerg Surg. 2016;42:571–84.
21. Altieri MS, Wright B, Peredo A, Pryor AD. Common weight loss procedures and their complications. Am J Emerg Med. 2018;36(3):475–479.
22. Warschkow R, Tarantino I, Folie P, Beutner U, Schmied BM, Bisang P, Schultes B, Thurnheer M. C-reactive protein 2 days after laparoscopic gastric bypass surgery reliably indicates leaks and moderately predicts mortality. J Gastrointest Surg. 2012;16:1128–35.
23. Chang SH, Freeman NLB, Lee JA, Stoll CR, Calhoun AJ, Eagon JC, Colditz GA. Early major complications after bariatric surgery in the USA, 2003–2014: a systematic review and meta-analysis. Obes Rev. 2018;19(4):529–537.

Bowel Obstructions in Bariatric Surgery Patients: How Are They Managed Differently from Other Surgical Patients?

123

Michael O'Keefe

Pearls and Pitfalls
- Obstructions occur due to strictures, adhesions, hernias, or complications related to prosthetic band placement.
- Obstructions occurring in early postoperative course often require surgical intervention.
- Consider internal hernias in any patient with severe, intractable abdominal pain or evidence of bowel obstruction and history of RYGB.
- CT imaging is an effective diagnostic modality but has a low sensitivity for internal hernias in Roux-en-Y gastric bypass patients.

As the prevalence of obesity increases, the number of bariatric surgeries performed annually has also increased. As such, clinicians can expect to encounter post-bariatric surgical patients in ever-increasing numbers. Laparoscopic sleeve gastrectomy, Roux-en-Y gastric bypass, and laparoscopic gastric banding comprise 90% of the procedures performed [1]. Obstruction is one the most common complications encountered after bariatric surgery [2].

The recognition and management of bowel obstructions in bariatric patients depends on the surgery performed, the time interval between surgery and symptom onset, and the clinician's understanding of the unique characteristics of obstruction in bariatric patients. Typically, patients present with nausea, vomiting (60–80%), cramping abdominal pain (80–100%), constipation/absence of flatus (80–90%), and abdominal distension (60%) [3]. The laboratory evaluation includes CBC with differential, chemistry panel and lactate. Although there is no reliable clinical or laboratory marker for ischemia, elevated serum lactate is sensitive but not specific for ischemic

bowel in patients with small bowel obstructions (sensitivity 90–100%, specificity 42–87%) [3]. Multiple imaging modalities are available to confirm a suspected diagnosis of small bowel obstruction, but computed tomography (CT) imaging is the most reliable and readily available. CT imaging is ideally performed with both oral and IV contrast to increase detection of obstruction [1]. Providers managing small bowel obstructions in patients with a history of bariatric surgery should consider early surgical consultation and intervention compared with other surgical patients [4]. Blind nasogastric tubes for decompression are usually not beneficial unless proximal obstruction of alimentary tract and may cause injury to anastomosis sites (Table 123.1).

Roux-en-Y Gastric Bypass

Bariatric surgery with Roux-en-Y gastric bypass (RYGB) has been and continues to be a commonly performed procedure for weight loss. Unfortunately, bowel obstruction is one of the most common causes of abdominal pain after Roux-en-Y gastric bypass, with an incidence of 3–5% [5, 6]. Early obstruction tends to result from technical complications with the Roux limb, such anastomotic stricture at the gastrojejunostomy or jejunojejunostomy sites, while delayed obstruction often is the result of adhesions or hernias [1]. Hwang et al. reported that the most common cause of obstruction was adhesions, accounting for 25% of obstructions in their series of 1715 bariatric patients [7].

The clinical presentation is dependent on the location of obstruction. Obstruction of the Roux limb or common channel (alimentary path) presents with classic symptoms of obstruction, including nausea, vomiting, abdominal pain, and distention (Fig. 123.1). Symptoms associated with stenosis of the proximal gastrojejunostomy include epigastric pain associated with progressive dysphagia and vomiting. Most strictures of the proximal anastomosis site occur within the first 90 days after surgery but may present beyond this time frame [2]. One study estimated the incidence of

M. O'Keefe
Division of Emergency Medicine, Duke University Medical Center, Durham, NC, USA
e-mail: michael.o'keefe@duke.edu

© Springer Nature Switzerland AG 2019
A. Graham, D. J. Carlberg (eds.), *Gastrointestinal Emergencies*, https://doi.org/10.1007/978-3-319-98343-1_123

Table 123.1 Bowel obstruction associated with bariatric surgeries

Surgery	Type of obstruction	Symptoms	Occurrence timing	Diagnosis	Treatment
Adjustable gastric band	ABG slippage	Nausea, vomiting, epigastric pain	Early – rare Late – increases with time	UGIS/CT oral contrast	Surgery with removal/repositioning of ABG
	Esophageal dilation	Nausea, vomiting, epigastric pain	Early	UGIS	Loosening of ABG; removal if failure
Sleeve gastrectomy	Stricture, gastric outlet obstruction	Nausea, vomiting, epigastric pain	Early postop	UGIS/CT scan	Based on location, Tx endoscopic or surgical conversion to Roux-en-Y
Gastric bypass	Anastomotic stricture	Pain, nausea, vomiting	Early	UGIS/CT oral contrast	Location dependent; endoscopic vs surgery
	Internal hernia	Intermittent pain	Late	Difficult, high false negative	Surgery consultation, closure of mesenteric gaps

Fig. 123.1 Obstruction of the Roux limb or common channel presents with classic symptoms of obstruction

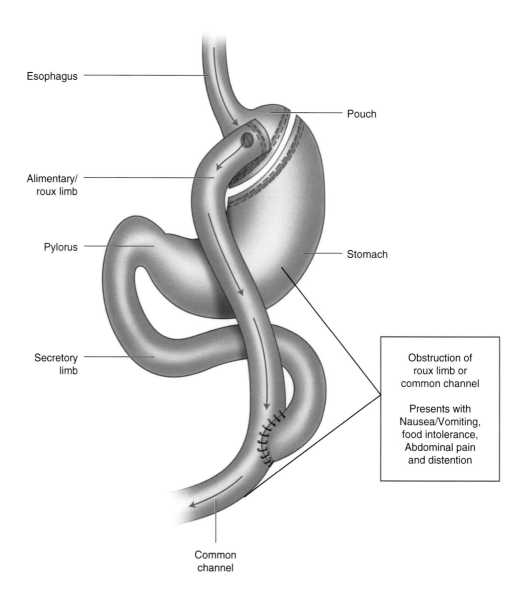

Esophagus

Pouch

Alimentary/ roux limb

Pylorus

Stomach

Secretory limb

Obstruction of roux limb or common channel

Presents with Nausea/Vomiting, food intolerance, Abdominal pain and distention

Common channel

gastrojejunal stricture requiring intervention as high as 7% [2]. Candy cane Roux syndrome occurs when a redundant proximal portion of the Roux limb twists, leading to obstruction and symptoms of nausea, vomiting, and early satiety [8]. CT is the study of choice for other sites of obstruction along the alimentary tract; however, if gastrojejunal stricture is suspected, upper endoscopy is preferred, offering both diagnosis and simultaneous intervention (e.g., balloon dilation).

The bypassed stomach is referred to as the gastric remnant and continues to produce mucus and gastric acid that combines with bile and pancreatic secretions and joins with the alimentary tract via the biliopancreatic limb. If the biliopancreatic limb is obstructed, then patients experience abdominal pain and fullness from distention of the gastric remnant as well as hiccups due to diaphragmatic irritation. Because the bypassed gastric remnant is no longer part of the alimentary tract, patients with biliopancreatic limb obstruction do not experience significant nausea or vomiting (Fig. 123.2). Obstruction due to stricture of the jejunojejunostomy is serious and may lead to rapid dilation of the remnant stomach, perforation, peritonitis, and rapid decline. Gastric remnant dilation is not always visible on plain abdominal radiographs; and if suspected, a CT with oral and IV contrast should be performed [9]. Treatment includes surgical or percutaneous decompression of the gastric remnant as well as addressing the cause of obstruction.

Internal Hernias

This specific type of obstruction involves herniation of bowel through a defect within the peritoneal cavity and is associated with a mortality rate up to 50% if untreated because of the high likelihood of bowel ischemia and necrosis [10]. While rare with an overall incidence of <1%, clinicians should maintain a higher clinical suspicion after specific bariatric surgeries and liver transplantation [10]. Both RYGB and biliopancreatic diversion with duodenal switch (BPD/DS) are predisposed to internal hernias due to the requisite weight loss increasing potential intra-abdominal space and the creation of iatrogenic mesenteric defects that allows the bowel to herniate through these defects (Fig. 123.3). In one series, internal hernias caused 41% of all obstructions [11]. To diminish this potential complication, some bariatric surgeons will close the mesenteric defects associated with

Fig. 123.2 Obstruction of biliopancreatic limb

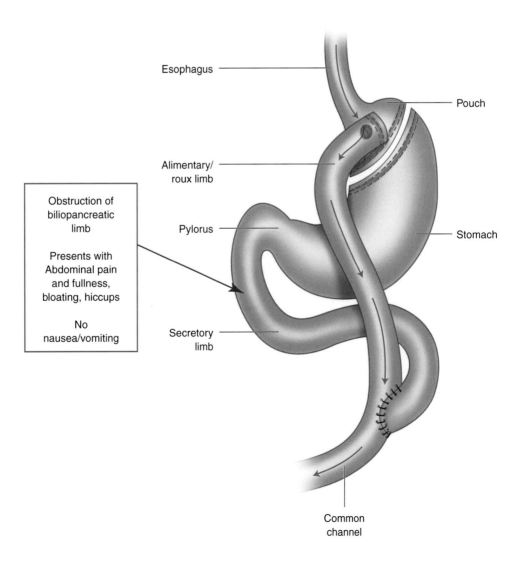

Obstruction of biliopancreatic limb

Presents with Abdominal pain and fullness, bloating, hiccups

No nausea/vomiting

Esophagus

Pouch

Alimentary/ roux limb

Pylorus

Stomach

Secretory limb

Common channel

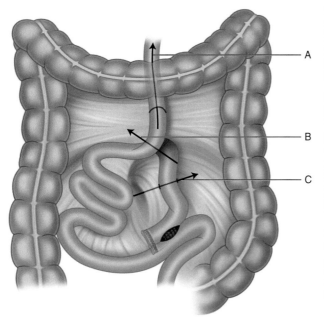

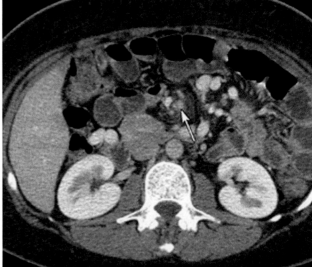

Fig. 123.3 Mesenteric defects after Roux-en-Y gastric bypass. (**a**) Petersen's defect is defined as the space between the Roux limb and the transverse mesocolon. (**b**) A defect is also present between the biliopancreatic and Roux limbs at the jejunojejunostomy. (**c**) If a retrocolic approach is used, a third defect in the transverse mesocolon is created

the surgical approach. A study performed at Mount Sinai found that closure of these defects resulted in a decreased incidence of internal hernias from 3.3% to 1.2% [2]. Internal hernias are not common in sleeve gastrectomy because of the difference in surgical technique.

The clinical presentation of obstruction from internal hernias is similar to that of small bowel obstructions from external hernias or adhesions. Patients experience abdominal pain in the midepigastrum with or without radiation to the back, pain relieved by leaning forward, colicky periumbilical abdominal pain, nausea, vomiting, low-grade fevers, and signs/symptoms of dehydration. Internal herniation of the mesenteric window at the level of the jejunojejunostomy often presents with localized pain to the left flank. Because of the high risk of ischemia and bowel necrosis, patients with prolonged bowel ischemia may describe severe abdominal pain out of proportion to physical examination.

Detection of internal hernias by CT imaging is difficult. In numerous studies, CT imaging was reported to have a low sensitivity (30–60%) and a high specificity (90.0%). The PPV and NPPV were found to be relatively low at 66.7% and 64.3%, respectively [12]. Internal hernias may intermittently become incarcerated and then spontaneously reduce; thus, imaging is best obtained while patient is symptomatic [11]. When performed during a bout of pain, CT with IV and oral contrast allows detection of bowel obstruction along with findings suggestive of internal herniation, such as abnormal location of encapsulated distended bowel loops, crowding of

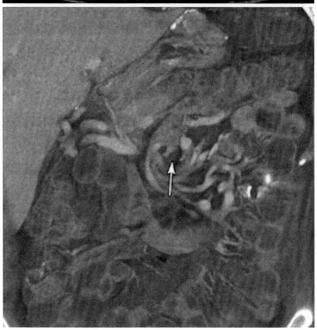

Fig. 123.4 The swirl or whirl sign on CT is seen approximately 80% of the time in patients with a Petersen hernia [13]

small bowel loops in hernia sac, and mesenteric vascular engorgement, crowding, or twisting [11]. In a study by Lockhart et al., the single best sign for detection of an internal hernia in laparoscopic RYGB patients was the "mesenteric swirl" [1]. Mesenteric swirl refers to a swirled appearance of either the mesenteric vessels or fat at the root of the small bowel mesentery (Fig. 123.4).

When detected, treatment involves discussion with bariatric surgeons for urgent exploratory laparoscopy to confirm the diagnosis, release incarcerated bowel, and close the mesenteric defects to prevent hernia recurrence [14]. A negative CT of the abdomen and pelvis in the patient with severe, persistent abdominal pain still constitutes a surgical emergency because internal hernias may not be distinguishable from obstruction due to adhesions and may not even be associated with bowel obstruction.

Sleeve Gastrectomy

Obstruction of the gastric sleeve may occur due to stenosis, twisting, or kinking, in the early postoperative period with postprandial nausea and vomiting. Diagnosis may be confirmed with upper GI series or CT with oral contrast. According to the location, treatment can be endoscopic with dilation or stent placement by GI or surgical conversion into a gastric bypass [4].

Adjustable Gastric Band

Early band obstruction (<30 days) causing esophagogastric pouch dilation is uncommon due to changes in the technical advances in gastric bands, occurring in 0.3–2.6% of LAGB placements [15]. However, band slippage with gastric obstruction is a common complication that occurs greater than 30 days from the procedure. Band slippage is movement of the band from its original position that causes the stomach to prolapse above or below the band [16]. Patients experience nausea, vomiting, dysphagia, and gastric reflux [17]. This diagnosis can be confirmed with history obtained from the patient and a plain upright abdominal radiograph (X-ray). Contrast imaging of the upper GI tract (esophagram) may help detect the rotation of the device, size of pouch, and herniated fundus (Refer to Chap. 126).

> **Suggested Resources**
> - BEAM ED. https://asmbs.org/resources/beam-ed.
> - Contival N, et al. Guiding the nonbariatric surgeon through complications of bariatric surgery. J Visc Surg. 2018;155(1):27–40. https://doi.org/10.1016/j.jviscsurg.2017.10.012. Epub 2017 Dec 23.

References

1. Riaz RM, et al. Multidetector CT imaging of bariatric surgical complications: a pictorial review. Abdom Radiol. 2016;41:174–88.
2. Herron D. Gastrointestinal obstruction after bariatric surgery. In: Nguyen NT, Blackstone RP, Morton JM, Ponce J, Rosenthal RJ, editors. The ASMBS textbook of bariatric surgery (2015). The ASMBS textbook of bariatric surgery: Volume 1: Bariatric surgery. New York: Springer. p. 228.
3. Cardaci MB, et al. Hiatal hernia containing alimentary limb and the gastric pouch: a rare cause of small bowel obstruction after Roux-en Y gastric bypass. Surg Obes Relat Dis. 2017;13:1929–31.
4. Sobinsky JD. Unusual cause of bowel obstruction after laparoscopic sleeve gastrectomy. Surg Obes Relat Dis. 2014;10:999–1001.
5. Carucci L, Turner M. Imaging after bariatric surgery for morbid obesity: roux-en-Y gastric bypass and laparoscopic adjustable gastric banding. Semin Roentgenol. 2009;44(4):283–96.
6. Lehnert B, Moshiri M, Osman S, Khandelwal S, Elojeimy S, Bhargava P, et al. Imaging of complications of common bariatric surgical procedures. Radiol Clin N Am. 2014;52(5):1071–86.
7. Hwang RF, Swartz DE, Felix EL. Cause of small bowel obstruction after laparoscopic gastric bypass. Surg Endosc. 2004;18:1631–5.
8. Aryaie AH, et al. Candy cane syndrome: an underappreciated cause of abdominal pain and nausea after Roux-en-Y gastric bypass surgery. Surg Obes Relat Dis. 2017;13:1501–5.
9. Levine MS. Imaging of bariatric surgery: normal anatomy and postoperative complications. Radiology. 2014;270(2):327–41.
10. Martin L, Merkle E, Thompson W. Review of internal hernias: radiographic and clinical findings. Am J Roentgenol. 2006;186(3):703–17.
11. Rogula T, Yenumula PR, Schauer PR. A complication of roux-en-Y gastric bypass: intestinal obstruction. Surg Endosc. 2007;21:1914–8.
12. Farukhi, Mohammad A, CT scan reliability in detecting internal hernia after gastric bypass. J Soc Laparoendosc Surg. 2017;21(4): e2017.00054.
13. Gaetke-Udager K, Wasnik A, Kaza R, Al-Hawary M, Maturen K, Cohan R. A guide to imaging in bariatric surgery. Emerg Radiol. 2014;21(3):309–19.
14. Quezada N, et al. High frequency of internal hernias after Roux-en-Y gastric bypass. Obes Surg. 2015;25(4):615–21.
15. Ren-Felding C, Allen J. Gastric banding complications: management. In: Nguyen N, et al., editors. The ASMBS textbook of bariatric surgery. New York: Springer; 2015. p. 249.
16. Carucci LR, Turner MA, Szucs RA. Adjustable laparoscopic gastric banding for morbid obesity: imaging assessment and complications. Radiol Clin N Am. 2007;45(2):261–74.
17. Snow JM, Severson PA. Complications of adjustable gastric banding. Surg Clin North Am. 2011;91(6):1249–64.

Gastrointestinal Bleeding in the Bariatric Patient: What Else Should I Consider?

124

Christina S. Houser and Julie T. Vieth

Pearls and Pitfalls
- Staple line bleeding occurs within 12–24 h postoperatively after gastric bypass or sleeve gastrectomy.
- Marginal ulcers can have an incidence as high as 52% in gastric bypass patients presenting with abdominal complaints.
- Band erosion occurs in approximately 1–3% of patients and typically presents with vague complaints.
- Hemodynamically stable patients require only fluid resuscitation and/or blood products for anemia.
- Endoscopy is the diagnostic standard for gastrointestinal bleeding in bariatric patients.

Gastrointestinal bleeding is a well-known complication of bariatric surgery. The majority of the available data focuses on gastrointestinal bleeding after Roux-en-Y gastric bypass (RYGB), sleeve gastrectomy, and gastric banding.

The clinician's evaluation of gastrointestinal bleeding in bariatric patients begins with an assessment of clinical stability, broad laboratory investigations, and tailored imaging studies based on the presumed cause of the bleeding. Similar to the management of gastrointestinal bleeding in non-bariatric patients, stabilization and management are dependent upon the hemodynamics of the patient, ranging from outpatient follow-up to medical resuscitation. Of note, emergent surgery plays a greater role in bariatric patients with postoperative bleeding. In general, unstable patients with acute, early, or late bleeding will often require a laparoscopy or laparotomy with concurrent intraoperative esophagogastroduodenoscopy (EGD); thus, early consultation with the patient's bariatric surgeon can facilitate care.

When considering the etiology of gastrointestinal bleeding in bariatric patients, it is helpful to categorize patients by (1) the bariatric procedure performed and (2) time elapsed since surgery.

- Acute bleeding complications occur in the first week (1–7 days).
- Early complications are defined as those that occur less than 30 days from the operation. Some experts will extend the early designation to 6 weeks postoperatively.
- Late complications are those that arise after 30 days (or 6 weeks), with chronic bleeding classified as >12 weeks postoperative.

Many patients will have history and physical exam findings of overt gastrointestinal bleeding including hematemesis, melena, or hematochezia. Evaluation of potential bleeding in bariatric patients can be challenging due to their body habitus, poor physiologic reserve, and new anatomy. Tachycardia, vague abdominal pain, nausea, and vomiting may indicate gastrointestinal bleeding or intra-abdominal bleeding in bariatric patients. Similar to anastomotic leaks with sepsis, tachycardia is a key indicator of bleeding in the bariatric patient. However, the pattern of tachycardia may help to distinguish between these two etiologies. Bleeding tends to have a cyclical pattern of tachycardia, while anastomotic leaks will maintain a steady tachycardia >120 beats per minute [1] (Fig. 124.1).

Furthermore, one should consider whether the cause of bleeding is intra-abdominal or intraluminal. Intra-abdominal bleeding is primarily a concern in the early postoperative period and is less likely to require reoperation compared to intraluminal [2]. Blood in the surgical drains, hypotension,

C. S. Houser (✉)
MedStar Washington Hospital Center, MedStar Georgetown University Hospital, Washington, DC, USA
e-mail: Christina.S.Houser@medstar.net

J. T. Vieth
Canton-Potsdam Hospital, Potsdam, NY, USA
e-mail: jvieth@cphospital.org

© Springer Nature Switzerland AG 2019
A. Graham, D. J. Carlberg (eds.), *Gastrointestinal Emergencies*, https://doi.org/10.1007/978-3-319-98343-1_124

Fig. 124.1 (**a**) Sustained
tachycardia >120 bpm in
anastomotic leak, (**b**) cyclical
tachycardia with bleeding in
RYGB patient [2]

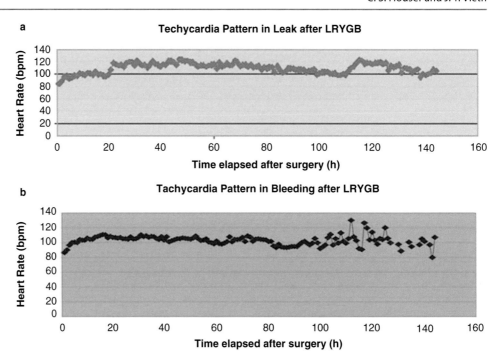

tachycardia, and decreasing hemoglobin/hematocrit without other source of bleeding would suggest an intra-abdominal etiology. Intraluminal bleeding presents with melena, hematemesis, or hematochezia.

The diagnostic standard for both early and late bleeds is endoscopy, as it affords the opportunity for simultaneous diagnosis and intervention [3–6]. If endoscopy does not reveal an obvious cause of intraluminal bleeding, then stable patients can be considered for a bleeding scan or less commonly angiography, as the source of bleeding is often from the jejunal branches of the superior mesenteric artery or gastric branches of the celiac artery [7]. Given that consultation with a specialist is required for endoscopy to be performed, it is reasonable for the clinician to obtain an intravenous and oral contrast-enhanced computed tomography (CT) and/or an upper gastrointestinal (UGI) series to further delineate the source of bleeding. CT may assist in determining intraluminal versus intra-abdominal bleeding [8]. CT may locate extraluminal bleeding or hematomas adjacent to anastomosis sites that cannot be seen on endoscopy [6]. Radiographic findings of GI bleeding include an intraluminal contrast blush or hyperattenuating clot, which can be present even in the absence of active bleeding [9]. It is important to remember that CT scans for bariatric patients with presumed gastrointestinal bleeding should include both intravenous and oral contrast.

Management of gastrointestinal bleeding in bariatric patients is dependent upon the hemodynamics of the patient. In hemodynamically stable patients, intravenous fluids and transfusion may be all that is necessary [3]. When determin-

ing the need for transfusion, it is important to remember that bariatric patients have a multitude of nutritional deficiencies that may contribute to anemia. Hemodynamically unstable patients require emergent imaging, including possible endoscopy [10]. In some cases, endoscopy may not be able to reach the source of bleeding, or the patient may be too unstable to undergo imaging, in which case emergent laparoscopy or laparotomy should be performed.

Roux-en-Y Gastric Bypass

Gastrointestinal bleeding after RYGB has an incidence of 0.6–3.7% [11].

Early, <30 Days Post-op

Bleeding in the early postoperative period is frequently due to hemorrhage at the staple line, visceral injury to the spleen or liver, abdominal wall/trocar site bleeding, or mesenteric vessel bleeding which typically occurs within the first 12–48 h postoperatively but has been described as late as postoperative day 42 [3, 10, 11]. Staple line bleeding has a higher incidence in laparoscopic RYGB compared with open RYGB due to multiple staple lines. Approximately 40% of staple line bleeds are from the gastric remnant, 30% are at the site of gastrojejunostomy, and 30% are at the jejunostomy [12].

Late, >30 Days Post-op

Late gastrointestinal bleeding after RYGB is frequently due to marginal ulcers. These ulcers typically occur at the gastrojejunal anastomosis and are thought to be secondary to the exposure of the jejunum to the acidity of gastric contents [13]. Since many patients are asymptomatic, the true incidence of marginal ulcers is difficult to determine, but it is estimated to range from 0.6% to 16%. In RYGB patients presenting with generalized abdominal complaints, the incidence of marginal ulcers can be as high as 52% [4]. Although less common, ulceration at the gastric pouch, bypassed stomach, and duodenum are also considerations as possible causes of late bleeding [3]. Risk factors for ulceration include the use of NSAIDs, smoking, gastrogastric fistulas, and the use of nonabsorbable sutures during the bypass procedure [11, 14]. A recently published retrospective cohort analysis of 253,765 patients with marginal ulcers in the setting of bariatric surgery demonstrated that *H. pylori* is an independent risk factor of marginal ulceration [15]. Preoperative testing and treatment may contribute to prevention. Previous smaller studies had not demonstrated this association [16, 17].

In a hemodynamically stable patient with minimal bleeding and good follow-up, oral proton pump inhibitor initiation may be all that is required in consultation with the bariatric surgeon if a marginal ulcer is suspected.

Adjustable Gastric Band

For bariatric patients who present with gastrointestinal bleeding after gastric banding, the clinician should consider perioperative hemorrhage in the early timeframe and band erosion in the late timeframe.

The incidence of band erosion is approximately 1%, although estimations range from 0.9% to 3.4% [11, 16, 17]. The mechanism of erosion is thought to be secondary to gastric necrosis from pressure, leading to the breakdown of the gastric lumen [18, 19]. Patients frequently present with symptoms of vague abdominal pain and weight gain [11]. Despite unimpressive symptoms, the clinician should have a low threshold to proceed with radiologic evaluation. Similar to RYGB patients, diagnostics may include upper gastrointestinal series, computed tomography, and/or endoscopy. Definitive treatment involves band deflation and/or readjustment and repair of the gastric lumen if necessary [11, 13].

Sleeve Gastrectomy

Gastrointestinal hemorrhage can occur in up to 6% of patients after gastric sleeve surgery [6]. In patients who have undergone sleeve gastrectomy, there are typically two sites of bleeding: the first is from gastric vessels along the dissection plane of the greater curvature of the stomach, and the second site is along the staple line [13]. In hemodynamically stable patients, this can be diagnosed with an intravenous and oral contrast-enhanced CT, and in hemodynamically unstable patients, emergent endoscopy is warranted for source control [6].

References

1. Bellorin O, Abdemur A, Sucandy I, Rosenthal R. Understanding the significance, reasons and patterns of abnormal vital signs after gastric bypass for morbid obesity. – PubMed – NCBI [Internet]. Ncbi.nlm.nih.gov. 2018 [cited 12 Jan 2018]. Available from: https://www.ncbi.nlm.nih.gov/m/pubmed/20582574/.
2. Fridman A, Szomstein S, Rosenthal RJ. Postoperative bleeding in the bariatric surgery patient. In: Nguyen N, Blackstone R, Morton J, Ponce J, Rosenthal R, editors. The ASMBS textbook of bariatric surgery. New York: Springer; 2015.
3. Rabl C, Peeva S, Prado K, James A, Rogers S, Posselt A, et al. Early and late abdominal bleeding after roux-en-Y gastric bypass: sources and tailored therapeutic strategies. Obes Surg. 2011;21(4):413–20.
4. Gumbs A, Duffy A, Bell R. Incidence and management of marginal ulceration after laparoscopic roux-Y gastric bypass. Surg Obes Relat Dis. 2006;2(4):460–3.
5. Puri V, Alagappan A, Rubin M, Merola S. Management of bleeding from gastric remnant after roux-en-Y gastric bypass. Surg Obes Relat Dis. 2012;8(1):e3–5.
6. Miao T, Kielar A, Patlas M, Riordon M, Chong S, Robins J, et al. Cross-sectional imaging, with surgical correlation, of patients presenting with complications after remote bariatric surgery without bowel obstruction. Abdom Imaging. 2015;40(8):2945–65.
7. Sidani S, Akkary E, Bell R. Catastrophic bleeding from a marginal ulcer after gastric bypass. J Soc of Laparoendosc Surg. 2013;17(1):148–51.
8. Kothari S. Bariatric surgery and postoperative imaging. Surg Clin N Am. 2011;91(1):155–72.
9. Guniganti P, Bradenham C, Raptis C, Menias C, Mellnick V. CT of gastric emergencies. Radiographics. 2015;35(7):1909–21.
10. Issa H, Al-Saif O, Al-Momen S, Bseiso B, Al-Salem A. Bleeding duodenal ulcer after roux-en-Y gastric bypass surgery: the value of laparoscopic gastroduodenoscopy. Ann Saudi Med. 2010;30(1):67–9.
11. Nguyen N, Wilson S. Complications of anti obesity surgery. Nat Clin Pract Gastroenterol Hepatol. 2007;4(3):138–47.
12. Heneghan H, Meron-Eldar S, Yenumula P, Rogula T, Brethauer S, Schauer P. Incidence and management of bleeding complications after gastric bypass surgery in the morbidly obese. Surg Obes Relat Dis. 2012;8(6):729–35.
13. Ellsmere J, Jones D, Chen W. Late complications of bariatric surgical operations [Internet]. Uptodate.com. 2017 [cited 12 Jan 2018]. Available from: https://www.uptodate.com/contents/late-complications-of-bariatric-surgical-operations.
14. Lewis K, Takenaka K, Luber S. Acute abdominal pain in the bariatric surgery patient. Emerg Med Clin North Am. 2016;34(2):387–407.
15. Schulman AR, Abougergi MS, Thompson CC. H. Pylori as a predictor of marginal ulceration: a nationwide analysis. Obesity. 2017;25(3):522–6.
16. Rawlins L, Rawlins MP, Brown CC, Schumacher DL. Effect on helicobacter pylori on marginal ulcer and stomal stenosis after roux-en-Y gastric bypass. Surg Obes Relat Dis. 2013;9(5):760–4.

17. Papasavas PK, Gagne DJ, Donnelly PE, Salgada J, Urbandt JE, Burton KK, Caushaj PF. Prevalence of helicobacter pylori infection and value of preoperative testing and treatment in patients undergoing laparoscopic roux-en-Y gastric bypass. Surg Obes Relat Dis. 2008;4(3):383–8.

18. Cappell M, Mogrovejo E, Desai T. Case report of patient presenting in shock from band penetration into stomach after LAGB surgery: diagnosis by emergency EGD after misdiagnosis by abdominal CT. Dig Dis Sci. 2016;61(11):3366–8.

19. Lehnert B, Moshiri M, Osman S, Khandelwal S, Elojeimy S, Bhargava P, et al. Imaging of complications of common bariatric surgical procedures. Radiol Clin N Am. 2014;52(5):1071–86.

What Is Dumping Syndrome? How Do I Diagnose and Treat Dumping Syndrome?

125

Zhaoxin Yang and Autumn Graham

Pearls and Pitfalls
- Dumping syndrome is a group of gastrointestinal and vasomotor symptoms which occurs when food reaches the small bowel too rapidly.
- Late symptoms result from hypoglycemia due to rapid insulin release.
- While the elimination of alternative diagnoses in combination with a high Sigstad score or Dumping Syndrome Rating Scale score is suggestive of dumping syndrome, definitive diagnosis is confirmed with a glucose tolerance test.
- Initial treatment is diet modification. Adjunct therapies such as somatostatin treatment have been found to alleviate symptoms when refractory to dietary changes.

Clinical Scenario

A patient with a history of Roux-en-Y gastric bypass surgery 3 months ago presents to the emergency department complaining of diarrhea and bloating. He is in no acute distress and has a benign abdominal exam. He has had similar symptoms in the past with negative imaging and medical workup. He asks if this could be a complication of his gastric bypass surgery.

Z. Yang (✉)
MedStar Georgetown University Hospital, Department of Emergency Medicine, Washington, DC, USA

A. Graham
Department of Emergency Medicine, MedStar Washington Hospital Center, MedStar Georgetown University Hospital, Washington, DC, USA

What is Dumping Syndrome?

Dumping syndrome refers to a constellation of gastrointestinal and vasomotor symptoms which occurs when food reaches the small bowel too rapidly. [Table 125.1] In addition to secreting digestive enzymes and mechanically breaking down food, the stomach controls the timing of nutrients released into the duodenum, e.g., a gatekeeper function [1]. In gastric bypass surgery, both structural and functional altercations of the stomach occur, such as removal of the pylorus. These changes allow rapid gastric emptying of large undigested food particles into the small bowel, contributing to the development of dumping syndrome.

Symptoms

Triggered by meals, the symptoms of dumping syndrome are classified as early or late. Early symptoms result from undigested hyperosmolar contents in the duodenum, causing a release of vasoactive agents, incretins, and glucose modulators [2]. This results in fluid shifting from intravascular compartments into the lumen. Early symptoms include gastrointestinal symptoms (e.g., early satiety, epigastric pain, diarrhea, nausea, cramping, and bloating) as well as systemic vasomotor symptoms (e.g., palpitations, tachycardia, fatigue, flushing, pallor, diaphoresis, lightheadedness, hypotension, and headache). Late symptoms occur between 1–3 h after ingestion [3]. These symptoms are due primarily to a transient hyperglycemia due to a large food bolus from a rapidly

Table 125.1 Symptoms of dumping syndrome

Early Symptoms
Gastrointestinal symptoms: abdominal pain, diarrhea, borborygmi, nausea, bloating
Vasomotor symptoms: flushing, palpitations, tachycardia, diaphoresis, hypotension, syncope
Late Symptoms
Hypoglycemia: hunger, weakness, confusion, syncope, tremor

© Springer Nature Switzerland AG 2019
A. Graham, D. J. Carlberg (eds.), *Gastrointestinal Emergencies*, https://doi.org/10.1007/978-3-319-98343-1_125

emptying stomach, followed by peak insulin secretion creating hypoglycemia hours following a meal.

How Do I Diagnose and Treat Dumping Syndrome?

Diagnosis

The differential diagnosis for dumping syndrome symptoms includes gastroparesis, irritable bowel syndrome, pancreatic insufficiency, celiac disease, VIPoma, and carcinoid syndrome. In the acute care setting, diagnosis is based on a pattern of symptoms in relationship with oral intake. In 1970, Sigstad et al. proposed a scoring system based on occurrence of symptoms in order to form a diagnostic index [3]. Positive predictive symptoms include 4 points for syncope or desire to sit/lie down; 3 points for dyspnea, lethargy, or palpitations; 2 points for restlessness or dizziness; and 1 point for headache, diaphoresis, nausea, or abdominal fullness. Inverse relationships with symptoms include −1 point for belching or - 4 points for vomiting. A score of >7 is suggestive of dumping syndrome whereas a score <4 suggests an alternative diagnosis [4]. A high Sigstad score in the setting of hypoglycemia is highly suggestive of dumping syndrome.

More recently, a self-assessment questionnaire, the Dumping Syndrome Rating Scale (DSRS), was created. There are 12 questions asking about patient's recent symptoms after a meal. Out of 129 patients, they found that after 1 and 2 years status post gastric bypass, 12% had persistent symptoms, with postprandial fatigue and desire to sit/lie down being the most common symptoms [5]. The DSRS can be easily accessed and given to patients who clinicians suspect of dumping syndrome.

Definitive diagnosis is made with a modified oral glucose tolerance test that can be done as an outpatient. Patients fast for 10 h overnight and then ingest 50 g of glucose. Pulse, blood pressure, glucose, and sometimes hematocrit is obtained before, during, and 30 min after ingestion. Overall, the test has a sensitivity, as high as 100% and specificity of 94% [6]. The best predictor of dumping syndrome is a rise in heart rate greater than ten beats per minute 30 min after 50 g glucose is ingested [6]. The rate of gastric emptying should be higher in patients with dumping syndrome, though it is neither sensitive nor specific [7]. However, these tests are rarely needed in an emergent setting.

Treatment

The initial management of dumping syndrome is dietary modifications. Recommendations include consuming smaller meals by dividing daily calorie intake into six meals and delaying liquids at least 30 min after meals [8]. Rapidly absorbable simple carbohydrates should also be avoided. Adjuncts to diet modification include pectin and guar gum, which slow down gastric emptying by increasing food viscosity [9]. Acarbose, which interferes with carbohydrate absorption in the small intestines, has also proven to relieve symptoms in small studies [10].

After dietary modifications, medications such as somatostatin analogs (e.g., octreotide) alleviate symptoms by delaying gastric emptying and small bowel transit time, as well as inhibiting gastric hormones and insulin secretion [11]. Multiple studies have evaluated both short- and long-term somatostatin therapies, with results showing sustained symptom control in patients refractory to dietary modifications [12]. In severe cases refractory to medical management, surgical interventions, such as narrowing of the anastomosis, conversion of the prior bariatric surgery, and using jejunostomy parenteral feeding, may help [13]. Follow-up with gastrointestinal specialists and the patient's bariatric surgeon is strongly recommended if dumping syndrome is suspected.

Summary

In summary, gastric bypass surgery can predispose patients to a constellation of symptoms known as dumping syndrome. Definitive diagnosis requires an oral glucose tolerance test, but ED clinicians can improve the quality of life for these patients by recommending dietary modifications and follow-up with gastroenterology and bariatric surgery.

Suggested Resources

- For patient information: https://www.medicalnews-today.com/articles/320479.php.
- For diagnostic scoring scales: https://www.wikidoc.org/index.php/Gastric_dumping_syndrome_screening.
- Tack J, et al. Pathophysiology, diagnosis and management of postoperative dumping syndrome. Nat Rev. Gastroenterol Hepatol. 2009;6:583–90.

References

1. Tack J. Pathophysiology, diagnosis and management of postoperative dumping syndrome. Nat Rev Gastroenterol Hepatol. 2009;6:583–90.
2. Tack J. Gastric motor disorders. Best Pract Res Clin Gastroenterol. 2007;21:633–44.
3. Sigstad H. A clinical diagnostic index in the diagnosis of the dumping syndrome. Changes in plasma volume and blood sugar after a test meal. Acta Med Scandinavica. 1970;188:479–86.

4. Service G. Hyperinsulinemic hypoglycemia with nesidioblastosis after gastric-bypass surgery. N Engl J Med. 2005;353:249–54.

5. Laurenius A. Dumping syndrome following gastric bypass: validation of the dumping syndrome rating scale. Obes Surg. 2013;23:740–55.

6. Van der Kleij F, Vecht J, Lamers C, Masclee AA. Diagnostic value of dumping provocation in patients after gastric surgery. Scand J Gastroenterol. 1996;31:1162–6.

7. Vecht J, Masclee A, Lamers C. The dumping syndrome: current insights into pathophysiology, diagnosis and treatment. Scand J Gastroenterol. 1997;223:21–7.

8. Abell T, Minocha A. Gastrointestinal complications of bariatric surgery: diagnosis and therapy. Am J Med Sci. 2006;331:214–8.

9. Harju E, Larmi T. Efficacy of guar gum in preventing the dumping syndrome. JPEN. 1983;7:470–2.

10. Lyons T, McLoughlin J, Shaw C, Buchanan K. Effect of acarbose on biochemical responses and clinical symptoms in dumping syndrome. Digestion. 1985;31:89–96.

11. Arts J. Efficacy of the long-acting repeatable formulation of the somatostatin analog octreotide in postoperative dumping. Clin Gastroenterol Hepatol. 2009;7:432–7.

12. Geer R. Efficacy of octreotide acetate in treatment of severe post-gastrectomy dumping syndrome. Ann Surg. 1990;212:678–87.

13. Woodward E, Deser P, Gasster M. Surgical treatment of the post-gastrectomy dumping syndrome. West J Surg Obstet Gynecol. 1955;63:567–73.

What Are the Complications of Gastric Banding? How Do I Diagnose and Treat Them in the Emergency Department?

126

Edward A. Descallar and Autumn Graham

Pearls and Pitfalls
- Most diagnosis will require a contrasted study of the upper GI tract.
- Important patient history includes meal volume, between meal snacks, and liquid consumption.
- Early diagnosis is crucial to preventing future complications.
- The two most common complications of LAGB are pouch dilation and band slippage.

Overall, laparoscopic adjustable gastric banding (LAGB) is a safe bariatric surgery with a 30 day morbidity of 3% but is associated with a delayed complication rate of 12% [1]. In 2011, the FDA expanded approval of the gastric band for patients with BMIs (body mass indexes) between 30 and 40 kg/m^2 with weight-related conditions. Despite LAGB's former popularity, approximately 50% of patients will require reoperation due to failed weight loss or intolerance of device, and therefore it currently accounts for only 5% of bariatric procedures performed [1]. The clinical presentation of most gastric banding complications is similar. Patients present with vomiting, dysphagia, reflux, abdominal pain, or failed weight loss. Most patients will require at least a screening single-view abdominal radiograph. In some instances, an upper GI series, lab work, endoscopy and surgical consultation are required to accurately diagnose the cause of their symptoms [2].

Complications of gastric banding vary depending on the time from the initial surgery. There are early postoperative complications that appear within 1 month following surgery and late postoperative complications that appear after 1 month. Early complications (<30-day morbidity) include gastric/esophageal perforation, bleeding, esophagogastric

Table 126.1 Complications of gastric banding

Early complications	Delayed complications
Gastric/esophageal perforation – Rare but typically occurs when a prior hiatal hernia changes the stomach anatomy	**Gastric prolapse**
	Port infection
	Band erosion
Bleeding – Most commonly from the spleen but has also been reported with patients with fatty livers and ensuring liver lacerations	**Port/tubing disconnection**
	Persistent GERD
Esophagogastric obstruction – Rare due to changes in the band device in recent years	
Port infection	

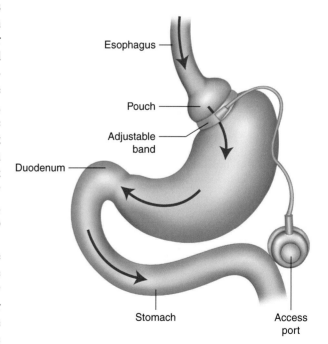

Fig. 126.1 Anatomic landmarks of gastric band procedure

obstruction, and port infection. Delayed or late complications (>30-day morbidity) include gastric prolapse, erosion, and port/tubing disconnection (Table 126.1, Fig. 126.1).

E. A. Descallar (✉) · A. Graham
Department of Emergency Medicine, MedStar Washington Hospital Center, MedStar Georgetown University Hospital, Washington, DC, USA

© Springer Nature Switzerland AG 2019
A. Graham, D. J. Carlberg (eds.), *Gastrointestinal Emergencies*, https://doi.org/10.1007/978-3-319-98343-1_126

Gastric or Esophageal Perforation

An optional component of the surgical placement of the adjustable gastric band is a probe that calibrates the volume of the gastric pouch and aids surgeons in the positioning of the band. This probe is inserted into the stomach via the mouth, and a 15–25 cm^3 balloon is inserted and then pulled against the gastric cardia. Employment of this procedure has been associated with esophageal and gastric perforation which may be identified intraoperatively or in the early postoperative course. It is more commonly employed in the peri-gastric technique compared with the more common "pars flaccida" technique. According to a meta-analysis conducted by the French National Agency for Health Evaluation, the growing use of the "pars flaccida" technique has lowered the incidence of iatrogenic perforation to 0.3% [3]. Patients present with chest pain, abdominal pain, tachycardia, and sepsis. While conservative medical treatment has been described, in most cases, operative management is necessary.

Band Obstruction/Esophagogastric Obstruction

Gastric pouch dilation with potential gastric necrosis and ischemia is rare, described in only 0.3–2.6% of LAGB placements [3]. Historically, rates of gastric obstruction occurred in up to 11% of patients. However, with the advent of newer bands with larger diameters and advances in surgical technique, the incidence of obstruction in the immediate postoperative period has decreased significantly [4]. Band obstruction or pouch dilation is suggested on radiograph by a vertical lie of the adjustable gastric band (AGB) and confirmed with an upper gastrointestinal series demonstrating obstruction. Management is usually surgical removal of the AGB, but some surgeons may attempt band repositioning [3].

Early Complications (<30 days from Procedure)

Gastric or Esophageal Perforation

Band slippage is a major complication that is usually considered a late complication of LAGB. The movement of the band from its original position causes the stomach to pro-

lapse above or below the band [5]. Regardless if the band slips posteriorly or more commonly anteriorly, patients experience varying degrees of obstruction and present with nausea, vomiting, dysphagia, and gastric reflux [6]. Noncompliance with a bariatric diet, such as overeating, increases the risk of gastric prolapse.

This diagnosis can be confirmed with history obtained from the patient and a plain upright abdominal radiograph (x-ray). Normal band placement is approximately 2 cm from the gastroesophageal junction creating a small pouch and limiting oral intake. On an upright abdominal radiograph, the gastric band should have a phi angle (angle between the vertical line of the spine and long axis of the gastric band) between 4 ° and 58 ° [4] (Fig. 126.2). An easier method of assessing the placement of the band is to determine if the band is "pointing" to the left shoulder (normal band placement), perpendicular to the spine or horizontal (abnormal band placement), or "pointing" to the left hip (abnormal band placement). Also, if the band creates an "O" sign on abdominal x-ray, then the band is not positioned correctly [5]. Contrast imaging of the upper GI tract (esophagram) may help detect the rotation of the device, size of pouch, and herniated fundus. Less commonly, the diagnosis is made with computed tomography or endoscopy, but these are not the preferred initial diagnostic modalities (Fig. 126.3).

Suspicion of ischemia or necrosis of the herniated gastric fundus should be high if the patient experiences severe pain given that band slippage alone rarely is associated with abdominal pain. Treatment is surgical revision so urgent surgical consultation is necessary. In the emergency department, deflation of the band may help alleviate symptoms and decrease the risk of continued tissue ischemia and necrosis [7] (Fig. 126.4).

Pouch Dilation

Pouch dilation, though not as severe as gastric band slippage, is the most common gastric banding postoperative complication [8]. This occurs with nonadherence to diet, usually with the consumption of poorly chewed food or large volumes of food [9]. Patients present with abdominal discomfort, food intolerance, early satiety, poor weight loss, or nausea/vomiting [10]. Pouch dilation can be diagnosed with a contrast-enhanced upper GI series. Treatment includes adherence to a bariatric diet, band deflation, band removal, or conversion to another bariatric surgery [11].

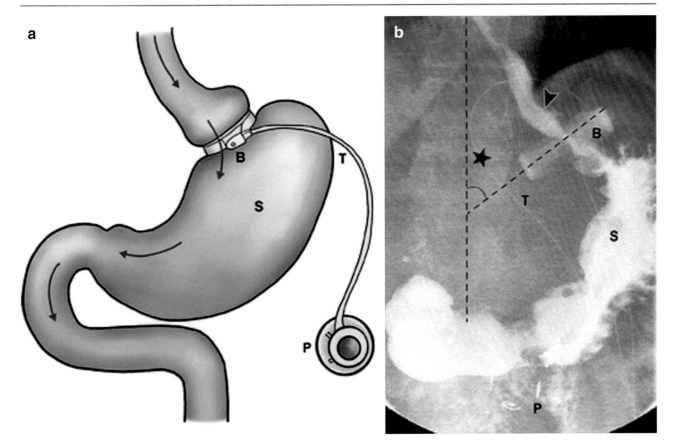

Fig. 126.2 (**a**) Illustration of normal anatomic placement of gastric band approximately 2 cm from GE junction. (**b**) Normal placement of gastric band on abdominal radiograph with oral contrast (esophagram) demonstrating a phi angle (*) between 4 ° and 58 ° as well as the band (**b**) pointing to the left shoulder (Gaetke-Udager et al. [12])

Band Erosion

Another serious adjustable gastric band complication is band erosion. It has been reported in approximately 0.2–32.6% of gastric bands placed and correlates with the surgical technique and experience of the surgeon [4]. Despite the seriousness of this complication, the presentation is often vague with chronic symptoms or patients may present asymptomatically and discover band erosion on routine endoscopy. Symptoms include delayed port infection (due to tracking of intragastric bacteria down the tubing to subcutaneous tissue around the port), increased appetite and decreased satiety despite maximal band adjustment, loss of fluid from device, abdominal pain, nausea/vomiting, fever, gastrointestinal bleeding, or sepsis [7]. Upper endoscopy is the diagnostic gold standard, but computed tomography, which is faster and readily available in most emergency departments, may aid the clinician in diagnosing this complication. Treatment involves immediate removal of the band by a bariatric surgeon as well as systemic antibiotics (Fig. 126.5).

Stomal Obstruction

Stomal obstruction is a complication that occurs more commonly in the early postoperative period but can be seen at any time following gastric band placement. It is normally caused by tissue edema, use of a band with insufficient diameter, nonadherence to diet modification, or swallowing unchewed food. Patients present with nausea, vomiting, and inability to tolerate oral intake. Diagnosis is confirmed with an upper GI series that shows no passage of contrast past the band. Treatment can range from nasogastric decompression

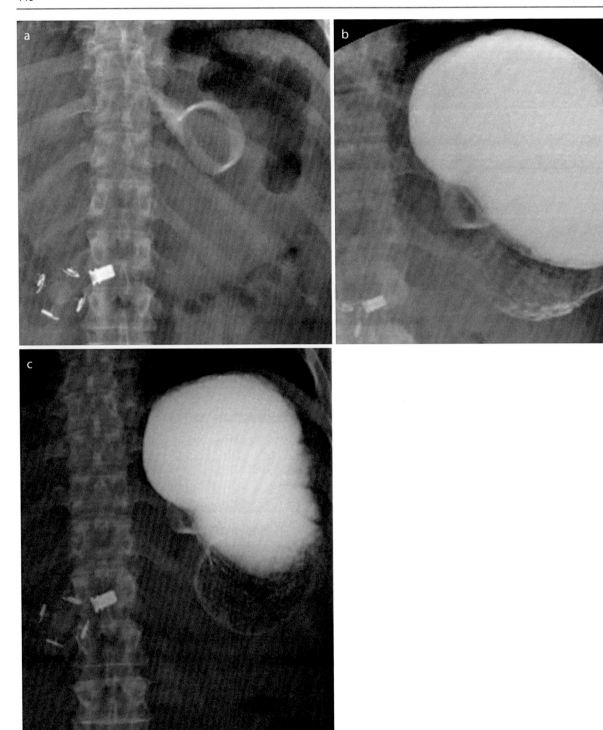

Fig. 126.3 Symptomatic slippage of gastric band. Frontal abdominal radiograph (**a**) shows abnormal tilting of the gastric band with en face orientation (the "O" sign), suggesting significant slippage, which is confirmed at contrast fluoroscopy (**b**) demonstrating a markedly dilated gastric pouch. A 2-h delayed radiograph (**c**) shows lack of emptying through the band, consistent with high-grade obstruction. (Reproduced from Gayer et al. [13] with automatic permission from Elsevier under the STM signatory guidelines)

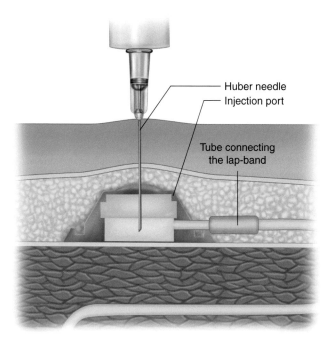

Huber needle
Injection port
Tube connecting
the lap-band

Fig. 126.4 Deflation of gastric band. Description: (1) insert a small amount of lidocaine once the port has been localized by palpation. (2) Cleanse the skin with chlorhexidine or betadine. (3) Stabilize port with the nondominant hand and then insert Huber needle to access the port. (4) Remove up to 5 cc of fluid to completely deflate the gastric band

if due to edema or surgical revision if obstruction persists after conservative management [12].

Reflux

GERD is a common complaint and presents similarly to reflux in patients without a gastric band. Causes of GERD in the LAGB patient include pouch dilation and poor diet compliance. Treatment consists of diet modification or medical management with use of proton pump inhibitors. If symptoms are attributed or suspected to be due to over-inflation of the balloon, the balloon can be deflated as described previously. If symptoms persist despite medical management, then surgical revision may be required [12, 13].

Port Disconnection/Infection

The adjustment port usually resides in the anterior abdominal wall, superficial to the rectus sheath. Its exact location varies due to surgeon preference but should be easily palpable. Pain at the port site, infection, disconnection, and inaccessibility may be complications faced by the acute care

Fig. 126.5 Erosion of gastric band into the lumen of the stomach. Abdominal CT images (**a, b**) in a patient with worsening abdominal pain and dysphagia show asymmetric gastric wall thickening along a portion of the band (a) and luminal gas immediately adjacent to another portion (**b**). Same-day upper endoscopy (**c**) confirmed erosion of the band into the gastric lumen, which required surgical exploration. (Reproduced from Gayer et al. [13] with automatic permission from Elsevier under the STM signatory guidelines)

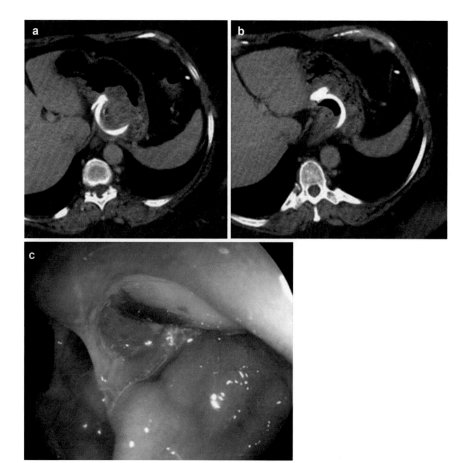

provider. Tube disconnection and inaccessibility of the port secondary to "flipped port" can be initially evaluated by the emergency medicine clinician with plain radiographs and then further management discussed with a bariatric surgeon. Delayed infected ports should be presumed to be due to band erosion until proven otherwise [4].

Due to the location of the port in the anterior abdominal wall, it may be difficult for the clinician to distinguish pain caused by the port versus intra-abdominal pathology, such as cholelithiasis or cholecystitis, if the port has been placed in the right upper quadrant. One technique to discriminate between anterior abdominal wall pain from the port and more serious pain originating from intra-abdominal disease is to sterilely inject a long-acting, local anesthetic agent around the port. If the pain resolves, then it is likely pain related to the port placement, and the patient can be safely referred to their bariatric surgeon for further evaluation of potential cutaneous nerve entrapment.

Summary

There must be a low threshold for obtaining imaging studies in patients who present with complaints following gastric banding. The rate of future complications can be decreased if diagnosed and treated early. It is strongly encouraged that clinicians consult with a bariatric surgeon prior to disposition of patients with gastric band complications.

Suggested Resource
- Ren-Felding C, Allen J. Gastric banding complications: management. In: Nguyen N, et al., editors. The ASMBS textbook of bariatric surgery. New York: Springer; 2015. p. 249.

References

1. Carelli AM, Youn HA, Kurian MS, Ren CJ, Fielding GA. Safety of the laparoscopic adjustable gastric band: 7-year data from a U.S. center of excellence. Surg Endosc. 2010;24(8):1819–23.
2. Lattuada E, Zappa MA, Mozzi E, Antonini I, Boati P, Roviaro GC. Injection port and connecting tube complications after laparoscopic adjustable gastric banding. Obes Surg. 2010;20(4):410–4.
3. Contival N, Menaham B, Gautier T, Le Roux Y, Alves A. Guiding the non-bariatric surgeon through complications of bariatric surgery. J Visc Surg. 2018;155:27–40.
4. Ren-Felding C, Allen J. Gastric banding complications: management. In: Nguyen N, et al., editors. The ASMBS textbook of bariatric surgery. New York: Springer; 2015. p. 249.
5. Carucci LR, Turner MA, Szucs RA. Adjustable laparoscopic gastric banding for morbid obesity: imaging assessment and complications. Radiol Clin N Am. 2007;45(2):261–74.
6. Snow JM, Severson PA. Complications of adjustable gastric banding. Surg Clin North Am. 2011;91(6):1249–64.
7. Kirshtein B, Lantsberg L, Mizrahi S, Avinoach E. Bariatric emergencies for non-bariatric surgeons: complications of laparoscopic gastric banding. Obes Surg. 2010;20(11):1468–78.
8. Eid I, Birch DW, Sharma AM, Sherman V, Karmali S. Complications associated with adjustable gastric banding for morbid obesity: a surgeon's guides. Can J Surg. 2011;54(1):61–6.
9. Louri N, Darwish B, Alkhalifa K. Stoma obstruction after laparoscopic adjustable gastric banding for morbid obesity: report of two cases and treatment options. Obes Rev. 2008;9(6):518–21.
10. Spivak H, Favretti F. Avoiding postoperative complications with the LAP-BAND system. Am J Surg. 2002;184(6B):31S–7S.
11. Hamdan K, Somers S, Chand M. Management of late postoperative complications of bariatric surgery. Br J Surg. 2011;98(10):1345–55.
12. Gaetke-Udager K, Wasnik A, Kaza R, Al-Hawary M, Maturen K, Cohan R. A guide to imaging in bariatric surgery. Emerg Radiol. 2014;21(3):309–19.
13. Gayer G, Lubner M, Bhalla S, Pickhardt P. Imaging of abdominal and pelvic surgical and postprocedural foreign bodies. Radiol Clin North Am. 2014;52(5):991–1027.

FAQs: Rapid Fire Answers to Pesky Clinical Questions – NGTs? Thiamine? PO Contrast? Nonsurgical Complications?

Erin Leiman

Key Concepts
- Blind placement of NG or OG tubes should not be performed routinely. For conclusive indication for NG tube placement, consider fluoroscopic guidance when an NG tube is definitively required.
- Fluid intake, including oral contrast, should be limited to 6 oz (177 mL) for patients with stomach-altering bariatric surgeries, such as Roux-en-Y gastric bypass and sleeve gastrectomy.
- Thiamine deficiency is a common nutritional deficit that can lead to Wernicke's encephalopathy in bariatric surgery patients.
- NSAIDs, aspirin, Plavix, and steroids have been associated with increased risk of marginal ulcers.
- Pulmonary embolism is the most common cause of death in bariatric surgery patients.

Use Caution with Blind Nasogastric Tube (NGT) Placement

Blind passage of nasogastric (NG) or orogastric (OG) tubes should not be routinely performed in bariatric surgery patients. Blind NG tube placement is contraindicated in the first 30 days after surgery. If attempted beyond the early postoperative period, clinicians should have a definitive indication and proceed with a clear understanding of the postsurgical anatomy. This procedure can lead to significant morbidity, especially in the Roux-en-Y gastric bypass (RYGB) population, and may be less helpful than in non-bypass patients especially when used for decompression [1].

A standard NG/OG tube is made with polyvinyl chloride (PVC) and is approximately 122 cm in length with the distal 8 cm containing multiple side holes, with the goal of the entire distal portion being contained within the stomach. Both NG and OG tubes are designed for a large and highly distensible stomach which can hold greater than 1600 mL of air volume with little to no increase in intragastric pressures [2]. In contrast, the gastric pouch following RYGB is only about 30 mL with a height of approximately 4 cm. Thus, the NG/OG tubes' proximal holes are in the esophagus, or the distal holes are in the Roux limb having traversed the gastroenterostomy and limiting decompression [3].

Furthermore, in contrast to the normal stomach, the post RYGB stomach contains several sites vulnerable to injury from an NG/OG tube, including the gastrojejunal anastomosis, the blind end of the Roux limb, as well as the proximal portion of the Roux limb which is thinner than the stomach wall. Serosal adhesions can develop and produce kinks in the Roux limb that prevent smooth forward passage of a tube.

The provider inserting the NG/OG tube must have knowledge of bypass anatomy and should never advance against resistance. Moreover, fluoroscopic guidance to allow for visualization of the tip of the tube should be considered along with use of softer more flexible tubes such as polyurethane or silicone if NG/OG tube placement is needed [1].

Limit Fluid Intake, Including Oral Contrast

The gastric pouch is about 15–30 mL in RYGB and approximately 100 mL in sleeve gastrectomy. Therefore, fluid intake, such as oral contrast or charcoal, should be limited to approximately 6 oz (177 mL) per the American Society of Bariatric Surgeons (ASBS) [4].

Consider Venous Thromboembolism (VTE) Beyond the Immediate Postoperative Period

Similar to other surgical procedures, venous thromboembolism remains a significant concern and is the most common cause of death after bariatric surgery [5]. The risk extends beyond the immediate postoperative period and up to a year after surgery. In one retrospective review of 17,434 bariatric

E. Leiman
Division of Emergency Medicine, Department of Surgery, Duke University Medical Center, Durham, NC, USA
e-mail: erin.leiman@duke.edu

A. Graham, D. J. Carlberg (eds.), *Gastrointestinal Emergencies*, https://doi.org/10.1007/978-3-319-98343-1_127

patients, the incidence of VTE during the index hospitalization for their bariatric procedure was 0.88%. The rate of VTE rose to 2.17% at one month and 2.99% at six months post-surgery [6].

Remember Bariatric Patients Have a High Risk of Thiamine Deficiency

If the procedure was intended to be malabsorptive, then nutritional complications are common, including deficiencies of iron, calcium, vitamins B1 (thiamine) and B12 (cobalalmin) as well as folate. Vitamin B1 deficiency often occurs in the first weeks to months after surgery due to its very short half-life in the body (9–18 days), while vitamin B12 deficiency may not manifest for months to years after surgery [7].

Vitamin B1 (thiamine) deficiency is thought to be a serious and major factor in the development of neurological complications (e.g., neuropathies, plexopathies, and myopathies) and Wernicke's encephalopathy after bariatric surgery. Wernicke's encephalopathy is characterized by the triad of ophthalmoplegia, confusion, and unsteady gait (ataxia). Korsakoff's syndrome is a combination of anterograde amnesia as well as retrograde amnesia combined with aphasia (inability to understand or express speech), apraxia (inability to perform specific purposeful actions), agnosia (inability to interpret sensations and recognize objects), and a deficit in executive functions. Cases of Wernicke's encephalopathy typically develop within 8–15 weeks after surgery [7]. It is important to note that B1 deficiency has been described in nearly all types of bariatric procedures not just malabsorptive procedures [7]. Therefore, thiamine should be administered if neurologic symptoms are present and prior to glucose administration in bariatric patients. Because thiamine is water-soluble, there is very low risk of systemic toxicity.

To replete thiamine [7]:

- Outpatient maintenance – multivitamins with 1.2 mg of thiamine orally and dietary recommendations to meet nutritional requirements
- If low suspicion of deficiency or short episode of GI symptoms – 10 mg orally daily
- If high suspicion of deficiency or prolonged nausea/vomiting/diarrhea – 100–250 mg IV daily
- If neurologic symptoms – 100–500 mg IV up to three times daily × 2–3 days followed by 250 mg IV until improvement and then 50–100 mg orally three times a day

Vitamin B12 (cobalamin) and folate deficiencies are common after bariatric surgery, especially Roux-en-Y gastric bypass (RYGB). In one study of 149 RYGB patients, 11% had low vitamin B12 levels postoperatively [8]. Clinical manifestations of B12 deficiency can range from vague symptoms of fatigue, cognitive slowness, glossitis, and irritability to overt symptoms of megaloblastic anemia and neuropsychiatric symptoms. In rare, severe cases, vitamin B12 deficiency has been linked to Guillain-Barre syndrome, characterized by ascending demyelinating polyneuropathy [8]. However, the time course of B12 deficiency usually progresses over months to years and only requires emergent intervention in advanced cases. Suspicion of mild to moderate vitamin B12 deficiency should be referred to the patient's primary care physician or bariatric surgeon for definitive diagnosis.

To replete vitamin B12 [7]:

- 250–500 mcg vitamin B12 by mouth daily or 500 mcg intranasally weekly
- If severe symptoms or unable to tolerate oral supplementation, 1000 mcg IM monthly

Gallstones Are Common After Bariatric Surgery and Ensuing Weight Loss

Gallstone formation is common and felt to be related to rapid weight loss, affecting up to nearly a third of postoperative bariatric patients [9]. Prophylactic treatment with ursodiol has been shown to reduce the incidence of gallstones. This is significant because access to the biliary tree via endoscopic retrograde cholangiopancreatography (ERCP) is nearly impossible after some bariatric surgeries. Thus, prophylactic cholecystectomy is routinely performed by some surgeons at the time of the bariatric procedure, but this is not a standard practice due to concerns regarding cost-effectiveness and complications [9].

Prescribe NSAIDs (Nonsteroidal Anti-inflammatory Medications), Aspirin, and Steroids with Caution

Similar to peptic ulcer disease, NSAIDs, aspirin, and steroids are risk factors for marginal ulcer development in bariatric patients. Diagnosis often requires esophagogastroduodenoscopy and is treated with proton pump inhibitors or topical agents like sucralfate. Refractory patients are often treated with misoprostol, and testing for *H. pylori* is a common practice both prior to bariatric surgery and postoperatively if there is concern for marginal ulceration [4].

Fear Anastomotic Leaks in the Early Postoperative Bariatric Patient

Anastomotic leaks are associated with high morbidity and mortality and are one of the leading causes of death after bariatric surgery. Given its availability, computed tomography (CT) is often the initial examination of choice. A CT scan is also able to evaluate for obstruction or intra-abdominal abscess [10, 11]. In order to opacify the gastric pouch and roux limb in the case of RYGB, oral contrast should be administered just prior to image acquisition [12]. An upper gastrointestinal (UGI) and small bowel follow-through can also demonstrate anastomotic leaks as well as assess for edema, ileus, and obstruction. Because of the concern for leak, the study should be completed with oral water-soluble contrast material, and if no leak is identified, then barium may be used to assess for more subtle leaks [10, 11].

Suggested Resources
- American Society of Metabolic and Bariatric Surgery. https://asmbs.org.
- BEAM-ED (Bariatric examination, Assessment, and Management in the Emergency Department), https://asmbs.org/resources/beam-ed.
- Nguyen N, Blackstone R, Morton J, Ponce J, Rosenthal R. The ASMBS textbook of bariatric surgery. New York: Springer.

References

1. Van Dinter TG, Lijo J, Guileyard JM, Fordtran JS. Intestinal perforation caused by insertion of a nasogastric tube later after gastric bypass. Proc Bayl Univ Med Cent. 2013;26(1):11–5.
2. McNally EF, Kelly JE, Ingelfinger FJ. Mechanism of belching: effects of gastric distention with air. Gastroenterology. 1964;46:254–9.
3. Alva S, Eisenberg D, Duffy A, Roberts K, Israel G, Bell R. Virtual three dimensional computed tomography assessment of the gastric pouch following laparoscopic Roux-Y gastric bypass. Obes Surg. 2008;18(4):364–6.
4. American Society for Metabolic and Bariatric Surgery. (n.d.). Retrieved from https://asmbs.org/.
5. Byrne TK. Complications of surgery for obesity. Surg Clin North Am. 2001;81:1181–93.
6. Steele K, Schweitzer M, et al. The long term risk of venous thromboembolism following bariatric surgery. Obes Surg. 2011;21:1371–6.
7. Goldenberg L, Pomp A. Management of nutritional complications. In: Nguyen N, Blackstone R, Morton J, Ponce J, Rosenthal R, editors. The ASMBS textbook of bariatric surgery. New York: Springer; 2015.
8. Toy S, Zarshenas N, Jorgensen J. Prevalence of nutrient deficiencies in bariatric patients. Nutrition. 2009;25(11–12):1150–6.
9. Sugarman HJ, Brewer WH, Shiffman ML, et al. Multicenter, placebo-controlled, randomized, double-blind, prospective trial of prophylactic ursodiol for the prevention of gallstone formation following gastric-bypass-induced rapid weight loss. Am J Surg. 1995;169:91–6.
10. Chandler RC, Srinivas G, Chintapalli KN, Schwesinger WH, Prasad SR. Imaging in bariatric surgery: a guide to postsurgical anatomy and common complications. AJR. 2008;190:122–35.
11. Carucci LR, Turner MA. Imaging after bariatric surgery for morbid obesity: Roux-en-Y gastric bypass and laparoscopic adjustable gastric banding. Semin Roentgenol. 2009;44(4):283–96.
12. Levine MS, Carucci LR. Imaging of bariatric surgery: normal anatomy and postoperative complications. Radiology. 2014;270:327–41.

Consultant Corner: Abdominal Pain in the Bariatric Patient

128

Essa M. Aleassa and Stacy Brethauer

Pearls and Pitfalls

- Adjustable gastric band complications include gastric perforation (early postoperative complication), band prolapse in which the distal stomach herniated up through the band, erosion of the band into the gastric lumen (typically occurs years after placement), and overtightening of the band causing an obstruction.
- Gastric ulcers are rare after sleeve gastrectomy.
- Internal herniation of the bowel through a mesenteric opening at the small bowel anastomosis or under the Roux limb mesentery is the most concerning scenario in a gastric bypass patient with severe abdominal pain.
- A nasogastric tube can be safely placed in a patient with a remote history of gastric bypass to decompress the Roux limb and decrease the risk of aspiration.

Introduction

Our practice setting is a tertiary referral center with a large volume of primary and revisional bariatric surgery operations. Our center is accredited as a bariatric surgery training facility. We are active in clinical and basic science research pertaining to bariatric and metabolic surgery.

E. M. Aleassa
Bariatric and Metabolic Institute, Cleveland Clinic Foundation, Cleveland, OH, USA

Department of Surgery, College of Medicine and Health Sciences, United Arab Emirates University, Al-Ain, United Arab Emirates

S. Brethauer (✉)
Bariatric and Metabolic Institute, Cleveland Clinic Foundation, Cleveland, OH, USA
e-mail: Brethas@ccf.org

Answers to Key Clinical Questions

1. What are the different types of bariatric procedures commonly performed?

Bariatric surgery is the most effective mean for weight loss and treating its metabolic complications. This has led to the wide acceptance of the procedure. Most commonly performed procedures in the United States are sleeve gastrectomy and Roux-en-Y gastric bypass (RYGB). Gastric banding went through phases where it initially was widely performed but has gradually fell out of favor due to its long-term complications and superiority of the other procedures. Adjustable gastric banding now represents about 5% of bariatric procedures performed.

It is essential to have some understanding of the post-bariatric surgery anatomy in order to understand the potential causes of abdominal pain after these procedures. Briefly, all procedures are almost exclusively performed laparoscopically. RYGB surgery involves creating a small proximal gastric pouch and two anastomoses (Fig. 128.1). The proximal jejunum is divided and the distal end brought up and anastomosed to the gastric pouch. The other (proximal) end of the divided jejunum is referred to as the biliopancreatic limb and is anastomosed about 150 cm downstream. The small bowel beyond this "Roux" anastomosis is referred to as the common channel where biliopancreatic juices and food mix and travel downstream. In sleeve gastrectomy, no anastomoses are created (Fig. 128.2). Rather, the stomach fundus and body are vertically resected leaving 20% of the stomach behind. The final sleeve resembles a tubular banana-shaped stomach that empties normally through the pylorus. Adjustable gastric banding involves placement of a silicon band around the stomach (Fig. 128.3). The inner circumference of the band is a circular balloon that is connected to tubing and a port to allow inflation or deflation with saline. Once the band is placed, it typically takes several "adjustments" to tighten the band enough to achieve the desired effect of decreased hunger and early satiety.

© Springer Nature Switzerland AG 2019
A. Graham, D. J. Carlberg (eds.), *Gastrointestinal Emergencies*, https://doi.org/10.1007/978-3-319-98343-1_128

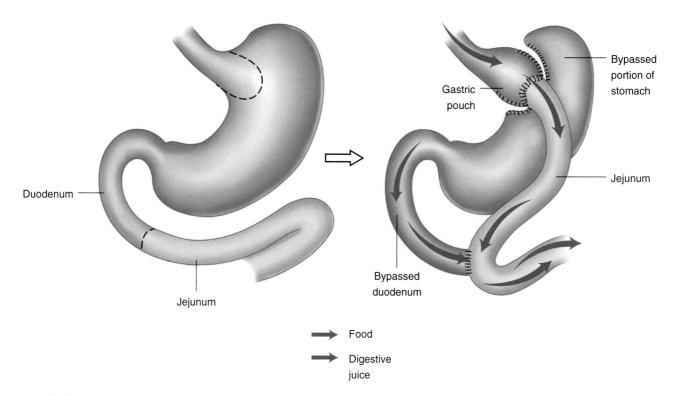

Fig. 128.1 Roux-en-Y gastric bypass (RYGB)

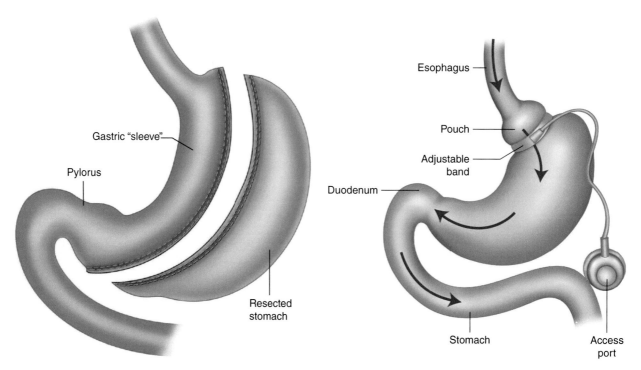

Fig. 128.2 Sleeve gastrectomy (SG)

Fig. 128.3 Gastric banding

2. What is the differential diagnosis of abdominal pain in a patient with a history of gastric banding?

Abdominal pain in the setting of a gastric band can be due to gastric perforation (early postoperative complication), band prolapse in which the distal stomach herniated up through the band, erosion of the band into the gastric lumen (typically occurs years after placement), and overtightening of the band causing an obstruction. A chronically overtight band can lead to dilation of the proximal stomach and esophagus and may cause chronic aspiration pneumonias and a "pseudo-achalasia" picture.

3. What is the differential diagnosis of abdominal pain in a patient with a history of sleeve gastrectomy?

Common causes of abdominal pain affecting the general population should be sought in patients with sleeve gastrectomy. Procedure-specific etiologies are gastroesophageal reflux disease, hiatal hernia, or stenosis of the gastric lumen. Gastric ulcers are rare after sleeve gastrectomy.

4. What is the differential diagnosis of abdominal pain in a patient with a history of Roux-en-Y gastric bypass?

Patients presenting with abdominal pain in the setting of a RYGB can potentially have an array of underlying diagnoses with different levels of urgency. It is best to stratify the differentials to either early (<30 days postoperatively) or late (>30 days postoperatively). Early causes of abdominal pain (aside from incisional pain) include small bowel obstruction at the level of the small bowel anastomosis, an incarcerated hernia at a laparoscopic port site or untreated hernia, or evolving abdominal sepsis secondary to an anastomotic leak or bowel perforation. Some patients present within the first 3 weeks with abdominal pain and failure of diet progression. In such cases, an anastomotic stenosis is a potential etiology. This is less of an emergency; however, it needs further evaluation. Typically, this is managed as an outpatient with endoscopic dilation and rarely required surgical intervention.

Late causes include small bowel obstruction due to internal hernias or adhesions, ulcers at the gastrojejunal anastomosis (marginal ulcer), small bowel intussusception, gallbladder disease, or other pathology unrelated to the gastric bypass. A rare cause of small bowel obstruction, often overlooked, is intussusception. It occurs usually after significant weight loss. Focal inflammation, adhesions, and long mesentery are few hypotheses for the pathophysiology of intussusception. The jejunojejunostomy is a common site of intussusception in gastric bypass patients as it can become dilated over time. Surgical consultation should be obtained in a symptomatic patient (pain) or if the intussusception is causing an obstruction.

Other causes for abdominal pain that should be in the differential list are marginal ulcers at the gastrojejunal anastomosis site. This is usually precipitated by smoking or taking nonsteroidal anti-inflammatory drugs (NSAIDs) after surgery. Smoking affects tissue perfusion at the anastomosis site and induces ulcers that progress to form strictures if not managed in a timely fashion. Occasionally, ulcers at the gastrojejunostomy can perforate, and this requires operative intervention as with any other gastric perforation. Non-bowel-related differentials for pain are postoperative adhesions, cholelithiasis, and nephrolithiasis. Gallstones are thought to occur due to rapid weight loss. The pathophysiology of nephrolithiasis is not well understood; however, it is believed to be secondary to hyperoxaluria as a result of increased intestinal absorption.

5. What are the key concerns regarding a patient with a SBO and history of RYGB?

Small bowel obstruction in the setting of RYGB can occur at any time point postoperatively and at different sites. Besides the laparoscopy port site, internal herniation of the bowel through a mesenteric opening at the small bowel anastomosis or under the Roux limb mesentery is the most concerning scenario in a gastric bypass patient with severe abdominal pain. These sites are commonly closed intraoperatively during the initial operation; however not every surgeon closes these defects, and even those that are closed can reopen after massive weight loss. Intermittent herniation or volvulus through these defects can also occur, and any gastric bypass patient who presents with intermittent severe abdominal pain should undergo CT imaging and a referral to a bariatric surgeon. Patients presenting with ongoing severe mid-abdominal pain require urgent evaluation, imaging, and referral to a surgeon, preferably a bariatric surgeon. Delay in diagnosing and treating an internal hernia can result in catastrophic loss of bowel or death.

Adhesive bowel obstructions can also occur after RYGB in patients who have had prior abdominal or pelvic surgery. It is important to understand that a small bowel obstruction in a gastric bypass patient cannot be managed in the same way as an adhesive bowel obstruction in a patient with normal anatomy. Because the biliopancreatic limb and excluded gastric remnant are now a blind end proximally, a distal obstruction can result in severe dilation of that limb and the remnant stomach. If untreated, perforation since that part of the gastrointestinal tract cannot be decompressed with a nasogastric tube may occur.

6. Is it safe to insert a nasogastric tube in a bariatric patient?

A nasogastric tube can be safely placed in a patient with a remote history of gastric bypass to decompress the Roux limb and decrease the risk of aspiration. In a patient who recently had a gastric bypass (within 30 days), a nasogastric tube should only be placed by the bariatric surgery team or the surgeon consulted on the case.

7. What is the approach to abdominal pain in a patient with a history of Roux-en-Y gastric bypass?

Our approach to abdominal pain in RYGB patients depends on the overall patient status and location of abdominal pain. It is important to involve a surgeon early in the care of the patient, preferably a bariatric surgeon if one is available.

It is imperative to get a comprehensive history of the presenting symptoms and the bariatric procedure performed. Details about the surgery should include the date, surgeon, center, perioperative course including complications, diet progression, adherence to postoperative prescriptions, current prescriptions, smoking habits, NSAID use amount of weight loss, and follow-ups.

Stable patients with epigastric abdominal pain and intolerance of food benefit from an upper endoscopy to rule out a marginal ulcer or stricture. Patients with mid-abdominal pain might have small bowel obstruction either due to an internal herniation, adhesions, or intussusception. These patients should have an abdominal CT scan with oral and IV contrast unless contraindicated. Performing a CT scan can help narrow down the diagnosis to further target the treatment, but even if the CT is normal, a patient with persistent pain should be seen by a bariatric surgeon. In these cases, a diagnostic laparoscopy is indicated to inspect the mesenteric defects or other causes of abdominal pain.

Suggested Resource
- BEAM ED. https://asmbs.org/resources/beam-ed.

Part XVII

Abdominal Pain and the Post-procedure Patient

How Do I Approach Pain or Bleeding After Upper Endoscopy?

Lauren Westover, Mohamed Hagahmed, Tracy M. Moore, and Adam Janicki

Pearls and Pitfalls
- Patients may present after an upper endoscopy with life-threatening conditions such as perforation or bleeding.
- Symptoms of perforation include chest pain, hoarseness, neck or back pain, dysphagia, odynophagia, dyspnea, hematemesis, subcutaneous emphysema, and peritonitis.
- Computed tomography is more sensitive than plain radiographs for diagnosing perforation.
- Management of perforation includes aggressive resuscitation, administration of antibiotics, and emergent surgical consultation.
- Early recognition of upper endoscopy-related hemorrhage is vital, and resuscitation with IV fluids and blood products should be initiated immediately.

Upper endoscopy is a procedure commonly performed to evaluate symptoms of dyspepsia, abdominal pain, dysphagia, gastroesophageal reflux, and suspected upper gastrointestinal (GI) bleeding [1]. In 2009, an estimated 6.9 million upper endoscopies were performed in the United States [2]. The procedure, whether performed for diagnostic or therapeutic purposes, is relatively safe and well-tolerated, with an overall complication rate of 0.13% and a mortality of 0.004% [3]. Minor post-procedural complications are often reported and include sore throat, abdominal discomfort, and chest pain [4]. Major adverse events occurring after diagnostic upper endoscopy, identified by the American Society for Gastrointestinal Endoscopy as cardiopulmonary events, infection, perforation, and bleeding, are rare [3].

Despite these reassuring statistics, patients often present to the acute care setting for evaluation of post-procedural symptoms. One study found that 2.5% of post-endoscopy patients sought emergency department care for throat discomfort and abdominal pain. Nearly half of these were ultimately hospitalized [5]. Another study cited a 1% incidence of hospital visits within 14 days of endoscopy, with abdominal pain (47%), GI bleeding (12%), and chest pain (11%) as chief complaints. The average time to presentation was 6 days post-procedure [6]. The acute care provider is often tasked with the initial evaluation and management of these patients and should consider low frequency and high morbidity and mortality complications during evaluation.

How Do I Approach Pain After Upper Endoscopy?

While perforation is the most feared complication of upper endoscopy, its presentation is quite rare, with rates between 1 in 2500 and 1 in 11,000 [7]. Presence of preexisting pathology such as esophageal stricture, Zenker's diverticulum, or malignancy increases the risk of perforation. Non-GI factors contributing to perforation include anterior cervical osteophytes and operator inexperience. Patients present with a multitude of complaints including neck pain, painful neck movement, dysphagia, chest pain, hoarseness, dyspnea, abdominal pain, nausea, vomiting, and fever. Some patients present ill-appearing and hemodynamically unstable; however, not all perforations are life-threatening [4].

Initial management should focus on maintaining a patent airway, providing adequate oxygenation, and fluid resuscitation. X-ray can be used as an initial test, as it is often readily available and evaluates for pneumothorax, pneumomediastinum, and intraperitoneal free air. If x-ray is unrevealing and suspicion remains high, further imaging is warranted, as plain films have a sensitivity of only 50–70%. CT is highly sensitive and specific and is useful for localizing the site of perforation [8, 9]. A small role may exist for fluoroscopy in

L. Westover (✉) · M. Hagahmed · T. M. Moore · A. Janicki
Department of Emergency Medicine, University of Pittsburgh Medical Center, Pittsburgh, PA, USA
e-mail: westoverll@upmc.edu; mooretm3@upmc.edu; janickiaj@upmc.edu

© Springer Nature Switzerland AG 2019
A. Graham, D. J. Carlberg (eds.), *Gastrointestinal Emergencies*, https://doi.org/10.1007/978-3-319-98343-1_129

diagnosing perforation, but this test may be challenging to obtain in the emergency setting. A water-soluble contrast swallow study has a sensitivity of 60–70% [9]. Barium studies are superior for detecting small perforations, with sensitivities up to 90%, but they can trigger a severe inflammatory response resulting in mediastinitis. Therefore, barium swallow should not be used as the primary diagnostic study for perforation [10–13].

Once diagnosed, perforation treatment entails no oral intake and broad-spectrum antibiotics covering aerobes and anaerobes. Antifungals may also be warranted, especially in the immunocompromised [10]. Early general or thoracic surgery consultation is key, as primary surgical repair is indicated in the majority of patients. Nasogastric tubes should only be placed in consultation with the treating surgeon [14].

Prompt surgical intervention is often warranted in patients showing signs of sepsis, hemodynamic instability, or heavily contaminated mediastinal, pleural, or peritoneal spaces. Surgery is also warranted in those failing more conservative therapy. Non-operative management may be indicated in patients who present early, are too sick or unstable for immediate surgical intervention, or have small cervical perforations that are surgically inaccessible [10, 15]. Patients should be admitted to an ICU for further management.

How Do I Approach Bleeding After Upper Endoscopy?

Bleeding is another high-risk complication of upper endoscopy. Patients that undergo therapeutic endoscopy or diagnostic endoscopy with biopsies are at greatest risk, as well as patients with coagulopathy, portal hypertension, or platelet count <20,000/μL. Standard aspirin and NSAID dosing, however, has not been shown to increase the risk of bleeding [3]. Patients may present with melena, hematemesis, anemia, or hemodynamic instability. Bleeding post-endoscopy is most commonly due to Mallory-Weiss tears that occur with retching during the procedure. They occur in less than 0.5% of diagnostic endoscopies [3, 16].

Evaluation and management of post-endoscopy bleeding center around stabilization and resuscitation, including airway protection as necessary, early large-bore IV access, serial hemoglobin measurements, and blood transfusion in hemodynamically compromised patients. Bleeding can be difficult to control in coagulopathic patients, and reversal agents, when indicated, should be administered early. Fresh frozen plasma, platelets, octreotide, and antibiotics should be considered in cirrhotic patients with severe bleeding. An intravenous proton pump inhibitor (PPI) such as pantoprazole should be given as a bolus followed by an infusion [17]. Although a recent meta-analysis found a mortality benefit associated with administration of tranexamic acid (TXA),

TXA did not improve outcomes when controlled for PPI administration and endoscopic therapy. Given its safety profile and low cost, TXA administration should be considered in unstable patients [18]. Early consultation with gastroenterology, interventional radiology, and/or surgery is generally required for definitive management of significant bleeding. Repeat upper endoscopy is the preferred procedure once the patient is stabilized [3]. Disposition will depend on the amount of bleeding and stability of the patient. With hemodynamic instability or active bleeding, intensive care unit admission is warranted.

While serious complications of upper endoscopy are rare, they do occur, and emergency providers must remain vigilant for signs of perforation and serious bleeding. A high index of suspicion is necessary given the array of minor complaints with which an acutely ill post-endoscopy patient can present. Aggressive resuscitation with an eye toward early specialty consultation in the ill post-procedural patient will frequently improve outcomes.

Suggested Resources
- The Unstable Patient with a Gastrointestinal Bleed. emDocs. Dec 2014. http://www.emdocs. net/unstable-patient-gi-bleed/.
- Massive GI bleeding. EM:RAP C3 core content. Apr 2016. https://www.emrap.org/episode/c3massivegi/c3massivegi.
- Coagulopathy management in the bleeding cirrhotic: Seven pearls and one crazy idea. EMCrit. Dec 2015.https://emcrit.org/pulmcrit/coagulopathy-bleeding-cirrhotic-inr/.

References

1. Lieberman DA, De Garmo PL, Fleischer DE, Eisen GM, Helfand M. Patterns of endoscopy use in the United States. Gastroenterology. 2000;118(3):619–24.
2. Peery AF, Dellon ES, Lund J, Crockett SD, McGowan CE, Bulsiewicz WJ, et al. Burden of Gastrointestinal Disease in the United States: 2012 update. Gastroenterology. 2012;143(5):1179–87.
3. American Society for Gastrointestinal Endoscopy. Adverse events of upper GI endoscopy. Gastrointest Endosc. 2012;76(4):707–18.
4. Riley S, Alderson D. Complications of gastrointestinal endoscopy. BSG Guidel Gastroenterol. 2006;(1):7–13.
5. Zubarik R, Eisen G, Mastropietro C, Lopez J, Carroll J, Benjamin S, Fleischer DE. Prospective analysis of complications 30 days after outpatient upper endoscopy. Am J Gastroenterol. 1999 Jun;94(6):1539–45.
6. Leffler DA, Kheraj R, Garud S, Neeman N, Nathanson LA, Kelly CP, Sawhney M, Landon B, Doyle R, Rosenberg S, Aronson M. The incidence and cost of unexpected hospital use after scheduled outpatient endoscopy. Arch Intern Med. 2010;170(19):1752–7.
7. Quine MA, Bell GD, McLoy RF, Matthews HR. Prospective audit of perforation rates following upper gastrointestinal endoscopy in two regions of England. Br J Surg. 1995;82:530–3.

8. Cho KC, Baker SR. Extraluminal air. Diagnosis and significance. Radiol Clin North Am. 1994;32(5):829.

9. Del Gaizo AJ, Lall C, Allen BC, Leyendecker JR. From esophagus to rectum: a comprehensive review of alimentary tract perforations at computed tomography. Abdom Imaging. 2014;39(4):802–23.

10. Kaman L, Iqbal J, Kundil B, Kochnar R. Management of Esophageal Perforation in adults. Gastroenterol Res. 2010;3(6):235–44.

11. Sarr MG, Pemberton JH, Payne WS. Management of instrumental perforations of the esophagus. J Thorac Cardiovasc Surg. 1982;84:211.

12. Bladergroen MR, Lowe JE, Postlethwait RW. Diagnosis and recommended management of esophageal perforation and rupture. Ann Thorac Surg. 1986;42:235.

13. Dodds WJ, Stewart ET, Vlymen WJ. Appropriate contrast media for evaluation of esophageal disruption. Radiology. 1982;144:439.

14. Shaffer HA Jr, Valenzuela G, Mittal RK. Esophageal perforation. A reassessment of the criteria for choosing medical or surgical therapy. Arch Intern Med. 1992;152:757.

15. Salo JA, Isolauri JO, Heikkila LJ, Merkkula HT, Heikkinen LO, Kivilaakso EO, Mattila SP. Management of delayed esophageal perforation with mediastinal sepsis. Esophagectomy or primary repair? J Thorac Cardiovasc Surg. 1993;106(6):1088.

16. Rolanda C, Caetano A, Dinis-Ribeiro M. Emergencies after endoscopic procedures. Best Pract Res Clin Gastroenterol. 2013;27:783–98.

17. Chan WH, Khin LW, Chung YF, Goh YC, Ong HS, Wang WK. Randomized controlled trial of standard versus high-dose intravenous omeprazole after endoscopic therapy in high-risk patients with acute peptic ulcer bleeding. Br J Surg. 2011;98:640.

18. Bennett C, Klingenberg SL, Langholz E, Gluud LL. Tranexamic acid for upper gastrointestinal bleeding. Cochrane Database Syst Rev. 2014;(11):CD006640.

How Do I Approach Pain or Bleeding After Colonoscopy?

130

W. Nathan Davis, Alejandro Negrete, and Adam Janicki

Pearls and Pitfalls

- The most common major complications after colonoscopy are perforation and bleeding.
- Emergent imaging should be considered for all patients presenting with pain after colonoscopy.
- Consider post-polypectomy syndrome in patients presenting with pain and no free air on imaging.
- Bleeding after colonoscopy is often minor but can occasionally be life-threatening.
- Complications after colonoscopy have been reported up to 42 days post-procedure.

Colonoscopy utilization for routine screening, diagnostic testing, and therapeutic intervention has increased significantly over the last 10 years [1–3]. Although colonoscopy complications are rare, ranging from 0.20% to 2.18%, this increased utilization has led to a growing number of patients presenting for emergency care with colonoscopy-related symptoms [4, 5]. Providers should assess for major, potentially life-threatening complications such as perforation, post-polypectomy syndrome, and massive bleeding.

How Do I Approach Pain After Colonoscopy?

Bowel perforation should be suspected in any patient with significant pain after colonoscopy. The frequency of iatrogenic perforation from colonoscopy ranges from 0.01% to 0.3% [4–8]. Only 42% of perforations from colonoscopy

W. N. Davis (✉) · A. Janicki
Department of Emergency Medicine, University of Pittsburgh Medical Center, Pittsburgh, PA, USA
e-mail: davisw3@upmc.edu; janickiaj@upmc.edu

A. Negrete
Case-Western Reserve University, Cleveland, OH, USA
e-mail: amn64@case.edu

are recognized during the procedure, and the presentation of a perforation can be delayed significantly, reported as far out as 42 days [9]. Perforations can occur via mechanical trauma, overdistention with insufflating gas, or therapeutic intervention such as electrocautery or polypectomy [10]. The risk of perforation significantly increases when an intervention is performed during colonoscopy [6]. The risk increases further in the elderly and those with intra-abdominal pathology (e.g., cancer or preexisting inflammatory pathology such as inflammatory bowel disease or diverticulitis) [11].

The most common presenting symptom for perforation is localized or generalized abdominal pain [9]. Some patients present with abdominal distention, leukocytosis, fever, peritonitis, or septic shock [9, 11]. Suspicion for perforation should prompt emergent radiographic evaluation. An upright abdominal x-ray may be utilized but has limited sensitivity for intraperitoneal free air [9]. Computed tomography (CT) is far more sensitive and can identify microperforations and retroperitoneal perforations [12]. Patients with perforation should be aggressively resuscitated and given broad-spectrum antibiotics with enteric gram-negative and anaerobic coverage [11]. Surgical consultation should be obtained early as definitive management is typically via operative procedure [13–15].

Post-polypectomy electrocoagulation syndrome, also known as post-polypectomy syndrome, should be suspected in patients presenting with symptoms suggestive of perforation (e.g., pain, peritoneal signs, fever, etc.) without radiographic evidence of perforation [6, 9]. Its reported frequency ranges from 0.009% to 0.1% [4, 6]. Post-polypectomy syndrome is a local peritonitis that most likely occurs secondary to transmural burns caused by electrocautery during polypectomy. Figure 130.1 shows post-polypectomy syndrome visualized with CT. Treatment is often nonsurgical, and providers should consider admission for IV antibiotics, serial abdominal examinations, and monitoring [6, 11].

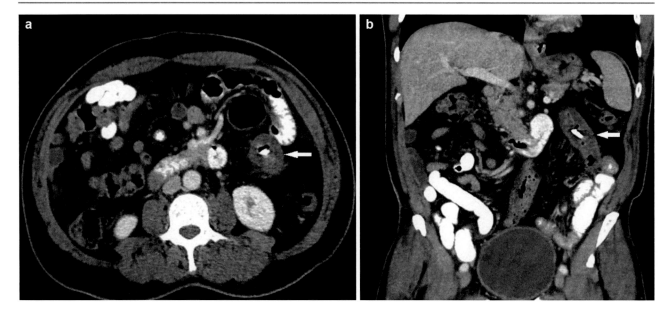

Fig. 130.1 Post-polypectomy syndrome visualized on CT. Axial image (**a**) and coronal image (**b**) show circumferential thickening and inflammation (arrows) in the descending colon at the site of polypec-tomy. Clip placed during polypectomy is seen in the colonic lumen at the site of inflammation

How Do I Approach Bleeding After Colonoscopy?

Post-colonoscopic hemorrhage is a potentially serious complication that the emergency provider may encounter. The frequency of bleeding after colonoscopy ranges between 0.05% and 0.87% [4–7]. In many cases, post-colonoscopic bleeding is minor and resolves spontaneously; however massive lower gastrointestinal hemorrhage may occur [11, 13]. Bleeding can also have a delayed presentation, with patients presenting as late as several weeks after the procedure [16]. Risk factors for bleeding include polypectomy and antico-agulation [6, 11]. In the event of a hemodynamically significant hemorrhage, stabilization with large-bore intravenous access, IV fluids, and blood product administration should be implemented. Failure of a minor/low volume bleed to resolve is approached similarly to other low-grade lower gastrointestinal bleeding episodes. Due to the potentially severe nature of post-colonoscopy bleeding, providers should consider admission for patients presenting with colonoscopy-related hemorrhage, even if it appears minor [11].

Other Complications

There are many other rare complications of colonoscopy that are beyond the scope of this chapter.

The two most common colonoscopy-related sedation complications are aspiration pneumonias and cardiovascular events such as myocardial infarctions and cerebrovascular accidents [4–6, 11].

Pneumothorax, splenic rupture, and iatrogenic volvulus have all been reported secondary to colonoscopy, as have intracolonic explosions due to electrocautery ignition of methane [6].

While these complications are generally recognized during or immediately post-procedure, they may present to the acute care setting as well.

Suggested Resources
- Kumar AS, Lee JK. Colonoscopy: advanced and emerging techniques - a review of Colonoscopic approaches to colorectal conditions. Clin Colon Rectal Surg. 2017;30(2):136–44. https://doi.org/10.1055/s-0036-1597312.
- Case Report: FAST detection of a rare colonoscopy complication. American College of Emergency Physicians: Emergency Ultrasound Section Newsletter. August 2012. https://www.acep.org/content.aspx?id=87317.

References

1. Lieberman DA, Williams JL, Holub JL, Morris CD, Logan JR, Eisen GM, et al. Colonoscopy utilization and outcomes 2000 to 2011. Gastrointest Endosc. 2014 Jul;80(1):133–43.
2. U.S. Preventive Services Task Force. Screening for colorectal cancer: recommendation statement. Am Fam Physician. 2017;95(4). Available from: http://www.aafp.org/afp/2017/0215/od1.html.
3. Lin JS, Piper MA, Perdue LA, Rutter CM, Webber EM, O'Connor E, et al. Screening for colorectal Cancer: updated evidence report

and systematic review for the US preventive services task force. JAMA. 2016;315(23):2576–94.

4. Ko CW, Riffle S, Michaels L, Morris C, Holub J, Shapiro JA, et al. Serious complications within 30 days of screening and surveillance colonoscopy are uncommon. Clin Gasteroentrol Hepatol. 2010;8(2):166–73. https://doi.org/10.1016/j.cgh.2009.10.007.

5. Louise W, Ajitha M, Gurkirpal S, Uri L. Low rates of gastrointestinal and non-gastrointestinal complications for screening or surveillance colonoscopies in a population-based study. Gastroenterology. 2018;154(3):540.e8–55.e8.   https://doi.org/10.1053/j.gastro.2017. 10.006.

6. ASGE Standards of Practice Committee, Fischer DA, Maple JT, Ben-Menachem T, Cash BD, Decker GA, Early DS, et al. Complications of colonoscopy. Gastrointest Endosc. 2011;74(4):745–52. https://doi.org/10.1016/j.gie.2011.07.025.

7. Levin TR, Zhao W, Conell C, Seeff LC, Manninen DL, Shapiro JA, et al. Complications of colonoscopy in an integrated health care delivery system. Ann Intern Med. 2006;145(12):880–6. https://doi.org/10.7326/0003-4819-145-12-200612190-00004.

8. Arora G, Mannalithara A, Singh G, Gerson LB, Triadafilopoulos G. Risk of perforation from a colonoscopy in adults: a large population-based study. Gastrointest Endosc. 2009;69(3):654–64. https://doi.org/10.1016/j.gie.2008.09.008.

9. Garbay JR, Suc B, Rotman N, Fourtanier G, Escat J. Multicentre study of surgical complications of colonoscopy. Br J Surg. 1996;83(1):42–4. https://doi.org/10.1002/bjs.1800830112.

10. Damore LJ, Rantis PC, Vernava AM, Longo WE. Colonoscopic perforations. Dis Colon Rectum. 1996 Nov;39(11):1308–14. https://doi.org/10.1007/bf02055129.

11. Green J. Guidelines on complications of gastrointestinal endoscopy. London: Br Soc Gastroenterol. 2006. http://f.i-md.com/medinfo/material/475/4ea7cdb844aebf27f87d9475/4ea7cdb844aebf27f87d9479.pdf.

12. Tiwari A, Sharma H, Qamar K, Sodeman T, Nawras A. Recognition of extraperitoneal colonic perforation following colonoscopy: a review of the literature. Case Rep Gastroenterol. 2017;11(1):256–64. https://doi.org/10.1159/000475750.

13. Johnson H. Management of major complications encountered with flexible colonoscopy. J Natl Med Assoc. 1993;85(12):916–20. PMID:8126742

14. Byeon JS. Colonic perforation: can we manage it endoscopically? Clin Endosc. 2013;46(5):495–9. https://doi.org/10.5946/ce.2013.46.5.495.

15. Raju GS, Saito Y, Matsuda T, Kaltenbach T, Soetikno R. Endoscopic management of colonoscopic perforations (with videos). Gastrointest Endosc. 2011;74(6):1380–8. https://doi.org/10.1016/j.gie.2011.08.007.

16. Singaram C, Torbey CF, Jacoby RF. Delayed postpolypectomy bleeding. Am J Gastroenterol. 1995;90(1):146–7. PMID: 7801918

How Do I Approach Pain After ERCP?

131

Robert M. Brickley and Kevin Vincent Leonard

Pearls and Pitfalls
- Abdominal pain following ERCP occurs in 20% of patients. Serious complications are rarer.
- The most common clinically significant complications following ERCP include pancreatitis, cholangitis, cholecystitis, hemorrhage, and perforation.
- Post-ERCP pancreatitis is probably underreported in the literature.
- Cholangitis and perforation are rare but associated with high morbidity and mortality.
- Laboratory investigation and appropriate imaging are often necessary to evaluate for these potentially serious complications.

Endoscopic retrograde cholangiopancreatography (ERCP) is a diagnostic and therapeutic procedure performed on patients with suspected biliary and/or pancreatic disease. Imaging modalities including magnetic resonance cholangiopancreatography (MRCP) and endoscopic ultrasound (EUS) have largely replaced ERCP for diagnosis, so most ERCP procedures are performed for therapeutic purposes with the intention of mechanically intervening on obstructive pathology [1, 2]. While ERCP can represent a safer alternative to surgery, the procedure is still associated with a 5–10% complication rate [3–5].

Although 50% of patients experience some pain during ERCP, nearly 20% of patients report moderate to severe pain following the procedure. Independent predictors of this include female gender, younger age (<50 years old), pre-cut endoscopic sphincterotomy (where the endoscopist cuts the ampulla prior to cannulation and contrast injection), use of a guide wire, and insertion of a self-expanding metal stent.

While not all pain is associated with a clinically significant complication, pain can be a sign of an adverse event [6]. The most common adverse events include pancreatitis (3.5–9.7%), cholangitis or cholecystitis (1.4–1.5%), hemorrhage (1.3–2.0%), and perforation (0.3–0.6%). Other miscellaneous events occur at a rate of 1.1–1.3% [4, 5, 7].

Post-ERCP pancreatitis (PEP) is the most common significant complication of ERCP and is thought to occur secondary to procedure-associated edema [8]. A recent review of 13,296 patients found the incidence was 9.7% (95%CI 8.6–10.7%) [7]. Risk factors for PEP include clinical suspicion of sphincter of Oddi dysfunction, history of PEP, age <50 years, female sex, multiple cannulation attempts, pancreatic sphincterotomy, pre-cut sphincterotomy, pneumatic dilation or ampullectomy, and multiple contrast injections into the pancreatic duct [5, 7, 9].

Amylase is elevated in 19% of patients after ERCP; however, only one quarter of patients with hyperamylasemia will have pancreatitis. Thus, pain associated with hyperamylasemia does not rule out other more serious post-procedural complications [10].

PEP is defined by typical symptoms in the setting of amylase or lipase elevation greater than three times the upper limit of normal at least 2 h after the procedure and/or in the setting of characteristic imaging findings. Gastroenterology literature commonly defines PEP by the need for greater than 2 days of pancreatitis-related hospitalization, likely resulting in an underestimate of PEP frequency [11].

In the acute care setting, PEP can be managed the same as any other acute pancreatitis, although repeat ERCP may be necessary if PEP is suspected to result from a pancreatic stent complication. A retrospective cohort study found that appropriate fluid resuscitation was associated with a significantly lower need for invasive intervention. The authors did not find a statistically significant decrease in local complications, persistent organ failure, or death [12].

Infectious complications have an incidence of only 1–2% but are associated with a mortality rate of 7.8% [4].

R. M. Brickley (✉) · K. V. Leonard
UPMC Department of Emergency Medicine, Pittsburgh, PA, USA
e-mail: brickleyrm@upmc.edu; leonardkv@upmc.edu

© Springer Nature Switzerland AG 2019
A. Graham, D. J. Carlberg (eds.), *Gastrointestinal Emergencies*, https://doi.org/10.1007/978-3-319-98343-1_131

Cholecystitis is reported to complicate only 0.5% of cases and should be treated in the usual fashion.

Cholangitis is one of the most serious complications of ERCP and is caused by failure to adequately drain the biliary tree. Cholangitis requires aggressive resuscitation, antibiotics, strong consideration of ICU admission, and early consultation for drainage with interventional radiology or gastroenterology [5, 6].

Bleeding is common during sphincterotomy but is usually addressed during the procedure. Hemorrhage that results in melena, hematemesis, >3 g hemoglobin drop, transfusion, or invasive intervention is rare and reported in only 4% of sphincterotomies and 1.3–2.0% of all ERCPs [4, 5, 7]. Bleeding can often be controlled endoscopically via injection of epinephrine, cauterization, or clips. Angiography and surgery are options for refractory bleeding [13].

Perforation has an incidence of 0.1–0.6% but is associated with a mortality rate of 9.9% [4]. Perforation can occur into the pancreaticobiliary tree, peritoneum, retroperitoneal space, or mediastinum. Perforations to the duodenum, stomach, and esophagus from the actual endoscopy are more likely to require surgical management than perforations due to sphincterotomies and guide-wire injuries, which are usually locally contained and can often be successfully managed with IV antibiotics and biliary stenting [14]. Concern for perforation necessitates gastroenterology and/or surgery consultation for appropriate management.

Other adverse events are more infrequent, complicating only 1.3% of cases. These include intestinal intramural injection of contrast or air, pneumothorax, biliary or pancreatic stent occlusion or impaction, as well as periprocedural events including allergic reactions and cardiovascular compromise [5].

Given the array of possible causes, it is imperative to investigate these relatively uncommon but potentially serious complications with appropriate laboratory studies and imaging tests. Specialty consultation is dictated by the clinical presentation. Early and aggressive resuscitation efforts, antibiotics for infection, and appropriate specialty consultation can decrease morbidity and mortality.

Suggested Resources
- American Society for Gastrointestinal Endoscopy. Adverse events associated with ERCP. Gastrointest Endosc. 2017;85:32–47.
- ERCP. MedLine Plus. April 2015. https://medlineplus.gov/ency/article/007479.htm.
- Episode 42: Mesenteric Ischemia and Pancreatitis (ERCP focus between minutes 50 and 57 of podcast). Emergency Medicine Cases. https://emergencymedicinecases.com/episode-42-mesenteric-ischemia-pancreatitis-3/.

References

1. Chandrasekhara V, Khashab MA, Muthusamy VR, Acosta RD, Agrawal D, Bruining DH, et al. Adverse events associated with ERCP. Gastrointest Endosc. 2017;85(1):32–47.
2. Early DS, Ben-Menachem T, Decker GA, Evans JA, Fanelli RD, Fisher DA, et al. Appropriate use of GI endoscopy. Gastrointest Endosc. 2012;75(6):1127–31.
3. Day LW, Lin L, Somsouk M. Adverse events in older patients undergoing ERCP: a systematic review and meta-analysis. Endosc Int Open. 2014;2(1):E28–36.
4. Andriulli A, Loperfido S, Napolitano G, Niro G, Valvano MR, Spirito F, et al. Incidence rates of post-ERCP complications: a systematic survey of prospective studies. Am J Gastroenterol. 2007;102(8):1781–8.
5. Freeman ML, Nelson DB, Sherman S, Haber GB, Herman ME, Dorsher PJ, et al. Complications of endoscopic biliary sphincterotomy. N Engl J Med. 1996;335(13):909–18.
6. Glomsaker TB, Hoff G, Kvaløy JT, Søreide K, Aabakken L, Søreide JA, et al. Patient-reported outcome measures after endoscopic retrograde cholangiopancreatography: a prospective, multicentre study. Scand J Gastroenterol. 2013;48(7):868–76.
7. Kochar B, Akshintala VS, Afghani E, Elmunzer BJ, Kim KJ, Lennon AM, et al. Incidence, severity, and mortality of post-ERCP pancreatitis: a systematic review by using randomized, controlled trials. Gastrointest Endosc. 2015;81(1):143–9.e9.
8. Szary NM, Al-Kawas FH. Complications of endoscopic retrograde cholangiopancreatography: how to avoid and manage them. Gastroenterol Hepatol (N Y). 2013;9(8):496–504.
9. Cotton PB, Garrow DA, Gallagher J, Romagnuolo J. Risk factors for complications after ERCP: a multivariate analysis of 11,497 procedures over 12 years. Gastrointest Endosc. 2009;70(1):80–8.
10. Wang P, Li ZS, Liu F, Ren X, Lu NH, Fan ZN, et al. Risk factors for ERCP-related complications: a prospective multicenter study. Am J Gastroenterol. 2009;104(1):31–40.
11. Cotton PB, Lehman G, Vennes J, Geenen JE, Russell RC, Meyers WC, et al. Endoscopic sphincterotomy complications and their management: an attempt at consensus. Gastrointest Endosc. 1991;37(3):383–93.
12. Singh VK, Gardner TB, Papachristou GI, Rey-Riveiro M, Faghih M, Koutroumpakis E, et al. An international multicenter study of early intravenous fluid administration and outcome in acute pancreatitis. United European Gastroenterol J. 2017;5(4):491–8.
13. Freeman ML. Complications of endoscopic retrograde cholangiopancreatography: avoidance and management. Gastrointest Endosc Clin N Am. 2012;22(3):567–86.
14. Enns R, Eloubeidi MA, Mergener K, Jowell PS, Branch MS, Pappas TM, et al. ERCP-related perforations: risk factors and management. Endoscopy. 2002;34(4):293–8.

How Do I Approach Pain After Liver Biopsy?

132

Robert M. Brickley and Heather A. Prunty

> **Pearls and Pitfalls**
> - Abdominal and shoulder pain are common after liver biopsy.
> - The most common serious complication of liver biopsy is hemorrhage.
> - Hypotension after liver biopsy may warrant empiric administration of blood products.
> - Pneumothorax and perforated abdominal viscera are rare but serious complications with high-associated morbidity and mortality.

Liver biopsy is generally a safe procedure with a low complication rate. Percutaneous biopsy with a 14–18G biopsy needle is the most common technique; however, transvenous biopsy may be performed when the percutaneous technique is contraindicated by coagulopathy or ascites. Surgical or laparoscopic biopsies are rare. Studies suggest that using ultrasound either for marking biopsy sites or for real-time guidance reduces complications including pain, but ultrasound has not yet gained universal acceptance [1]. The mortality rate from liver biopsy (0.05–0.2%) is elevated by underlying pathology and comorbidities [2–5].

Pain after liver biopsy is the most common complication [6–9]. One study showed pain severity and prevalence peaked at 30 min after needle removal. 39% of patients still experienced pain 24 h later. Additional studies have highlighted the role of psychosocial factors in post-liver biopsy pain, with pre-procedure anxiety and history of intravenous drug abuse highly associated with post-procedure pain and the need for analgesia [6, 7].

While pain may be common, acute evaluation of pain after liver biopsy should focus on evaluating for high-risk complications including hemorrhage, pneumothorax, and visceral perforation. Varying definitions of complications are described in the literature, but published major complication rates range from 0.22% to 1.06%. The most common clinically significant complication after liver biopsy is hemorrhage, but numerous other complications have been reported, including pneumothorax, hemothorax, bile peritonitis, biloma (late), infection (bacteremia, abscess, sepsis), hemobilia, neuralgia, and ventricular arrhythmia with transjugular approach [1, 4, 5, 8–13]. About 60% of major complications present within the first 2 h of biopsy, while 83–96% present within 24 h. Case reports document patients presenting with major intraperitoneal hemorrhage >2 weeks after the procedure [4, 9, 14–16].

If there is clinical suspicion for a major complication from liver biopsy, lab work including complete blood count, complete metabolic panel, coagulation studies, and type and screen are recommended. Chest X-ray, ultrasound (bedside or formal), and/or CT imaging should be considered based on clinical suspicion. Supportive care with fluid resuscitation and pain control should be initiated. Table 132.1 shows common complications of liver biopsy, as well as their appropriate workup and treatment.

Hemorrhage requiring transfusion, embolization, or surgical intervention is rare, occurring in 0.3–0.6% of proce-

Table 132.1 Common Complications of Liver Biopsy

Complication	Presentation	Diagnostic study	Treatment
Hemorrhage	Pain, +/− tachycardia, and/or hypotension	Ultrasound and/or CT	Blood products, angiographic embolization, or observation
Pneumothorax	Chest pain, dyspnea	Chest X-ray	Thoracostomy or observation
Bile leak/ biloma	Pain (delayed), liver panel abnormalities	CT +/− HIDA scan	Percutaneous drain or ERCP stent placement
Visceral perforation	Pain	CT	Surgical consultation

R. M. Brickley (✉) · H. A. Prunty
UPMC Department of Emergency Medicine, Pittsburgh, PA, USA
e-mail: brickleyrm@upmc.edu; pruntyh2@upmc.edu

© Springer Nature Switzerland AG 2019
A. Graham, D. J. Carlberg (eds.), *Gastrointestinal Emergencies*, https://doi.org/10.1007/978-3-319-98343-1_132

dures [2–4, 9, 12, 14, 17]. A recent large retrospective study of 18,947 image-guided percutaneous biopsies of multiple organs (about 1/3 of which were liver biopsies) found that hemorrhage most commonly manifests as pain (61%) or hemodynamic instability (42%) [14]. Persistent abdominal pain, especially in the setting of tachycardia and/or hypotension, should prompt acute care providers to consider life-threatening post-biopsy hemorrhage and arrange for transfusion of blood products. Ultrasound may be used as an initial test, but if clinical suspicion persists, CT is recommended. Size and location of the bleed, as well as response to early resuscitation, will guide subsequent management. If the patient fails to respond to resuscitation, emergent angiography with embolization or exploratory surgery is warranted. The presence of a subcapsular hematoma without associated vital sign abnormalities or new anemia rarely requires intervention. Observation and repeat hemoglobin measurement are recommended.

Bile leak and bilomas can present in a delayed fashion and should be suspected in patients with pain in addition to abnormal liver chemistries. Cholescintigraphy can be useful for diagnosis if computed tomography is unrevealing. Concern for bile leak should prompt interventional radiology consultation for percutaneous drainage or gastroenterology consultation for ERCP with stenting to decompress the biliary tree [18].

While liver biopsy itself is generally a safe procedure, patients often have significant associated comorbidities and may present after biopsy with unrelated complaints. Regardless, complications after liver biopsy, including hemorrhage, pneumothorax, and visceral perforation (with gallbladder perforation being the most common), are associated with high morbidity and mortality. They require appropriate laboratory studies and imaging tests, with specialty consultation as dictated by the clinical presentation.

> **Suggested Resource**
> - Friedman LS. Controversies in liver biopsy: who, where, when, how, why? Curr Gastroenterol Rep. 2004;6:30–6.
> - Rockley DC, Caldwell SH, Goodman ZD, Nelson RC, Smith AD. American Association for the Study of Liver Diseases Position Paper: liver biopsy. Hepatology. 2009;49:1017–44.

References

1. Rockey DC, Caldwell SH, Goodman ZD, Nelson RC, Smith AD. Diseases AAftSoL.Liver biopsy. Hepatology. 2009;49(3):1017–44.
2. Myers RP, Fong A, Shaheen AA. Utilization rates, complications and costs of percutaneous liver biopsy: a population-based study including 4275 biopsies. Liver Int. 2008;28(5):705–12.
3. West J, Card TR. Reduced mortality rates following elective percutaneous liver biopsies. Gastroenterology. 2010;139(4):1230–7.
4. Boyum JH, Atwell TD, Schmit GD, Poterucha JJ, Schleck CD, Harmsen WS, et al. Incidence and risk factors for adverse events related to image-guided liver biopsy. Mayo Clin Proc. 2016;91(3):329–35.
5. Kalambokis G, Manousou P, Vibhakorn S, Marelli L, Cholongitas E, Senzolo M, et al. Transjugular liver biopsy--indications, adequacy, quality of specimens, and complications--a systematic review. J Hepatol. 2007;47(2):284–94.
6. Riley TR. Predictors of pain medication use after percutaneous liver biopsy. Dig Dis Sci. 2002;47(10):2151–3.
7. Eisenberg E, Konopniki M, Veitsman E, Kramskay R, Gaitini D, Baruch Y. Prevalence and characteristics of pain induced by percutaneous liver biopsy. Anesth Analg. 2003;96(5):1392–6. table of contents.
8. Van Thiel DH, Gavaler JS, Wright H, Tzakis A. Liver biopsy. Its safety and complications as seen at a liver transplant center. Transplantation. 1993;55(5):1087–90.
9. Piccinino F, Sagnelli E, Pasquale G, Giusti G. Complications following percutaneous liver biopsy. A multicentre retrospective study on 68,276 biopsies. J Hepatol. 1986;2(2):165–73.
10. Weigand K. Percutaneous liver biopsy: retrospective study over 15 years comparing 287 inpatients with 428 outpatients. J Gastroenterol Hepatol. 2009;24(5):792–9.
11. McGill DB, Rakela J, Zinsmeister AR, Ott BJ. A 21-year experience with major hemorrhage after percutaneous liver biopsy. Gastroenterology. 1990;99(5):1396–400.
12. Seeff LB, Everson GT, Morgan TR, Curto TM, Lee WM, Ghany MG, et al. Complication rate of percutaneous liver biopsies among persons with advanced chronic liver disease in the HALT-C trial. Clin Gastroenterol Hepatol. 2010;8(10):877–83.
13. van der Poorten D, Kwok A, Lam T, Ridley L, Jones DB, Ngu MC, et al. Twenty-year audit of percutaneous liver biopsy in a major Australian teaching hospital. Intern Med J. 2006;36(11):692–9.
14. Atwell TD, Spanbauer JC, McMenomy BP, Stockland AH, Hesley GK, Schleck CD, et al. The timing and presentation of major hemorrhage after 18,947 image-guided percutaneous biopsies. AJR Am J Roentgenol. 2015;205(1):190–5.
15. Reichert CM, Weisenthal LM, Klein HG. Delayed hemorrhage after percutaneous liver biopsy. J Clin Gastroenterol. 1983;5(3):263–6.
16. Kowdley KV, Aggarwal AM, Sachs PB. Delayed hemorrhage after percutaneous liver biopsy. Role of therapeutic angiography. J Clin Gastroenterol. 1994;19(1):50–3.
17. Kitchin DR, Del Rio AM, Woods M, Ludeman L, Hinshaw JL. Percutaneous liver biopsy and revised coagulation guidelines: a 9-year experience. Abdom Radiol (NY). 2017;43(6):1494–501.
18. Fricker Z, Levy E, Kleiner D, Taylor JG, Koh C, Holland SM, et al. Case series: biliary leak after transjugular liver biopsy. Am J Gastroenterol. 2013;108(1):145–7.

How Do I Approach the Peritoneal Dialysis Patient with Pain/Fever?

133

Andrew Victory and Emily Lovallo

Pearls and Pitfalls
- Abdominal pain and cloudy effluent are suggestive of peritonitis, and empiric treatment with antibiotics is indicated.
- Exit-site infections are a common cause of peritonitis, with similar organisms isolated.
- Mechanical obstructions of the catheter can be relieved with push/pull saline or tissue plasminogen activator.
- Constipation can cause catheter migration. Adding a bowel regimen can improve effluent drainage.
- Complications of renal failure such as hyperkalemia and volume overload may require emergent stabilization and temporary transition to hemodialysis.

While the majority of end-stage renal disease patients who present for acute care receive hemodialysis, around 10% use peritoneal dialysis (PD) for renal replacement therapy. Since PD occurs at home in a medically unsupervised setting, most PD patients are highly reliable and well connected to their nephrologists. In preparation for PD initiation, a Tenckhoff catheter is surgically implanted into the peritoneum to facilitate instillation and drainage of dialysate. Patients are trained to present at the first sign of infection and/or other complication. The PD patient with abdominal pain or other PD-related complaint should be approached with a broad differential diagnosis.

Infection rates are reported at 0.24–1.66 episodes/patient/year (including peritonitis and exit site infections) [1]. Risks for peritonitis include methicillin-resistant *S. aureus* (MRSA) carrier status, exit-site infection, poor hand hygiene, lower socioeconomic status, and poor PD technique [1, 2]. Cloudy effluent can be the first manifestation of peritonitis, even before pain, with or without fever or other signs of infection. When PD-associated peritonitis causes pain, the pain is typically diffuse and non-focal and can be associated with rebound tenderness [1].

When peritonitis is suspected, effluent should be sent for cell count, gram stain, and culture. Blood culture bottles can be used to collect 10–20 mL of dialysate effluent for culture [3]. Specifics of how to obtain the dialysate sample will vary depending on equipment and timing of last dialysis. This should be discussed with nephrology. See the "Suggested Resources" section of this chapter for one region's protocol for collection of peritoneal dialysate.

Cloudy effluent with other findings such as pain, fever, leukocytosis, or peritoneal effluent white blood cells >100/hpf should be treated for presumed peritonitis with antibiotics until cultures return negative [1]. Gram-positive coverage should be provided by intraperitoneal (IP) vancomycin, which has been shown to have higher rates of cure than intravenous vancomycin, although data is sparse. Gram-negative coverage should be provided with an IP third-generation cephalosporin, although intravenous (IV) administration is indicated if the patient appears systemically ill. Treatment should continue for a minimum of 2 weeks. In the case of recurrent peritonitis or failure to clear effluent by day 5, fungal infection and bacterial colonization of the catheter should be considered and discussed with the nephrologist [4, 5].

Hemodynamically stable patients can be treated as outpatients; however, inability to obtain and administer home IP antibiotics may prompt admission or observation for treatment initiation.

Erythema, purulence, or focal pain at the site of the catheter tunnel or cuff is suggestive of an exit-site infection (ESI). PD patients generally require prophylaxis for *S. aureus* infection with daily topical mupirocin at the exit site, and MRSA carriers generally receive treatment to eliminate colonization. Up to 85% of cases of *S. aureus* peritonitis are culture-positive at the exit site, and the majority are associated with clinical exit-site infections [2]. Additionally, 15.9% of patients with ESI develop peritonitis within 15 days [6]. *S. aureus* and

A. Victory (✉) · E. Lovallo
UPMC Department of Emergency Medicine, Pittsburgh, PA, USA
e-mail: victoryas@upmc.edu; lovalloem2@upmc.edu

© Springer Nature Switzerland AG 2019
A. Graham, D. J. Carlberg (eds.), *Gastrointestinal Emergencies*, https://doi.org/10.1007/978-3-319-98343-1_133

Pseudomonas are the most common bacteria causing peritonitis associated with ESI. Twenty percent of ESI-associated peritoneal infections are fungal or polymicrobial [7]. In the absence of peritonitis, ESI treatment is similar to treatment of other skin infections. In appropriately selected patients, treatment with oral cephalexin is reasonable. Coverage should be expanded to cover *MRSA* (clindamycin) and/or *Pseudomonas* (fluoroquinolones) based on local sensitivities and clinical suspicion [8]. Evidence of ESI with underlying abscess should be evaluated by a surgeon for drainage and may necessitate catheter removal.

PD patients may occasionally complain of pleuritic pain, which should prompt computed tomography (CT), as the indwelling catheter can cause intestinal perforation and free air leading to diaphragmatic irritation. However, a small amount of free air is not necessarily pathologic, as the dialysate may contain dissolved gasses that come out of solution after instillation [8].

Chronic abdominal pain or bowel obstruction in a PD patient can suggest encapsulating peritoneal sclerosis (EPS). Thickening and calcification of the peritoneum with fibrous band development can predispose to bowel obstruction. Contrast CT imaging is diagnostic and shows peritoneal enhancement and calcification with or without obstruction. The mortality rate of EPS is 37.5–56%. Patients must be transitioned to hemodialysis, and steroids are often initiated. Surgical consultation for possible enterolysis should be considered [9].

Acute care providers will also likely encounter mechanical complications of PD. Patients have difficulty instilling or draining dialysate, which is indicative of catheter malpositioning or obstruction. Low output flow is typically caused by pericatheter leak, malposition, or obstruction of the catheter by fibrin deposition. Case reports have demonstrated successful catheter clearance by instilling 1 mg/mL tissue plasminogen activator (t-PA) into the entire available volume of the catheter for 1 h if unable to clear the obstruction by manual push/pull with saline [10].

Tenckhoff catheters can migrate from a normal dependent pelvic position, become dislodged through the subcutaneous tract, or become entangled in omental tissue. On abdominal X-ray, a catheter tip facing in a superior direction may be corrected by a laxative bowel regimen to improve constipation and unload the sigmoid colon, subsequently allowing the catheter to fall back into the pelvis. If plain film radiography does not show an obvious etiology for catheter failure, CT with intraperitoneal gastrografin contrast may be utilized to evaluate catheter tip location. It may demonstrate the catheter tip lodged in adhesions or wrapped in omentum [11]. Kinked or malpositioned catheters which fail conservative management typically require manipulation under fluoroscopy or surgical replacement [12].

Acute care providers should evaluate for sequelae of ESRD, including hyperkalemia and fluid overload, as these may prompt emergent intervention and/or temporary transition to hemodialysis [13].

Suggested Resources

- Collection of peritoneal dialysis fluid sample for cell count and culture. Prince of Whales/Sydney-Sydney Eye Hospitals and Health Services. August 2016. https://www.aci.health.nsw.gov.au/__data/assets/word_doc/0006/249081/Collection_of_PD_fluid_for_cell_count_and_culture_2013.docx.
- Emergencies in the dialysis patient. Relias. May 2012. https://www.ahcmedia.com/articles/77642-emergencies-in-the-dialysis-patient.
- Episode 92.0 – Dialysis emergencies. Core EM. April 2017. https://coreem.net/podcast/episode-92-0/. Discussion on peritoneal dialysis beginning at 6 min and 25 sec.

References

1. Akoh JA. Peritoneal dialysis associated infections: an update on diagnosis and management. World J Nephrol. 2012;1(4):106–22.
2. Segal JH, Messana JM. Prevention of peritonitis in peritoneal dialysis. Semin Dial. 2013;26(4):494–502.
3. Li PK, Szeto CC, Piraino B, de Arteaga J, Fan S, Figueiredo AE, Fish DN, Goffin E, Kim YL, Salzer W, Struijk DG, Teitelbaum I, Johnson DW. ISPD peritonitis recommendations: 2016 update on prevention and treatment. Perit Dial Int. 2016;36(5):481–508.
4. Ballinger AE, Palmer SC, Wiggins KJ, Craig JC, Johnson DW, Cross NB, Strippoli GFM. Treatment for peritoneal dialysis-associated peritonitis. Cochrane Database of Systematic Reviews. 2014;4: Art. No: CD005284.
5. Cho Y, Johnson DW. Peritoneal dialysis-related peritonitis: towards improving evidence, practices and outcomes. Am J Kidney Dis. 2014;64(2):278–89.
6. van Diepen ATN, Tomlinson GA, Jassal SJ. The association between exit site infection and subsequent peritonitis among peritoneal dialysis patients. Clin J Am Soc Nephrol. 2012;7(8):1266–71.
7. Mehrotra R, Singh H. Peritoneal dialysis-associated peritonitis with simultaneous exit-site infection. Clin J Am Soc Nephrol. 2013;8(1):126–30.
8. Li PK, Szeto CC, Piraino B, Bernardini J, Figueiredo AE, Gupta A, Johnson DW, Juijper EJ, Lye WC, Salzer W, Schaefer F, Struijk DG. Peritoneal dialysis-related infections recommendations: 2010 update. Perit Dial Int. 2010;30(4):393–423.
9. Ekim M, Fitöz S, Yagmurlu A, Ensari A, Yüksel S, Acar B, Özçakar ZB, Kendirli T, Bingöler B, Yalçinkaya F. Encapsulating peritoneal sclerosis in paediatric peritoneal dialysis patients. Asian Pac Soc Neph. 2005;10:341–3.
10. Sahani MM, Mukhtar KN, Boorgu R, Leehey DJ, Popli S, Ing TS. Tissue plasminogen activator can effectively declot peritoneal dialysis catheters. Am J Kid Dis. 2000;36(3):675–6.
11. Stuart S, Booth TC, Cash CJC, Hameeduddin A, Goode JA, Harvey C, Malhotra A. Complications of continuous ambulatory peritoneal dialysis. Radiographics. 2009;29(2):441–60.
12. Beig AA, Marashi SM, Asadabadi HR, Sharifi A, Zarch ZN. A novel method for salvage of malfunctioning peritoneal dialysis catheter. Urol Ann. 2014;6(2):147–51.
13. Kim JE, Park SJ, Oh JY, Kim JH, Lee JS, Kim PK, Shin JI. Noninfectious complications of peritoneal dialysis in Korean children: a 26-year single-center study. Yonsei Med J. 2015;56(5):1359–64.

G-Tube Troubleshooting: When Is It Unsafe to Replace? What Is the Best Way to Verify Placement? What Is the Best Approach to Bleeding/Pain/Drainage/Blockage?

Andrew Victory and Alanna Peterson

Pearls and Pitfalls/Key Concepts
- Dislodged percutaneous endoscopic gastrostomy tubes (PEG tubes) and gastrostomy tubes (G-tubes) with mature tracts can frequently be replaced or reinserted at the bedside.
- Most PEG/G-tube complications that present within 14 days of initial placement should be evaluated in concert with the specialist who placed it.
- Low-volume upper gastrointestinal bleeding associated with a PEG/G-tube can be managed with a proton pump inhibitor.
- A PEG/G-tube bumper placed too tightly can cause gastric pressure necrosis or buried bumper syndrome.
- The push/pull technique using either warm water or pancreatic enzymes with sodium bicarbonate can help relieve tube obstruction.

Many patients who present for acute care have alternate methods of feeding. The most common is the gastrostomy tube (G-tube), which is placed surgically by either laparotomy or laparoscopy. Endoscopic methods are used to place a percutaneous endoscopic gastrostomy tubes (PEG tubes) from within the gastric lumen. Management of the two is similar, with a few exceptions as detailed below. While these procedures provide excellent enteral access for medication and nutrition, numerous early and late complications occur.

When Is It Unsafe to Replace a G-Tube?

Dislodgment is the most common complication seen in PEG/G-tube patients, with 5.3–12.8% of tubes dislodging during their period of intended use [1].

Length of time since tube placement must be considered prior to reinsertion, as a mature gastrocutaneous fistula may not have formed during the first 14 days after placement. Studies have shown safety and success with manual reinsertion of a dislodged tube after this 2-week window [2]. In those who are severely malnourished, delayed healing may push this timeframe to 1 month from original placement [3].

Early dislodgment of the tube (within 7 days of original placement) may lead to an open gastrostomy site, which requires emergent surgical consultation. The open gastrostomy site is effectively an intraperitoneal gastric perforation. Dislodgement of the immature tube between 7 days and 14 days requires consultation with the surgeon or gastroenterologist who placed it. These tubes should be replaced in the operating room or endoscopy suite because there is a higher risk of accidental peritoneal placement.

When a mature gastrocutaneous tract is present, providers should work to minimize the period of dislodgment, as the tract can begin healing, form strictures, or fully close within hours. If the tract has matured and the patient presents in a timely fashion, the tube can be replaced by the acute care provider without consultation. The first attempt at replacement should be with a tube the same size as the one that dislodged. If unsuccessful, a smaller tube may be attempted. If a G-tube is not available, the tract can be maintained with a Foley catheter that can be used for medications and feeding in the interim [4].

What Is the Best Way to Verify G-Tube Placement?

Confirmation of successful replacement is performed by gastric content aspiration and/or injection of water-soluble contrast and verification with abdominal X-ray. In both adults

A. Victory (✉) · A. Peterson
UPMC Department of Emergency Medicine, Pittsburgh, PA, USA
e-mail: victoryas@upmc.edu; petersona2@upmc.edu

© Springer Nature Switzerland AG 2019
A. Graham, D. J. Carlberg (eds.), *Gastrointestinal Emergencies*, https://doi.org/10.1007/978-3-319-98343-1_134

and children with mature tracts, tube replacement does not require confirmatory imaging if gastric contents are successfully aspirated. However, confirmatory imaging should be obtained in patients with traumatic tube dislodgment or replacement, clinical concern for a malpositioned tube, or inability to aspirate gastric contents. Imaging is also indicated if a tube was replaced through an immature tract [5, 6].

What Is the Best Approach to Bleeding?

Irritation and erosion of the surrounding gastric endothelium by the G-tube can cause bleeding. Presentations include bloody discharge from the tube, hematemesis, melena, and/or hematochezia with or without abdominal pain.

Early bleeding (0–3 days) is likely a surgical complication and should be managed with typical resuscitation measures and early consultation with the placing physician. Extra-luminal bleeding may occur due to injury of the abdominal vasculature and may produce retroperitoneal bleeding or an abdominal wall hematoma. Early bleeding may produce hemodynamic instability, and severe bleeding may require endoscopy or embolization [7].

Late presentation (>2 weeks) low-volume bleeding can be managed conservatively with outpatient follow-up (surgery or gastroenterology) and a proton pump inhibitor, which is more effective than a histamine-2 blocker [8]. Local bleeding in the tract can often be managed with direct pressure at the site.

What Is the Best Approach to Pain?

Abdominal pain is a common complaint in the emergency care setting, and there are a few additional considerations for those with G-tubes in place.

Pain may be caused by gastritis or ulceration, as a bumper that is drawn too tightly may cause pressure necrosis internally or on the skin. Loosening the bolster can relieve discomfort and allow healing. The area of skin pressure necrosis requires frequent dressing changes [3].

Pain and pressure sensation with a palpable mass at the insertion site is suggestive of buried bumper syndrome, in which the tube is partially dislodged and stuck in the abdominal wall due to migration of the internal bumper into the soft tissue. Continued use of a tube in this position can lead to blockage, peristomal leak, local infection, and even peritonitis [9]. Buried bumper syndrome requires tube removal and likely admission for IV hydration, replacement of the tube by a specialist, and IV antibiotics if evidence of infection is present [10].

What Is the Best Approach to Drainage?

The G-tube creates a gastrocutaneous fistula, which can result in the skin surrounding the tube developing chronic changes from exposure to gastric contents. While a small amount of granulation tissue is normal, the skin can also become irritated and macerated due to leakage of gastric acid. The best management includes quality wound care with frequent dressing changes and ensuring an appropriately sized tube. Tubes should generally not be upsized in the acute care setting. Patients should be referred to specialists for this procedure.

Skin site infections have a reported prevalence of 5–25% [9]. Cellulitic changes require systemic antibiotics with consideration of the patient's immune status and local MRSA prevalence. Early infections, less than 30 days after placement, should be treated as hospital associated and should receive broad spectrum antibiotics [11].

What Is the Best Approach to Blockage?

PEG or G-tube blockage will prevent tube usage and is a common reason for emergency care. Approximately 45% of patients develop blockage of a tube during its lifetime [3]. Patients may require IV hydration and medications until enteral access is regained.

The first step in unclogging is manually kneading the tube to break up concretions. This should be followed by a push/pull technique using warm water to mobilize the obstruction [9]. If unsuccessful, providers can dissolve one crushed pancreatic enzymes tablet and one crushed sodium bicarbonate tablet (650 mg) in 10–20 mL of warm water. The fluid is instilled into the obstructed tube for 30 min, and another attempt is made to clear the tube with a push/pull technique. If necessary, this procedure can be repeated 3 times [12].

Suggested Resources
- EM in 5 – Feeding tube replacement – https://emin5.com/2015/10/25/feeding-tube-replacement/.
- emDocs – Troubleshooting G-tubes & J-tubes: Common scenarios/Tips & Tricks – http://www.emdocs.net/troubleshooting-g-tubes-j-tubes-common-scenarios-tips-tricks/.

References

1. Rosenberger LH, Newhook T, Schirmer B, Sawyer RG. Late accidental dislodgement of a percutaneous endoscopic gastrostomy tube: an underestimated burden on patients and the health care system. Surg Endosc. 2011;25(10):3307–11.
2. Mincheff TV. Early dislodgement of percutaneous and endoscopic gastrostomy tube. J S C Med Assoc. 2007;103(1):13–5.

3. Schrag SP, Sharma R, Jaik NP, Seamon MJ, Lukaszczyk JJ, Martin ND, Hoey BA, Stawicki SP. Complications related to percutaneous endoscopic gastrostomy (PEG) tubes. A comprehensive clinical review. J Gastrointestin Liver Dis. 2007;16(4):407–18.
4. Metussin A, Sia R, Bakar S, Chong VH. Foley catheters as temporary gastrostomy tubes. Soc Gastroent Nurses Assoc. 2016;39(4):273–7.
5. Jacobson G, Brokish PA, Wrenn K. Percutaneous feeding tube replacement in the ED- Are confirmatory x-rays necessary? Am J Emerg Med. 2009;27(5):519–24.
6. Showalter CD, Kerrey B, Spellman-Kennebeck S, Timm N. Gastrostomy tube replacement in a pediatric ED: frequency of complications and impact of confirmatory imaging. Am J Emerg Med. 2012;30(8):1501–6.
7. Seo N, Shin JH, Ko GY, Gwon DI, Kim JH, Sung KB. Incidence and management of bleeding complications following percutaneous radiologic gastrostomy. Korean J Radiol. 2012;13(2):174–81.
8. Dharmarajan TS, Yadav D, Adiga GU, Kokkat A, Pitchumoni CS. Gastrostomy, esophagitis, and gastrointestinal bleeding in older adults. J Am Med Dir Assoc. 2004;5(4):228–32.
9. Rahnemai-Azar AA, Rahnemaiazar AA, Naghshizadian R, Kurtz A, Farkas DT. Percutaneous endoscopic gastrostomy: indications, technique, complications and management. World J Gastroenterol. 2014;20(24):7739–51.
10. Geer W, Jeanmonod R. Early presentation of buried bumper syndrome. West J Emerg Med. 2013;14(5):421–3.
11. Duarte H, Santos C, Capelas ML, Fonseca J. Peristomal infection after percutaneous endoscopic gastrostomy: a 7-year surveillance of 297 patients. Arq Gastroenterol. 2012;49(4):255–8.
12. Tubes UPMC presbyterian shadyside policies and procedures: unclogging enteral feeding tubes (P-PEF 14). Pittsburgh: University of Pittsburgh Medical Center; 2010.

Consultant Corner: Abdominal Pain and the Post-procedure Patient

135

Patrick D. Webb

Introduction

Patrick D. Webb, M.D., is an attending physician with the Centers for Gastroenterology in Fort Collins, Colorado. He trained in internal medicine from 2004 to 2007 at Naval Medical Center San Diego (NMCSD). Following a chief resident year, he completed a fellowship in Gastroenterology at NMCSD from 2008 to 2011. After serving as an active duty physician, Dr. Webb transitioned to private practice in 2018. His practice includes advanced endoscopy, including endoscopic ultrasound and endoscopic retrograde cholangiopancreatography (ERCP).

Answers to Key Clinical Questions

1. How do I approach pain after upper endoscopy?

When pain after upper endoscopy leads to unscheduled acute care, the pain is typically related to a specific intervention performed during the procedure. Most endoscopists provide the patient or family with a copy of the procedure report. Acute care providers should review this document, as it may give clues regarding potential diagnoses. In some instances, it may help spare patients from unnecessary testing, and in others it may increase the provider's suspicion for major complications.

Delayed presentations of perforation (greater than 2 h after endoscopy) are among the most feared complications of upper endoscopy. The vast majority of perforations are related to dilation or device placement (i.e., esophageal stent). Esophageal perforations can be categorized as contained or non-contained. The former is treated with IV antibiotics, withholding oral intake, and observation. The later typically requires surgical repair. When evaluating for esophageal perforation, chest x-ray is typically the first imaging study ordered. If this is negative, computed tomography of the chest with oral contrast (which is frequently diluted) is usually indicated. When suspicion for esophageal perforation is high, consultation with radiology, cardiothoracic surgery, and gastroenterology may help determine the optimal imaging approach. Timely diagnosis is important, as some perforations can be managed non-operatively with placement of fully covered self-expanding metal stents (FCSEMS), but these can only be placed during a brief window post-perforation.

P. D. Webb
Centers for Gastroenterology, Fort Collins, CO, USA

© Springer Nature Switzerland AG 2019
A. Graham, D. J. Carlberg (eds.), *Gastrointestinal Emergencies*, https://doi.org/10.1007/978-3-319-98343-1_135

A more comprehensive list of causes of post-endoscopy pain includes:

1. Perforation (secondary to)
   (a) Esophageal dilation
   (b) Esophageal stent placement
   (c) Cervical esophageal perforation with intubation of the esophagus
   (d) Free peritoneal perforation
2. Intervention-related complications
   (a) Post-polypectomy syndrome
   (b) Esophageal banding
   (c) Mucosal resections
3. Cardiopulmonary events
4. Pneumothorax
5. Exacerbation of pain related to the patients' initial complaint that led to endoscopy

Pain unrelated to the endoscopy (i.e., acute pancreatitis, chest wall pain, etc.) should also be considered.

Following exclusion of high-risk complications (i.e., perforation, pneumothorax), the majority of patients can be reassured and provided with analgesics that target the patient's chief complaint. For instance, sore throat or chest discomfort caused by local irritation may be treated with 2–5% topical lidocaine. Dyspeptic symptoms may be treated with a proton pump inhibitor or Carafate. Nonsteroidal anti-inflammatory drugs should be avoided in patients with an active peptic ulcer or recent polypectomy because of the bleeding risk.

Acute care providers should have a low threshold for contacting the endoscopist who performed the procedure to discuss the case.

2. How do I approach pain after colonoscopy?

Pain following colonoscopy can vary from excessive bloating from air insufflation to perforation. Bleeding can equally vary from mild anorectal bleeding due to scope trauma to severe post-polypectomy hemorrhage. Gastroenterologists frequently discharge patients or their families with colonoscopy reports, and reviewing these reports may give acute care providers clues to potential complications.

The major causes of pain following colonoscopy include perforation, post-polypectomy syndrome, excessive air insufflation, and solid organ injury.

Perforation is typically recognized at the time of or immediately following colonoscopy. An acute abdominal series and/or computed tomography should be the initial study. Perforation can be caused by either direct injury from the scope or an intervention during the procedure (i.e., polypectomy). Initial treatment is broad-spectrum antibiotics, pain control, and IV fluids. Consultation with general surgery and a gastroenterologist is mandatory.

Post-polypectomy syndrome can occur following the use of electrocautery and is thought to be a transmural "burn." It mimics diverticulitis in many cases and is typically treated with IV antibiotics, fluids, bowel rest, and observation. Patients often have a mild leukocytosis. Imaging should be done to rule out perforation.

Excessive air insufflation is not uncommon post colonoscopy, and patients with chronic bowel conditions are predisposed to have post-procedural pain due to the air insufflation alone. Imaging is likely to show diffusely distended large and small intestines but no evidence of perforation. Treatment is reassurance. Having the patient go onto his or her hands and knees to perform a "cat-cow" maneuver may help.

Solid organ injury is a very rare complication produced by shear forces on extra-luminal organs. Splenic, liver, and renal injuries have been described.

3. How do I approach bleeding after colonoscopy?

Bleeding after colonoscopy is approached similarly to other episodes of lower gastrointestinal bleeding. Non-procedure-related sources should be considered. Clinically significant bleeding needs to be recognized early to avoid delays in resuscitative efforts. Patient variables will influence many decisions. For example, bleeding is more concerning in a patient who recently restarted his or her systemic anticoagulation after polypectomy.

The majority of post-colonoscopy bleeding is secondary to polypectomy, and the clinical significance is related to the size/methods used to remove the lesion and the anticoagulation status of the patient. The majority of patients will require admission for observation, lab monitoring, and repeat colonoscopy to aid in diagnosis and treatment. Patients with minor, non-hemodynamically significant bleeding with reassuring labs are potential candidates for discharge in the right clinical situation.

4. How do I approach pain after ERCP?

Pain following endoscopic retrograde cholangiopancreatography (ERCP) that causes a patient to seek unscheduled emergency care should be approached carefully and methodically. ERCPs are almost always performed for therapeutic indications, and the procedure may involve biliary sphincterotomy, dilation, and stent placement. Other interventions may also take place during ERCP. Given the therapeutic nature of the procedure, there is a higher risk that the pain could be related to a serious complication. As with the upper endoscopy and colonoscopy, the procedure report may provide valuable clues to potential procedural complications.

Post-ERCP pancreatitis (PEP) occurs in 3–20% of ERCPs. PEP typically presents within 0–8 h of the procedure, but delayed presentations can occur days later. The presenting symptoms are typical of any pancreatitis, and the diagnosis still requires two of three elements: lipase >3 times the upper limit of normal, pain consistent with pancreatitis, and imaging consistent with pancreatitis. Most patients will undergo computed tomography of the abdomen with contrast, as the differential diagnosis includes both perforation and PEP. Treatment is the same for any acute pancreatitis and should involve fluid resuscitation with lactated ringers. PEP patients are generally admitted to the hospital or placed in observation status.

Another cause of pain following ERCP is perforation, which is divided into free duodenal perforation and peri-ampullary perforation. The former is typically caused by the endoscope exerting excessive force on the duodenum and is frequently recognized immediately. Peri-ampullary perforations are typically related to sphincterotomy, and a pre-cut sphincterotomy is associated with a higher risk of peri-ampullary perforation. This type of perforation can occur retroperitoneally or intraperitoneally. Intraperitoneal perforations generally have free intraperitoneal air on imaging and require immediate consultation with general surgery. Retroperitoneal perforations are approached differently, and many can be managed conservatively with bowel rest, IV antibiotics, and pain control. Consultation with general surgery and gastroenterology is mandatory for all patients with diagnosed or suspected ERCP-related perforation.

Besides PEP and perforation, cholangitis may cause pain following ERCP. Cholangitis should remain high in the differential diagnosis, especially for patients with underlying malignancy and/or primary sclerosing cholangitis (PSC). Cholangitis following ERCP is typically related to underdrained obstructed biliary segments. The endoscopist is very mindful of this potential complication and tries to minimize the risk of it. Other potential causes involve malfunctioning or migrated biliary stents. Cholangitis represents a medical emergency, and patients generally require high level of care (i.e., medical ICU) and should have access to interventional radiology services.

When other causes have been ruled out, providers should consider the possibility that the patient's pain may be due an underlying chronic condition. This can be seen in patients with chronic pancreatitis who have recently undergone stricture dilation or stent placement. However, many patients with chronic pancreatitis undergoing repeat ERCPs are better equipped to "handle" their pain following ERCP, so their presentation for unscheduled care should increase the provider's level of concern.

5. How do I approach pain after liver biopsy?

A patient presenting for acute care following liver biopsy should be approached with care given the invasive nature of the test and the fact that liver biopsy is typically performed on patients with underlying chronic liver disease.

The liver's sensory fibers are primarily located on Glisson's capsule. Any patient undergoing a liver biopsy should expect to have some pain for 2–3 days, which is typically experienced in the right upper quadrant and can radiate to the right shoulder. Two serious causes of pain include liver hematomas and bilomas.

Hematomas may be discovered with ultrasound and/or cross-sectional imaging. They rarely require intervention as long as they are small and the patient has a reassuring set of vital signs and laboratory workup. If there is hypotension or new anemia, surgery consultation and computed tomography with intravenous contrast should be obtained.

A biloma is a rare complication from liver biopsy and is typically a delayed finding. It may present several days to weeks after biopsy, and patients may have icterus and/or jaundice. Some patients will require percutaneous drainage, but this is not an emergent intervention. Gastroenterology consultation should be obtained, as this team will guide potential interventions.

Though liver biopsies are generally performed using bedside ultrasound, there is a low risk for adjacent organ puncture. The right kidney, intestine, gallbladder, lung, and diaphragm may all be injured. Gallbladder injury is generally recognized immediately, as bile peritonitis ensues and the patient becomes very uncomfortable. When lung puncture occurs, patients may develop pneumothorax.

Patients may also develop cellulitis or musculoskeletal injury secondary to transcutaneous liver biopsy.

Suggested Resources
- American Society for Gastrointestinal Endoscopy. Adverse events associated with ERCP. Gastrointest Endosc. 2017;85:32–47.
- Kumar AS, Lee JK. Colonoscopy: advanced and emerging techniques – a review of colonoscopic approaches to colorectal conditions. Clin Colon Rectal Surg. 2017;30(2):136–44. https://doi.org/10. 1055/s-0036-1597312.
- Rockley DC, Caldwell SH, Goodman ZD, Nelson RC, Smith AD, American Association for the Study of Liver Diseases Position Paper. Liver biopsy. Hepatology. 2009;49:1017–44.

What Causes of Chronic Abdominal Pain, Both Common and Uncommon, Should Be Considered and Investigated by the Emergency Medicine Provider?

Joseph Izzo and Janet Smereck

Pearls and Pitfalls
- Chronic abdominal pain has many potential etiologies that may be missed; the underlying cause should be identified when considering treatment.
- Vascular, obstructive, and metabolic causes of chronically recurring abdominal pain may have devastating consequences if diagnoses and treatments are delayed.
- Anterior cutaneous nerve entrapment syndromes (ACNES) are often overlooked; point tenderness of the rectus muscle that worsens with lifting of the head or legs (Carnett's sign) is a characteristic.
- The diagnosis of malignancy as a cause of chronic abdominal pain may be considered although not established in the ED; symptoms including fevers, a change in bowel habits, jaundice, and unintentional weight loss should lead to more in-depth investigation.
- Functional disorders, including narcotic bowel syndrome and opioid-seeking behaviors, are commonplace in the ED setting but should be considered a diagnosis of exclusion.

Chronic abdominal pain is defined as continuous or intermittent abdominal discomfort lasting for 6 months or longer [1]. Approximately 5% of ED patients have a presenting complaint of abdominal pain, and an estimated 20–30% of these visits fall in the category of chronic or recurrent pain [2]. In one database analysis, chronic abdominal pain accounted for 4% of serial or repeated visits to the ED [3]. Chronic undifferentiated abdominal pain should not be considered a distinct clinical entity; it is important to be aware of serious and potentially life-threatening causes of chronic abdominal pain. Categorical etiologies of chronic abdominal pain are described, both common and commonly missed, with the goal of appropriate management and disposition.

What Causes of Chronic Abdominal Pain Should the Emergency Medicine Provider Consider?

Inflammatory conditions, such as Crohn's disease and ulcerative colitis, present with recurrent pain episodes relating to disease flares or sequelae from strictures, adhesions, and fistulas. Clues to the diagnoses include fever, localized tenderness, and diarrheal stools, often with blood. Extraintestinal symptoms are common and include ophthalmologic (uveitis, episcleritis), dermatologic (erythema nodosum, pyoderma gangrenosum), and rheumatologic manifestations [4]. Surgery may be required for complications such as intestinal obstruction, perforation, and fistula formation (e.g., perianal, entero-entero-cutaneous, and entero-cutaneous fistulas).

Motility disorders result from the dysfunction of normal peristalsis and commonly require endoscopy or dynamic imaging studies to confirm the diagnosis. Gastroparesis, a syndrome of chronic recurrent flares of vomiting, bloating, and abdominal pain, stems from decreased gastric emptying without evident mechanical obstruction [5, 6]. Complications of diabetes mellitus and gastric surgeries (Roux-en-Y or partial gastrectomy for peptic ulcer, especially with concurrent vagotomy) may lead to delayed gastric emptying. Gastroparesis syndrome is often idiopathic or relating to chronic opioid use [7]. Specific management strategies include dietary changes to promote gut motility, including increase in dietary fiber, and prokinetic agents [5].

Chronic intestinal pseudo-obstruction (CIPO) is often misinterpreted as bowel obstruction and may lead to unnecessary surgical intervention. Intestinal dilatation, as a result of impaired motility due to neuropathies or myopathies, is without a transition or lead point which distinguishes CIPO

J. Izzo · J. Smereck (✉)
Department of Emergency Medicine, MedStar Georgetown University Hospital, Washington, DC, USA

© Springer Nature Switzerland AG 2019
A. Graham, D. J. Carlberg (eds.), *Gastrointestinal Emergencies*, https://doi.org/10.1007/978-3-319-98343-1_136

from true obstruction. Weight loss and malnutrition are common, secondary to food avoidance [8].

Obstructive causes of abdominal pain include hernias, both external and internal, adhesions from inflammation or surgical scarring, and neoplastic disease. Paramount importance should be placed on investigating hernia that previously was reducible. Gastric outlet obstruction may result from scarring of untreated peptic ulcer disease, damage from caustic substances, or malignancy, including gastric and pancreatic cancers [9, 10]. Patients typically present with pain in the epigastrium, postprandial emesis (often projectile vomiting), and weight loss [11].

Hepatobiliary disorders responsible for chronic recurrent abdominal pain episodes include chronic pancreatitis, infectious hepatitis, hepatic capsular stretching due to malformations and neoplastic disease, and, rarely, choledocholithiasis [1].

Genitourinary disorders may cause intermittent pain, such as with endometriosis, leiomyomatosis, and ovarian cysts, or chronic unremitting pain, as with obstructive uropathy and genitourinary malignancies.

Vascular etiologies are uncommon but should be considered in patients with episodic/recurrent abdominal pain.

- Chronic mesenteric ischemia (CMI), also referred to as "abdominal angina," presents with symptoms often referred to as "splanchnic syndrome": postprandial pain, weight loss, epigastric bruit, and food avoidance. The syndrome occurs from stenosis of one or more of the splanchnic vessels: celiac, superior mesenteric, and inferior mesenteric arteries [12]. CMI usually results from atherosclerotic arterial insufficiency, although vasculitis from autoimmune conditions such as scleroderma may also produce ischemic symptoms [12, 13].
- Median arcuate ligament syndrome (MALS), also known as celiac artery compression syndrome or Dunbar syndrome, is a specific form of mesenteric artery stenosis, occurring when the median arcuate ligament compresses the celiac trunk [14].
- Superior mesenteric artery (SMA) syndrome occurs when the SMA compresses the third portion of the duodenum against the aorta [15].
- Symptoms of portal vein thrombosis (PVT) include abdominal pain and distension; the syndrome is associated with chronic liver disease and thrombophilias [16].
- Not uncommonly, recurrent abdominal pain from sickle cell crises is due to microvessel occlusion and infarcts of viscera and mesentery from sickling of erythrocytes [17].
- A rare condition, intermittent splenic torsion or "wandering spleen," has been reported in the setting of splenomegaly and ligamentous laxity allowing torsion on the vascular pedicle, creating ischemic pain [18].

Abdominal wall pain is associated with hernias and nerve entrapment syndromes. Abdominal wall hernias may be present in the inguinal or umbilical regions, as well as along prior incisional sites. Various nerve entrapment syndromes are documented, including anterior cutaneous nerve entrapment syndrome (ACNES), first described in 1926 by Carnett. ACNES occurs when terminal branches of lower intercostal nerves become entrapped between abdominal muscles [19]. Carnett's sign of point tenderness along the distribution of the rectus muscle, worsened by lifting the head with legs straightened, should raise suspicion for the syndrome [20]. Trigger point injections are both diagnostic and therapeutic, although surgical excision may be required [21, 22]. C-section-related nerve entrapment syndromes have also been described with similar management [23].

Rare metabolic disorders causing chronic or recurrent abdominal pain are seldom diagnosed in the ED setting. Familial Mediterranean fever (FMF) is characterized by recurrent bouts of fever, arthralgias and abdominal pain in persons with a positive family history [1]. Chronically recurring abdominal pain is the most common presenting symptom of the intermittent porphyrias, which are genetically mediated disorders of heme biosynthesis. Potentially life-threatening attacks of severe abdominal pain, nausea, seizures, delirium, and psychiatric symptoms can be triggered by premenstrual hormonal changes, infections, specific medications (notably phenobarbital and phenytoin), alcohol, and fasting [24–26]. Lead poisoning may also present with recurring or chronic abdominal pain and nausea [27].

What Serious Causes of Chronic or Recurrent Abdominal Pain Should Be Considered?

Serious causes of chronic or recurrent abdominal pain include conditions typically having acute presentations but rarely having a more indolent course.

- Chronic appendicitis has an estimated incidence of 1.5% of all cases of appendicitis, with higher complication rates of perforation and abscess formation [28].
- Serious vascular phenomena which may be a source of chronic abdominal pain include aortic aneurysm, chronic aortic dissection, and chronic vena cava perforation from filter migration [29, 30].
- Neoplastic causes are vast and include visceral organ, neuroendocrine, and genitourinary mass lesions which may cause intermittent unremitting pain. Pancreatic, hepatic, and biliary primary or metastatic malignancy, gastric lymphoma, and peritoneal carcinomatosis have indolent courses associated with chronic abdominal pain. Although the diagnosis of malignancy is not established in the ED setting, patients presenting with symptoms such

as significant change in bowel habits, new anemia, jaundice, and unexplained weight loss should lead the clinician to more in-depth investigation and close referral.

Functional abdominal pain disorders should be considered diagnoses of exclusion – *irritable bowel syndromes, narcotic bowel syndrome,* and *opioid-seeking behavior.* *Irritable bowel syndrome (IBS)* represents a cluster of symptoms including abdominal discomfort and altered bowel habits, without structural or laboratory abnormalities, often commonly with comorbid psychosocial factors [31]. The Rome Foundation has offered consensus guidelines to assist with diagnosis of IBS: recurrent abdominal pain on average at least 1 day/week over a course of 3 months, associated with constipation, diarrhea, or both [32, 33].

Narcotic bowel syndrome is characterized by the presence of chronic, recurrent abdominal pain in patients typically taking opioids on a long-term basis, typically associated with escalating doses of narcotic pain medicines. Some studies estimate the prevalence of the disorder is 4% of all patients taking narcotics. Patients will have opioid-induced gastrointestinal symptoms such as constipation or pseudo-obstruction [34]. Awareness of the well-documented association between chronic abdominal pain and history of abuse, particularly childhood sexual abuse, allows the clinician to approach opiate-dependent patients with a practical sense of compassion [35].

Tables 136.1 and 136.2 summarize conditions associated with chronic abdominal pain.

Table 136.1 Gastrointestinal conditions producing chronic abdominal pain

Inflammatory bowel diseases (Crohn's, ulcerative colitis)
Gastroparesis
Chronic intestinal pseudo-obstruction
Gastric outlet obstruction
Chronic pancreatitis
Hepatitis
Chronic mesenteric ischemia
Median arcuate ligament syndrome
Portal vein thrombosis
Sickle cell anemia
Anterior cutaneous nerve entrapment syndrome (ACNES)
Familial Mediterranean fever
Intermittent porphyrias
Lead poisoning
Irritable bowel syndromes (IBS)
Narcotic bowel syndrome

Table 136.2 Serious "don't miss" diagnoses associated with chronic abdominal pain

Appendicitis
Bowel obstruction, strangulated hernia
Mesenteric ischemia
Aortic aneurysm and dissection

References

1. Zackowski S. Chronic recurrent abdominal pain. Emerg Med Clin North Am. 1998;16(4):877–94.
2. Tack J, Talley N, Camilleri M, Holtmann G, Malagelada JR, Stanghellini V. Functional gastroduodenal disorders. Gastroenterol. 2006;130:1466–79.
3. Cook L, Knight S, Junkins E, Mann NC, Dean JM, Olson LM. Repeat patients to the emergency department in a statewide database. Acad Emerg Med. 2004;11:256–63.
4. Levine JS, Burakoff R. Extraintestinal manifestations of inflammatory bowel disease. Gastroenterol Hepatol. 2011;7(4):235–41.
5. Stein B, Everhart KK, Lacy BE. Gastroparesis: a review of current diagnosis and treatment options. J Clin Gastroenterol. 2015;49(7):550–8.
6. Parkman HP, Hasler WL, Fisher RS. American Gastroenterological Association technical review on the diagnosis and treatment of gastroparesis. Gastroenterology. 2004;127(5):1592–622.
7. Soykan I, Sivri B, Sarosiek I, Kiernan B, McCallum RW. Demography, clinical characteristics, psychological and abuse profiles, treatment, and long-term follow-up of patients with gastroparesis. Dig Dis Sci. 1998;43(11):2398–404.
8. Bernardi MP, Warrier S, Lynch AC, Heriot AG. Acute and chronic pseudo-obstruction: a current update. ANZ J Surg. 2015;85(10):709–14.
9. Wong YT, Brams DM, Munson L, Sanders L, Heiss F, Chase M, Birkett DH. Gastric outlet obstruction secondary to pancreatic cancer: surgical vs endoscopic palliation. Surg Endosc. 2002;16(2):310–2.
10. Tendler DA. Malignant gastric outlet obstruction: bridging another divide. Am J Gastroenterol. 2002;97(1):4–6.
11. Chowdhury A, Dhali GK, Banerjee PK. Etiology of gastric outlet obstruction. Amer J Gastroenterol. 1996;91(8):1679.
12. Barret M, Martineau C, Rahmi G, Pellerin O. Chronic mesenteric ischemia: a rare cause of chronic abdominal pain. Am J Med. 2015;128(12):1363.
13. Kolkman JJ, Geelkerken RH. Diagnosis and treatment of chronic mesenteric ischemia: an update. Best Pract Res Clin Gastroenterol. 2017;31(1):49–57.
14. Kallus SJ, Singhal P, Palese C, Smith JP, Haddad N. Median arcuate ligament syndrome: an unusual cause of chronic abdominal pain. Neuroenterology. 2016;4:235916, 6 pages. 10.4303/ne/235916.
15. Hlnas JR, Gore RM, Ballantyne GH. Superior mesenteric artery syndrome: diagnostic criteria and therapeutic approaches. Am J Surg. 1984;148:4–6.
16. Farmer A, Saadeddin A, Holt CE, Bateman JM, Ahmed M, Syn WK. Portal vein thrombosis in the district general hospital: management and clinical outcomes. Eur J Gastroenterol Heopatol. 2009;21(5):517–21.
17. Ahmed S, Shahid R, Russo L. Unusual causes of abdominal pain: sickle cell anemia. Best Pract Res Clin Gastroenterol. 2005;19(2):297–310.
18. Ho CL. Wandering spleen with chronic torsion in a patient with thalassaemia. Singap Med J. 2014;55(12):2002–4.
19. Costanza C, Longstreth G, Liu A. Chronic abdominal wall pain: clinical features, health care costs and long term outcome. Gastroenterol. 2012;6(2):300–8.
20. van Assen T, Brouns J, Scheltinga MR, Roumen RM. Incidence of abdominal pain due to the anterior cutaneous nerve entrapment syndrome in an emergency department. Scand J Trauma Resusc Emerg Med. 2015;23(19):1–6.
21. Oor JE, Ünlü Ç, Hazebroek EJ. A systematic review of the treatment for abdominal cutaneous nerve entrapment syndrome. Am J Surg. 2016;212(1):165–74.

22. Thome J, Egeler C. Abdominal cutaneous nerve entrapment syndrome (ACNES) in a patient with a pain syndrome previously assumed to be of psychiatric origin. World J Biol Psychiatry. 2006;7(2):116–8.

23. Loos MJ, Scheltinga MR, Mulders LG. The Pfannenstiel incision as a source of chronic pain. Gynecologie. 2008;111(4):839–46.

24. Herrick A, McColl K. Acute intermittent porphyria. Best Pract Res Clin Gastroenterol. 2005;19(2):235–49.

25. Karim Z, Lyoumi S, Nicolas G, Deybach JC, Gouya L, Puy H. Porphyrias: a 2015 update. Clin Res Hepatol Gastroenterol. 2015;39(4):412–25.

26. Liu Y, Lien W, Fang C, Lai TI, Chen WJ, Wang HP. ED presentation of acute porphyria. Am J Emerg Med. 2005;23:164–7.

27. Tsai M, Huang S, Cheng S. Lead poisoning can be easily misdiagnosed as acute porphyria and nonspecific abdominal pain. Case Rep Emerg Med. 2017;9050713, 4 pages. Accessed online 01/19/2018.

28. Shah S, Gaffney R, Dykes T, Goldstein J. Chronic appendicitis: an often forgotten cause of recurrent abdominal pain. Am J Med. 2013;126:e7–8.

29. Yuan S, Tager S. Acute onset of chronic aortic dissection presenting as abdominal pain. Kardiol Pol. 2009;67(2):168–71.

30. Zelivianskaia A, Boddu P, Samee M. Chronic abdominal pain from inferior vena cava filter strut perforation: a case report. Am J Med. 2016;129(3):e5–7.

31. Chey WD, Kurlander J, Eswaran S. Irritable bowel syndrome: a clinical review. JAMA. 2015;313(9):949–58.

32. Kellow JE. A practical evidence-based approach to the diagnosis of the functional gastrointestinal disorders. Am J Gastroenterol. 2010;105(4):743–6.

33. Schmulson MJ, Drossman DA. What is new in Rome IV. J Neurogastroenterol Motil. 2017;23(2):151–63.

34. Grover C, Wielo E, Close RJ. Narcotic bowel syndrome. J Emerg Med. 2012;43(6):992–5.

35. Drossman D. Abuse, trauma and GI illness: is there a link? Am J Gastroenterol. 2011;106(1):14–25.

What "Red Flags" Should the Emergency Clinician Be Aware of When Evaluating the Patient with Chronic Abdominal Pain?

Herman Kalsi and Janet Smereck

> **Pearls and Pitfalls**
> - About half of chronically recurring abdominal pain cases are believed to be functional in nature.
> - Historical red flags include fever, pain that awakens from sleep, sudden change in character of pain, anorexia, dysphagia, unintentional weight loss, dyspnea, change in stool caliber for >3 weeks, increase in abdominal girth, persistent vomiting, blood in stool or urine, jaundice, diffuse edema, testicular pain, postcoital bleeding, or possibility of pregnancy.
> - On physical examination, fever, tachycardia, jaundice, edema, and focal tenderness are concerning findings.
> - Approach each patient encounter without bias, and consider commonly missed conditions.
> - Malingering, although a possibility, should be a diagnosis of exclusion.

Chronic abdominal pain (CAP) is abdominal pain that persists either continuously or intermittently for longer than 6 months [1]. Approximately 2% of adults are thought to have CAP at some point in their lives [2]. While the vast majority of CAP is confined to the genitourinary and gastrointestinal systems, a few systemic disorders such as porphyria, lead poisoning, and migraine equivalents may present with CAP and respond to specific therapies. It is important to keep a broad differential when approaching chronic abdominal pain, as half of cases of chronically recurring abdominal pain are believed to be functional, without demonstrable pathologic abnormality [1, 3, 4].

"Red Flags" for Acute Pathology

The history should elicit information regarding pain location, quality, duration, timing, and frequency of recurrence of symptoms as well as any relieving or aggravating factors. A diet history should be obtained including potential allergens and milk products, as lactose intolerance can cause chronic abdominal discomfort. A focused evaluation should give particular attention to "red flag" signs and symptoms. The following symptoms should heighten suspicion for an acute on chronic or new potentially life-threatening process: *fever, pain that awakens from sleep, sudden change in character of pain, anorexia, dysphagia, unintentional weight loss, dyspnea, change in stool caliber for > 3 weeks, increase in abdominal girth, persistent vomiting, blood in stool or urine, jaundice, diffuse edema, testicular pain, postcoital bleeding, and possibility of pregnancy* [1, 4, 5].

On physical examination, the presence of fever or tachycardia in the setting of abdominal pain should heighten the suspicion of an acute process. The presence of jaundice, pallor, and peripheral edema can also be indicative of gastrointestinal illness which requires in-depth evaluation. In particular, focal areas of tenderness on the abdominal exam, with "peritoneal signs" of involuntary guarding and rebound tenderness, or the presence of palpable abdominal masses, should prompt further evaluation in the setting of abdominal pain.

Table 137.1 summarizes the "red flag" symptoms and signs which should be the subject of particular attention in patients with chronic abdominal pain.

"Red Flags" for Opiate Seeking

It is incumbent on the emergency care provider to evaluate and treat pain in the emergency department (ED), but the use of opioids is not mandatory. Indeed, narcotic bowel syndrome leads to chronic abdominal pain as well as constipation [6]. Although many studies have suggested that pain is

H. Kalsi · J. Smereck (✉)
Department of Emergency Medicine, MedStar Georgetown University Hospital, Washington, DC, USA

© Springer Nature Switzerland AG 2019
A. Graham, D. J. Carlberg (eds.), *Gastrointestinal Emergencies*, https://doi.org/10.1007/978-3-319-98343-1_137

Table 137.1 "Red flag" symptoms and signs in chronic abdominal pain

Symptom	Sign
Fever	Fever
Change in pattern of pain	Tachycardia
Dysphagia or odynophagia	Jaundice
Anorexia	Pallor
Unintentional weight loss	Focal abdominal tenderness, involuntary guarding
Dyspnea	
Increased abdominal girth	Palpable mass, organomegaly
Dark or maroon stool	Ascites
Persistent change in caliber of stool	Peripheral edema/anasarca
Postcoital bleeding	
Hematuria	
Testicular pain	
Possibility of pregnancy	

Table 137.2 "Red flags" for narcotic seeking or malingering in chronic abdominal pain

Vague descriptions of pain and medical history; extraneous issues discussed at length
Request for specific narcotic medications and doses, request for parenteral medication
Multiple drug allergies, often allergies to all analgesics except for requested medication
Exaggeration of pain severity (10 out of 10 or greater than 10 out of 10 pain)
Multiple ED visits and multiple controlled substance prescriptions from multiple providers

undertreated in the ED, opiate seeking for non-therapeutic purposes is estimated to occur in as many as 20% of all ED visits [7–10]. Patients with chronic pain may present to the ED due to worsening pain or acute flares of pain. It is difficult to assess chronic, persistent pain as there is often no objective evidence for active disease or unhealed injury, and autonomic changes such as tachycardia that accompany acute pain are typically absent in chronic pain [5].

When confronted with inconsistencies in the history or physical exam that raise the possibility malingering, all other possible diagnoses must generally be considered before classifying a patient as "drug seeking." Patients with drug-seeking behavior frequently claim to have had a prescription lost or stolen, request a specific narcotic by name and dosage, request parenteral narcotics, report intolerance or allergies to nonnarcotic analgesics, describe a textbook list of symptoms or be unable to describe actual symptoms, exaggerate the severity of symptoms (reporting "10 out of 10" pain or greater than "10 out of 10" pain), and have visits to multiple clinicians within a short period of time for pain issues [7, 9, 10].

Table 137.2 outlines the "red flag" indicators of narcotic seeking or malingering. That being stated, it nevertheless is incumbent on the emergency care provider to approach every patient with an unbiased approach, as malingering is a diagnosis of exclusion [11–13].

References

1. Zackowski S. Chronic recurrent abdominal pain. Emerg Med Clin North Am. 1998;16(4):877–94.
2. Tolba R, Shroll J, Kanu A, Rizk M. Ch 2. The epidemiology of chronic abdominal pain. In: Kapural L, editor. Chronic abdominal pain: an evidence-based, comprehensive guide to clinical management. New York: Springer; 2015. p. 13–24. https://doi.org/10.1007/978-1-4939-1992-5, 2.
3. Hauser W, Layer P, Henningsen P, Kruis W. Functional bowel disorders in adults. Dtsch Artebl Int. 2012;109(5):83–94.
4. Hansen G. Management of chronic pain in the acute care setting. Emerg Med Clin North Am. 2005;23:307–38.
5. Jones R, Charlton J, Latinovic R, Gulliford M. Alarm symptoms and identification of non-cancer diagnoses in primary care: cohort study. BMJ. 2009;339:b3094.
6. Grover C, Wielo E, Close RJ. Narcotic bowel syndrome. J Emerg Med. 2012;43(6):992–5.
7. Grover C, Elder J, Close R, Curry S. How frequently are "classic" drug-seeking behaviors used by drug-seeking patients in the emergency department? West J Emerg Med. 2012;13(5):416–21.
8. Moore TM, Jones T, Browder JH, et al. A comparison of common screening methods for predicting aberrant drug-related behavior among patients receiving opioids for chronic pain management. Pain Med. 2009;10:1426–33.
9. McNabb C, Foot C, Ting J, et al. Diagnosing drug-seeking behavior in an adult emergency department. Emerg Med Australas. 2006;18:138–42.
10. Todd K. Pain and prescription monitoring programs in the emergency department. Ann Emerg Med. 2010;56(1):24–6.
11. Rupp T, Delaney KA. Inadequate analgesia in emergency medicine. Ann Emerg Med. 2004;43:494–503.
12. Tamayo-Sarver JH, Dawson NV, Cydulka RK, et al. Variability in emergency physician decision making about prescribing opioid analgesics. Ann Emerg Med. 2004;43:483–93.
13. Wilson JE, Pendleton JM. Oligoanalgesia in the emergency department. Am J Emerg Med. 1989;7:620–3.

What Is the Role of Imaging and Reimaging in Patients with Chronic Abdominal Pain?

138

Theodore Katz and Janet Smereck

Pearls and Pitfalls
- Functional syndromes are a common cause of chronic abdominal pain.
- Red-flag symptoms can help indicate the need to consider serious underlying diagnoses.
- Existing evidence is limited, but there appears to be little value in repeating CT-scans after previous negative imaging in patients with chronically recurring abdominal pain.

Assessing the patient with chronic abdominal pain is a challenging task for the emergency medicine provider. A crucial decision in the care of these patients is whether to pursue diagnostic imaging. Computerized tomography (CT) is a frequently performed study and is the modality of choice for patients with undifferentiated abdominal pain. However, due to the chronicity of symptoms, many of these patients have undergone imaging previously, and the question arises as to when to reimage. No consensus guidelines exist as to when imaging or reimaging is indicated in chronic abdominal pain.

Narrowing down the scope of differential diagnoses is crucial and should drive all imaging decisions. If indicated, imaging should be used to assess for a particular diagnosis, rather than for screening. The American College of Radiology Appropriateness Criteria can provide guidance in deciding on an imaging modality when a particular diagnosis is deemed likely [1] (https://www.acr.org/Clinical-Resources/ACR-Appropriateness-Criteria).

Studies indicate that functional syndromes, especially irritable bowel syndrome (IBS), are a frequent cause of chronic abdominal pain and have a low likelihood of under-lying structural disease that would be identified with imaging [2–5]. A recent review article examining the evidence for imaging in patients with IBS found a low rate of structural disease in patients who fulfilled the Rome III symptom-based criteria for IBS and did not have symptoms concerning for other organic disease [6].

The presence of certain "red-flag symptoms" should raise concern for underlying organic disease. Although there exists no definitive list of red-flag symptoms, those commonly cited in the literature include abnormal vital signs, anemia, weight loss, bloody stools, age greater than 50 years, symptoms causing awakening from sleep, and antibiotic usage [7–11]. However, these symptoms do not consistently correlate with underlying disease. One study examined the association of various red-flag symptoms and organic disease, specifically gastrointestinal malignancies, IBD, and malabsorption. The authors used the red-flag symptoms of bloody stools, symptoms causing nocturnal awakening, weight loss, antibiotic usage, family history of colon cancer, and age over 50 years. None of these symptoms, when examined individually, were found to have a positive predictive value (PPV) greater than 10% for one of the selected organic diseases, likely due to the high baseline prevalence of red-flag symptoms in their patient population. For instance, the presence of bloody stools had only a 2.4% PPV for detecting GI cancer [11]. Even in the presence of particular red-flag symptoms, imaging may often not be indicated in the acute care setting; rather, referral to a specialist for endoscopy or colonoscopy may be more prudent in certain situations [8].

Another challenge facing providers is the decision to obtain reimaging in patients with chronic abdominal pain. One study examined the value of repeat abdominal CT-scans in patients with prior negative CT-scans. This retrospective study included patients presenting to the ED on two or more occasions with non-traumatic abdominal pain, undergoing CT-imaging of their abdomen on each visit. The positivity rate (findings on imaging that reasonably explained the patient's pain) for first-time CT-imaging was 22.5%, with

T. Katz (✉) · J. Smereck
Department of Emergency Medicine, MedStar Georgetown University Hospital, Washington, DC, USA

© Springer Nature Switzerland AG 2019
A. Graham, D. J. Carlberg (eds.), *Gastrointestinal Emergencies*, https://doi.org/10.1007/978-3-319-98343-1_138

positivity rates falling to 8.4% after one prior negative CT-scan and just 4.9% after two prior negative CT-scans. However, findings such as leukocytosis or an APACHE II score greater than 5 were associated with higher rates of positivity on repeat imaging [12]. More research is needed, but this study indicates repeat CT-imaging of the abdomen after prior negative CT-scans appear to have limited value in the vast majority of patients.

Summary

As with acute abdominal pain, the goal of care in chronic abdominal pain is to exclude "don't miss" diagnoses and then identify treatable etiologies when possible [13]. With selected patients, a careful examination, observation, and re-evaluation can exclude cases that require urgent intervention and, by inference, CT-imaging, thus sparing the patient unnecessary radiation and testing.

Suggested Resources
- American College of Radiology Appropriateness Criteria: https://www.acr.org/Clinical-Resources/ ACR-Appropriateness-Criteria.
- Nojkov B, Duffy MC, Cappell MS. Utility of repeated abdominal CT scans after prior negative CT scans in patients presenting to ER with non-traumatic abdominal pain. Dig Dis Sci. 2013;58:1074–83.

References

1. American College of Radiology Appropriateness Criteria. 2017. Available at: https://www.acr.org/Quality-Safety/ Appropriateness-Criteria.
2. Wallander MA, Johansson S, Ruigomez A, Garcia Rodriguez LA. Unspecified abdominal pain in primary care: the role of gastrointestinal morbidity. Int J Clin Pract. 2007;61:1663–70.
3. Drossman DA, Li Z, Andruzzi E, Temple RD, Talley NJ, Thompson WG, et al. U.S. householder survey of functional gastrointestinal disorders. Prevalence, sociodemography, and health impact. Dig Dis Sci. 1993;38:1569–80.
4. Jones R, Lydeard S. Irritable bowel syndrome in the general population. BMJ. 1992;304:87–90.
5. Tolba R, Shroll J, Kanu A, Rizk MK. The epidemiology of chronic abdominal pain. In: Kapural L, editor. Chronic abdominal pain. New York: Springer; 2015. p. 13–24.
6. O'Conor O, McSweeney S, McWilliams S, O'Neill S, Shanahan F, Quigley EM, et al. Role of radiological imaging in irritable bowel syndrome: evidence-based review. Radiology. 2012;262:485–94.
7. Mendelson R. Imaging for chronic abdominal pain in adults. Aust Prescr. 2015;38:49–52.
8. Brandt L, Chey W, Foxx-Orenstein A, Schiller LR, Schoenfeld PS, Spiegel BM, et al. An evidence-based position statement on the management of irritable bowel syndrome. AJG. 2009;104:S1–S35.
9. Tack J, Talley N, Camilleri M, Holtmann G, Malagelada JR, Stanghellini Y. Functional gastroduodenal disorders. Gastroenterol. 2006;130:1466–79.
10. Jones R, Charlton J, Latinovic R, Gulliford M. Alarm symptoms and identification of non-cancer diagnoses in primary care: cohort study. BMJ. 2009;339:b3094.
11. Whitehead WE, Palsson OS, Feld AD, Levy RL, Von Korff M, Turner MJ, et al. Utility of red flag symptom exclusions in the diagnosis of irritable bowel syndrome. AP&T. 2006;24:137–46.
12. Nojkov B, Duffy MC, Cappell MS. Utility of repeated abdominal CT scans after prior negative CT scans in patients presenting to ER with nontraumatic abdominal pain. Dig Dis Sci. 2013;58:1074–83.
13. Schifeling C, Williams D. Appropriate use of imaging for acute abdominal pain. JAMA Int Med. 2017;177(12):1853.

Is There Any Benefit to Obtaining a Pelvic Ultrasound After a Negative CT of the Abdomen/Pelvis in a Woman with Chronic Abdominal Pain?

139

Janet Smereck and Kerri Layman

Pearls and Pitfalls
- "Red flags" in the history indicative of serious disease processes include age greater than 50 years, fever, unexplained weight loss, hematuria, postcoital bleeding, postmenopausal bleeding, and deep dyspareunia.
- Pelvic ultrasonography has the potential to yield important diagnoses in the woman with chronic pelvic pain, detecting conditions which may be missed by CT.
- Ovarian torsion is generally regarded as an acutely painful condition, but a more chronic course is possible. Due to a dual blood supply, color Doppler flow may still be present on ultrasound of a torsed ovary.

The female patient with chronic pelvic pain presents unique diagnostic challenges for the emergency care provider. Chronic pelvic pain is defined in the literature as noncyclic pain related to the pelvic organs lasting more than 6 months [1–4]. Symptom intensity may range from mild to severe and may be gynecologic, gastrointestinal, urologic, or neuropathic in origin [5, 6]. In the absence of a specifically identified etiology, chronic pelvic pain is often regarded as a functional disorder, which is a diagnosis of exclusion in the emergency care setting.

The incidence of chronic pelvic pain in women (excluding dysmenorrhea) is reported in 4–24% of adult women [7,

8]. It is incumbent on the emergency care provider to establish or exclude a serious cause, so as to initiate the appropriate therapeutic pathway.

"Red flags" in the history suggestive of potentially serious disease processes include age greater than 50 years, presence of fever, unexplained weight loss, hematuria, postcoital bleeding, postmenopausal bleeding, and deep dyspareunia [1, 9]. Historical features of significance include pain quality. For example, cramping pain may be indicative of irritable bowel syndrome or partial bowel obstruction. Chronic dysuria or hematuria may indicate infection, neoplasm, or interstitial cystitis. Pain that fluctuates in intensity with the menstrual cycle may indicate endometriosis or adenomyosis, the latter tending to present later in reproductive life (mid-40s or older) [10]. Prior abdominal surgery or infection may produce painful pelvic adhesions. Pain described as burning or electric may be due to pelvic floor or abdominal wall nerve entrapment, which may be identified by reproduction of symptoms with abdominal wall muscle contraction, the Carnett's sign [2, 4, 11]. Of significance, positive correlation with post-traumatic stress disorders and childhood sexual abuse is frequently found in women presenting with chronic pelvic pain [12]. Table 139.1 summarizes conditions associated with chronic pelvic pain.

Value of Ultrasonography in Evaluation of Chronic Abdominal/Pelvic Pain

Recommendations for diagnostic imaging in female patients with chronic pelvic pain are derived from literature crossing multiple specialties, including gastroenterology, urology, obstetrics/gynecology, general surgery, emergency medicine, rehabilitation, and radiology. Plain films are of limited utility but may show ureteral or adnexal calcifications or air fluid levels, indicative of bowel dilatation or obstruction. Computerized tomography (CT) is a frequently performed study and is the modality of choice for patients with undifferentiated abdominal pain. If CT of the abdomen/pelvis is

J. Smereck (✉)
Department of Emergency Medicine, MedStar Georgetown University Hospital, Washington, DC, USA

K. Layman
Department of Emergency Medicine, MedStar Washington Hospital Center & MedStar Georgetown University Hospital, Washington, DC, USA
e-mail: Kerri.L.Layman@medstar.net

© Springer Nature Switzerland AG 2019
A. Graham, D. J. Carlberg (eds.), *Gastrointestinal Emergencies*, https://doi.org/10.1007/978-3-319-98343-1_139

Table 139.1 Conditions associated with female chronic pelvic pain

Gynecologic
Endometriosis
Adenomyosis
Uterine leiomyoma
Ovarian cyst/polycystic ovary syndrome
Pelvic congestion syndrome
Chronic ovarian torsion
Chronic salpingitis/tubo-ovarian abscess
Urologic
Ureteral stone
Urinary tract infection
Interstitial cystitis
Gastrointestinal
Irritable bowel syndrome
Diverticulitis
Chronic appendicitis
Sigmoid or cecal colonic neoplasm
Abdominal/pelvic wall
Inguinal hernia
Pelvic adhesion
Pelvic floor laxity
Nerve entrapment

negative or nondiagnostic, ultrasonography may reveal significant pelvic pathology. Ultrasound (US) is considered the initial imaging modality of choice in the woman with pelvic pain, both acute and chronic [13].

US is the preferred investigative tool for suspected adnexal or uterine disease [14]. A number of conditions associated with chronic pelvic pain, including adenomyosis, leiomyomas, and small pelvic masses (< 4 cm in diameter) including endometriosis and ovarian neoplasms, are readily detectable by transvaginal ultrasonography but often missed on CT [15, 16]. Pelvic congestion syndrome (PCS), the presence of varices in the pelvic veins, is a recognized and treatable cause of chronic pelvic pain, best diagnosed with duplex US [17, 18]. The presence of ovarian vein >5–6 mm is diagnostic, and US may show reversed venous flow on color Doppler after Valsalva [19].

Importantly, duplex ultrasonography is necessary to detect ovarian torsion, which may present with intermittent or chronic pain symptoms. Ovarian torsion is generally regarded as an acutely painful condition, but a more chronic course has been reported; it may occur in a normal ovary but often occurs in the presence of ovarian enlargement due to large cystic lesions (particularly dermoid), neoplasm, or endometrial implant. Torsion of an ovary around its vascular pedicle is a gynecologic emergency; due to a dual blood supply, color Doppler flow may still be present in ovarian torsion, complicating diagnosis [20, 21]. A positive "whirlpool sign" is considered the most definitive finding for ovarian torsion [22]. For clinicians skilled in point-of-care ultrasound (POCUS), bed-side US (both transabdominal and transvaginal) allows faster diagnosis, improving time to consultation, treatment, or discharge [23].

Summary

In summary, pelvic ultrasonography has the potential to yield important diagnoses in the woman with chronic pelvic pain, detecting conditions which may be missed by CT. Emergency care providers should consider US to be the imaging study of choice when evaluating the female patient with chronic pelvic pain.

Case Example: Chronic Pelvic Pain

A 60-year-old woman presented to the emergency department (ED) with right lower abdominal pain and bloating, which she stated had been present for intermittently for several years and had become more severe in the preceding few days. The pain was described as dull and aching, with occasional nausea, but no change in bowel habits, dysuria, or vaginal bleeding. She was postmenopausal for at least 10 years and had two pregnancies delivered vaginally over 30 years in the past. She had undergone appendectomy at age 9. On examination, the patient was afebrile and appeared mildly uncomfortable. Her abdomen was obese and soft with moderate tenderness in the suprapubic region and bilateral lower quadrants, without peritoneal signs. Bimanual pelvic examination revealed mild diffuse tenderness without abnormal vaginal bleeding or discharge. There was no palpable mass, but body habitus restricted a complete assessment of adnexal and uterine size. CT of the abdomen and pelvis revealed scattered colonic diverticuli without evidence for acute inflammation. The uterus and adnexa were described as "normal" on CT imaging. Transvaginal ultrasound was then performed which revealed a 3.5 cm right fundal fibroid with signs of cystic degeneration. Endometrial thickness was 4 mm. There was no adnexal enlargement and color flow to the ovaries was normal. The patient expressed satisfaction for having her symptoms addressed with objective testing; she was referred to outpatient gynecology for further management of uterine leiomyoma.

References

1. Vercellini P, Somigliana E, Vigano P, Abbiati A, Barbara G, Fedele L. Chronic pelvic pain in women: etiology, pathogenesis and diagnostic approach. Gynecol Endocrinol. 2009;25(3):149–58.

2. Speer L, Mushkbar S, Erbele T. Chronic pelvic pain in women. Am Fam Physician. 2016;93(5):380–7.

3. Engeler DS, Baranowski AP, Dinis-Oliveira P, Elneil S, Hughes J, Messelink EJ, et al. The 2013 EAU guidelines on chronic pelvic pain: is management of chronic pelvic pain a habit, a philosophy, or a science? 10 years of development. Eur Urol. 2013;64(3):431–9.

4. Stein SL. Chronic pelvic pain. Gastroenterol Clin N Am. 2013;42(4):785–800.

5. Reiter RC. Occult somatic pathology in women with chronic pelvic pain. Clin Obstet Gynecol. 1990;33(1):154–60.

6. Zackowski S. Chronic recurrent abdominal pain. Emerg Med Clin North Am. 1998;16(4):877–94.

7. Latthe P, Latthe MC, Say L, Gulmezoglu M, Khan KS. WHO systemic review of prevalence of chronic pelvic pain: a neglected reproductive health morbidity. BMC Public Health. 2006;6:177.

8. Ahangari A. Prevalence of chronic pelvic pain among women: and updated review. Pain Physician. 2014;17(2):E141–7.

9. Ferrero S, Ragni N, Remorgida V. Deep dyspareunia: causes, treatments, and results. Curr Opin Obstet Gynecol. 2008;20(4):394–9.

10. Parazzini F, Mais V, Cipriani S, Busacca M, Venturini P. GISE. Determinants of adenomyosis in women who underwent hysterectomy for benign gynecological conditions: results from a prospective multicentric study in Italy. Eur J Obstet Gynecol Reprod Biol. 2009;143(2):103–6.

11. Mui J, Allaire C, Williams C, Yong PJ. Abdominal wall pain in women with chronic pelvic pain. J Obstet Gynaecol Can. 2016;38(2):154–9.

12. Farley M, Patsalides B. Physical symptoms, posttraumatic stress disorder, and healthcare utilization of women with and without childhood physical and sexual abuse. Psychol Rep. 2002;89:595–606.

13. Amirbekian S, Hooley R. Ultrasound evaluation of pelvic pain. Radiol Clin North Am. 2014;52(6):1215–35.

14. Juhan V. Chronic pelvic pain: an imaging approach. Diagn Interv Imaging. 2015;96(10):997–1007.

15. Khatri G, Khan A, Raval G, Chhabra A. Diagnostic evaluation of chronic pelvic pain. Phys Med Rehabil Clin N Am. 2017;28(3):477–500.

16. Benjamin-Pratt AR, Howard FM. Management of chronic pelvic pain. Minerva Ginecol. 2010;62(5):447–65.

17. Liddle AD, Davies AH. Pelvic congestion syndrome: chronic pelvic pain caused by ovarian and internal iliac varices. Phlebology. 2007;22(3):100–4.

18. Rane N, Leyon JJ, Littlehales T, Ganeshan A, Crowe P, Uberoi R. Pelvic congestion syndrome. Curr Probl Diagn Radiol. 2013;42(4):135–40.

19. Ganeshan A, Upponi S, Hon L, Uthappa MC, Warakaulle DR, Uberoi R. Chronic pelvic pain due to pelvic congestion syndrome: the role of diagnostic and interventional radiology. Cardiovasc Intervent Radiol. 2007;30(6):1105–11.

20. Ssi-Yan G, Rivain AL, Trichot C, Morcelet MC, Prevot S, Deffieux X, et al. What every radiologist should know about adnexal torsion. Emerg Radiol. 2018;25(1):51–9.

21. Lourenco A, Swenson D, Tubbs R, Lazarus E. Ovarian and tubal torsion: imaging findings on US, CT and MRI. Emerg Radiol. 2014;21(2):179–87.

22. Vijayaraghavan SB. Sonographic whirlpool sign in ovarian torsion. J Ultrasound Med. 2004;23(12):1643–9.

23. Sohoni A, Bosley J, Miss JC. Bedside ultrasonography for obstetric and gynecologic emergencies. Crit Care Clin. 2014;30(2):207–26.

Is Laboratory Data Helpful in the Workup of Chronic Abdominal Pain?

140

Janet Smereck

Pitfalls and Pearls
- Female patients of childbearing age presenting with abdominal or pelvic pain (unless prior hysterectomy) benefit from a pregnancy test. Testing should not be omitted in patients who report tubal ligation and contraceptive use or deny engaging in sexual activity.
- The complete blood count (CBC) demonstrates leukocytosis in only about half of patients who present with serious abdominal pathology.
- Sterile pyuria may be present in over 70% of patients with serious intra-abdominal infections.
- An elevated serum lactate level has high sensitivity for mesenteric ischemia.
- Abnormalities of liver function tests may not signify a gastrointestinal disease process, such as hyperbilirubinemia in Gilbert syndrome and hemolytic anemias and hyperlipasemia in Gullo syndrome and renal failure.

The primary goal in the acute care setting when evaluating chronic abdominal pain is to establish or exclude serious causes, so as to initiate the appropriate therapeutic pathway. As chronicity does not necessarily rule out severity of disease, laboratory testing is frequently used to detect acute or previously overlooked disease processes. While the literature is robust with guidelines for evidenced-based diagnostic tools in patients with acute abdominal complaints, there is sparse data to guide the emergency care provider for patients with chronic abdominal pain [1]. Laboratory studies are of limited utility in the evaluation of most cases of chronic abdominal pain, but specific testing is recommended in a number of clinical circumstances.

J. Smereck
Department of Emergency Medicine, MedStar Georgetown University Hospital, Washington, DC, USA

Human Chorionic Gonadotropin (hCG)

A pregnancy test should be considered for all female patients of childbearing age presenting with abdominal pain, whether acute or chronic, unless prior hysterectomy [2]. Patient self-reports of routine birth control use, normal menstrual history, absence of sexual activity, or negative home pregnancy tests do not preclude the necessity of hCG testing. Studies examining pregnancy rates in patients with abdominal pain reporting "no chance" of pregnancy report positive pregnancies in 2–11% of cases [3, 4]. Point-of-care (POC) urine pregnancy testing expedites management with accuracy rates equivalent to the clinical laboratory [5, 6]. False-positive serum hCG results are rarely reported and may signal the presence of heterophilic antibodies, which can be excluded by performing urine testing. Gestational trophoblastic disease may also produce false-positive hCG results [7].

Complete Blood Count

As an index of inflammation or infection, the white blood cell (WBC) count lacks sensitivity in patients with chronic abdominal pain. Leukocytosis is found in about half of all patients with serious abdominal pathology [8, 9]. A low hemoglobin and hematocrit may indicate chronic anemia or blood loss, while a high hemoglobin may indicate dehydration with hemoconcentration.

Urinalysis

Urinalysis is considered a useful diagnostic test in the evaluation of abdominal pain, with or without urinary symptoms [10]. Pyuria may indicate urinary tract infection but may also be present in conditions that cause peritoneal irritation, such as diverticulitis, inflammatory bowel disease, and abscesses. Sterile pyuria has been reported in over 70% of patients with serious intra-abdominal conditions including appendicitis

© Springer Nature Switzerland AG 2019
A. Graham, D. J. Carlberg (eds.), *Gastrointestinal Emergencies*, https://doi.org/10.1007/978-3-319-98343-1_140

and diverticulitis [11]. Of note, the absence of pyuria does not exclude renal abscess or pyelonephritis [12].

Hematuria is suggestive of renal or ureteral calculi but also found in a number of chronic conditions including malignancies, renal cysts, and vascular anomalies. Nutcracker syndrome, a rare anomaly of renal vascular compression between the abdominal aorta and superior mesenteric artery, is characterized by chronic abdominal pain and hematuria [13]. Interstitial cystitis (IC), a chronic sterile inflammatory disease of the bladder of unknown etiology, is characterized by chronic bladder pain and urinary urgency [14]. Hematuria is found in up to 30% of patients with IC [15].

Comprehensive Metabolic Panel (CMP)

A CMP (basic metabolic panel plus liver function testing) is a frequently ordered to screen for systemic disease, such as diabetes, renal insufficiency, or electrolyte abnormalities. In general, routine sampling of liver function studies in patients with chronic diffuse abdominal pain without signs or symptoms of liver or gallbladder involvement is of low utility. For patients with right upper quadrant pain, an elevated bilirubin level has high specificity for biliary tract inflammation or obstruction [16].

Lipase

Acute pancreatitis is characterized by lipase elevation three or more times the upper limit of normal. However, chronic pancreatitis is not reliably diagnosed by laboratory tests readily available in the emergency department [17]. With chronic pancreatitis, lipase may not be elevated, and other markers for exocrine insufficiency require lengthy processes, such as stool collection over a period of days for fecal fat measurements [18]. Furthermore, lipase elevations may be present in disease processes unrelated to pancreatitis. Renal insufficiency, critical illness such as the shock state, and idiopathic hyperlipasemia (Gullo syndrome) may cause significant elevations of serum lipase [17].

Inflammatory Markers

Lactate levels are often considered a surrogate for disease severity. Lactate level elevation has high sensitivity for mesenteric ischemia, as well as peritonitis and acute pancreatitis [18]. Inflammatory markers such as C-reactive protein (CRP) may be elevated in a number of conditions causing chronic abdominal pain, including inflammatory bowel diseases, perforated diverticulitis, appendicitis, and gynecologic disorders, including salpingitis and tubo-ovarian abscess. However, CRP has low discriminatory value in differentiating urgent from non-urgent conditions in patients with abdominal pain [19].

Metabolic Disorders

Rare metabolic disorders causing chronic or recurrent abdominal pain are seldom diagnosed in the ED setting. Chronically recurring abdominal pain is the most common presenting symptom of the intermittent porphyrias, which are genetically mediated disorders in heme biosynthesis [20, 21]. Diagnosis involves genetic analysis and urine tests for porphobilinogen; dark or red urine may be observed at the bedside [20, 22]. Lead poisoning may also present with recurring or chronic abdominal pain, nausea, and weakness; microcytic anemia is characteristic and diagnosis is made by serum assay [23].

Summary

The selective use of laboratory testing may alert the emergency care provider to the possibility of an acute exacerbation of a chronic abdominal complaint, detect a previously overlooked etiology for a chronic abdominal syndrome, or reveal a new disease process unrelated to the chronic condition. The emergency clinician must strive both to consider urgent diagnoses and avoid low-yield or repetitive testing when ordering laboratory studies in the evaluation of chronic abdominal pain.

References

1. Gans S, Pols M, Stoker J, Boermeester M. Guideline for the diagnostic pathway in patients with acute abdominal pain. Dig Surg. 2015;32(1):23–31.
2. Olshaker J. Emergency department pregnancy testing. J Emerg Med. 1996;14(1):59–65.
3. Ramoska E, Sacchetti A, Nepp M. Reliability of patient history in determining the possibility of pregnancy. Ann Emerg Med. 1989;18(1):48–50.
4. Strote J, Chen G. Patient self assessment of pregnancy status in the emergency department. Emerg Med J. 2006;23(7):554–7.
5. Lazarenko G, Dobson C, Enokson R, Brant R. Accuracy and speed of urine pregnancy tests done in the emergency department: a prospective study. CJEM. 2001;3(4):292–5.
6. Gottlieb M, Wnek K, Moskoff J, Christian E, Bailitz J. Comparison of result times between urine and whole blood point-of-care pregnancy testing. West J Emerg Med. 2016;17(4):449–53.
7. Committee on Gynecologic Practice. Avoiding inappropriate clinical decisions based on false-positive human chorionic gonatropin test. ACOG Committee Opinion No. 278, November 2002, reaffirmed 2017. Accessed online 11/2/2017.
8. Young G. CBC or not CBC? That is the question. Ann Emerg Med. 1986;15(3):367–71.

9. Gans S, Atema J, Stoker J, Toorenvliet BR, Laurell H, Boermeester MA. C-reactive protein and white blood cell count as triage test between urgent and nonurgent conditions in 2961 patients with acute abdominal pain. Open Access Med. 2015;94(9):1–9.

10. Nagurney J, Brown D, Chang Y, Sane S, Wang AC, Weiner JB. Use of diagnostic testing in the emergency department for patients presenting with non-traumatic abdominal pain. J Emerg Med. 2003;25(4):363–71.

11. Goonewardene S, Persad R. Sterile pyuria: a forgotten entity. Ther Adv Urol. 2015;7(5):295–8.

12. Conley S, Frumkin K. Acute lobar nephronia: a case report and literature review. J Emerg Med. 2014;46(5):624–6.

13. Policha A, Lamparello P, Sadek M, Berland T, Maldonado T. Endovascular treatment of nutcracker syndrome. Ann Vasc Surg. 2016;36:e1–295e7.

14. Kelada E, Jones A. Interstitial cystitis. Arch Gynecol Obstet. 2007;275(4):223–9.

15. Gomes C, Sanchez-Ortiz R, Harris C, Wein AJ, Rovner ES. Significance of hematuria in patients with interstitial cystitis: review of radiographic and endoscopic findings. Urology. 2001;57(2):262–5.

16. Fargo M, Grogan S, Saguil A. Evaluation of jaundice in adults. Am Fam Physician. 2017;95(3):164–8.

17. Hameed A, Lam V, Pleass H. Significant elevations of serum lipase not caused by pancreatitis: a systemic review. HPB (Oxford). 2015;17(2):99–112.

18. Duggan S, Chonchubhair H, Lawal O, O'Connor DB, Conlon KC. Chronic pancreatitis: a diagnostic dilemma. World J Gastroenterol. 2016;22(7):2304–13.

19. Andersen L, Mackenhauer J, Roberts J, Berg KM, Cocchi MN, Donnino MW. Etiology and therapeutic approach to elevated lactate. Mayo Clin Proc. 2014;88(10):1127–40.

20. Herrick A, McColl K. Acute intermittent porphyria. Best Pract Res Clin Gastroenterol. 2005;19(2):235–49.

21. Karim Z, Lyoumi S, Nicholas G, Deybach JC, Gouya L, Puy H. Porphyrias: a 2015 update. Clin Res Hepatol Gastroenterol. 2015;39(4):412–25.

22. Liu Y, Lien W, Fang C, Lai TI, Chen WJ, Wang HP. ED presentation of acute porphyria. Am J Emerg Med. 2005;23:164–7.

23. Tsai M, Huang S, Cheng S. Lead poisoning can be easily misdiagnosed as acute porphyria and nonspecific abdominal pain. Case Rep Emerg Med. 2017; ID 9050713, 4 pages. Accessed online 01/19/2018.

Non-opioid Management of Chronic Abdominal Pain

141

Zachary Repanshek

Pearls and Pitfalls
- Chronic abdominal pain is a difficult clinical scenario for patients and physicians.
- Opioid pain medications should not routinely be used for chronic abdominal pain and may in fact worsen the condition.
- Narcotic bowel syndrome is a condition of unexplained abdominal pain requiring escalating doses of opioid medication.
- Treatment of abdominal pain should be directed toward underlying cause when possible.

Abdominal pain is the second most common medical complaint in patients presenting to US emergency departments (EDs) [1]. While the majority of these presentations are acute, emergency care providers are also called upon to manage patients who present with chronic abdominal pain.

Chronic abdominal pain is typically defined as intermittent or persistent abdominal pain which lasts longer than 6 months in duration [2]. The exact prevalence of chronic abdominal pain is unknown, and the list of potential etiologies is immense [3]. Patients experiencing chronic abdominal pain may have significant morbidity and decrease in quality of life. They frequently undergo extensive diagnostic testing and spend large amounts of time in healthcare facilities. This can also provide a challenge to physicians, as in many cases no organic pathology is ever found and treatment is ineffective.

As with other types of chronic pain, patients with chronic abdominal pain who fail other analgesic modalities are often prescribed narcotic pain medications. The Centers for Disease Control and Prevention (CDC) has issued guidelines for prescribing opioids for chronic pain. These guidelines state: "Non-pharmacologic therapy and non-opioid pharmacologic therapy are preferred for chronic pain. Clinicians should consider opioid therapy only if expected benefits for both pain and function are anticipated to outweigh risks to the patient" [4]. There is little evidence to support opioid use for chronic abdominal pain [3, 5]. There are well-established risks of harm, however, not limited to addiction and diminished gastrointestinal motility. Given this, there is little reason to anticipate benefits would outweigh risks, as outlined in the CDC guidelines. Opioid pain medications should not routinely be used for chronic abdominal pain and may in fact worsen the condition.

Narcotic bowel syndrome (NBS) is a condition of unexplained abdominal pain requiring escalating doses of opioid medication. Patients with NBS may frequently present to EDs looking for treatment of their pain, making this an important condition for emergency physicians to be aware. NBS can be diagnosed in a patient with chronic or frequently recurring abdominal pain who (1) is taking high doses of narcotic pain medication; (2) notes marked worsening of pain when narcotic dose is decreased and improvement when high doses are reinstituted; (3) has progression of the frequency, duration, and severity of pain; and (4) has no other explanation for the pain [6].

The pathology of NBS is cyclical, as illustrated in Fig. 141.1. A patient with unexplained abdominal pain is started on opioid pain medications, which cause a decrease in gastrointestinal motility, leading to nausea, bloating, constipation, and, subsequently, worsening abdominal pain. Increasing doses of pain medications are required to treat this worsening pain. As dosages are increased, opioid receptors may become less responsive, leading to hyperalgesia and dependence [7].

Z. Repanshek
Lewis Katz School of Medicine, Temple University Hospital, Philadelphia, PA, USA
e-mail: Zachary.repanshek2@tuhs.temple.edu

© Springer Nature Switzerland AG 2019
A. Graham, D. J. Carlberg (eds.), *Gastrointestinal Emergencies*, https://doi.org/10.1007/978-3-319-98343-1_141

NARCOTIC BOWEL SYNDROME

Chronic Abdominal Pain

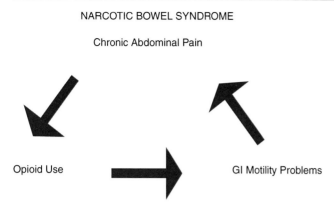

Fig. 141.1 Narcotic bowel syndrome

The ultimate treatment of NBS involves cessation of opioid medications. However, this must be done on a long-term basis with both non-pharmacological and psychosocial support and typically requires opioid detoxification. This will be outside of the practice for most emergency physicians. For NBS patients presenting to the ED, the most critical point is to avoid using opioid medications and thus exacerbating the condition. Physicians should treat related symptoms, such as using promotility antiemetics for nausea and laxatives and stool softeners for constipation. Referrals to gastroenterology and substance detoxification centers are both appropriate steps. Emergency physicians should recognize signs of opioid withdrawal and manage these symptoms with clonidine, antidiarrheal medications, and benzodiazepines as necessary. Discussing with the patient their condition and the risk of worsening with opioid use is an important intervention, as patients are often given little explanation for their symptoms [6, 7].

As with acute abdominal pain, when a suspected cause for chronic abdominal pain can be determined, treatment should be directed toward that etiology. Centrally mediated gastrointestinal pain, formally known as "functional abdominal pain," is nearly continuous abdominal pain that limits daily functioning, without other structural disorder or associated gastrointestinal dysfunction [8]. Psychiatric comorbidity is frequently present,

and pharmacologic treatment may include tricyclic antidepressants (TCAs), selective serotonin reuptake inhibitors (SSRIs), and serotonin-norepinephrine reuptake inhibitors (SNRIs), although these agents are not generally prescribed in the ED. Patients should be referred for psychological evaluation as well, especially if coexisting mental illness is suspected [5, 8, 9].

Abdominal wall pain is estimated to be the cause in 2–3% of patients with chronic abdominal pain [10]. Pain is typically very well localized and well circumscribed at the lateral border of the rectus abdominis muscle. Pain with palpation at this area is usually worsened with tensing of the abdominal wall muscles, a maneuver known as the Carnett's test. Acute treatment involves a local trigger point injection of anesthetic, sometimes combined with a corticosteroid [5, 10]. While this is currently done primarily by gastroenterologists, it is a technique that could feasibly be performed safely by emergency physicians on patients presenting with worsening of chronic abdominal wall pain. Improvement with a trigger point injection is considered to be diagnostic for abdominal wall pain [5, 10].

Inflammatory bowel disease, irritable bowel syndrome (IBS), and functional dyspepsia may also be sources of chronic pain. Inflammatory bowel disease, such as Crohn's disease and ulcerative colitis, may be initially diagnosed by an emergency physician, typically by computed tomography. In this scenario, patients should be referred to gastroenterology for definitive treatment, but initiation of corticosteroids may provide symptom relief [11]. IBS is associated with other gastrointestinal dysfunction, such as constipation or diarrhea. First-line treatment of abdominal pain and bloating in these patients is typically antispasmodic agents, such as dicyclomine. Dietary modification, probiotics, and treatment of the disorder of defecation should also be considered [12]. Functional dyspepsia, presenting with dyspeptic symptoms without findings of esophagitis, ulcer disease, or malignancy on esophagogastroduodenoscopy (EGD), can be treated with dietary changes, histamine-2 receptor antagonists (H-2 blockers), and proton pump inhibitors (PPIs) [13]. Table 141.1 summarizes the chronic abdominal pain syndromes and recommended non-opiate therapies.

Table 141.1 Common causes of chronic abdominal pain and recommended pharmacologic treatments

Cause of pain	Treatment	Pearls
Acute exacerbation of chronic abdominal pain	**Nondissociative, low-dose ketamine** < 1 mg/kg IV infusion	The data supporting low-dose ketamine (LDK) for abdominal pain in the acute setting does exist. The use of ketamine to treat chronic pain is certainly on the rise, but is still somewhat controversial. In one analysis of 11 studies of patients with both acute and chronic pain, LDK was found to be comparable but not superior to opioids. It proposed that ketamine infusion may be applicable to opioid-tolerant patients with "acute intractable exacerbations of acute pain" due to a potential "re-sensitizing" mechanism to their opioid regimen [15]
Centrally mediated gastrointestinal pain: Nearly continuous, limits daily function. No associated structural abnormality or gastrointestinal dysfunction	**TCAs** Nortriptyline 10–25 mg PO daily **SSRIs, SNRIs** Duloxetine 30 mg PO daily **Psychological referral**	TCAs are the most studied antidepressant class. A meta-analysis (2014) found a benefit in patients with painful functional gastrointestinal disorders [16]. Anticholinergic and antihistamine side effects more pronounced in amitriptyline compared to nortriptyline. Consider another treatment option if pregnant, liver disease, treated for psychiatric illness, or allergy to medication. SSRIs do not have a role in the treatment of abdominal pain unless a psychiatric component such as depression or anxiety also exists. SNRIs have no proven benefit on acute pain, but studies suggest improvement in chronic pain with fewer side effects compared to TCAs [16]

Table 141.1 (continued)

Cause of pain	Treatment	Pearls
Abdominal wall pain Well-localized pain Positive Carnett's test	**Trigger point injection** **Lidocaine topical/patch**	Prescription lidocaine patches (lidocaine 5% patch) is indicated for postherpetic neuralgia, neuropathic pain (not sciatica) and osteoarthritis that has failed at least three prescription medications. Without insurance, lidocaine patches cost approximately $500 for 30 topical film patches. Often, insurance companies require preauthorization. Over-the-counter lidocaine patches (lidocaine 4% patch) are available
Inflammatory bowel disease Gastrointestinal dysfunction Bloody diarrhea Colonoscopy findings	**Corticosteroids** **GI referral for anti-inflammatory or immune modulator therapy**	
Irritable bowel syndrome Altered bowel habits Bloating, cramping	**Antispasmodics** Dicyclomine 10–20 mg q8 h **Dietary modification**	Dicyclomine (Bentyl) is an antispasmodic and anticholinergic agent that decreases GI hypermotility associated with IBS and ulcerative colitis. Studies prescribing between 10 mg and 40 mg 3–4 times a day reported statistically significant improvement in global assessment for IBS compared to placebo, but patients experienced high rates (up to 70%) of anticholinergic side effects. Safety data is not available for doses > 80 mg per day. Other antispasmodic agents such as mebeverine (not available in the USA) have similar efficacy but fewer side effects. Other agents such as lubiprostone and linaclotide have shown promise in clinical trials. Lubiprostone (Amitiza) is FDA approved for IBS with constipation in adult women as well as opioid-induced constipation, 8 mcg orally 2 times a day. [14]
Functional dyspepsia Dyspeptic symptoms Normal EGD	**H-2 blockers** **PPIs** **Dietary modification**	While long-term use has been associated with unintended consequences such as susceptibility to enteric infections, coronary artery disease, hypomagnesemia, kidney disease, a Cochrane review demonstrated a relative risk reduction in symptoms of 14% compared to placebo in patients with functional dyspepsia [17]

Suggested Resources

- CDC guideline for prescribing opioids for chronic pain (fact sheet). https://www.cdc.gov/drugoverdose/pdf/Guidelines_Factsheet-a.pdf.
- Narcotic bowel syndrome emergency medicine literature of note. http://www.emlitofnote.com/?p=1348.
- Narcotic bowel syndrome: an important diagnosis you may not have heard of http://www.thepoisonreview.com/2011/07/07/narcotic-bowel-syndrome-an-important-diagnosis-you-may-not-have-heard-of-i-hadnt/.

References

1. Bhuiya FA, Pitts SR, McCaig LF. Emergency department visits for chest pain and abdominal pain: United States, 1999–2008. NCHS Data Brief. 2010;43:1–8.
2. Tolba R, Shroll J. The epidemiology of chronic abdominal pain. In: Kapural L, editor. Chronic abdominal pain: an evidence-based, comprehensive guide to clinical management. New York: Springer; 2015.
3. Wang D. Opioid medications in the management of chronic abdominal pain. Curr Pain Headache Rep. 2017;21(9):40.
4. Centers for Disease Control and Prevention Public Health Service U S Department of Health and Human Services. Guideline for prescribing opioids for chronic pain. J Pain Palliat Care Pharmacother. 2016;30(2):138–40.
5. Camilleri M. Management of patients with chronic abdominal pain in clinical practice. Neurogastroenterol Motil. 2006;18(7):499–506.
6. Grover CA, Wiele ED, Close RJ. Narcotic bowel syndrome. J Emerg Med. 2012;43(6):992–5.
7. Farmer AD, Gallagher J, Bruckner-Holt C, Aziz Q. Narcotic bowel syndrome. Lancet Gastroenterol Hepatol. 2017;2(5):361–8.
8. Keefer L, Drossman DA, Guthrie E, Simrén M, Tillisch K, Olden K, Whorwell PJ. Centrally mediated disorders of gastrointestinal pain. Gastroenterology. 2016;150(60):1408–19.
9. Drossman DA. Severe and refractory chronic abdominal pain: treatment strategies. Clin Gastroenterol Hepatol. 2008;6(9):978–82.
10. Koop H, Koprdova S, Schürmann C. Chronic abdominal wall pain. Dtsch Arztebl Int. 2016;113(4):51–7.
11. Mowat C, Cole A, Windsor A, Ahmad T, Arnott I, Driscoll R, Mitton S, Orchard T, Rutter M, Younge L, Lees C, Ho GT, Satsangi J, Bloom S, IBD Section of the British Society of Gastroenterology. Guidelines for the management of inflammatory bowel disease in adults. Gut. 2011;60(5):571–607.
12. American College of Gastroenterology Task Force on Irritable Bowel Syndrome, Brandt LJ, Chey WD, Foxx-Orenstein AE, Schiller LR, Schoenfeld PS, Spiegel BM, Talley NJ, Quigley EM. An evidence-based position statement on the management of irritable bowel syndrome. Am J Gastroenterol. 2009;104(Suppl 1):S1–35.
13. Talley NJ. Functional dyspepsia: new insights into pathogenesis and therapy. Korean J Intern Med. 2016;31(3):444–56.

What Discharge Instructions and Follow-Up Planning Should Patients with Chronic Abdominal Pain Be Given?

142

Stephen Shaheen

Pearls and Pitfalls
- Even with negative testing, acknowledge the patient's symptoms in a positive, encouraging, and supportive manner.
- Remain vigilant for overlooked causes of abdominal pain, especially when multiple work-ups have been negative. Intimate partner violence, depression, and stress have been shown to worsen and provoke symptoms.
- While there is a high rate of psychiatric comorbidities with chronic abdominal pain, not all patients with this complaint carry a secondary mental health diagnosis.
- Engage the patient and family to develop a reasonable discharge that accounts for pain control, follow-up, and very explicit return instructions.
- Avoid narcotics and benzodiazepines – there is good data to support high abuse potential and a multitude of side effects directly worsening abdominal pain.
- Utilize multidisciplinary teams when available, including case management, social work, and therapists, to build a care plan.

Abdominal pain is the leading chief complaint seen in the Emergency Department (ED), with approximately 8% of yearly visits as recorded by the National Hospital Ambulatory Medical Care Survey in 2014. There is incomplete data on the breakdown between acute and chronic complaints, likely related to conflicting definitions [1]. Chronic abdominal pain is a complicated, multifactorial presenting complaint. After appropriate diagnosis and treatment has been completed, dis-

position remains complex and requires analysis of the patient's current care plan, ambulatory medical providers, medical comprehension, and support system, as well as hospital and local resources.

What Is the Patient's Motivation for Their Visit?

Research has shown that while there is a socioeconomic component, a large number of patients presenting to the ED with repeat visits have the necessary follow-up and medical home but become frustrated with the wait time for their outpatient appointments or identify their current symptoms as "acute" [2–4]. No obvious outliers have been identified with regard to insurance type or payment method [5]. If frequent user characteristics are identified, consultation with case management and social work may be warranted to help construct a viable care plan with a specialist and pain management team. In practice, these coordinated care programs for frequent ED users have had varying success. [6, 7]

Understanding the motivation for a presentation is especially important in chronic abdominal pain to help guide discharge and prevent unnecessary return or admission. Chronic abdominal pain is often dismissed in the emergency department as a purely psychologic pathology. This diagnosis is often accompanied by mental health comorbidities such as anxiety and depression [8, 9]. Epidemiologic studies reveal the possibility that a large percentage of patients with this complaint suffer from poorly controlled organic causes or functional gastrointestinal disorders (e.g., irritable bowel syndrome) [10–12]. However, leading researchers are continuing to find actual neurohormonal linkages between the brain and digestive system [13].

Although this chapter will not focus on workup and diagnosis, it is important to acknowledge that, although there can be significant overlap between mental health disorders and chronic complaints, we do not fully understand all elements of pain syndromes. In addition, psychiatric disorders or

S. Shaheen
Duke University Medical Center, Durham, NC, USA
e-mail: stephen.shaheen@duke.edu

© Springer Nature Switzerland AG 2019
A. Graham, D. J. Carlberg (eds.), *Gastrointestinal Emergencies*, https://doi.org/10.1007/978-3-319-98343-1_142

manifestations are pathologies which result in symptoms. Because of previously mentioned comorbidities, screening for increased stressors and safety at home should be considered [14, 15].

Communicating with Patients

A safe discharge from the ED relies on a trusting relationship between the provider and patient. Admission of internal biases is important to acknowledge. Cultural beliefs need to be taken into account. While some patients have secondary intention or gain, the role of the physician is to provide the best way forward for a presenting complaint. Discussion with the patient should focus on the current workup and objective findings. Acknowledgement of the perception of symptoms helps the patient feel that their issues are being addressed. The discharge plan should be realistic and involve any family or support persons who are present. Identification of support structures and inclusion of family can improve buy-in to a plan of care.

If the workup revealed an organic cause of disease, data and referral should be sent to the primary care provider for follow-up. Suspicion for specific diagnoses should also prompt referral to the appropriate specialty service, including gastroenterology, gynecology, urology, and general surgery. Psychiatry consultation, unless immediately indicated, is best left to outpatient colleagues because implications can elicit immediate negative connotations for the patient and undermine any plan set in motion. When a referral is requested by a patient, judgment should be as to whether the request is valid and with merit. If not, the best course is to permit management guidance by a primary care physician. Maintenance of a "hub-and-spoke" model with one team (most likely gastroenterology) or primary care provider as the central manager helps with communication, prevention of unnecessary return visits, and "doctor shopping."

Negotiating Pain Management

One of the most difficult conflicts for the emergency medicine provider is with regard to pain control and prescriptions upon discharge. To begin, any medications written should fall within the guidelines for an individual's credentialing, hospital policy, and prescriber's comfort level. Inquiry about pain management contracts can be broached, if applicable.

Identifiable or likely causes of abdominal pain necessitate the directed intervention. Patients can be started on adjunctive medications like H2-blocking agents, proton-pump inhibitors, and antacids. If no organic cause has been found, over-the-counter peripherally acting analgesics such as acetaminophen and nonsteroidal anti-inflammatory drugs (NSAIDs) are unlikely to attain symptom alleviation.

When possible, narcotic pain medications should be avoided. Opioids have shown little to no efficacy for long-term pain control [16]. In addition, opioids have a poor side effect profile for nonorganic abdominal pain, especially when a psychologic component is present. In the long term, narcotic use can worsen pain, as with narcotic bowel syndrome (NBS) [17]. The abuse potential with narcotics is well-documented. In light of recent opioid misuse trends and new CDC guidelines and recommendations, any prescriptions should be for the smallest dose and shortest course possible [18, 19]. An honest and practical discussion with the patient about these high-risk medications and the reasons to avoid them may help facilitate discharge [20]. Benzodiazepines, as with narcotics, have a limited role because of high risk for abuse and dangerous side effects.

Although not likely within the scope of practice within the ED, several agents have been promising in the long-term control of nonorganic chronic abdominal pain. Tricyclic antidepressants (TCAs) and selective serotonin reuptake inhibitors (SSRIs) act as modulators of related neurohormonal pathways. Anticonvulsants and neuropathic pain medications (e.g., gabapentin) have not been shown to have efficacious qualities [21–23]. Some patients will benefit from cognitive therapy and biofeedback as part of a comprehensive plan [24].

Discharge Instructions

Discharge instructions should be clear and focused, identify objective measurements (i.e., lab work, imaging), and highlight the lack of positive findings. Reasons for return should be explicit, avoiding nebulous and generic terms, to aid in recognition of urgent conditions and to establish boundaries and appropriate use of the ED. The patient should always know that they can present for evaluation, at any time, without consequence. However, limitations as to the scope of ED practice in the diagnosis of chronic conditions and performance of diagnostic procedures can be discussed as part of the referral process. When able, the provider should personally review the instructions with the patient, family, and nursing staff, to establish clear communication and avoid misunderstanding.

Suggested Resources
- Kapural L. Chronic abdominal pain. New York: Springer; 2015.
- Feldman M. Chap 12: Chronic abdominal pain. In: Sleisenger and Fordtran's gastrointestinal and liver disease. Philadelphia: Elsevier Saunders; 2016. p. 174–85.

References

1. Center for Disease Control and Prevention: National Center for Health Statistics. National Hospital Ambulatory Medical Care Survey: 2014 emergency department summary tables. Atlanta; 2014.
2. Lucas RH, Sanford SM. An analysis of frequent users of emergency care at an Urban University Hospital. Ann Emerg Med. 1998;32(5):563–8.
3. Purdie FR, Honigman B, Rosen P. The chronic emergency department patient. Ann Emerg Med. 1981;10(6):298–301.
4. Birmingham L, Cochran T, Frey J, Stiffler K, Wilber S. Emergency department use and barriers to wellness: a survey of emergency department frequent users. BMC Emerg Med. 2016;17(1):16.
5. Fuda KK, Immekus R. Frequent users of Massachusetts emergency departments: a statewide analysis. Ann Emerg Med. 2006;48(1):9–16.
6. Grover CA, Crawford E, Close RJ. The efficacy of case management on emergency department frequent users: an eight-year observational study. J Emerg Med. 2016;51(5):595–604.
7. Soril LJ, Leggett LE, Lorenzetti DL, Noseworthy TW, Clement FM. Reducing frequent visits to the emergency department: a systematic review of interventions. PLoS One. 2015;10(4):e0123660.
8. Shelby G, Shirkey K, Sherman A, Beck J, Haman K, Shears A, et al. Functional abdominal pain in childhood and long-term vulnerability to anxiety disorders. Pediatrics. 2013;132(3):475–82.
9. Simons L, Sieberg C, Claar R. Anxiety and functional disability in a large sample of children and adolescents with chronic pain. Pain Res Manag. 2012;17(2):93–7.
10. Keefer L, Drossman D, Guthrie E, Simrén M, Tillisch K, Olden K, et al. Centrally mediated disorders of gastrointestinal pain. Gastroenterology. 2016;150(6):1408–19.
11. Drossman D, Li Z, Andruzzi E, Temple R, Talley N, Grant Thompson W, et al. U. S. householder survey of functional gastrointestinal disorders. Dig Dis Sci. 1993;38(9):1569–80.
12. Bharucha A, Chakraborty S, Sletten C. Common functional gastroenterological disorders associated with abdominal pain. Mayo Clin Proc. 2016;91(8):1118–32.
13. Mayer E, Tillisch K. The brain-gut Axis in abdominal pain syndromes. Annu Rev Med. 2011;62(1):381–96.
14. Creed F, Craig T, Farmer R. Functional abdominal pain, psychiatric illness, and life events. Gut. 1988;29(2):235–42.
15. Drossman D. Sexual and physical abuse and gastrointestinal illness: review and recommendations. Ann Intern Med. 1995;123(10):782.
16. Wang D. Opioid medications in the management of chronic abdominal pain. Curr Pain Headache Rep. 2017;21(9):40.
17. Drossman D, Szigethy E. The narcotic bowel syndrome: a recent update. Am J Gastroenterol Suppl. 2014;2(1):22–30.
18. Chou R, Fanciullo GJ, Fine PG, et al. Clinical guidelines for the use of chronic opioid therapy in chronic noncancer pain. J Pain. 2009;10(2):113–30. Spine J 2010;10(4):355–356.
19. Dowell D, Haegerich T, Chou R. CDC guideline for prescribing opioids for chronic pain — United States, 2016. MMWR Recomm Rep. 2016;65(1):1–49.
20. Drossman D. Severe and refractory chronic abdominal pain: treatment strategies. Clin Gastroenterol Hepatol. 2008;6(9):978–82.
21. Ford A, Talley N, Schoenfeld P, Quigley E, Moayyedi P. Efficacy of antidepressants and psychological therapies in irritable bowel syndrome: systematic review and meta-analysis. Gut. 2008;58(3):367–78.
22. Chao G, Zhang S. A meta-analysis of the therapeutic effects of amitriptyline for treating irritable bowel syndrome. Intern Med. 2013;52(4):419–24.
23. Drossman D. Beyond tricyclics: new ideas for treating patients with painful and refractory functional gastrointestinal symptoms. Am J Gastroenterol. 2009;104(12):2897–902.
24. Weinland S, Morris C, Dalton C, Hu Y, Whitehead W, Toner B, et al. Cognitive factors affect treatment response to medical and psychological treatments in functional bowel disorders. Am J Gastroenterol. 2010;105(6):1397–406.

Consultant Corner: Chronic Abdominal Pain

Sandra Quezada

Pearls and Pitfalls
- Colitis, malignancy, functional abdominal pain syndromes/irritable bowel syndromes, and adhesions from prior surgical procedures are commonly established diagnoses with specific therapeutic options.
- For patients without a treatable underlying cause who have had chronic need for potent analgesia, mesenteric nerve block can be effective.

Introduction

Dr. Quezada practices at the University of Maryland School of Medicine in downtown Baltimore. Their patient population is largely urban, although many of their patients also live in rural and suburban settings. Their patients are also as diverse as are the city of Baltimore and the state of Maryland, which are 63% Black or African American and 9.2% Latino, respectively. They work in both the inpatient and outpatient setting, also serving the veteran population at the Baltimore VA Medical Center. They treat patients presenting with a variety of gastrointestinal diseases, with a focus on managing inflammatory bowel disease.

Answers to Key Clinical Questions:

1. In what time frame should patients with chronic abdominal pain be referred to a gastroenterologist?
The patient presenting to the emergency department with chronic abdominal pain presents difficulties in diagnosis and management; input from a specialist in gastroenterology may yield important missed diagnoses which are best established with specialty procedures such as endoscopy, ERCP, and video capsule enteroscopy. The incidence of serious missed diagnoses is associated with increasing age. For patients presenting with chronic abdominal pain, referral to a gastroenterologist for follow-up within approximately 2 weeks is recommended.

2. Computerized tomography (CT) is a frequently performed study and is the modality of first choice for patients with undifferentiated abdominal pain. What is the role of MRI in workup of chronic abdominal pain?
Magnetic resonance imaging (MRI) is also a valuable option in patients who may have already accumulated a high burden of radiation exposure due to multiple prior CT scans. In addition, for patients with elevated alkaline phosphatase and bilirubin levels suggestive of biliary ductal pathology, an MRCP (magnetic resonance cholangiopancreatography) can provide detailed imaging that more clearly specifies whether ERCP is indicated. Given ERCP is not without its inherent risk, in these cases, an MRCP can either prevent an unnecessary procedure or justify the need to proceed.

3. What are the top diagnoses that are considered in patients presenting to you with chronic abdominal pain?
Chronic abdominal pain has many potential etiologies; the underlying cause should be identified when possible to best guide treatment. Colitis, malignancy, functional abdominal pain syndromes/irritable bowel syndromes, and adhesions from prior surgical procedures are commonly established diagnoses with specific therapeutic options. Food intolerances most often present with bloating, with or without diarrhea. It is uncommon for food intolerances to cause chronic abdominal pain. In older patients with history of vascular pathology, chronic mesenteric ischemia is a less likely but serious cause that should be considered, particularly when other explanations have been excluded.

S. Quezada
Division of Gastroenterology and Hepatology, University of Maryland School of Medicine, Baltimore, MD, USA
e-mail: squezada@som.umaryland.edu

© Springer Nature Switzerland AG 2019
A. Graham, D. J. Carlberg (eds.), *Gastrointestinal Emergencies*, https://doi.org/10.1007/978-3-319-98343-1_143

4. Any suggestions for pain management?

Analgesia for chronic abdominal pain can be a challenge but is best guided by understanding the underlying cause. Certainly, if the pain is due to inflammation, malignancy, or ischemia, treating the underlying disorder should significantly alleviate symptoms. In cases where the pain is due to a functional abdominal pain syndrome such as irritable bowel syndrome or adhesive disease, a thoughtful discussion between patient and provider should take place, to discuss the risks and benefits of different methods of analgesia. Nonsteroidal anti-inflammatory drugs (NSAIDs) can be helpful in the short term but if used consistently over extended periods can increase risk of peptic ulcer disease and inflammatory complications of the bowel. Acetaminophen does not confer these risks and used in moderation can be helpful, provided the patients are educated about risks of hepatotoxicity and even hepatic failure if consumed in large doses. Narcotics should be avoided in the treatment of chronic abdominal pain, as extended use of these drugs may not only lead to medication tolerance and dependence but is also associated with narcotic bowel syndrome, which can result in significant constipation and abdominal pain, resulting in counterproductive effects. For patients without a treatable underlying cause who have had chronic need for potent analgesia, mesenteric nerve block can be effective. Finally, consideration of integrative medicine strategies including yoga, acupuncture, and relaxation techniques may also be helpful for some patients.

Index

© Springer Nature Switzerland AG 2019

A. Graham, D. J. Carlberg (eds.), *Gastrointestinal Emergencies*, https://doi.org/10.1007/978-3-319-98343-1